Medical Microbiology and Immunology

Medical Microbiology and Immunology

Editor: Addison Boyd

AMERICAN
MEDICAL PUBLISHERS
www.americanmedicalpublishers.com

AMERICAN
MEDICAL PUBLISHERS
www.americanmedicalpublishers.com

Cataloging-in-Publication Data

Medical microbiology and immunology / edited by Addison Boyd.
p. cm.
Includes bibliographical references and index.
ISBN 979-8-88740-252-9
1. Medical microbiology. 2. Immunology. 3. Clinical immunology. I. Boyd, Addison.
QR46 .M43 2023
616.01--dc23

American Medical Publishers,
41 Flatbush Avenue,
1st Floor, New York,
NY 11217, USA

ISBN 979-8-88740-252-9 (Hardback)

Contents

Preface

This book has been an outcome of determined endeavour from a group of educationists in the field. The primary objective was to involve a broad spectrum of professionals from diverse cultural background involved in the field for developing new researches. The book not only targets students but also scholars pursuing higher research for further enhancement of the theoretical and practical applications of the subject.

Microbiology refers to the scientific study of microorganisms, such as viruses, fungi and bacteria. One of the subsets of microbiology is medical microbiology, which is focused on the prevention, diagnosis and treatment of various infectious diseases. It studies microbes for finding out their clinical applications to improve human health. Immunology is a branch of biology and medicine, which includes the study of immune systems in every organism. Protozoa, bacteria and viruses cause various diseases, such as tuberculosis, leishmaniasis, malaria and dengue fever. Medical microbiology and immunology are interlinked, as the microbes which cause disease, trigger an immune reaction and control the immune system during the infection. An integrated approach of medical microbiology and immunology is focused on understanding the response of the immune system towards the infection in the host organisms. This book elucidates the concepts and innovative models around prospective developments with respect to medical microbiology and immunology. It will serve as a valuable source of reference for graduate and post graduate students.

It was an honour to edit such a profound book and also a challenging task to compile and examine all the relevant data for accuracy and originality. I wish to acknowledge the efforts of the contributors for submitting such brilliant and diverse chapters in the field and for endlessly working for the completion of the book. Last, but not the least; I thank my family for being a constant source of support in all my research endeavours.

Editor

1

The Impact of *Helicobacter pylori* Urease upon Platelets and Consequent Contributions to Inflammation

Adriele Scopel-Guerra [1†], Deiber Olivera-Severo [1,2†], Fernanda Staniscuaski [1,3], Augusto F. Uberti [1,4], Natália Callai-Silva [1], Natália Jaeger [5], Bárbara N. Porto [5] and Celia R. Carlini [6]*

[1] Center of Biotechnology, Universidade Federal do Rio Grande do Sul, Porto Alegre, Brazil, [2] Department of Biology, Universidade Regional Integrada do Alto Uruguai e das Missões, São Luiz Gonzaga, Brazil, [3] Department of Molecular Biology and Biotechnology, Institute of Biosciences, Universidade Federal do Rio Grande do Sul, Porto Alegre, Brazil, [4] Institute of Biology, Universidade Federal de Pelotas, Pelotas, Brazil, [5] Institute of Biomedical Research, Pontifícia Universidade Católica do Rio Grande do Sul, Porto Alegre, Brazil, [6] Brain Institute (BRAINS-InsCer), Pontifícia Universidade Católica do Rio Grande do Sul, Porto Alegre, Brazil

***Correspondence:**
Celia R. Carlini
celia.carlini@pucrs.br

† These authors have contributed equally to this work.

Gastric infection by *Helicobacter pylori* is considered a risk factor for gastric and duodenal cancer, and extragastric diseases. Previous data have shown that, in a non-enzymatic way, *H. pylori* urease (HPU) activates neutrophils to produce ROS and also induces platelet aggregation, requiring ADP secretion modulated by the 12-lipoxygenase pathway, a signaling cascade also triggered by the physiological agonist collagen. Here we investigated further the effects on platelets of recombinant versions of the holoenzyme HPU, and of its two subunits (HpUreA and HpUreB). Although HpUreA had no aggregating activity on platelets, it partially inhibited collagen-induced aggregation. HpUreB induced platelet aggregation in the nanomolar range, and also interfered dose-dependently on both collagen- and ADP-induced platelet aggregation. HPU-induced platelet aggregation was inhibited by antibodies against glycoprotein VI (GPVI), the main collagen receptor in platelets. Flow cytometry analysis revealed exposure of P-selectin in HPU-activated platelets. Anti-glycoprotein IIbIIIa (GPIIbIIIa) antibodies increased the binding of FITC-labeled HPU to activated platelets, whereas anti-GPVI did not. Evaluation of post-transcriptional events in HPU-activated platelets revealed modifications in the pre-mRNA processing of pro-inflammatory proteins, with increased levels of mRNAs encoding IL-1β and CD14. We concluded that HPU activates platelets probably through its HpUreB subunit. Activation of platelets by HPU turns these cells into a pro-inflammatory phenotype. Altogether, our data suggest that *H. pylori* urease, besides allowing bacterial survival within the gastric mucosa, may have an important, and so far overlooked, role in gastric inflammation mediated by urease-activated neutrophils and platelets.

Keywords: inflammation, mRNA processing, IL-1β, lipoxygenase inhibitors, CD14, GPVI, collagen receptor, platelet aggregation

INTRODUCTION

Diseases caused by *Helicobacter pylori* have a great impact on public health, since this bacterium colonizes the gastric mucosa of half of the world's population, with a higher prevalence in the poorer countries (Parkin, 2004). *Helicobacter pylori* is a major cause of gastric and duodenal pathologies (Ferlay et al., 2013) and it was classified as the first carcinogenic bacterium by the World Health Organization more than 2 decades ago (IARC, 1994). Urease produced by *H. pylori* enables bacterial colonization of the gastric mucosa by catalyzing the hydrolysis of urea into carbon dioxide and ammonia, thereby causing a local pH increase and alterations of the mucus properties that favor the pathogen's survival (Perrais et al., 2014). Urease-negative strains of *H. pylori* were unable to infect the gastric mucosa of germfree piglets, ferrets, or mice (Hu and Mobley, 1990; Eaton et al., 1991; Andrutis et al., 1995).

Helicobacter pylori urease (HPU) accounts for ~10% of total cell protein content (Suzuki et al., 2007). HPU is a large protein, consisting of a dodecameric organization of two subunits (HpUreA, 26.5 kDa; HpUreB, 61.7 kDa; Ha et al., 2001). Structure vs. activity relationships of the non-enzymatic properties of ureases have been so far poorly characterized (Carlini and Ligabue-Braun, 2016). It has been reported that HpUreB interacts with CD74 on gastric epithelial cells inducing IL-8 production (Beswick et al., 2006) and it also binds to Th17 lymphocytes (Zhang et al., 2011). A monopartite nuclear localization signal is present in HpUreA (sequence $_{21}$KKRKEK$_{26}$), and the protein is able to target the nuclei of COS-7 (Lee et al., 2012) and of AGS gastric epithelial cells, causing alterations of the cellular morphology (Lee et al., 2015). Additionally, *H. pylori* secreted outer membrane vesicles (OMVs) contain urease-related proteins, including HpUreA and HpUreB (Olofsson et al., 2010). Incubation of AGS gastric epithelial cells with *H. pylori* OMVs promoted the translocation of HpUreA into the cell cytoplasm and nuclear localization of the protein (Olofsson et al., 2010).

Epidemiological studies have shown that *H. pylori* infection correlates positively with several extragastric pathologies, such as intestine bowel diseases, cardiovascular and cerebrovascular diseases (Franceschi et al., 2015; Goni and Franceschi, 2016; Kyburz and Muller, 2017). Several hematological diseases such as primary immune thrombocytopenia, iron deficiency anemia, childhood leukemia, and coagulation disorders have been associated with *H. pylori* infection (Papagiannakis et al., 2013). The role of this pathogen (Christodoulou et al., 2011) and of its virulence factors in these extragastric diseases is still controversial, requiring further studies (Muhammad et al., 2017).

We have previously reported that canatoxin (Carlini and Guimaraes, 1981), an isoform of *Canavalia ensiformis* urease (Follmer et al., 2001), presents biological properties that are independent of its enzyme activity, including neurotoxicity, activation of blood platelets (Carlini and Guimaraes, 1981; Carlini et al., 1985; Ghazaleh et al., 1997) and *in vivo* pro-inflammatory activity (Benjamin et al., 1992; Carlini and Ligabue-Braun, 2016; Olivera-Severo et al., 2017). We have also demonstrated that a recombinant HPU activated platelets through a lipoxygenase-mediated pathway, leading to exocytosis of dense granules and release of adenosine diphosphate (ADP), which then promoted platelet aggregation (Wassermann et al., 2010). Independently of its enzyme activity, HPU displays a potent lipoxygenase-dependent chemotactic effect on neutrophils, both *in vivo* and *in vitro*, causing cell migration in levels comparable to those induced by fMLP (Uberti et al., 2013). HPU activated human neutrophils eliciting extracellular ROS production and protected neutrophils as well as cultured gastric epithelial cells against apoptosis, interfering on the levels of mitochondrial proteins regulating this process (Uberti et al., 2013; Olivera-Severo et al., 2017). Recently we reported on the angiogenic potential of HPU, a property that could have implication in the invasion and metastization of gastric tumors (Olivera-Severo et al., 2017).

Platelets are anucleated cells involved, aside of hemostasis and thrombi formation, in physiological processes such as tissue regeneration, angiogenesis, inflammation and immunity (Jurk and Kehrel, 2005; Farndale, 2009; Vieira-de-Abreu et al., 2012). Platelets store distinct compounds in granules that, once released, contribute to the immune response (Vieira-de-Abreu et al., 2012) and they produce IL-1β, a pro-inflammatory cytokine (Lindemann et al., 2001; Morrell et al., 2014). IL-1β is considered a platelet agonist, which acts through an autocrine loop to link thrombosis and immunity, signaling to endothelial cells and promoting neutrophil adhesion (Brown et al., 2013). Platelet activation leads to a sustained synthesis of the pro-IL-1β protein, which accumulates in the platelets' cytosol until cleavage to release the cytokine (Lindemann et al., 2001). Platelets interact with components of the subendothelial matrix, with different immune cells and many pathogens (Clemetson, 2011; Morrell et al., 2014) and participate in cancer metastasis (Jurk and Kehrel, 2005; Farndale, 2009). Platelets signal the innate immune system through the release of microparticles and NET formation (Italiano et al., 2010; Carestia et al., 2016). These various characteristics of platelets enable a large spectrum of possible cell interactions and modulation by different membrane receptors (Cimmino and Golino, 2013; Thomas and Storey, 2015).

Collagen, the main component of the subendothelial matrix, promotes adhesion and activation of platelets. Several platelet collagen receptors are involved in these events (Clemetson and Clemetson, 2001). Among them, glycoprotein VI (GPVI), a member of the immunoglobulin superfamily of receptors (Clemetson et al., 1999; Jandrot-Perrus et al., 2000), plays a crucial role in the responses of platelets to collagen. GPVI participates in platelet adhesion to the subendothelium matrix and triggers a collagen-induced activation, resulting in a thromboxane A_2- and ADP-mediated aggregation thus providing a procoagulant surface for thrombin formation (Moroi et al., 1989; Nieswandt et al., 2001; Nieswandt and Watson, 2003). Collagen binding to GPVI receptor involves signaling through the 12-lipoxygenase pathway (Coffey et al., 2004a,b). On the other hand, when platelets are exposed to low collagen doses, activation through GPVI leads to a secretory phenotype accompanied by release of their dense- and alpha granules' contents, but without changing the platelets into their prothrombotic state (Ollivier et al., 2014).

In this study, we aimed to elucidate the mechanism underlying the activation of platelets exposed to an enzymatically active HPU holoenzyme and to its subunits HpUreA and HpUreB. To that aim, we performed aggregation assays and investigated the roles of platelet's glycoprotein VI and IIbIIIa in HPU-induced and subunits-induced responses. Furthermore, we analyzed expression of P-selectin and the processing of pre-mRNAs in platelets treated with these proteins.

MATERIALS AND METHODS

Helicobacter pylori Urease (HPU)

A recombinant *Helicobacter pylori* urease (HPU) was produced by heterologous expression in *Escherichia coli* BL21 (DE3)-RIL transformed with a PGEM-T-easy (Promega) plasmid carrying the whole urease operon (kindly provided by Dr. Barbara Zambelli, Universitá di Bologna, Italy). HPU was purified from bacterial extracts according to Olivera-Severo et al. (2017). Protein homogeneity was checked by 0.1% sodium dodecyl sulfate 10% polyacrylamide gel electrophoresis (SDS-PAGE) (Figure S1A). Previous to the experiments, a 0.5 mg protein.mL^{-1} solution was dialyzed against 20 mM sodium phosphate 150 mM sodium chloride, pH 7.5 (PBS 7.5), and the buffer from the last dialysis change was used as a negative control in the bioassays.

Fluorescent HPU was prepared by incubation of a 1.0 mg.mL^{-1} solution of urease with 0.1% fluorescein isothiocyanate (FITC) in PBS 7.5 for 60 min at 4°C. The mixture was exhaustively dialyzed against PBS 7.5 and then applied into a Fast-Desalting column (Amersham Biosciences) to remove any unbound FITC (Wassermann et al., 2010).

Helicobacter pylori Urease Isolated Subunits

The subunits of *Helicobacter pylori* urease, HpUreA and HpUreB, were produced in *Escherichia coli* BL21 (DE3)-RIL transformed with pET101/D-TOPO (Thermo Fisher Scientific) plasmids containing the cDNA encoding each of the subunits (a generous gift from Dr Cesare Montecucco, Universitá di Padova, Italy). Bacteria were grown in Luria broth with the antibiotics chloramphenicol (Sigma Aldrich, USA; 40 μg.mL^{-1}) and ampicillin (Sigma Aldrich, USA; 100 μg.mL^{-1}) for maintenance of the plasmids. The His-tagged subunits HpUreA and HpUreB were purified from bacterial extracts as follows: after cultivation, cells were harvested by centrifugation, suspended in extraction buffer (20 mM sodium phosphate, 500 mM sodium chloride, 5 mM imidazole, pH 7) and lysed using an ultrasonic homogenizer (10 pulses of 30 s) in an ice bath. After centrifugation (20 min, 20,000 × g, 4°C), the homogenates were submitted to Ni^{2+} affinity chromatography on a 5 mL Chelating Sepharose Fast Flow column (GE Healthcare Life Sciences). After removal of the unbound proteins, the column was eluted stepwise with 300 mM imidazole in 20 mM sodium phosphate, 500 mM sodium chloride, pH 7.0 to obtain HpUreA- and HpUreB-enriched fractions. For the last step of purification, the fractions from the Ni^{2+}-affinity step were concentrated in Amicon devices with 10 kDa cut-off (Millipore, Belford, MA, USA), applied into a Superdex S200 Hi-load column mounted in a Akta Purifier system (GE Healthcare Life Sciences), equilibrated in PBS 7.5. The protein fractions were analyzed by SDS-PAGE and by Western blots (Figure S1B), pooled and concentrated in Amicon devices (10 kDa cut-off) to a concentration of 0.5 mg.mL^{-1}.

Protein Determination

The protein content of samples was determined by absorbance at 280 nm, or by the Coomassie dye binding method (Bradford, 1976).

Urease Activity

The urea hydrolyzing activity of HPU was measured by the alkaline nitroprussiate method (Weatherburn, 1967) using ammonium sulfate as reference, to follow the purification of the holoenzyme.

Platelet Aggregation

Rabbit platelets were used in the aggregation assays. Animal care and handling followed international guidelines and all protocols were approved by the institutional Ethics Committee (UFRGS process 721.217). Platelet aggregation assays were performed essentially as described by Wassermann et al. (2010) using two different turbidimetric assays. For platelet aggregation assays performed in a plate reader (SpectraMax® M3, Molecular Devices), agonists were added to 100 μL aliquots of PRP, without or with inhibitors, to make 150 μL final reaction volume in 96 wells flat bottom plates, with absorbance readings at 650 nm every 11 s during 20 min. For platelet aggregation using a Lummi-aggregometer (Chrono-Log Corp.), after pre-incubation of PRP (300 μL) for 2 min under continuous stirring at 37°C, aggregation was triggered by addition of the agonist (maximal volume 30 μL) and the reaction was registered during 10 min. In both assays, platelet's response was quantified as area under the aggregation tracings. Response to the physiological agonist collagen (bovine tendon, 50 μg.mL^{-1}) or ADP (10 μM) (final concentrations) was taken as positive control of platelet activation.

In some of the experiments, platelets were pre-incubated at room temperature without stirring with HPU subunits, inhibitors or antibodies before addition of the platelet agonist: eicosanoid synthesis inhibitors esculetin (0.5 and 1 mM) and indomethacin (75–300 μM); antibodies against platelet glycoproteins GPVI or IIbIIIa, or anti-platelet cell markers (see the following sections for more details).

Platelet Isolation

Peripheral human blood of healthy volunteers was obtained in the presence of 0.313% (w/v) sodium citrate. Written informed consent was obtained from the participants of this study. All procedures regarding blood collection and handling were conducted in strict accordance to Brazilian legislation (Law no. 6.638/1979) and were approved by the institutional Ethics Committee (UFRGS process 721.217).

Human platelets were isolated according to Ollivier et al. (2014) with some modifications; briefly, a platelet-rich plasma (PRP) was separated from whole blood by centrifugation at 200 g for 15 min. For flow cytometry assays (see below), the platelets were pelleted from PRP by an additional centrifugation step (800 × g, 10 min), and washed 3 times (800 × g, 10 min) with a modified Tyrode's buffer (3.6 mM citric acid, 0.5 mM glucose, 0.5 mM KCl, 0.1 mM $MgCl_2$, 10.3 mM NaCl, 2 mM $CaCl_2$ pH 6.5). After the third wash, the platelets were suspended in the reaction buffer (5 mM HEPES, 12 mM $NaHCO_3$, 137 mM NaCl, 2 mM KCl, 2 mM $CaCl_2$, 0.3 mM NaH_2PO_3, 1 mM $MgCl_2$, 5.5 mM glucose, pH 7.4). For quantitative PCR, washed platelets were immunolabeled as CD61 positive cells and separated in a MidiMACS LS column (Miltenyi Biotec) according to manufacturer's instructions.

RNA Extraction and cDNA Synthesis

For RNA extraction, the isolated platelets were suspended in reaction buffer to a final cell concentration of 10^7.mL^{-1}. Platelets were incubated with 50 μg.mL^{-1} collagen or 100 nM urease, HpUreA or HpUreB, in reaction buffer, without stirring (to avoid aggregation), at 37°C, for 30, 90, and 180 min. Total RNA was extracted immediately after the stimuli, using TriZol reagent (Ludwig Biotec), following the manufacturer's instructions. cDNA synthesis from total RNA was performed with the High-Capacity cDNA Reverse Transcription kit (Applied Biosystens/ThermoFischer Scientific), following the manufacturer's instructions, using random primers.

Pro-Inflammatory Expression Profile Analysis

Real time quantitative PCR was performed to compare CD14, interleukin-1 beta (IL-1β), cyclooxygenase-2 (COX-2), intercellular adhesion molecule 1 (ICAM-1), and inducible nitric oxide synthase (iNOS) genes expression levels in platelets challenged by collagen, the holoenzyme HPU, and by the HpUreA and HpUreB subunits, in three different time intervals at 37°C, without stirring. The beta actin gene was used (Zsori et al., 2013) to normalize the RNA content of the samples. Gene specific primers were designed to span exon junctions (Table S1). Reactions were carried in an Eco thermocycler (Illumina), using the qPCR-Sybr Green kit (Ludwig Biotec), and following the parameters: 95°C for 5 min (initial denaturation), 40 cycles at 95°C for 10 s (denaturation), 60°C for 15 s (annealing), 72°C for 15 s (extension). Melting curves were performed at the end of each reaction, with temperatures ranging from 55 to 95°C (increments of 0.1°C/s). All cDNA samples were diluted 1:5. Reactions were carried out in technical quadruplicates from two independent biological replicates. Results were analyzed by the $2^{-\Delta\Delta C_T}$ method (Livak and Schmittgen, 2001).

Flow Cytometry Analysis

Platelets (5 μL of PRP) kept at 37°C without stirring were stimulated with 100 nM or 300 nM HPU, 25 μg.mL^{-1} collagen, for 1, 5, and 10 min. Resting platelets (negative controls, no addition) and stimulated platelets in 50 μL of reaction buffer were stained with FITC-labeled anti-CD42 (GP1b) (1:25) (Abcam) and PerCP-labeled anti-CD62P (P-selectin) (1:5) (Abcam) antibodies for 20 min, at room temperature in the dark. After the incubation period, platelets were fixed with 1% paraformaldehyde. Platelets were identified by gating on platelets' size on the basis of forward scatter (FSC) and side scatter (SSC), followed by CD42 expression, a platelet marker. A total of 20,000 events were analyzed for MFI/percentage of CD62P expression. Data were acquired using a FACSCanto II flow cytometer (Becton Dickinson) with BD FACSDiva software and analyzed by Flowjo® vX.

In another set of experiments, platelets were previously treated with polyclonal anti-GPVI (1:10) (Santa Cruz Biotech) or monoclonal anti-IIbIIIa (1:10) (Santa Cruz Biotech) for 20 min at room temperature and then stimulated with 100 nM FITC-conjugated HPU for 1, 5, and 10 min at 37°C. Platelets not treated with the antibodies nor exposed to HPU served as negative controls. After the incubation period, cells were fixed with 1% paraformaldehyde. Platelets were identified as described before. A total of 50,000 events were analyzed for percentage of FITC-positive cells. Data were acquired using a FACSCanto II (Beckton Dickinson) with BD FACSDiva software and analyzed by Flowjo® vX.

Statistical Analysis

The statistical significance of the differences between two groups was assessed using the unpaired Student's *t*-test. For multiple comparisons a two-way analysis of variance (ANOVA) was performed, and the Tukey *post hoc* test was used to calculate significance. GraphPad Prism6 software (San Diego, CA, USA) was used to perform statistical analysis. Statistically significance was set at p-value ≤ 0.05. Data in graphs represent mean ± standard error of the mean (SEM) of at least three experiments, unless otherwise stated.

RESULTS

Effects of HPU Subunits on Platelet Aggregation

Our previous study has shown that HPU induces aggregation of rabbit platelets in nanomolar concentrations (Wassermann et al., 2010). To test if the isolated subunits also induce this effect, HpUreA and HpUreB were tested as platelet agonists. While HpUreB induced platelet aggregation in a dose dependent manner (**Figures 1A,B**), HpUreA had no activity under the same conditions. As reported for HPU, aggregation induced by HpUreB in rabbit platelets also depends on the production of lipoxygenase-derived eicosanoids (**Figures 1C,D**), as indicated by the inhibitory effect of esculetin, which blocks the platelet 12-lipoxygenase, and by the potentiating effect of the cyclooxygenase inhibitor, indomethacin (**Figures 1E,F**) (Wassermann et al., 2010). To investigate whether the isolated subunits could interfere in the aggregation triggered by the physiological agonists collagen or ADP, the platelets were previously incubated without stirring with HpUreA or HpUreB, and then challenged with the agonists (**Figure 2**). Surprisingly, considering the lack of direct effect of HpUreA, both subunits caused a dose-dependent inhibition of platelets' response to the agonists (**Figure 2A**). HpUreB was more effective than HpUreA in inhibiting platelet's response to collagen or ADP (**Figure 2B**). Moreover, HpUreB apparently interfered in the second wave of aggregation, abruptly

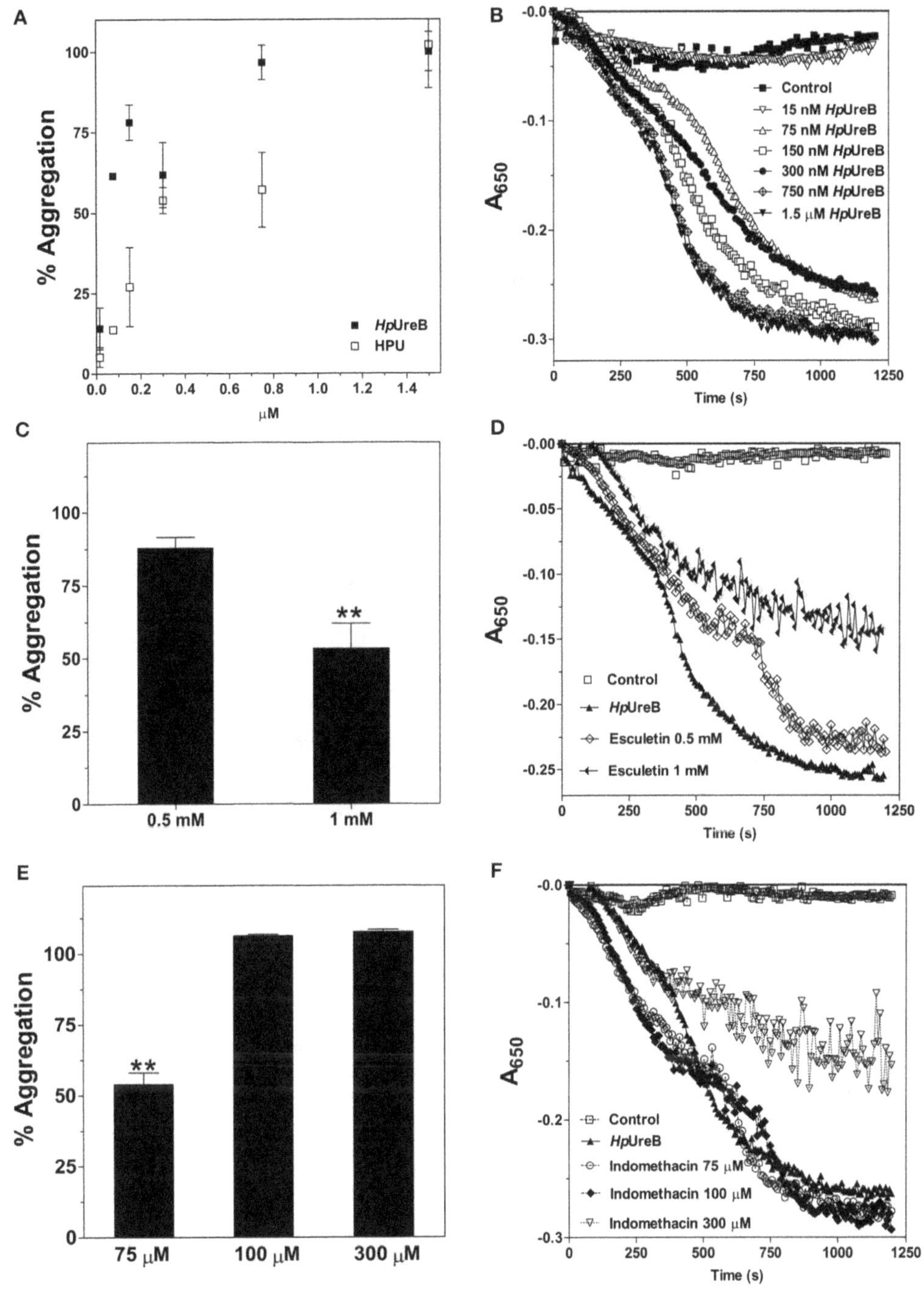

FIGURE 1 | Effects of HPU subunits on platelet aggregation. **(A,B)** HpUreB induces platelet aggregation in a dose dependent manner. **(A)** Aggregation of rabbit platelets was induced with the indicated final concentrations of HPU (open symbols, results taken from Wassermann et al., 2010) and HpUreB (closed symbols, this work). Aggregation induced by HPU or HpUreB at 1.2–1.4 μM was considered 100%. **(B)** Superimposed tracings of aggregation induced by different HpUreB concentrations as measured in the plate reader. **(C–E)** HpUreB-induced platelet aggregation depends on lipoxygenase-derived eicosanoid(s). Platelets were pretreated with the inhibitors of eicosanoids synthesis, esculetin (a 12-lipoxygenase inhibitor) **(C,D)** and indomethacin (a cyclooxygenase inhibitor) **(E,F)** at room temperature for 5 min without stirring. Aggregation was triggered by addition of 750 nM HpUreB (time zero), and after 2 min at 37°C stirring was turned on. Platelets response was monitored on SpectraMax M3 plate reader, with readings at 650 nm every 7 s for 20 min. Superimposed individual tracings of typical experiments are shown in **(B,D,F)**. Aggregation responses were quantified as area under the tracings using SotfMax Pro 5.4.1 **(A,C,E)**. Data are expressed as means ± SEM. Statistical significance was determined by ANOVA followed by Tukey-Kramer test. Values of $^{**}p < 0.01$.

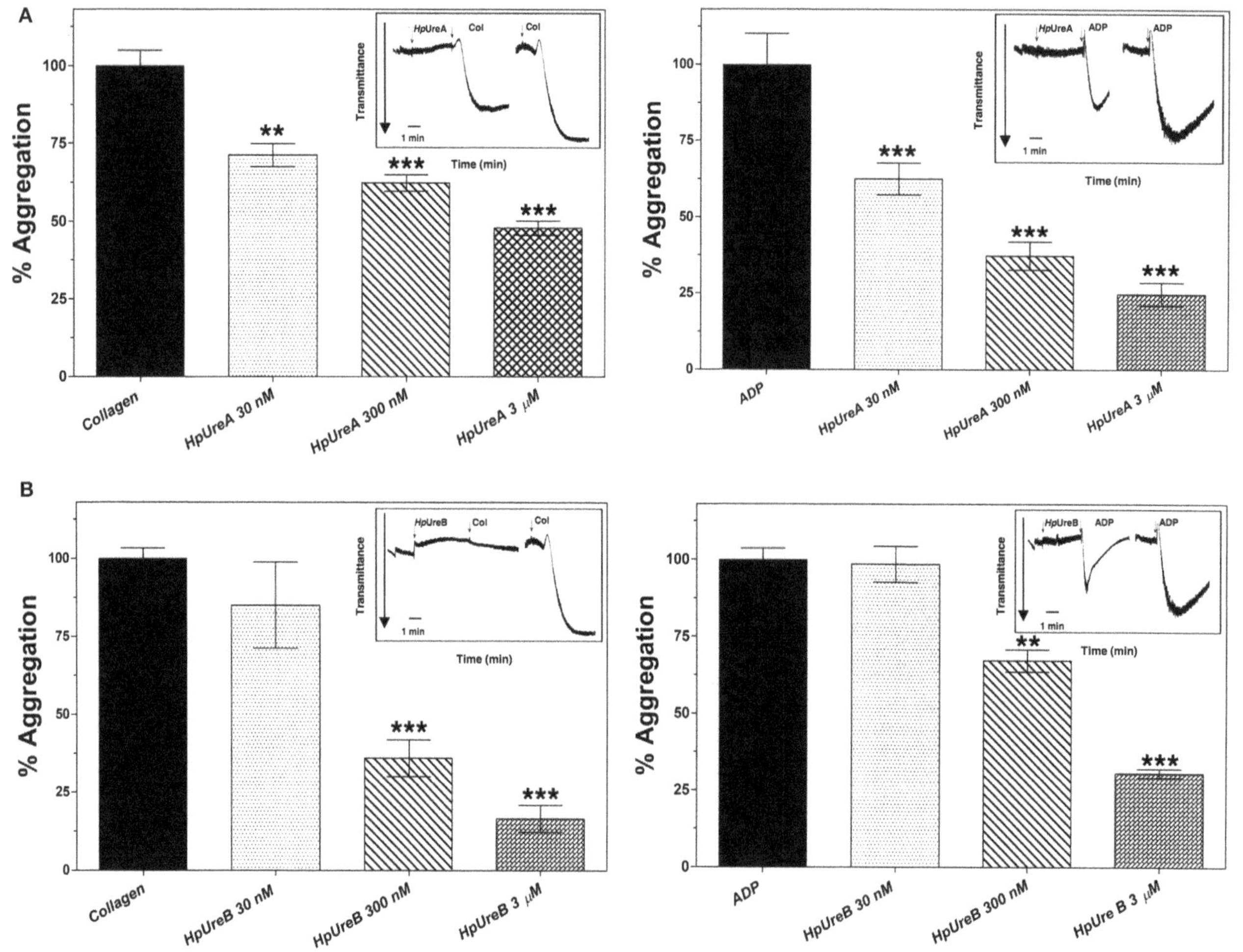

FIGURE 2 | HPU isolated subunits interfere on platelet aggregation triggered by collagen or ADP. Pretreatment with HpUreA **(A)** or HpUreB **(B)** interferes in a dose-dependent manner on the response of rabbit platelets to the physiological agonists collagen (left panels) and ADP (right panels). Platelets were pre-incubated for 5 min at 37°C without stirring with increasing concentrations of HpUreA or HpUreB. Aggregation was then triggered with collagen (50 μg.mL^{-1}) or 10 μM ADP. The results are expressed as a percentage of maximum aggregation produced by collagen or ADP. Aggregation was monitored in a plate reader SpectraMax® M3 (Molecular Devices), with readings every 11 s for 20 min at 650 nm. Typical recordings of the aggregation responses are shown in the insets. In all panels, the aggregation responses were quantified as area under the tracings using SoftMax Pro 5.4.1. Data are expressed as means ± SEM. Statistical significance was determined by ANOVA followed by Tukey-Kramer test. Values of $^{**}p < 0.01$, $^{***}p < 0.001$.

blocking the progression of aggregation in response to released ADP (**Figure 2B**, right panel), an effect not seen in HpUreA-treated platelets. HpUreA and HpUreB also interfered in the HPU-induced platelet aggregation (**Figure 3**). While 1 μM HpUreB had a synergistic effect on platelets activated by 300 nM HPU, increasing the aggregation response by 150% (**Figure 3A**), 1 μM HpUreA decreased the aggregation response by 75% (**Figure 3B**).

HPU Interaction with Platelet Membrane Receptors

Activation of human platelets by 100 and 300 nM HPU induced P-selectin exposure in a subpopulation of these cells (**Figure 4A**). This effect occurred immediately after addition of HPU and persisted for at least 10 min. Other signs of activation were also seen, such as increase in the cellular size and membrane complexity (Figure S4). Previously we have hypothesized (see Wassermann et al., 2010) that, in rabbit platelets, HPU may recruit the same signaling pathway triggered by collagen. Considering that anti-GPVI antibodies almost completely blocked HPU-induced aggregation (Figure S2), here we investigated whether HPU interacts with platelets receptors. For that aim pretreatments of human platelets with either anti-GPVI, the main collagen receptor, or anti-GPIIbIIIa, implicated in platelets' activation by fibrinogen and von Willebrand factor, were carried out. Surprisingly, after blockade of GPIIbIIIa by the antibodies, there was an increase in HPU binding to platelets (**Figure 4B**, left panel). We could not observe reactivity of the employed commercial polyclonal anti-GPIIaIIIb antibodies against HpUreB under our experimental conditions (Figure S3). Nonetheless, the signs of platelet activation (increased cell size) could no longer be seen, thereby confirming that HPU-induced

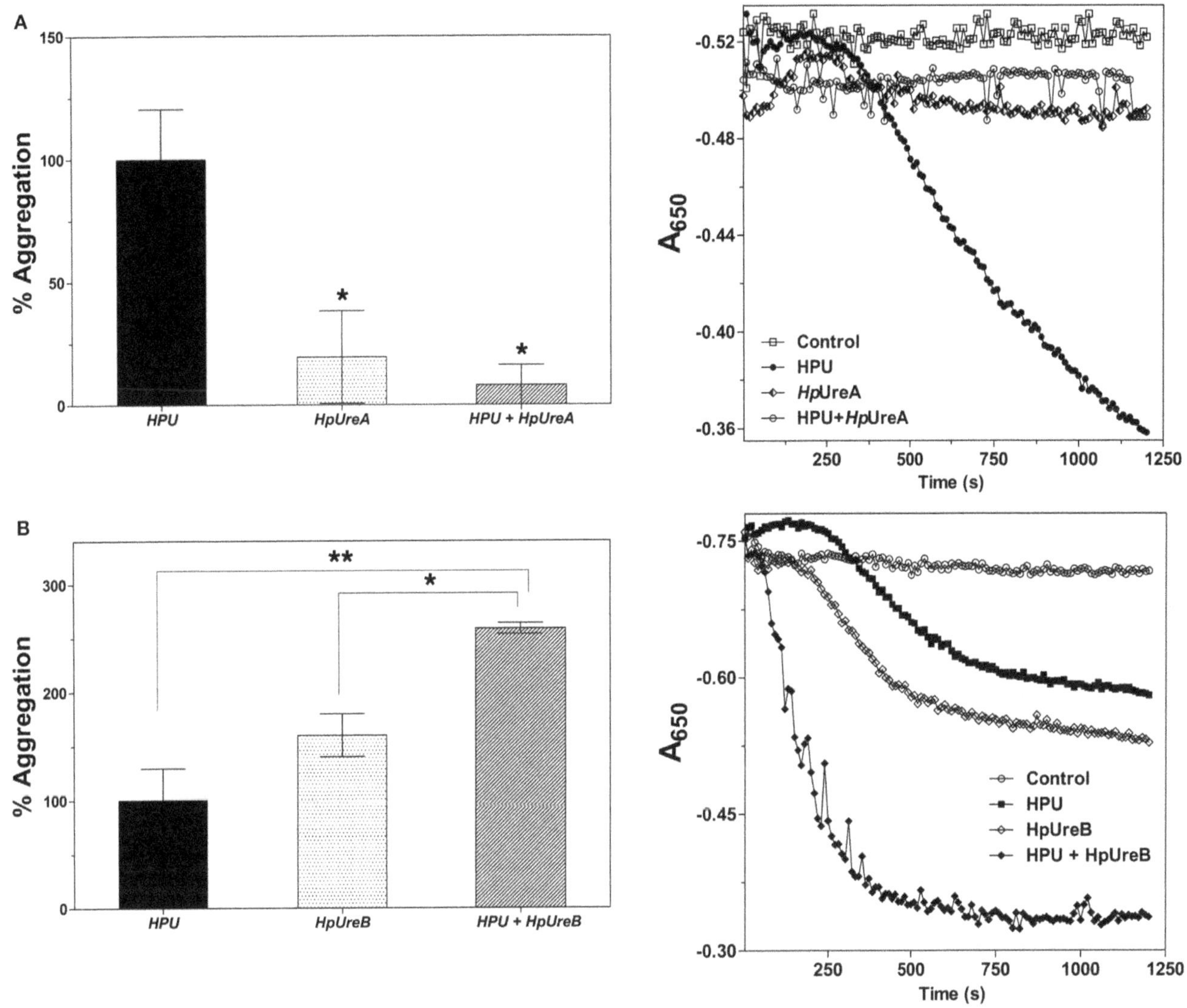

FIGURE 3 | HPU subunits interfere on HPU-induced platelet aggregation. Pretreatment of rabbit platelets with HpUreA **(A)** or HpUreB **(B)** interferes on platelet aggregation induced by 300 nM HPU. Platelets were pre-incubated for 5 min at 37°C without stirring with 1 μM HpUreA or HpUreB and then challenged with 300 nM HPU. Platelets' responses are expressed as percentage of the maximum aggregation produced by HPU (left panels). Aggregation was monitored in a plate reader SpectraMax® M3 (Molecular Devices), with readings every 11 s for 20 min at 650 nm. Superimposed tracings of individual experiments are shown in the right panels. The aggregation responses were quantified as area under the tracings (SoftMax Pro 5.4.1). Data are expressed as means ± SEM. Statistical significance was determined by ANOVA followed by Tukey-Kramer test. Values of $^*p < 0.05$, $^{**}p < 0.01$.

platelet activation somehow involves binding to the platelet membrane, if not directly to, at least in the vicinity of, this physiologically relevant receptor. On the other hand, the binding of FITC-labeled HPU to platelets was not affected by either mono- or polyclonal antibodies against GPVI (**Figure 4B**, right panel).

Urease and Its Subunits Modify Pre-mRNA Processing in Platelets

To evaluate the processing of pre-mRNA in platelets, qPCR analysis was performed after platelets treatment with HPU or its subunits. Collagen-activated platelets were used as positive controls. Collagen increased the IL-1β mRNA processing levels (**Figure 5A**), peaking at 30 min of treatment and then gradually decreasing to reach levels below the controls in 3 h-treated platelets. Differently, HPU-treated platelets decreased the process in the short treatment (30 min) and then gradually increased IL-1β pre-mRNA processing to reach, after a 3 h treatment, levels similar to those seen in collagen-treated platelets at 30 min (**Figure 5A**). Exposure of platelets to either HPU's subunits modified the IL-1β mRNA processing, but with different patterns as compared to that produced by the holoenzyme. The time-course of HpUreA's effect was similar to that seen in collagen-exposed platelets. On the other hand, treatment of platelets with HpUreB inhibited IL-1β mRNA processing in all tested times (**Figure 5B**).

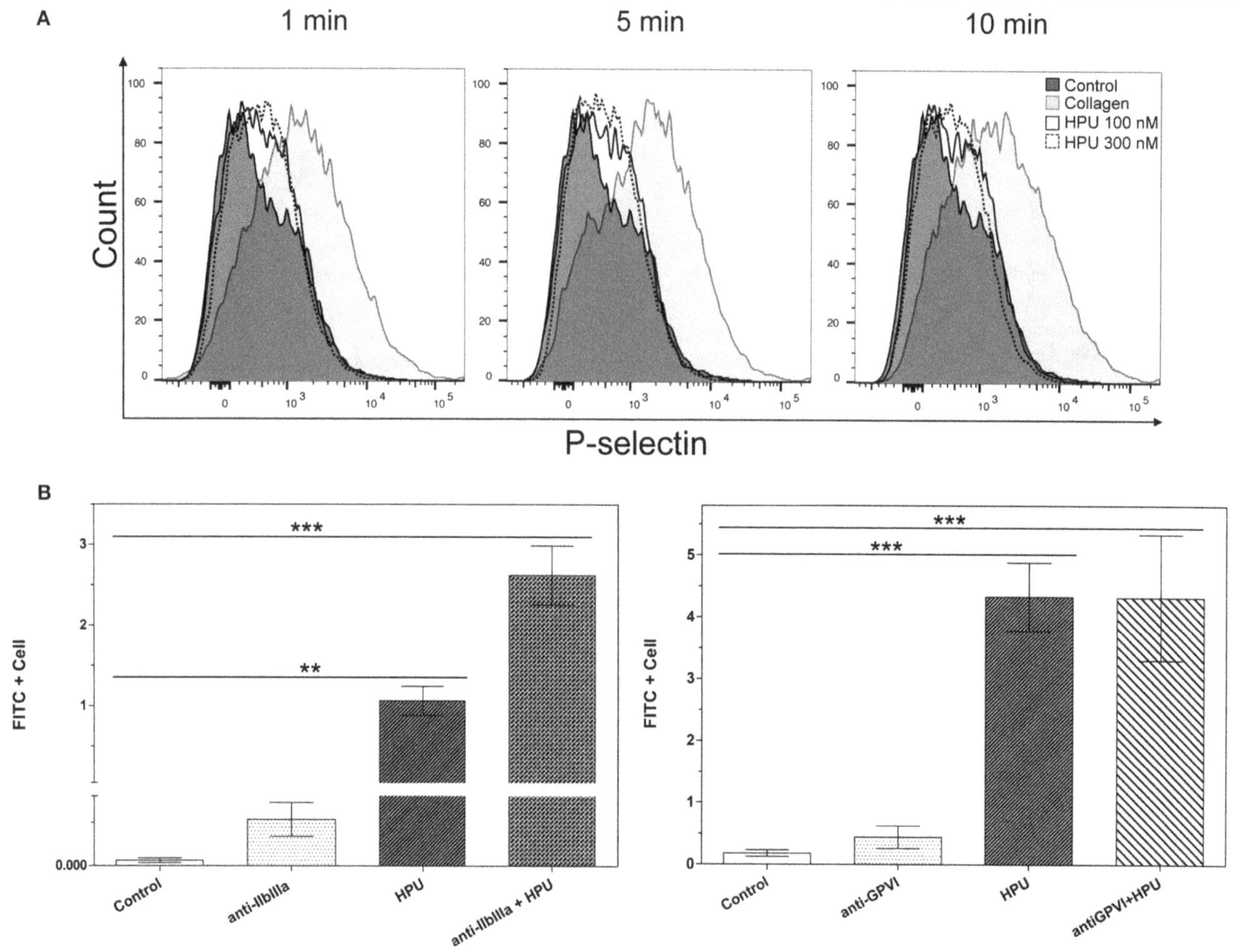

FIGURE 4 | Urease interaction with platelet membrane receptors. Representative flow cytometry histograms of P-selectin exposure on platelets' membranes of non-treated (control), collagen- or HPU-treated cells, at three different times (1, 5, and 10 min), are shown in **(A)**. The bar graph in **(B)** shows the mean percentage of FITC positive cells. Platelets were pre-treated with anti-GPVI or anti-IIbIIIa for 20 min and then challenged with 50 nM FITC-labeled HPU. Data are means ± SEM. Statistical significance was determined by ANOVA followed by Tukey-Kramer test. Values of $^{**}p < 0.01$, $^{***}p < 0.001$.

Contrasting with the inhibition observed in collagen-treated platelets (**Figure 5C**), the processing of CD14 mRNA was greatly enhanced (about 100-fold) in HPU-treated plateletes (30 min). The levels gradually decreased to reach levels still 4-fold higher than in resting platelets with 3 h of HPU treatment. Similar to the inhibition patterns seen in collagen-stimulated platelets, HpUreA or HpUreB inhibited the processing of CD14 mRNA up to 1.5 h after treatment, returning to control levels after 3 h (**Figure 5D**). Neither HPU nor its subunits interfered on the processing of pre-mRNA of COX-2, ICAM-1, or iNOS under the tested conditions.

DISCUSSION

The association of *H. pylori* infection, a pathogen with a global dispersal, with several extragastric pathologies has not gone unnoticed. Besides its well established role in stomach diseases, gastric and duodenal cancer (Ferlay et al., 2013), epidemiological studies have associated this bacterial infection with cardiovascular and thromboembolic conditions (Manolakis et al., 2007; Papagiannakis et al., 2013) and other extragastric diseases (Franceschi et al., 2015; Goni and Franceschi, 2016; Kyburz and Muller, 2017). The potential contribution of the very abundant bacterial urease to the pathogenesis of these extragastric diseases in *H. pylori* positive patients has been so far mostly overlooked.

Microbial and plant ureases have many non-enzymatic properties, mostly based on induction of exocytosis and recruitment of eicosanoids pathways, among which are neurotoxicity and pro-inflammatory activity (Carlini and Ligabue-Braun, 2016). One of these non-enzymatic properties of ureases, regardless of their source and quaternary structures, is their ability to induce aggregation of blood platelets (Follmer et al., 2004; Carlini and Ligabue-Braun, 2016). This platelet-aggregating effect of ureases is due to their exocytosis-inducing activity which leads to the release of

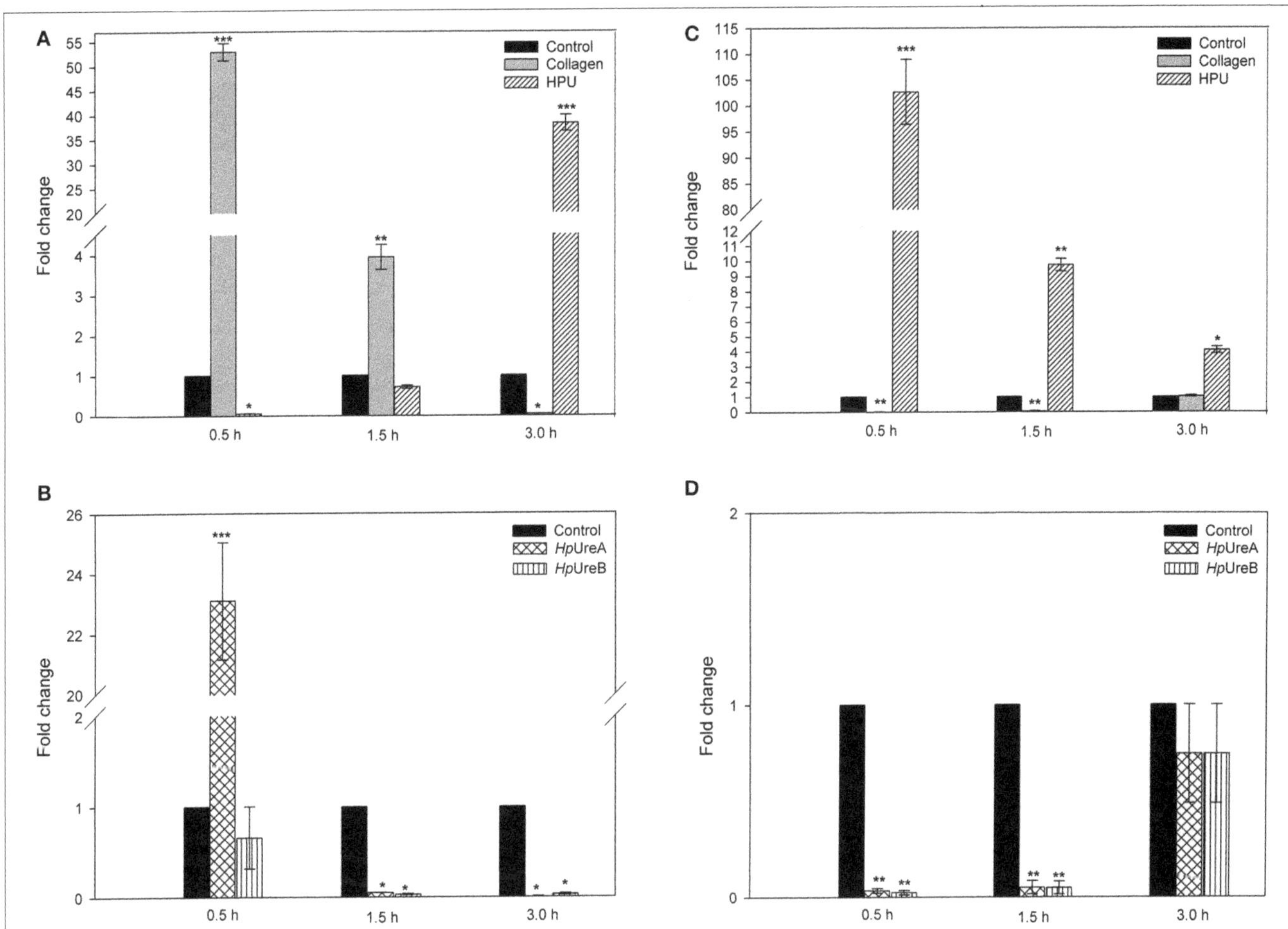

FIGURE 5 | HPU and its isolated subunits modify human platelet's mRNA processing. Platelets were treated with 50 μg.mL^{-1} of collagen, 100 nM HPU, 100 nM HpUreA, or 100 nM HpUreB for 0.5, 1.5, and 3 h at 37°C, without stirring. Untreated platelets were taken as the negative control. mRNA processing was evaluated by RT qPCR using primers designed to span exon junctions. **(A,B)** IL-1β mRNA processing. **(C,D)** CD 14 mRNA processing. Results are shown as means ± SEM of three independent biological replicates, performed in quadruplicates. A *t*-test was performed to compare treatments with the control (buffer). Values of $^*p < 0.05$, $^{**}p < 0.01$, $^{***}p < 0.001$.

ADP from platelets' dense granules, and requires the eicosanoid 12-hydroxy-peroxy-eicosatetraenoic acid (12-HPETE), produced by the platelet 12-lipoxygenase (Carlini et al., 1985; Olivera-Severo et al., 2006a,b; Wassermann et al., 2010). These data suggested that platelet aggregation induced by HPU resembles that of collagen-activated platelets through its GPVI receptor, a response reported to also require 12-HPETE synthesis by the activated platelets (Coffey et al., 2004a,b). Back then, we hypothesized that ureases and collagen may recruit similar or overlapping signaling cascades to exert their actions in platelets (Wassermann et al., 2010).

Here, we aimed to deepen the knowledge on how HPU interacts with platelets. Recombinant versions of HPU, and of its two subunits, HpUreA and HpUreB, were produced and platelet aggregation assays, flow cytometry and quantitative PCR were used to analyze how these proteins affect platelets' physiology.

In Wassermann et al. (2010), we reported that 1 μM HPU induced maximal aggregation of rabbit platelets. The response of rabbit platelets to HPU involved the 12-lipoxygenase, as it could be blocked by esculetin, and the eicosanoid 12-HETE, an oxidized derivative of 12-HPETE, was detected in the medium (Wassermann et al., 2010). Here we showed that HpUreB induces rabbit platelet aggregation in the same molar range as that of the holoenzyme. In contrast HpUreA, even in a 10-fold greater concentration had no platelet aggregating activity. This result reinforces the non-enzymatic nature of the platelet-activating property of HPU, since HpUreB has no enzymatic activity (Ha et al., 2001; Suzuki et al., 2007). Platelets' response to HpUreB required production of lipoxygenase-derived eicosanoids, as could be deduced from the dose-dependent inhibitory effect of esculetin (**Figures 1C,D**). The fact that pretreatment of platelets with the cyclooxygenase inhibitor indomethacin enhanced platelets' reactivity to HpUreB (**Figures 1E,F**) is expected for a lipoxygenase-mediated process, in a condition of increased availability of arachidonic acid, which is the substrate of both enzymes (Wassermann et al., 2010). These data can be interpreted as HpUreB being the HPU's domain active on platelets, and corroborates previous findings showing that this effect does not require the enzyme's ureolytic activity.

Pre-incubation of platelets with either one of the HPU's subunits inhibited, in a dose-dependent manner, the aggregation response to collagen or ADP (**Figure 2**). These data indicate that (1) although not inducing platelet aggregation, HpUreA also interacts with platelets; (2) HPU binds to platelets' membranes through at least two binding sites, one present in each of its subunits; (3) the isolated subunits bind to platelets in the same sites as does HPU itself; and (4) the binding of HPU's subunits partially blocks physiological functions of platelets. While an explanation for these observations is not trivial, the data clearly indicated that the binding sites and/or the type of binding to platelet membrane of the two subunits are quite different, implying that distinct mechanisms of action may underly their effects on platelets. The reason why pre-incubation with either HPU's subunits inhibited the platelet aggregation promoted by collagen or ADP is unclear, considering their effects on HPU-induced aggregation (**Figure 3**). HpUreA inhibited HPU-induced aggregation, which is consistent to its binding to platelets with an antagonist-like behavior. This effect may be related to fact that ureases insert themselves into lipid bilayers thereby affecting membrane physicochemical properties (Piovesan et al., 2014; Micheletto et al., 2016). On the other hand, HpUreB probably interacts specifically with some platelet receptor, as it induces aggregation *per se*, and it acted synergistically with HPU to amplify the aggregating effect (**Figure 3**).

Activation of human platelets (constitutively positive for CD42, or glycoprotein 1b) by HPU in comparison to collagen was studied by flow cytometry following the expression of P-selectin (CD62P) (**Figure 4**). Platelets are known to modulate their degranulation and release of specific granules according to the stimulus (Jonnalagadda et al., 2012). For instance, collagen-activated platelets, when in low concentrations of the agonist, can degranulate and release their granular contents without a significant exposure of P-selectin (Ollivier et al., 2014). Here we demonstrated that HPU-stimulated human platelets, despite their low expression of P-selectin, show signs of activation, and eventually aggregate under favorable conditions.

Fibrinogen binding to GPIIbIIIa is a requirement for ADP-induced platelet aggregation. We have previously reported that platelet aggregation induced by canatoxin required ADP release and the presence of fibrinogen (Carlini et al., 1985; Follmer et al., 2001). Here we showed that pre-treatment of platelets with antibodies against GPIIbIIIa enhanced the binding of FITC-labeled HPU to the cells (**Figure 4B**, left panel). Altogether, these results implicate the involvement of GPIIbIIIa in the ADP-dependent platelet-aggregating effect of ureases. Muhammad et al. (2017) reviewed the mechanisms by which *H. pylori* infection could lead to cardiovascular and thromboembolic diseases, emphasizing that a cross-reactivity between HpUreB and GPIIIa could be the link associating *H. pylori* infection to immune thrombocytopenia. Bai et al. (2009) produced monoclonal antibodies against a recombinant HpUreB and showed that these antibodies cross-reacted with GPIIIa from normal platelets and partially inhibited aggregation induced by ADP. The binding motif recognized by the monoclonal anti-HpUreB in the platelet GPIIIa was not identified. This cross-reactivity of HpUreB and GPIIIa may be implicated in our observation that platelets pre-treated with anti-GP IIbIIIa bound more FITC-labeled HPU than did unstimulated platelets (**Figure 4B**). The lack of effect of the anti-GPVI antibodies in preventing HPU binding to platelets does not go against our previous hypothesis that HPU (**Figure 4B**, right panel), and now including HpUreB, share with collagen a lipoxygenase-mediated pathway of platelet activation (Wassermann et al., 2010). However, binding to GPVI seems not to be the feature that explains the similarity of platelets' response to these agonists.

It is well known that platelets participate in the inflammatory process by modulating the activity of other inflammatory cells (Thomas and Storey, 2015; Koenen, 2016). We have previously demonstrated that HPU displays pro-inflammatory activity in the mouse paw edema model, causing an intense eicosanoid-dependent neutrophil infiltration in the tissues (Uberti et al., 2013). In the same study, HPU showed a non-enzymatic, lipoxygenase-dependent, chemotactic effect on human neutrophils, and induced extracellular production of reactive oxygen species (ROS) by the activated cells (Uberti et al., 2013). Our data reinforced results obtained by other groups showing that purified HPU elicited the production of ROS and inflammatory cytokines by human macrophages and primary monocytes *in vitro* (Harris and Granger, 1996; Shimoyama et al., 2003), induced transendothelial migration of T cells (Enarsson et al., 2005) and increased the expression of inducible NO synthase (Gobert et al., 2002). All these activities of HPU contribute to tissue inflammation and injury. Here we investigated whether activation of human platelets by HPU leads to a pro-inflammatory phenotype of these cells.

Platelets have reservoirs of pre-mRNA that are processed into the corresponding mRNA upon stimulation (Denis et al., 2005). Treatment of platelets with collagen, HPU, HpUreA, or HpUreB, modified their processing of IL-1β and CD14 pre-mRNAs, each protein producing effects with a distinct kinetics. Collagen and HpUreA had similar time pattern for stimulation of IL-1β pre-mRNA processing, with peaks at 30 min after treatment and then decreasing to levels below control after 3 h (**Figures 5A,B**). The slower but persistent effect of HPU of increasing IL-1β production 3 h after treatment confirms that this protein changes platelets into a pro-inflammatory phenotype. Further studies are necessary to confirm if the pre-mRNA processing changes observed here impact as well the platelets' protein levels of IL-1β and CD-14 after exposure to HPU.

Zhang et al. (2009) reported that platelets express TLR4, CD14 and MyD88, the signaling pathway triggered in response to lipopolysaccharides (LPS), as described in other cell types (Funda et al., 2001). CD14 is a co-receptor of various Toll-like receptors (TRLs) present in hematopoietic and non-hematopoietic cells that recognizes PAMPs (pathogen-associated molecular patters), triggering the innate immune response and participating in inflammation (Zanoni and Granucci, 2013). Distinct from collagen and the subunits HpUreA and HpUreB, that lowered CD14 pre-mRNA processing below control levels, HPU greatly enhanced the processing of CD14 mRNA (**Figure 5**). This result suggests that HPU activates at least part of the signaling pathway triggered by LPS, and the increased expression of CD14 in HPU-activated platelets corroborates their phenotype conversion into pro-inflammatory cells. The absence of CD14 expression in unstimulated platelets, or in platelets stimulated by collagen under normal physiological conditions, in contrast to the increased levels after HPU stimulus, resembles the reaction of intestinal mucosal cells, which only show increased expression levels of CD14 associated to inflammatory processes (Funda et al., 2001).

Similar to cell activation through LPS where a role of CD14 in the induction of TNF-α, IL-1β, IL-6, and IL-8 expression has been identified (Dentener et al., 1993; Schumann et al., 1994), here we hypothesize that CD14 expression may be modulating the IL-1β levels in platelets stimulated with HPU. This does not occur when platelets are stimulated with collagen, HpUreA or HpUreB. It has been described that platelets stimulated by LPS (Brown and McIntyre, 2011) or dengue virus (Hottz et al., 2013) process IL-1β pre-mRNA and that once stimulated, these cells release microparticles loaded with IL-1β by a mechanism not yet completely elucidated (Hottz et al., 2013). If HPU-stimulated platelets also release microparticles containing IL-1β, that could be delivered nearby endothelial cells or immune cells responsive to IL-1β, such as macrophages and lymphocytes, will be a subject of future studies.

The natural existence of any urease's subunits in a free state has never been described thus the relevance of the biological effects described here for HpUreA or HpUreB is uncertain. On the other hand this study provided valuable insights into the structure vs. activity relationships of HPU concerning its effects on platelets. While it became clear that HpUreB carries the major "platelet-active" domain of HPU, the contributions of HpUreA to the platelet activating effect of HPU are less clear. The antagonistic effect of HpUreA against aggregation induced by the physiological agonists ADP and collagen, proved its interaction with platelets' membranes. Moreover only HpUreA increased IL-1β pre-mRNA processing like HPU did. Thus both HPU subunits contribute to the protein's effect on platelets although in different ways. Another evidence of the existence of two platelet binding sites in HPU is the fact that both of its subunits competed with HPU, partially blocking the aggregating effect of the holoenzyme. In alignment with this conclusion, other studies by our group performed with the isolated subunits of the tri-chained *Proteus mirabilis* urease have identified a "platelet-activating" domain in one of its small subunits whose sequence is homologous to the C-terminal half of HpUreA (Broll V, unpublished results).

In summary, in this work we have shown that HPU and its subunits affect platelet physiology in ways that may contribute to the pathogenicity of *H. pylori* by other mechanisms besides enabling bacterial survival in the gastric lumen. The pro-inflammatory phenotype of HPU-activated platelets implies altered participation of these cells in many physiological processes, possibly contributing to the development of the extragastric diseases associated to *H. pylori* infection. Altogether our results reinforce the importance of microbial ureases, acting also in non-enzymatic ways, as a virulence factor of pathogenic microorganisms.

AUTHOR CONTRIBUTIONS

AS-G and DO-S planned and conducted experiments on the interactions of urease and its subunits with platelets; AS-G, DO-S, and AFU planned and conducted platelet aggregation assays; AS-G, DO-S, AFU, and NC-S produced the recombinant proteins; AS-G and FS planned and conducted mRNA processing experiments; NJ and BP conducted flow cytometry assays; AS-G, DO-S, FS, NJ, and CC have written and revised the manuscript; CC has conceived and coordinated this study.

FUNDING

This work was supported by Brazilian agencies Coordenação de Pessoal de Nível Superior (CAPES, Edital 63/2010 Toxinologia, proj. 1205/2011; Edital PosDoc-SUS 2909/2010, proj. 054/2010) and Conselho Nacional de Desenvolvimento Científico e Tecnológico (CNPq, Edital Universal Proc. No. 475908/2012-0 and No. 446052/2014-1). AS-G was a recipient of a CAPES Ph.D. fellowship.

ACKNOWLEDGMENTS

The authors acknowledge Barbara Zambelli, PhD, from Universitá di Bologna, Italy, and Cesare Montecucco, PhD, Universitá di Padova, Italy, for kindling providing the holoprotein (HPU) and HPU's isolated chains constructs.

REFERENCES

Andrutis, K. A., Fox, J. G., Schauer, D. B., Marini, R. P., Murphy, J. C., Yan, L., et al. (1995). Inability of an isogenic urease-negative mutant stain of *Helicobacter mustelae* to colonize the ferret stomach. *Infect. Immun.* 63, 3722–3725.

Bai, Y., Wang, Z., Bai, X., Yu, Z., Cao, L., Zhang, W., et al. (2009). Cross-reaction of antibody against *Helicobacter pylori* urease B with platelet glycoprotein IIIa and its significance in the pathogenesis of immune thrombocytopenic purpura. *Int. J. Hematol.* 89, 142–149. doi: 10.1007/s12185-008-0247-4

Benjamin, C. F., Carlini, C. R., and Barja-Fidalgo, C. (1992). Pharmacological characterization of rat paw edema induced by canatoxin, the toxic protein from *Canavalia ensiformis* (jack bean) seeds. *Toxicon* 30, 879–885. doi: 10.1016/0041-0101(92)90386-J

Beswick, E. J., Pinchuk, I. V., Minch, K., Suarez, G., Sierra, J. C., Yamaoka, Y., et al. (2006). The *Helicobacter pylori* urease B subunit binds to CD74 on gastric epithelial cells and induces NF-kappaB activation and interleukin-8 production. *Infect. Immun.* 74, 1148–1155. doi: 10.1128/IAI.74.2.1148-1155.2006

Bradford, M. M. (1976). A rapid and sensitive method for the quantitation of microgram quantities of protein utilizing the principle of protein-dye binding. *Anal. Biochem.* 72, 248–254. doi: 10.1016/0003-2697(76)90527-3

Brown, G. T., and McIntyre, T. M. (2011). Lipopolysaccharide signaling without a nucleus: kinase cascades stimulate platelet shedding of proinflammatory IL-1β-rich microparticles. *J. Immunol.* 186, 5489–5496. doi: 10.4049/jimmunol.1001623

Brown, G. T., Narayanan, P., Li, W., Silverstein, R. L., and McIntyre, T. M. (2013). Lipopolysaccharide stimulates platelets through an IL-1β autocrine loop. *J. Immunol.* 191, 5196–5203. doi: 10.4049/jimmunol.1300354

Carestia, A., Kaufman, T., and Schattner, M. (2016). Platelets: new bricks in the building of neutrophil extracellular traps. *Front. Immunol.* 7:271. doi: 10.3389/fimmu.2016.00271

Carlini, C. R., and Guimaraes, J. A. (1981). Isolation and characterization of a toxic protein from *Canavalia ensiformis* (jack bean) seeds, distinct from concanavalin A. *Toxicon* 19, 667–675. doi: 10.1016/0041-0101(81)90104-5

Carlini, C. R., Guimaraes, J. A., and Ribeiro, J. M. (1985). Platelet release reaction and aggregation induced by canatoxin, a convulsant protein: evidence for the involvement of the platelet lipoxygenase pathway. *Br. J. Pharmacol.* 84, 551–560. doi: 10.1111/j.1476-5381.1985.tb12940.x

Carlini, C. R., and Ligabue-Braun, R. (2016). Ureases as multifunctional toxic proteins: A review. *Toxicon* 110, 90–109. doi: 10.1016/j.toxicon.2015.11.020

Christodoulou, D. K., Milionis, H. J., Pappa, P., Katsanos, K. H., Sigounas, D., Florentin, M., et al. (2011). Association of *Helicobacter pylori* infection with cardiovascular disease–is it just a myth? *Eur. J. Intern. Med.* 22, 191–194. doi: 10.1016/j.ejim.2010.11.010

Cimmino, G., and Golino, P. (2013). Platelet biology and receptor pathways. *J. Cardiovasc. Transl. Res.* 6, 299–309. doi: 10.1007/s12265-012-9445-9

Clemetson, J. M., Polgar, J., Magnenat, E., Wells, T. N., and Clemetson, K. J. (1999). The platelet collagen receptor glycoprotein VI is a member of the immunoglobulin superfamily closely related to FcalphaR and the natural killer receptors. *J. Biol. Chem.* 274, 29019–29024. doi: 10.1074/jbc.274.41.29019

Clemetson, K. J. (2011). The role of platelets in defence against pathogens. *Hamostaseologie* 31, 264–268. doi: 10.5482/ha-1152

Clemetson, K. J., and Clemetson, J. M. (2001). Platelet collagen receptors. *Thromb. Haemost.* 86, 189–197.

Coffey, M. J., Coles, B., Locke, M., Bermudez-Fajardo, A., Williams, P. C., Jarvis, G. E., et al. (2004a). Interactions of 12-lipoxygenase with phospholipase A2 isoforms following platelet activation through the glycoprotein VI collagen receptor. *FEBS Lett.* 576, 165–168. doi: 10.1016/j.febslet.2004.09.007

Coffey, M. J., Jarvis, G. E., Gibbins, J. M., Coles, B., Barrett, N. E., Wylie, O. R., et al. (2004b). Platelet 12-lipoxygenase activation via glycoprotein VI: involvement of multiple signaling pathways in agonist control of H(P)ETE synthesis. *Circ. Res.* 94, 1598–1605. doi: 10.1161/01.RES.0000132281.78948.65

Denis, M. M., Tolley, N. D., Bunting, M., Schwertz, H., Jiang, H., Lindemann, S., et al. (2005). Escaping the nuclear confines: signal-dependent pre-mRNA splicing in anucleate platelets. *Cell* 122, 379–391. doi: 10.1016/j.cell.2005.06.015

Dentener, M. A., Bazil, V., Von Asmuth, E. J., Ceska, M., and Buurman, W. A. (1993). Involvement of CD14 in lipopolysaccharide-induced tumor necrosis factor-alpha, IL-6 and IL-8 release by human monocytes and alveolar macrophages. *J. Immunol.* 150, 2885–2891.

Eaton, K. A., Brooks, C. L., Morgan, D. R., and Krakowka, S. (1991). Essential role of urease in pathogenesis of gastritis induced by *Helicobacter pylori* in gnotobiotic piglets. *Infect. Immun.* 59, 2470–2475.

Enarsson, K., Brisslert, M., Backert, S., and Quiding-Jarbrink, M. (2005). *Helicobacter pylori* induces transendothelial migration of activated memory T cells. *Infect. Immun.* 73, 761–769. doi: 10.1128/IAI.73.2.761-769.2005

Farndale, R. W. (2009). Platelet glycoprotein VI as a mediator of metastasis. *J. Thromb. Haemost.* 7, 1711–1712. doi: 10.1111/j.1538-7836.2009.03566.x

Ferlay, J., Steliarova-Foucher, E., Lortet-Tieulent, J., Rosso, S., Coebergh, J. W., Comber, H., et al. (2013). Cancer incidence and mortality patterns in Europe: estimates for 40 countries in 2012. *Eur. J. Cancer* 49, 1374–1403. doi: 10.1016/j.ejca.2012.12.027

Follmer, C., Barcellos, G. B., Zingali, R. B., Machado, O. L., Alves, E. W., Barja-Fidalgo, C., et al. (2001). Canatoxin, a toxic protein from jack beans (*Canavalia ensiformis*), is a variant form of urease (EC 3.5.1.5): biological effects of urease independent of its ureolytic activity. *Biochem. J.* 360(Pt 1), 217–224. doi: 10.1042/0264-6021:3600217

Follmer, C., Real-Guerra, R., Wasserman, G. E., Olivera-Severo, D., and Carlini, C. R. (2004). Jackbean, soybean and Bacillus pasteurii ureases: biological effects unrelated to ureolytic activity. *Eur. J. Biochem.* 271, 1357–1363. doi: 10.1111/j.1432-1033.2004.04046.x

Franceschi, F., Gasbarrini, A., Polyzos, S. A., and Kountouras, J. (2015). Extragastric Diseases and *Helicobacter pylori*. *Helicobacter* 20(Suppl. 1), 40–46. doi: 10.1111/hel.12256

Funda, D. P., Tuckova, L., Farre, M. A., Iwase, T., Moro, I., and Tlaskalova-Hogenova, H. (2001). CD14 is expressed and released as soluble CD14 by human intestinal epithelial cells *in vitro*: lipopolysaccharide activation of epithelial cells revisited. *Infect. Immun.* 69, 3772–3781. doi: 10.1128/IAI.69.6.3772-3781.2001

Ghazaleh, F. A., Francischetti, I. M., Gombarovits, M. E., and Carlini, C. R. (1997). Stimulation of calcium influx and platelet activation by canatoxin: methoxyverapamil inhibition and downregulation by cGMP. *Arch. Biochem. Biophys.* 339, 362–367. doi: 10.1006/abbi.1997.9898

Gobert, A. P., Mersey, B. D., Cheng, Y., Blumberg, D. R., Newton, J. C., and Wilson, K. T. (2002). Cutting edge: urease release by *Helicobacter pylori* stimulates macrophage inducible nitric oxide synthase. *J. Immunol.* 168, 6002–6006. doi: 10.4049/jimmunol.168.12.6002

Goni, E., and Franceschi, F. (2016). *Helicobacter pylori* and extragastric diseases. *Helicobacter* 21(Suppl. 1), 45–48. doi: 10.1111/hel.12340

Ha, N. C., Oh, S. T., Sung, J. Y., Cha, K. A., Lee, M. H., and Oh, B. H. (2001). Supramolecular assembly and acid resistance of *Helicobacter pylori* urease. *Nat. Struct. Biol.* 8, 505–509. doi: 10.1038/88563

Harris, N. R., and Granger, D. N. (1996). Mechanisms underlying enhanced capillary filtration induced by platelet-activating factor. *Am. J. Physiol.* 270(1 Pt 2), H127–133.

Hottz, E. D., Lopes, J. F., Freitas, C., Valls-de-Souza, R., Oliveira, M. F., Bozza, M. T., et al. (2013). Platelets mediate increased endothelium permeability in dengue through NLRP3-inflammasome activation. *Blood* 122, 3405–3414. doi: 10.1182/blood-2013-05-504449

Hu, L. T., and Mobley, H. L. (1990). Purification and N-terminal analysis of urease from *Helicobacter pylori*. *Infect. Immun.* 58, 992–998.

IARC (1994). Schistosomes, liver flukes and *Helicobacter pylori*. IARC Working Group on the Evaluation of Carcinogenic Risks to Humans. Lyon, 7–14 June 1994. *IARC Monogr. Eval. Carcinog. Risks Hum.* 61, 1–241.

Italiano, J. E. Jr., Mairuhu, A. T., and Flaumenhaft, R. (2010). Clinical relevance of microparticles from platelets and megakaryocytes. *Curr. Opin. Hematol.* 17, 578–584. doi: 10.1097/MOH.0b013e32833e77ee

Jandrot-Perrus, M., Busfield, S., Lagrue, A. H., Xiong, X., Debili, N., Chickering, T., et al. (2000). Cloning, characterization, and functional studies of human and mouse glycoprotein VI: a platelet-specific collagen receptor from the immunoglobulin superfamily. *Blood* 96, 1798–1807.

Jonnalagadda, D., Izu, L. T., and Whiteheart, S. W. (2012). Platelet secretion is kinetically heterogeneous in an agonist-responsive manner. *Blood* 120, 5209–5216. doi: 10.1182/blood-2012-07-445080

Jurk, K., and Kehrel, B. E. (2005). Platelets: physiology and biochemistry. *Semin. Thromb. Hemost.* 31, 381–392. doi: 10.1055/s-2005-916671

Koenen, R. R. (2016). The prowess of platelets in immunity and inflammation. *Thromb. Haemost.* 116, 605–612. doi: 10.1160/TH16-04-0300

Kyburz, A., and Muller, A. (2017). *Helicobacter pylori* and Extragastric Diseases. *Curr. Top. Microbiol. Immunol.* 400, 325–347. doi: 10.1007/978-3-319-50520-6_14

Lee, J. H., Jun, S. H., Baik, S. C., Kim, D. R., Park, J. Y., Lee, Y. S., et al. (2012). Prediction and screening of nuclear targeting proteins with nuclear localization signals in *Helicobacter pylori*. *J. Microbiol. Methods* 91, 490–496. doi: 10.1016/j.mimet.2012.10.004

Lee, J. H., Jun, S. H., Kim, J. M., Baik, S. C., and Lee, J. C. (2015). Morphological changes in human gastric epithelial cells induced by nuclear targeting of *Helicobacter pylori* urease subunit A. *J. Microbiol.* 53, 406–414. doi: 10.1007/s12275-015-5085-5

Lindemann, S., Tolley, N. D., Dixon, D. A., McIntyre, T. M., Prescott, S. M., Zimmerman, G. A., et al. (2001). Activated platelets mediate inflammatory signaling by regulated interleukin 1beta synthesis. *J. Cell Biol.* 154, 485–490. doi: 10.1083/jcb.200105058

Livak, K. J., and Schmittgen, T. D. (2001). Analysis of relative gene expression data using real-time quantitative PCR and the 2(-Delta Delta C(T)) Method. *Methods* 25, 402–408. doi: 10.1006/meth.2001.1262

Manolakis, A., Kapsoritakis, A. N., and Potamianos, S. P. (2007). A review of the postulated mechanisms concerning the association of *Helicobacter pylori* with ischemic heart disease. *Helicobacter* 12, 287–297. doi: 10.1111/j.1523-5378.2007.00511.x

Micheletto, Y. M. S., Moro, C. F., Lopes, F. C., Ligabue-Braun, R., Martinelli, A. H. S., Marques, C. M., et al. (2016). Interaction of jack bean (Canavalia ensiformis) urease and a derived peptide with lipid vesicles. *Colloids Surf. B Biointerf.* 145, 576–585. doi: 10.1016/j.colsurfb.2016.05.063

Moroi, M., Jung, S. M., Okuma, M., and Shinmyozu, K. (1989). A patient with platelets deficient in glycoprotein VI that lack both collagen-induced aggregation and adhesion. *J. Clin. Invest.* 84, 1440–1445. doi: 10.1172/JCI114318

Morrell, C. N., Aggrey, A. A., Chapman, L. M., and Modjeski, K. L. (2014). Emerging roles for platelets as immune and inflammatory cells. *Blood* 123, 2759–2767. doi: 10.1182/blood-2013-11-462432

Muhammad, J. S., Zaidi, S. F., Saeed, S. A., and Ishaq, M. (2017). Current status of *Helicobacter pylori* association with haematological and cardiovascular diseases: a mini review. *J. Pak. Med. Assoc.* 67, 907–911.

Nieswandt, B., Brakebusch, C., Bergmeier, W., Schulte, V., Bouvard, D., Mokhtari-Nejad, R., et al. (2001). Glycoprotein VI but not alpha2beta1 integrin is essential for platelet interaction with collagen. *EMBO J.* 20, 2120–2130. doi: 10.1093/emboj/20.9.2120

Nieswandt, B., and Watson, S. P. (2003). Platelet-collagen interaction: is GPVI the central receptor? *Blood* 102, 449–461. doi: 10.1182/blood-2002-12-3882

Olivera-Severo, D., Uberti, A. F., Marques, M. S., Pinto, M. T., Gomez-Lazaro, M., Figueiredo, C., et al. (2017). A new role for *Helicobacter pylori* urease: contributions to angiogenesis. *Front. Microbiol.* 8:1883. doi: 10.3389/fmicb.2017.01883

Olivera-Severo, D., Wassermann, G. E., and Carlini, C. R. (2006a). *Bacillus pasteurii* urease shares with plant ureases the ability to induce aggregation of blood platelets. *Arch. Biochem. Biophys.* 452, 149–155. doi: 10.1016/j.abb.2006.06.001

Olivera-Severo, D., Wassermann, G. E., and Carlini, C. R. (2006b). Ureases display biological effects independent of enzymatic activity: is there a connection to diseases caused by urease-producing bacteria? *Braz. J. Med. Biol. Res.* 39, 851–861. doi: 10.1590/S0100-879X2006000700002

Ollivier, V., Syvannarath, V., Gros, A., Butt, A., Loyau, S., Jandrot-Perrus, M., et al. (2014). Collagen can selectively trigger a platelet secretory phenotype via glycoprotein VI. *PLoS ONE* 9:e104712. doi: 10.1371/journal.pone.0104712

Olofsson, A., Vallstrom, A., Petzold, K., Tegtmeyer, N., Schleucher, J., Carlsson, S., et al. (2010). Biochemical and functional characterization of *Helicobacter pylori* vesicles. *Mol. Microbiol.* 77, 1539–1555. doi: 10.1111/j.1365-2958.2010.07307.x

Papagiannakis, P., Michalopoulos, C., Papalexi, F., Dalampoura, D., and Diamantidis, M. D. (2013). The role of *Helicobacter pylori* infection in hematological disorders. *Eur. J. Intern. Med.* 24, 685–690. doi: 10.1016/j.ejim.2013.02.011

Parkin, D. M. (2004). International variation. *Oncogene* 23, 6329–6340. doi: 10.1038/sj.onc.1207726

Perrais, M., Rousseaux, C., Ducourouble, M. P., Courcol, R., Vincent, P., Jonckheere, N., et al. (2014). *Helicobacter pylori* urease and flagellin alter mucin gene expression in human gastric cancer cells. *Gastric Cancer* 17, 235–246. doi: 10.1007/s10120-013-0267-5

Piovesan, A. R., Martinelli, A. H., Ligabue-Braun, R., Schwartz, J. L., and Carlini, C. R. (2014). *Canavalia ensiformis* urease, Jaburetox and derived peptides form ion channels in planar lipid bilayers. *Arch. Biochem. Biophys.* 547, 6–17. doi: 10.1016/j.abb.2014.02.006

Schumann, R. R., Rietschel, E. T., and Loppnow, H. (1994). The role of CD14 and lipopolysaccharide-binding protein (LBP) in the activation of different cell types by endotoxin. *Med. Microbiol. Immunol.* 183, 279–297. doi: 10.1007/BF00196679

Shimoyama, T., Fukuda, S., Liu, Q., Nakaji, S., Fukuda, Y., and Sugawara, K. (2003). *Helicobacter pylori* water soluble surface proteins prime human neutrophils for enhanced production of reactive oxygen species and stimulate chemokine production. *J. Clin. Pathol.* 56, 348–351. doi: 10.1136/jcp.56.5.348

Suzuki, H., Hibi, T., and Marshall, B. J. (2007). *Helicobacter pylori*: present status and future prospects in Japan. *J. Gastroenterol.* 42, 1–15. doi: 10.1007/s00535-006-1990-z

Thomas, M. R., and Storey, R. F. (2015). The role of platelets in inflammation. *Thromb. Haemost.* 114, 449–458. doi: 10.1160/TH14-12-1067

Uberti, A. F., Olivera-Severo, D., Wassermann, G. E., Scopel-Guerra, A., Moraes, J. A., Barcellos-de-Souza, P., et al. (2013). Pro-inflammatory properties and neutrophil activation by *Helicobacter pylori* urease. *Toxicon* 69, 240–249. doi: 10.1016/j.toxicon.2013.02.009

Vieira-de-Abreu, A., Campbell, R. A., Weyrich, A. S., and Zimmerman, G. A. (2012). Platelets: versatile effector cells in hemostasis, inflammation, and the immune continuum. *Semin. Immunopathol.* 34, 5–30. doi: 10.1007/s00281-011-0286-4

Wassermann, G. E., Olivera-Severo, D., Uberti, A. F., and Carlini, C. R. (2010). *Helicobacter pylori* urease activates blood platelets through a lipoxygenase-mediated pathway. *J. Cell. Mol. Med.* 14, 2025–2034. doi: 10.1111/j.1582-4934.2009.00901.x

Weatherburn, M. W. (1967). Phenol-hypochlorite reaction for determination of ammonia. *Anal. Chem.* 39 , 971–974. doi: 10.1021/ac60252a045

Zanoni, I., and Granucci, F. (2013). Role of CD14 in host protection against infections and in metabolism regulation. *Front. Cell. Infect. Microbiol.* 3:32. doi: 10.3389/fcimb.2013.00032

Zhang, G., Han, J., Welch, E. J., Ye, R. D., Voyno-Yasenetskaya, T. A., Malik, A. B., et al. (2009). Lipopolysaccharide stimulates platelet secretion and potentiates platelet aggregation via TLR4/MyD88 and the cGMP-dependent protein kinase pathway. *J. Immunol.* 182, 7997–8004. doi: 10.4049/jimmunol.0802884

Zhang, J. Y., Liu, T., Guo, H., Liu, X. F., Zhuang, Y., Yu, S., et al. (2011). Induction of a Th17 cell response by *Helicobacter pylori* Urease subunit B. *Immunobiology* 216, 803–810. doi: 10.1016/j.imbio.2010.12.006

Zsori, K. S., Muszbek, L., Csiki, Z., and Shemirani, A. H. (2013). Validation of reference genes for the determination of platelet transcript level in healthy individuals and in patients with the history of myocardial infarction. *Int. J. Mol. Sci.* 14, 3456–3466. doi: 10.3390/ijms14023456

2

A New Role for *Helicobacter pylori* Urease: Contributions to Angiogenesis

Deiber Olivera-Severo[1,2†], Augusto F. Uberti[1,3†], Miguel S. Marques[4,5,6], Marta T. Pinto[4,5], Maria Gomez-Lazaro[4,7], Céu Figueiredo[4,5,6], Marina Leite[4,5†] and Célia R. Carlini[1,8*†]*

[1] Center of Biotechnology, Universidade Federal Rio Grande do Sul, Porto Alegre, Brazil, [2] Biology Department, Universidade Regional Integrada do Alto Uruguai e das Missões, São Luiz Gonzaga, Brazil, [3] Institute of Biology, Universidade Federal de Pelotas, Pelotas, Brazil, [4] i3S, Instituto de Investigação e Inovação em Saúde, University of Porto, Porto, Portugal, [5] Ipatimup-Institute of Molecular Pathology and Immunology of the University of Porto, Porto, Portugal, [6] Faculty of Medicine of the University of Porto, Porto, Portugal, [7] INEB - Instituto Nacional de Engenharia Biomédica, University of Porto, Porto, Portugal, [8] Brain Institute (BRAINS-InsCer), Pontifícia Universidade Católica do Rio Grande do Sul, Porto Alegre, Brazil

***Correspondence:**
Célia R. Carlini
celia.carlini@pucrs.br
Marina Leite
mleite@ipatimup.pt

† These authors have contributed equally to this work.

Helicobacter pylori is a pathogen involved in gastric diseases such as ulcers and carcinomas. *H. pylori's* urease is an important virulence factor produced in large amounts by this bacterium. In previous studies, we have shown that this protein is able to activate several cell types like neutrophils, monocytes, platelets, endothelial cells, and gastric epithelial cells. Angiogenesis is a physiological process implicated in growth, invasion and metastization of tumors. Here, we have analyzed the angiogenic potential of *H. pylori* urease (HPU) in gastric epithelial cells. No cytotoxicity was observed in AGS, Kato-III, and MKN28 gastric cell lines treated with 300 nM HPU, as evaluated by the 3-(4,5-Dimethylthiazol-2-yl)-2,5-diphenyltetrazolium bromide (MTT) assay. As we previously reported in neutrophils, treatment with 300 nM HPU also had an anti-apoptotic effect in gastric epithelial cells leading to a 2.2-fold increase in the levels of Bcl-X_L after 6 h, and a decrease of 80% in the content of BAD, after 48 h, two mitochondrial proteins involved in regulation of apoptosis. Within 10 min of exposure, HPU is rapidly internalized by gastric epithelial cells. Treatment of the gastric cells with methyl-β-cyclodextrin abolished HPU internalization suggesting a cholesterol-dependent process. HPU induces the expression of pro-angiogenic factors and the decrease of expression of anti-angiogenic factors by AGS cells. The angiogenic activity of HPU was analyzed using *in vitro* and *in vivo* models. HPU induced formation of tube-like structures by human umbilical vascular endothelial cells in a 9 h experiment. In the chicken embryo chorioallantoic membrane model, HPU induced intense neo-vascularization after 3 days. In conclusion, our results indicate that besides allowing bacterial colonization of the gastric mucosa, *H. pylori*'s urease triggers processes that initiate pro-angiogenic responses in different cellular models. Thus, this bacterial urease, a major virulence factor, may also play a role in gastric carcinoma development.

Keywords: *Helicobacter pylori*, urease, endocytosis, vasculogenesis, angiogenesis

INTRODUCTION

Helicobacter pylori is a Gram-negative bacterium that infects more than half of the world's population and it is the major cause of gastroduodenal diseases, such as gastritis, peptic ulcers, and gastric cancer (IARC, 1994). *H. pylori* infection was responsible for 770,000 new cases of gastric cancer worldwide in 2012 (Plummer et al., 2016). Gastric cancer is the third most common cause of cancer-related deaths worldwide according to GLOBOCAN 2012 database, and risk factors include smoking, obesity, diet and bacterial infections, most importantly, *H. pylori* infection (Ferlay et al., 2013).

This bacterium produces large amounts of urease, an important virulence factor involved in a series of processes that allow bacteria to colonize and induce a strong inflammatory response in the gastric epithelium. HPU enzymatic activity causes hydrolysis of urea into ammonia, thereby neutralizing the acid environment of the stomach (Marshall et al., 1990), leading to altered properties of the gastric mucous layer (Perrais et al., 2014). HPU is a large protein, consisting of a dodecameric organization of two subunits (UreA, 26.5 kDa; UreB, 61.7 kDa; Ha et al., 2001). Its smaller subunit UreA was found to localize in the nuclei of cultured gastric epithelial cells, leading to altered morphology of AGS cells (Lee et al., 2012, 2015). Additionally, both HPU subunits, UreA and UreB, were observed inside outer membrane vesicles secreted by *H. pylori* and vesicles derived from pathogenic bacteria are often involved in toxin delivery to the host (Olofsson et al., 2010). By a mechanism not yet fully understood, HPU is also involved in the dysregulation of gastric epithelial tight junctions (Wroblewski et al., 2009) and independently of its enzyme activity, it promotes activation of neutrophils both *in vivo* and *in vitro* conditions (Uberti et al., 2013; Carlini and Ligabue-Braun, 2016).

Angiogenesis, the formation of new blood vessels from the pre-existing vasculature, is essential for tumor growth, invasion, and metastatic dissemination and it plays a central role in the progression of gastric cancer by providing nutrients and oxygen (Hanahan and Weinberg, 2011; De Palma et al., 2017; Macedo et al., 2017). *H. pylori* infection can induce and modulate the synthesis of angiogenic and invasive factors in gastric cancer cells (Kitadai, 2010), and gastritis *H. pylori*-positive patients have an increased number of blood vessels in the gastric mucosa compared to *H. pylori*-negative patients (Yeo et al., 2006). Recently, Liu et al. (2016) showed that *H. pylori* colonization correlated to the depth of tumor invasion and higher stage metastasis. VEGF is overexpressed in *H. pylori*-positive patients and gastric cancer tumors (Okines et al., 2011). However, VEGF overexpression is a poor prognosis indicator of increased angiogenesis in gastric cancer, suggesting that different factors may be involved in this process (Pinto et al., 2017).

Here, we seek to investigate whether HPU plays a role in the angiogenesis process induced by *H. pylori.*

Abbreviations: b-FGF2, fibroblast growth factor; CAM, chorioallantoic membrane model; EG-VEGF, endocrine gland-derived vascular endothelial growth factor; GFP, green fluorescent protein; HB-EGF, heparin- binding epidermal growth factor-like growth factor; HPU, *Helicobacter pylori* urease; HUVECs, human umbilical vascular endothelial cells; IGFBP, insulin-like growth factor-binding proteins; IL-1β, interleukin 1β; mβCD, methyl-β-cyclodextrin; MTT, 3-(4,5-dimethylthiazol-2-yl)-2,5-diphenyltetrazolium bromide; NRG1-B1, neuroglin; PF-4, platelet factor-4; PTX3, pentraxin-3; TSAII, trypticase soy agar with 5% sheep blood; VEGF, vascular endothelial growth factor.

MATERIALS AND METHODS

Cell Culture

Human AGS (ATCC®CRL-1739™), AGS-Ecad (Oliveira et al., 2009), Kato-III (ATCC®HTB-103™), MKN28 (JCRB0253™) were maintained in RPMI 1640 medium with GlutaMAX™ (Invitrogen, Thermo Fisher Scientific, Inc., Waltham, MA, United States) supplemented with 10% fetal bovine serum (FBS, HyClone™, GE Healthcare Life Sciences, Logan, UT, United States), 200 IU/mL penicillin G-200 μg/mL streptomycin sulfate (Invitrogen) at 37°C under 5% CO_2 humidified atmosphere. Human umbilical vein endothelial cells (HUVECs; HUV-EC-C, ATCC®CRL1730™) were maintained in Medium 199 (M199) with Earle's salts, stable glutamine, and 25 mM HEPES buffer (Biowest, Nuaillé, France) supplemented with 10% FBS, 100 IU-100 μg/mL Penicillin G-Streptomycin Sulfate (Gibco), 100 μg/mL Heparin (Sigma-Aldrich, St. Louis, MO, United States), and 30 μg/mL Endothelial Mitogen (ECGS) (BioMedical Technologies, Inc., Stoughton, MA, United States), in gelatin-coated (Sigma-Aldrich, St. Louis, MO, United States) tissue-culture Petri dishes (TPP® Plastic Products AG, Trasadingen, Switzerland), at 37°C under 5% CO_2 humidified atmosphere.

Bacterial Strain and Growth Conditions

Bacteria were grown for 48 h at 37°C under a microaerophilic atmosphere (GENbox microaer; bioMérieux S.A., Marcy l'Etoile, France) in Trypticase™ Soy Agar with 5% sheep blood (TSAII; Becton, Dickinson and Company, Franklin Lakes, NJ, United States). Experiments were performed with *H. pylori* strain 26695 (ATCC®700392™; *cag* PAI$^+$).

HPU Purification

Helicobacter pylori bacteria grown for 48 h in TSAII (40 plates) were harvested in phosphate buffer (20 mM NaH_2PO_4, pH 7.5) and lysed by ultrasound (Ultrasonic Homogenizer 4710; 10 pulses of 30 s in ice bath). After centrifugation (20 min, 20,000 × *g*, 4°C), the supernatant was processed according to a previously published protocol to obtain purified HPU (Wassermann et al., 2010). Protein purity was assessed by gel electrophoresis in 10% polyacrylamide gels containing 0.1% sodium dodecyl sulfate (SDS-PAGE).

Immunofluorescence and Microscopy

Immunofluorescence studies and analysis by laser scanning confocal microscopy were performed using a PL APO 63× NA 1.40 oil objective (Spectral Confocal Microscope Leica TCS-SP5; Leica Microsystems, Mannheim, Germany). The images were combined and merged using ImageJ (Schneider et al., 2012) with the plugin Bio-Formats (Linkert et al., 2010). For immunocytochemistry, after treatment with 100 nM

HPU for 5, 15, and 45 min, the AGS cells were fixed with 4% paraformaldehyde (Polysciences, Warrington, PA, United States), washed with phosphate buffered saline (PBS), and permeabilized with ice-cold 100% methanol. Cells were incubated with the primary rabbit polyclonal antibody anti-UreB and mouse monoclonal antibody anti-Early Endosome Antigen 1 (EEA1) (Santa Cruz Biotechnology, Dallas, TX, United States). The secondary antibodies Alexa Fluor 488 goat anti-rabbit IgG and Alexa Fluor 596 goat anti-mouse (Thermo Fisher Scientific) were used to monitor the location of UreB and EEA1. 4′,6-diamidino-2-phenylindole (DAPI) was used to visualize the nuclei (0.1 mg/mL, Molecular Probes, Eugene, OR, United States).

For live cell experiments, AGS cells were previously transfected with Lampl-GFP (donated by Dr. Allan Levey, Emory University) using Lipofectamine 2000 transfection reagent (Invitrogen) according to manufacturer's recommendations. HPU was covalently tagged with Texas Red (Sulforhodamine 101 acid chloride; Sigma–Aldrich).

Helicobacter pylori urease incubated with Texas Red (0.5 mg/mL) during 1 h, at 4°C, with continuous stirring. This sample was then exhaustively dialyzed against 20 mM phosphate buffer, pH 7.0, and gel-filtrated using a De-Salting column (Sigma–Aldrich) to remove any excess of free dye.

Cholesterol Depletion

Cholesterol was depleted in AGS cells by incubation with 5 mg/mL mβCD (Sigma–Aldrich) in serum-free medium at 37°C under 5% CO_2 for 60 min (Hutton et al., 2010). This treatment did not affect cell viability as assessed by the trypan blue exclusion test (Strober, 2001).

Cell Viability Assay

The viability of the gastric epithelial cells upon HPU treatment was evaluated using the MTT assay 3-(4,5-Dimethylthiazol-2-yl)-2,5-diphenyltetrazolium bromide (M2128) (Sigma–Aldrich), according to manufacturer's instructions. Cells were seeded at a density of 1.5×10^5 cells/well in 96-well plates, and then incubated with 300 nM HPU or PBS for 24 h. After incubation, 20 μL of MTT solution (5 mg/mL) was added to each well and incubated for 150 min at 37°C. The media was carefully removed and 150 μL MTT solvent (4 mM HCl, 0.1% NP40, in isopropanol) was added to the wells. The absorbance was measured at 570 nm in a plate reader (SpectraMax M3, Molecular Devices, Sunnyvale, CA, United States). The experiments were performed in triplicates.

Analysis for Apoptosis-Related Proteins by Western Blot

Two different administrations schedules were used for HPU incubation in AGS cells. To investigate an "acute" effect of the protein, two doses of 300 nM HPU were added to the medium at 0 and 2 h, and the experiment was concluded after 6 h of total incubation. To simulate a "chronic" effect, cells received three doses of HPU, with additions of freshly diluted HPU (300 nM) at 0, 6 and 24 h time-points and the experiment was terminated after 48 h. Cell lysates from both groups were prepared, denatured in sample buffer (50 mM Tris-HCl, pH 6.8, 1% SDS, 5% 2-mercaptoethanol, 10% glycerol, 0.001% bromophenol blue) and heated in a boiling water bath for 3 min. Samples (30 μg total protein) were resolved in 10% SDS-PAGE gels and proteins were transferred to polyvinylidene difluoride (PVDF) membranes (Hybond-P, Amersham Pharmacia Biotech). Rainbow markers (Thermo Fisher Scientific, Inc.) were run in parallel to estimate molecular masses. Membranes were blocked with Tween-Tris buffered saline (TBS) (20 mM Tris-HCl, pH 7.5, 500 mM NaCl, 0.1% Tween-20) containing 1% bovine serum albumin (BSA) and probed with rabbit monoclonal antibodies: anti-Bcl-X_L (Cell Signaling Technology, Danvers, MA, United States, 1:500) and anti-BAD (Cell Signaling Technology, 1:500). Secondary antibodies (anti-rabbit, 1:20,000) coupled to horseradish peroxidase were from Jackson ImmunoResearch Laboratories, Inc. (West Grove, PA, United States). The protein bands were visualized using a chemiluminescence detection kit (Millipore, Billerica, MA, United States). The levels of protein expression were quantified using the software ImageJ and normalized against β-actin as an endogenous control.

Human Angiogenesis-Related Proteins

The Human Angiogenesis Array Kit (Proteome Profiler™-ARY007 Array, R&D Systems, Inc., Minneapolis, MN, United States) was used to detect the expression of angiogenesis-related proteins in cellular extracts from AGS cells treated with 300 nM HPU for 9 h in comparison with PBS-treated cells, as control. The array was performed once according to manufacturer's instructions, using a pool of cellular lysates from three independent experiments, containing 300 μg of total protein.

Endothelial Cell Capillary-Like Tube Formation Assay

Human umbilical vascular endothelial cells were seeded in 96-wells plates coated with 100 μL of growth factor-reduced Matrigel™ (Corning®Inc., Tewksbury, MA, United States) in serum-free RPMI 1640 GlutaMax medium (Gibco) at a density of 6×10^4 cells per well in the presence of 300 nM HPU or PBS (control) for a total of 9 h. HUVECs were allowed to stabilize for 3 h in a cell culture incubator at 37°C with 5% CO_2 humidified atmosphere. The formation of endothelial network was then followed in the center of each well using a Leica DMI 6000 time-lapse microscope (Leica Microsystems, Germany) for 6 h, with a 10x magnification and z-stacks of 2.08 μm were acquired every 30 min. The number of tubes and branching points per microscopic field were automatically quantified using Angiogenesis analyzer plugin (Carpentier, 2012) for ImageJ software (Schneider et al., 2012).

Chicken Embryo Chorioallantoic Membrane Angiogenesis Assay

The chicken embryo CAM model was used to evaluate angiogenic activity of HPU as previously described (Teresa Pinto et al., 2016).

HPU (50 nM, $N = 16$; 100 nM, $N = 12$ and 500 nM, $N = 14$), 2.78 μM of b-FGF2 (positive control, $N = 14$) and PBS/vehicle (negative control, $N = 16$) were tested. Briefly, fertilized chick (*Gallus gallus*) eggs obtained from commercial sources were incubated horizontally at 37.8°C in a humidified atmosphere and referred as embryonic day (E). On E3, a square window was opened in the shell after removal of 2–2.5 mL of albumen to allow detachment of the developing CAM. The window was sealed with a transparent adhesive tape and the eggs returned to the incubator. On E10, 10 μL of test solution were placed on the top of growing CAM into a 3 mm silicon ring under sterile conditions. The eggs were re-sealed and returned to the incubator for three more days. After removing the ring, the CAM was excised from the embryos, photographed *ex ovo* under a stereoscope, at 20x magnification (Olympus, SZX16 coupled with a DP71 camera). The number of new vessels (less than 15 μm diameter) growing radially toward the ring area was counted in a blind fashion manner. Statistical analysis was performed as described below.

Statistical Analysis

The statistical significance of the differences between two groups was assessed using the unpaired Student's *t*-test and for multiple comparisons it was performed a two-way analysis of variance (ANOVA) followed by Dunnett's multi-comparison post hoc test, used to calculate significance. GraphPad Prism6 software (San Diego, CA, United States) was used to perform statistical analysis. Statistically significance was set at p-value ≤ 0.05. Data in graphs represent average ± standard error of the mean (SEM) of at least three experiments, unless otherwise stated.

RESULTS

HPU Is Not Cytotoxic to Gastric Epithelial Cells

To address whether purified HPU could affect cell proliferation and viability of gastric epithelial cell lines we performed the MTT cell proliferation assay. The incubation of AGS, Kato-III, and MKN28 cells with 300 nM HPU for 24 h does not interfere with the proliferation rate, nor with the cell viability of gastric cell lines, as indirectly measured in the MTT assay (**Figure 1A**). Further, the levels of Bcl-X_L, an anti-apoptotic protein, and the levels of BAD, a pro-apoptotic protein, were evaluated by western blot in AGS cells after incubation with HPU under two experimental conditions. One of them aimed to simulate an "acute" effect of HPU (6 h of treatment), and the other a "chronic" effect (48 h of treatment) (**Figures 1B,C**). HPU induced

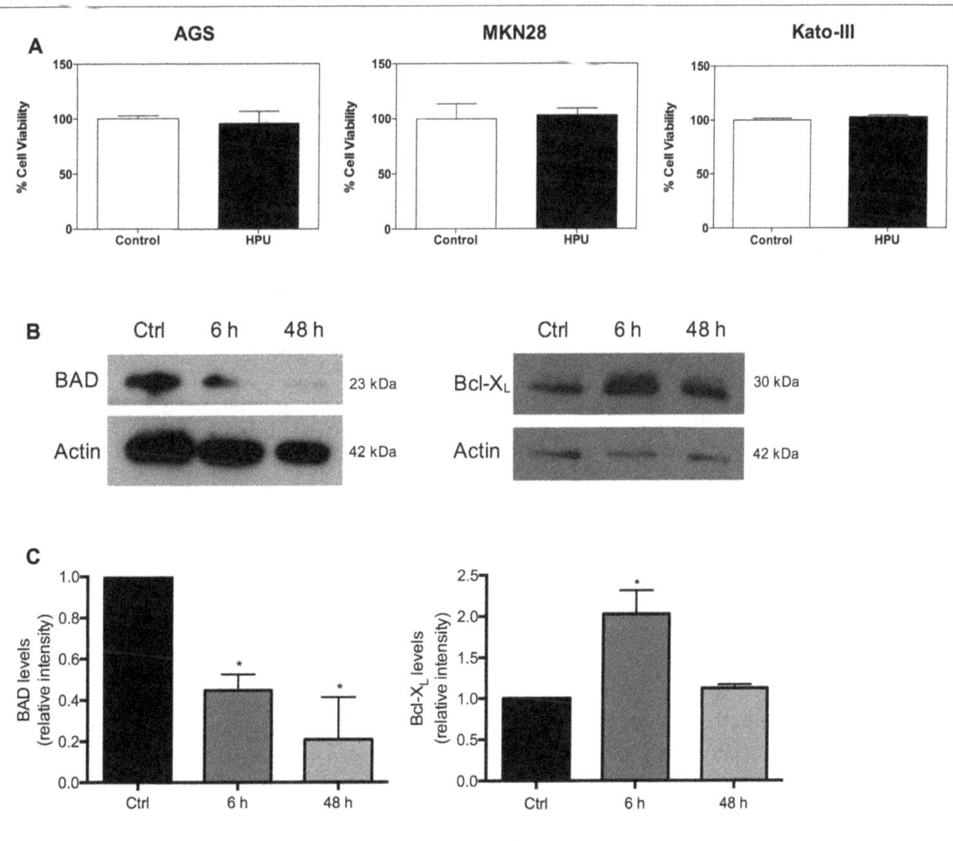

FIGURE 1 | *Helicobacter pylori* urease is not cytotoxic to gastric epithelial cell lines. **(A)** Effect of HPU in cell proliferation and viability of AGS, Kato-III, and MKN28 cell lines incubated with 300 nM HPU or PBS for 24 h, was evaluated by the MTT assay. **(B)** Levels of pro- and anti-apoptotic proteins in AGS cells treated with daily freshly added 300 nM HPU for 6 h ("acute" exposure), and for 48 h ("chronic" exposure). **(C)** Cell lysates were analyzed for the cytoplasmic content of BAD (left panel) and Bcl-X_L (right panel) by Western blot. Results shown are means ± SEM, $N = 3$; $^*p \leq 0.05$ was considered statistically significant.

a significant decrease in the expression levels of BAD in both "acute" and "chronic" conditions when compared to untreated cells, of 55 and 80%, respectively. The levels of Bcl-X_L, on the other hand, increased almost 100% relative to untreated cells, but only in the "acute" model of stimulation.

HPU Is Internalized by Gastric Epithelial

To explore if HPU is internalized by gastric epithelial cells, we treated AGS cells with HPU and performed confocal immunofluorescence microscopy. After 15 min of incubation, HPU detected with an anti-UreB antibody and an Alexa-488-conjugated secondary antibody was found on the plasma membrane, and some molecules were already in the cytoplasm (**Figure 2A**). After 45 min post-stimulation, HPU was still seen in a specific area of the plasma membrane (**Figure 2B**), suggesting that the internalization process may occur via specific receptors or cellular structures. Next, to gain insight of HPU's internalization route, AGS cells were analyzed at shorter periods of treatment for co-localization of HPU and early endosomes, by confocal immunofluorescence microscopy. As shown in **Figures 2C,D**, during the initial steps of internalization HPU co-localizes with EEA1-positive early endosomes. After 10 min, a co-localization with Lamp1 was observed, suggesting the progression of HPU sorting to late endosomes/lysosomes (**Figures 2E,F**).

In order to investigate the involvement of cholesterol in the binding and endocytosis of HPU, AGS cells were treated with mβCD, a cholesterol scavenger, previously to treatment with HPU. **Figures 2G,H** show that binding of HPU to the cell membrane depends on cholesterol, suggesting that HPU internalization probably occurs through cholesterol-rich plasma membrane structures, such as lipid rafts.

HPU Induces Angiogenesis

To investigate the involvement of HPU in angiogenesis we performed the endothelial cell tube formation assay. The addition of 300 nM HPU induced the formation of tube-like structure by HUVECs, after 9 h of treatment (**Figure 3A**). Quantification of the total number of tubes and branching points per microscopic field showed a significantly higher number of both structures in HPU-treated HUVECs than in control, the PBS-treated HUVECs (**Figure 3B**).

Further, to evaluate the role of HPU in an *in vivo* angiogenesis model we used the chick embryo CAM assay. All tested concentrations of HPU (50, 100, and 300 nM) induced a strong angiogenic response comparable to the positive control (b-FGF2) and a significantly higher angiogenic response than the negative control, as measured by the number of new blood vessels formed (**Figures 3C,D**). Together, the data from the *in vitro* and *in vivo* angiogenesis assays indicate that HPU can act as a pro-angiogenic factor in *H. pylori* infections.

HPU Reshapes the Expression of Angiogenic Factors

To characterize the angiogenic profile of gastric epithelial cells upon treatment with HPU we performed an antibody

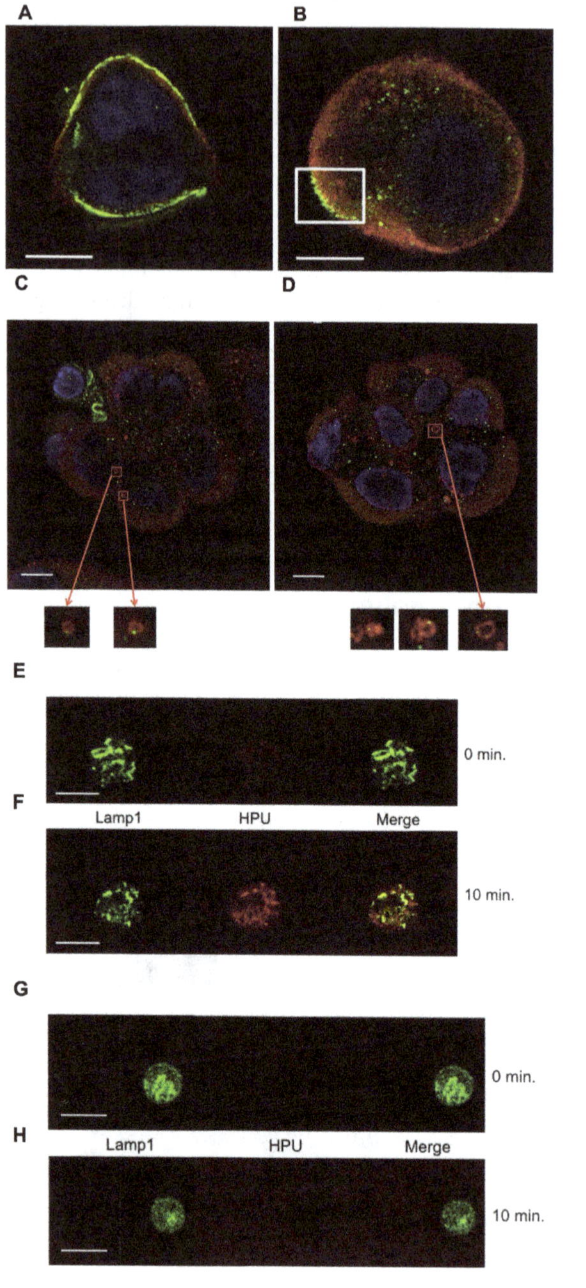

FIGURE 2 | Internalization of HPU by gastric epithelial cells occurs through a classic endocytic pathway and is dependent on cholesterol. **(A,B)** Confocal immunofluorescence microscopy showing internalization of HPU in AGS cells treated with 100 nM HPU. Cells were fixed, permeabilized and processed for the detection of HPU, using an antibody against urease (Ure-B subunit) stained with Alexa-488-conjugated secondary antibody (green), and for the detection of early endosomes, using an antibody for EEA-1 with Alexa-596-conjugated antibody (red). A representative result is shown for cells fixed after 15 min **(A)** and after 45 min **(B)** of treatment with HPU, at 37°C. **(C,D)** Colocalization (yellow) of HPU (green) and EEA1-positive endosomes (red) in AGS cells treated with HPU for 5 min at 37°C evaluated by confocal microscopy. **(C,D)** Show different sections of the same cell agglomerate. Inserts are 100x original magnifications depicting EEA1-positive endosomes (anti-EEA-1 antibody and Alexa-596 secondary antibody) containing HPU (anti-UreB antibody labeled with Alexa-488 secondary antibody)

(Continued)

FIGURE 2 | Continued
next to the plasma membrane. **(E–G)** Endocytosis of HPU involves Lamp1-positive endosomes and is impaired upon cholesterol depletion. **(E,F)** AGS cells were transfected with a Lamp1-GFP plasmid prior to the addition of TexasRed-labeled HPU at 100 nM. **(G,H)** Transfected cells were pre-treated with 5 mg/mL mβCD, for 1 h, washed, and then treated with 100 nM TexasRed-labeled HPU. After approximately 1 min of contact of the cells with HPU, the detection of fluorescence by confocal microscope was started and the time point called 0 min. Scale bars 10 μm.

angiogenesis array, using cellular extracts of AGS cells treated with 300 nM HPU and its untreated counterparts, pooled from three independent experiments. The effect of treatment of AGS cells with HPU on the expression of molecules involved in angiogenesis was then analyzed. The increased expression of angiogenin, angiopoietin-1, angiopoietin-2, EG-VEGF, endoglin, HB-EGF, IGFBP-1, IGFBP-2, IGFBP-3, IL-1β, neuroglin-B1 (NRG1-B1) and pentraxin-3 (PTX3), well-known pro-angiogenic factors and the decrease of anti-angiogenic factors platelet factor 4 (PF4), serpin B5, serpin F1 and vasohibin, were detected in the array assay, confirming the participation of HPU in angiogenesis-related processes (**Figure 4**).

DISCUSSION

Estimates are that *H. pylori* infection accounts for 5.5% gastroduodenal cancer worldwide and for more than 60% of all gastric cancer cases (Correa and Piazuelo, 2011). The infection by *H. pylori* causes damage of gastric tissues in humans, with epithelial cell cytoplasmic vacuolization and disorganization of gastric glands in the mucosa (Kusters et al., 2006). Ulcers due to gastritis in *H. pylori* infected patients have a typically slow healing process (Brzozowski et al., 1999). Previous studies using different models of endothelial cells *in vitro* have indicated that angiogenesis, a process that enhances microcirculation and is critical to recover to wounded tissue, is impaired by *H. pylori* infection (Kim et al., 2004; Tobin et al., 2008). Kim et al. (2004) have demonstrated that treatment of HUVECs with a water extract of *H. pylori* significantly inhibited capillary tube formation and decreased the expression of VEGF and angiopoietin.

Several damages seen in gastric tissues infected with *H. pylori* have been ascribed to the vacuolating toxin, VacA. For example, Tobin et al. (2008) reported that a conditioned medium obtained from a VacA-positive *H. pylori* strain inhibited bovine aortic endothelial cell functions through a VacA-dependent nitric oxide reduction mechanism. This conditioned medium reduced cell proliferation, tube formation and migration, effects that were blocked by the VacA inhibitor 5-nitro-2-(3-phenylpropylamino)benzoic acid. Moreover, no such effects were observed in cells treated with a VacA-negative *H. pylori*- or *Escherichia coli*-conditioned media (Tobin et al., 2008). VacA is known to associate with lipid rafts and is internalized by gastric cells (Gauthier et al., 2005). Moreover, VacA is known to reach the cytoplasm and promote vacuolization and affect mitochondrial function in gastric epithelial cells by mechanisms not yet fully characterized (Palframan et al., 2012).

On the other hand, other *H. pylori*-derived proteins promote angiogenesis and contribute to tumor invasiveness and growth. *H. pylori* heat shock protein 60 (HSP60) has been reported to play a role in tumor aggressiveness (Li et al., 2014) and to display proangiogenic activity in HUVECs (Lin et al., 2010). Cyclooxygenase-2 has also been implicated in angiogenesis and tumor invasiveness due to *H. pylori* (Chang et al., 2005). Here we demonstrate that HPU, a crucial virulence factor that allows bacterial survival and colonization of gastric mucosa, also plays a role in processes that underlie tumor growth in the stomach of infected patients.

Searching for a better understanding of how HPU exerts its pro-angiogenic effects, we have monitored the cytotoxicity of the purified urease on three gastric cell lines and studied its internalization by AGS cells. Incubation with 300 nM HPU for 24 h has not interfered in cell proliferation rates or in the cell viability of AGS, Kato-III, and MKN28 cells. This is a relatively high protein concentration considering the dose range (10–500 nM) of HPU which activates other cell types, such as platelets (Wassermann et al., 2010) and neutrophils (Uberti et al., 2013).

HPU's internalization is evident about 5 min following its addition to AGS cells. This internalization seems to be a receptor- or structure-specific process since we could observe an increased density of HPU-immunoreactive molecules in a particular region of the plasma membrane after 45 min of incubation, when most of the protein had already been endocytosed (**Figure 2B**). The lack of binding and internalization of HPU after treatment of AGS cells with the cholesterol scavenger mβCD indicates that specific plasma membrane regions, such as cholesterol-rich lipid rafts could be involved in this process. It has been reported that *H. pylori* takes advantage of cholesterol-rich lipid rafts to induce responses in epithelial cells, such as the activation of NF-κB and expression of IL-8 (Hutton et al., 2010). Particularly relevant to *H. pylori* pathogenesis is its type IV secretion system, which delivers CagA and VacA into the gastric cell and interacts with lipid rafts (Schraw et al., 2002; Lai et al., 2008).

As shown in **Figures 2C,D**, HPU co-localized with early endosomes, positives for the marker EEA1. Early endosomes are the first endocytic compartment to accept incoming cargo after internalization from the plasma membrane and their primary function is the sorting of internalized molecules to different intracellular locations (Marko et al., 2010).

Lamp-1 is a marker found in either late endosomes or lysosomes, as a glycoprotein present in the cytoplasmic face of these organelles (Cook et al., 2004). **Figure 2F** shows that 10 min after the addition of HPU to AGS cells, the protein could be localized in structures containing Lamp-1, suggesting that the urease may be directed to a degradation route. The intracellular fate of HPU beyond this point was not investigated in this study. On the other hand, as an invasive bacterium, *H. pylori* induces autophagy in gastric epithelial cells, a process that results in the sequestration of cytosolic components within double-membrane vesicles called autophagosomes (Terebiznik et al., 2009). These vesicles fuse with lysosomes to become autophagolysosomes,

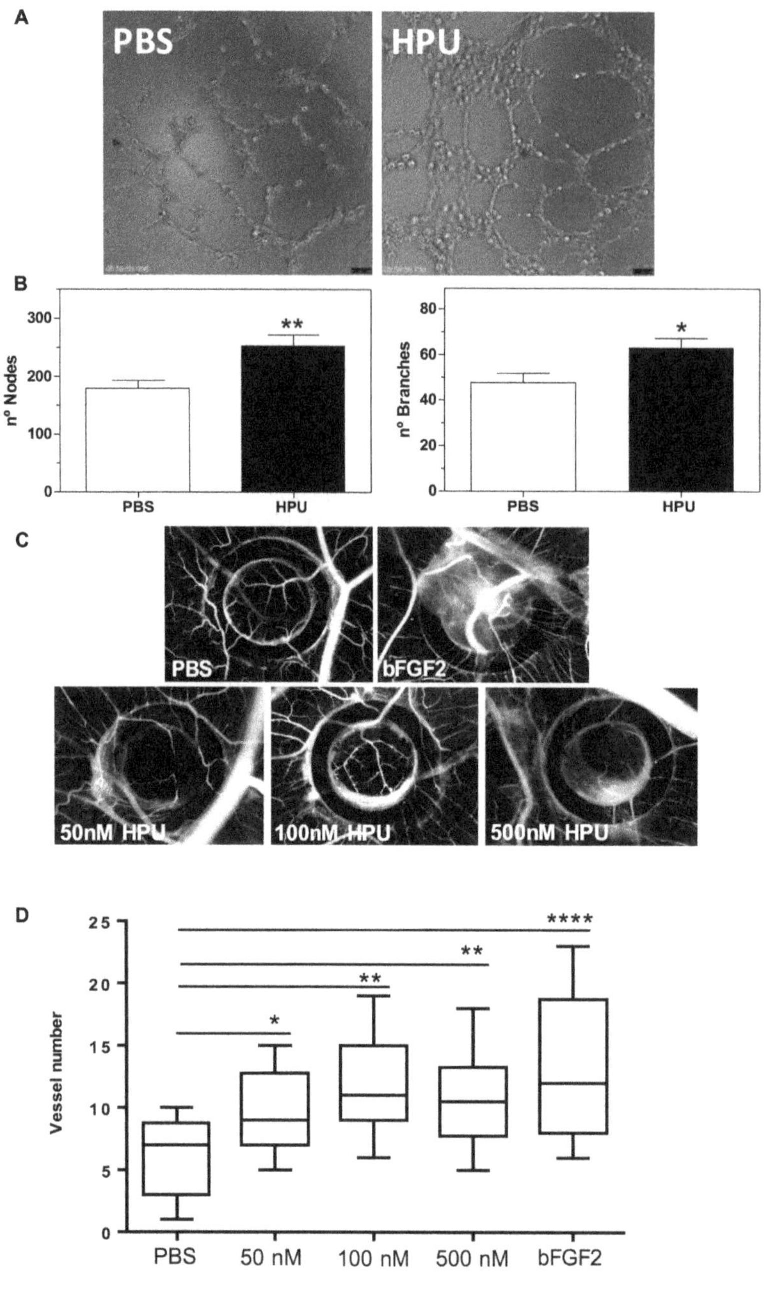

FIGURE 3 | *Helicobacter pylori* urease induces an angiogenic response both *in vitro* and *in vivo* models. **(A,B)** Effect of HPU in the induction of tube-like structures by HUVECs. **(A)** Representative micrographs showing the endothelial network formed by HUVECs exposed to 300 nM HPU after 9 h of treatment in comparison with that of untreated cells. **(B)** Quantification of the number of nodes and branches points formed per microscopic field of three independent experiments, using the plugin Angiogenesis Analyzer from the ImageJ software. Data are presented as mean ± SEM, $^{**}p$ <0.005 and $^{*}p < 0.01$ *versus* control, unpaired two-tail *t*-test. **(C,D)** Angiogenenic response induced by HPU on the *in vivo* CAM Assay. **(C)** Representative photomicrographs of new blood vessel formation are shown per condition (original magnification 20x). Analysis of HPU-induced angiogenesis was performed through quantification of the number of new vessels in controls and experimental conditions. **(D)** Number of new vessels in the CAM after 72 h incubation with 10 μL of 50, 100, and 500 nM HPU; PBS (negative control) and 10 μL of a 2.78 μM solution of b-FGF2 (positive control). Data regarding 12–16 fertilized eggs per condition is depicted on the box plot graph. ANOVA analysis, followed by Dunnett's multi-comparison test, demonstrated significant differences between groups. $^{****}p < 0.0001$, $^{**}p < 0.005$, and $^{*}p < 0.05$.

in which the vesicle contents are degraded by lysosomal hydrolases. *H. pylori* was reported to modulate and subvert this process preventing the formation of autophagolysosomes, thereby allowing bacterial proliferation (Greenfield and Jones, 2013). It has also been described that *H. pylori* induces the fusion of phagosomes, generating large less-acidic compartments called megasomes, which are necessary for intracellular bacterial survival. The formation of megasomes was shown to be

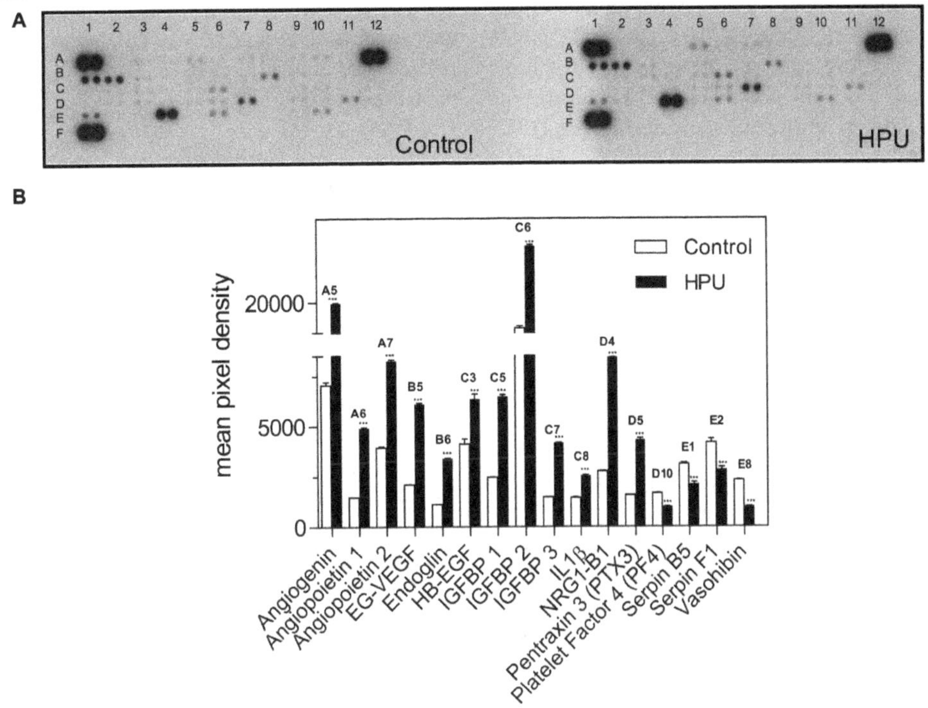

FIGURE 4 | Effect of HPU on the expression levels of angiogenesis-related proteins. **(A)** Angiogenic array membranes obtained with cellular extracts from AGS cells treated or untreated with 300 nM HPU for 9 h. **(B)** Profile of angiogenic factors generated from the array membranes. The values in the bar graph represent the mean of pixel density of the two spots of the array ±SEM from one experiment, using pooled cellular extracts from three independent experiments; $^{***}p < 0.001$ *versus* control, unpaired two-tailed *t*-test.

HPU-dependent (Schwartz and Allen, 2006). As suggested by the HPU-like immunoreactivity localized in Lamp1-positive compartments, the protein itself or fragments of it after lysosomal hydrolysis, may have a role in the regulation of the fusion of lysosomes and autophagosomes.

The strong inflammatory response of gastric epithelial cells to *H. pylori* infection results in an intense infiltration of the gastric mucosa by polymorphonuclear leukocytes, macrophages, and lymphocytes. The degree of mucosal damage correlates with the degree of neutrophil infiltration (D'Elios et al., 2007). *H. pylori* was shown to induce apoptosis of gastric epithelial cells both *in vivo* and *in vitro* (Cover et al., 2003). Our group has previously shown that HPU activates human neutrophils and delays their apoptosis by altering the expression of pro- and anti-apoptotic proteins (Uberti et al., 2013). Here, we showed that purified HPU tested on three different gastric cancer epithelial cell lines increased their survival and inhibited apoptosis by modulation of the levels of Bcl-X_L, an anti-apoptotic protein, and of BAD, a pro-apoptotic protein. This result goes in line with the hypothesis of a cancer promoting effect of HPU, that could add to or potentiate the action of other tumor-inducing factors produced by the bacterium.

The production of high cytokine levels by gastric cells upon *H. pylori* infection has been reported (Fiorentino et al., 2013), accompanied by activation of matrix metalloproteinase 10 via EGFR and ERK-mediated pathways (Costa et al., 2016). To evaluate the participation of HPU in tumorigenic processes related to *H. pylori*, we investigated the role of this protein in angiogenesis by measuring the expression of molecules involved in this phenomenon using an array analysis, and *in vitro* tubulogenesis and *in vivo* angiogenesis models.

The capillary-like tube forming assay and the Chicken embryo CAM assay are two well-accepted *in vitro* and *in vivo* models in angiogenesis studies (Kim et al., 2004; Teresa Pinto et al., 2016). Platelet factor-4 (PF-4/CXCL4) was reported to inhibit angiogenesis using the CAM assay (Maione et al., 1990). Studies demonstrating down-regulation of VEGF and angiopoietin receptors in HUVECs by *H. pylori* employed a capillary tube formation assay (Kim et al., 2004). Here, we showed that purified HPU induced angiogenesis in both *in vitro* and *in vivo* models. Addition to the CAM of 1–5 picomoles of HPU produced a strong angiogenic effect equivalent to that obtained for 27.8 picomoles of b-FGF2, the positive control (**Figure 3D**). Thus, the angiogenic stimulus provided by HPU is about 10–15-fold more potent than that of b-FGF2.

It has been shown that the array analysis of molecules participating in angiogenesis in AGS cells after treatment with 300 nM HPU led to an increased expression of pro-angiogenic factors such as angiogenin (Miyake et al., 2015), angiopoietins 1 and 2 (Jones et al., 2001; Zhou et al., 2009), EG-VEGF, also known as prokineticin-1 (Goi et al., 2004; Alfaidy et al., 2014), HB-EGF (Ito et al., 2001; Mehta et al., 2008), endoglin (Ollauri-Ibanez et al., 2017), IGFBP 1, 2 and 3, considered as endothelial tumor markers (Hintz et al., 1991; Lee et al., 2000; Le Jan et al., 2006), IL-1β (Kaluz and Van Meir, 2011; Christofides et al., 2015), NRG1-B1 (Gemberling et al., 2015), and PTX3 (Stallone et al., 2014). The same experiment showed contrasting results regarding the expression of anti-angiogenic factors in HPU-treated AGS cells, revealing decrease in the levels of PF-4 (Maione et al., 1990; Vandercappellen et al., 2011), serpin B5 and serpin F1 (Cher et al., 2003; Law et al., 2006), and vasohibin-1 (Sato, 2013).

CONCLUSION

The set of results presented here allow us to conclude that *H. pylori*'s urease, a well-recognized virulence factor for its enzymatic property that allows bacterial survival in the stomach mucosa, displays a potent and so far overlooked pro-angiogenic activity on gastric epithelial cells. Altogether with its platelet- and neutrophil-activating properties and pro-inflammatory activity, which are independent of its enzyme nature, HPU has potential to contribute in other ways to the pathogenesis of diseases caused by *H. pylori*. The data also emphasize the multifunctional character of this protein and throw light on the need of new approaches to better understand the pathologies associated with *H. pylori*.

AUTHOR CONTRIBUTIONS

DO-S: planning and conducting the angiogenesis experiments; AU: planning and conducting the cell viability and internalization experiments; MSM: conducting immunofluorescence and cell transfection with GFP-Lamp1 plasmid; MTP: conducting and analysis of CAM assay; MG-L: conducting immunofluorescence experiments; DO-S, AU, CF, ML, and CC: have written and revised the manuscript; ML (in Portugal) and CC (in Brazil) have coordinated this study.

FUNDING

This work was supported by FEDER funds through Portugal 2020, NORTE 2020, and COMPETE 2020 programs (NORTE-01-0145-FEDER-000029; POCI-01-0145-FEDER-007274), and by Fundação para a Ciência e a Tecnologia grants (FCT/CNPq-Proc° 4.4.1.00 and FCT/CAPES- FCT/4805/28/5/2014/S to ML) and fellowships (SFRH/BD/95631/2013 to MSM; SFRH/BPD/33420/2008 and SFRH/BPD/110065/2015 to ML). The Brazilian agencies Coordenação de Pessoal de Nível Superior (CAPES, Edital 63/2010 Toxinologia, proj.1205/2011; Edital CAPES/FCT proj 386/14) and Conselho Nacional de Desenvolvimento Científico e Tecnológico (CNPq, Edital Universal Proc.N° 475908/2012-0 and N° 446052/2014-1) provided financial support to CC and fellowships (CAPES/PDSE/11164-12-3/2012 to AU; CAPES-FCT/BEX: 8207/14-3/2014 to DO-S).

ACKNOWLEDGMENT

The authors acknowledge the support of the i3S Scientific Platforms b.IMAGE for laser scanning confocal microscopy and the *In vivo* CAM Assays Unit.

REFERENCES

Alfaidy, N., Hoffmann, P., Boufettal, H., Samouh, N., Aboussaouira, T., Benharouga, M., et al. (2014). The multiple roles of EG-VEGF/PROK1 in normal and pathological placental angiogenesis. *Biomed Res. Int.* 2014:451906. doi: 10.1155/2014/451906

Brzozowski, T., Konturek, P. C., Konturek, S. J., Kwiecien, S., Pajdo, R., Karczewska, E., et al. (1999). Water extracts of *Helicobacter pylori* delay healing of chronic gastric ulcers in rats: role of cytokines and gastrin-somatostatin link. *Digestion* 60, 22–33. doi: 10.1159/000007585

Carlini, C. R., and Ligabue-Braun, R. (2016). Ureases as multifunctional toxic proteins: a review. *Toxicon* 110, 90–109. doi: 10.1016/j.toxicon.2015.11.020

Carpentier, G. (2012). *ImageJ Contribution: Angiogenesis Analyzer. ImageJ News* 1.47e. Available at: http://image.bio.methods.free.fr/ImageJ/?Angiogenesis-Analyzer-for-ImageJ

Chang, Y.-J., Wu, M.-S., Lin, J.-T., and Chen, C.-C. (2005). *Helicobacter pylori*-induced invasion and angiogenesis of gastric cells is mediated by cyclooxygenase-2 induction through TLR2/TLR9 and promoter regulation. *J. Immunol.* 175, 8242–8252. doi: 10.4049/jimmunol.175.12.8242

Cher, M. L., Biliran, H. R. Jr., Bhagat, S., Meng, Y., Che, M., Lockett, J., et al. (2003). Maspin expression inhibits osteolysis, tumor growth, and angiogenesis in a model of prostate cancer bone metastasis. *Proc. Natl. Acad. Sci. U.S.A.* 100, 7847–7852. doi: 10.1073/pnas.1331360100

Christofides, A., Kosmopoulos, M., and Piperi, C. (2015). Pathophysiological mechanisms regulated by cytokines in gliomas. *Cytokine* 71, 377–384. doi: 10.1016/j.cyto.2014.09.008

Cook, N. R., Row, P. E., and Davidson, H. W. (2004). Lysosome associated membrane protein 1 (Lamp1) traffics directly from the TGN to early endosomes. *Traffic* 5, 685–699. doi: 10.1111/j.1600-0854.2004.00212.x

Correa, P., and Piazuelo, M. B. (2011). *Helicobacter pylori* infection and gastric adenocarcinoma. *US Gastroenterol. Hepatol. Rev.* 7, 59–64.

Costa, A. M., Ferreira, R. M., Pinto-Ribeiro, I., Sougleri, I. S., Oliveira, M. J., Carreto, L., et al. (2016). *Helicobacter pylori* activates matrix metalloproteinase 10 in gastric epithelial cells via EGFR and ERK-mediated pathways. *J. Infect. Dis.* 213, 1767–1776. doi: 10.1093/infdis/jiw031

Cover, T. L., Krishna, U. S., Israel, D. A., and Peek, R. M. Jr. (2003). Induction of gastric epithelial cell apoptosis by *Helicobacter pylori* vacuolating cytotoxin. *Cancer Res.* 63, 951–957.

D'Elios, M. M., Amedei, A., Cappon, A., Del Prete, G., and de Bernard, M. (2007). The neutrophil-activating protein of *Helicobacter pylori* (HP-NAP) as an immune modulating agent. *FEMS Immunol. Med. Microbiol.* 50, 157–164. doi: 10.1111/j.1574-695X.2007.00258.x

De Palma, M., Biziato, D., and Petrova, T. V. (2017). Microenvironmental regulation of tumour angiogenesis. *Nat. Rev. Cancer* 17, 457–474. doi: 10.1038/nrc.2017.51

Ferlay, J., Soerjomataram, I., Ervik, M., Dikshit, R., Eser, S., Mathers, C., et al. (2013). *GLOBOCAN 2012 v1.0, Cancer Incidence and Mortality Worldwide: IARC CancerBase No. 11.* Lyon: International Agency for Research on Cancer.

Fiorentino, M., Ding, H., Blanchard, T. G., Czinn, S. J., Sztein, M. B., and Fasano, A. (2013). *Helicobacter pylori*-induced disruption of monolayer permeability and proinflammatory cytokine secretion in polarized human gastric epithelial cells. *Infect. Immun.* 81, 876–883. doi: 10.1128/IAI.01406-12

Gauthier, N. C., Monzo, P., Kaddai, V., Doye, A., Ricci, V., and Boquet, P. (2005). *Helicobacter pylori* VacA cytotoxin: a probe for a clathrin-independent and Cdc42-dependent pinocytic pathway routed to late endosomes. *Mol. Biol. Cell* 16, 4852–4866. doi: 10.1091/mbc.E05-05-0398

Gemberling, M., Karra, R., Dickson, A. L., and Poss, K. D. (2015). Nrg1 is an injury-induced cardiomyocyte mitogen for the endogenous heart regeneration program in zebrafish. *eLife* 4:e05871. doi: 10.7554/eLife.05871

Goi, T., Fujioka, M., Satoh, Y., Tabata, S., Koneri, K., Nagano, H., et al. (2004). Angiogenesis and tumor proliferation/metastasis of human colorectal cancer cell line SW620 transfected with endocrine glands-derived-vascular endothelial growth factor, as a new angiogenic factor. *Cancer Res.* 64, 1906–1910. doi: 10.1158/0008-5472.CAN-3696-2

Greenfield, L. K., and Jones, N. L. (2013). Modulation of autophagy by *Helicobacter pylori* and its role in gastric carcinogenesis. *Trends Microbiol.* 21, 602–612. doi: 10.1016/j.tim.2013.09.004

Ha, N. C., Oh, S. T., Sung, J. Y., Cha, K. A., Lee, M. H., and Oh, B. H. (2001). Supramolecular assembly and acid resistance of *Helicobacter pylori* urease. *Nat. Struct. Biol.* 8, 505–509. doi: 10.1038/88563

Hanahan, D., and Weinberg, R. A. (2011). Hallmarks of cancer: the next generation. *Cell* 144, 646–674. doi: 10.1016/j.cell.2011.02.013

Hintz, R. L., Bock, S., Thorsson, A. V., Bovens, J., Powell, D. R., Jakse, G., et al. (1991). Expression of the insulin like growth factor-binding protein 3 (IGFBP-3) gene is increased in human renal carcinomas. *J. Urol.* 146, 1160–1163. doi: 10.1016/S0022-5347(17)38031-X

Hutton, M. L., Kaparakis-Liaskos, M., Turner, L., Cardona, A., Kwok, T., and Ferrero, R. L. (2010). *Helicobacter pylori* exploits cholesterol-rich microdomains for induction of NF-kappaB-dependent responses and peptidoglycan delivery in epithelial cells. *Infect. Immun.* 78, 4523–4531. doi: 10.1128/IAI.00439-10

IARC (1994). *Schistosomes, Liver Flukes and Helicobacter pylori. IARC Working Group on the Evaluation of Carcinogenic Risks to Humans.* Lyon: IARC.

Ito, Y., Takeda, T., Higashiyama, S., Sakon, M., Wakasa, K. I., Tsujimoto, M., et al. (2001). Expression of heparin binding epidermal growth factor-like growth factor in hepatocellular carcinoma: an immunohistochemical study. *Oncol. Rep.* 8, 903–907. doi: 10.3892/or.8.4.903

Jones, N., Iljin, K., Dumont, D. J., and Alitalo, K. (2001). Tie receptors: new modulators of angiogenic and lymphangiogenic responses. *Nat. Rev. Mol. Cell Biol.* 2, 257–267. doi: 10.1038/35067005

Kaluz, S., and Van Meir, E. G. (2011). At the crossroads of cancer and inflammation: ras rewires an HIF-driven IL-1 autocrine loop. *J. Mol. Med.* 89, 91–94. doi: 10.1007/s00109-010-0706-2

Kim, J. S., Kim, J. M., Jung, H. C., and Song, I. S. (2004). *Helicobacter pylori* down-regulates the receptors of vascular endothelial growth factor and angiopoietin in vascular endothelial cells: implications in the impairment of gastric ulcer healing. *Dig. Dis. Sci.* 49, 778–786. doi: 10.1023/B:DDAS.0000030089.76514.e4

Kitadai, Y. (2010). Cancer-stromal cell interaction and tumor angiogenesis in gastric cancer. *Cancer Microenviron.* 3, 109–116. doi: 10.1007/s12307-009-0032-9

Kusters, J. G., van Vliet, A. H., and Kuipers, E. J. (2006). Pathogenesis of *Helicobacter pylori* infection. *Clin. Microbiol. Rev.* 19, 449–490. doi: 10.1128/CMR.00054-05

Lai, C. H., Chang, Y. C., Du, S. Y., Wang, H. J., Kuo, C. H., Fang, S. H., et al. (2008). Cholesterol depletion reduces *Helicobacter pylori* CagA translocation and CagA-induced responses in AGS cells. *Infect. Immun.* 76, 3293–3303. doi: 10.1128/IAI.00365-08

Law, R. H., Zhang, Q., McGowan, S., Buckle, A. M., Silverman, G. A., Wong, W., et al. (2006). An overview of the serpin superfamily. *Genome Biol.* 7:216. doi: 10.1186/gb-2006-7-5-216

Le Jan, S., Le Meur, N., Cazes, A., Philippe, J., Le Cunff, M., Leger, J., et al. (2006). Characterization of the expression of the hypoxia-induced genes neuritin, TXNIP and IGFBP3 in cancer. *FEBS Lett.* 580, 3395–3400. doi: 10.1016/j.febslet.2006.05.011

Lee, J. H., Jun, S. H., Baik, S. C., Kim, D. R., Park, J. Y., Lee, Y. S., et al. (2012). Prediction and screening of nuclear targeting proteins with nuclear localization signals in *Helicobacter pylori*. *J. Microbiol. Methods* 91, 490–496. doi: 10.1016/j.mimet.2012.10.004

Lee, J. H., Jun, S. H., Kim, J.-M., Baik, S. C., and Lee, J. C. (2015). Morphological changes in human gastric epithelial cells induced by nuclear targeting of *Helicobacter pylori* urease subunit A. *J. Microbiol.* 53, 406–414. doi: 10.1007/s12275-015-5085-5

Lee, O. H., Bae, S. K., Bae, M. H., Lee, Y. M., Moon, E. J., Cha, H. J., et al. (2000). Identification of angiogenic properties of insulin-like growth factor II in in vitro angiogenesis models. *Br. J. Cancer* 82, 385–391. doi: 10.1054/bjoc.1999.0931

Li, X. S., Xu, Q., Fu, X. Y., and Luo, W. S. (2014). Heat shock protein 60 overexpression is associated with the progression and prognosis in gastric cancer. *PLOS ONE* 9:e107507. doi: 10.1371/journal.pone.0107507

Lin, C.-S., He, P.-J., Hsu, W.-T., Wu, M.-S., Wu, C.-J., Shen, H.-W., et al. (2010). *Helicobacter pylori*-derived heat shock protein 60 enhances angiogenesis via a CXCR2-mediated signaling pathway. *Biochem. Biophys. Res. Commun.* 397, 283–289. doi: 10.1016/j.bbrc.2010.05.101

Linkert, M., Rueden, C. T., Allan, C., Burel, J. M., Moore, W., Patterson, A., et al. (2010). Metadata matters: access to image data in the real world. *J. Cell Biol.* 189, 777–782. doi: 10.1083/jcb.201004104

Liu, N., Zhou, N., Chai, N., Liu, X., Jiang, H., Wu, Q., et al. (2016). *Helicobacter pylori* promotes angiogenesis depending on Wnt/beta-catenin-mediated vascular endothelial growth factor via the cyclooxygenase-2 pathway in gastric cancer. *BMC Cancer* 16:321. doi: 10.1186/s12885-016-2351-9

Macedo, F., Ladeira, K., Longatto-Filho, A., and Martins, S. F. (2017). Gastric cancer and angiogenesis: is VEGF a useful biomarker to assess progression and remission? *J. Gastric Cancer* 17, 1–10. doi: 10.5230/jgc.2017.17.e1

Maione, T. E., Gray, G. S., Petro, J., Hunt, A. J., Donner, A. L., Bauer, S. I., et al. (1990). Inhibition of angiogenesis by recombinant human platelet factor-4 and related peptides. *Science* 247, 77–79. doi: 10.1126/science.1688470

Marko, J., Mahak, S., Juliati, R., and Steve, C. (2010). The early endosome: a busy sorting station for proteins at the crossroads. *Histol. Histopathol.* 25, 99–112.

Marshall, B. J., Barrett, L. J., Prakash, C., McCallum, R. W., and Guerrant, R. L. (1990). Urea protects *Helicobacter* (*Campylobacter*) *pylori* from the bactericidal effect of acid. *Gastroenterology* 99, 697–702. doi: 10.1016/0016-5085(90)90957-3

Mehta, V. B., Zhou, Y., Radulescu, A., and Besner, G. E. (2008). HB-EGF stimulates eNOS expression and nitric oxide production and promotes eNOS dependent angiogenesis. *Growth Factors* 26, 301–315. doi: 10.1080/08977190802393596

Miyake, M., Goodison, S., Lawton, A., Gomes-Giacoia, E., and Rosser, C. J. (2015). Angiogenin promotes tumoral growth and angiogenesis by regulating matrix metallopeptidase-2 expression via the ERK1/2 pathway. *Oncogene* 34, 890–901. doi: 10.1038/onc.2014.2

Okines, A. F. C., Reynolds, A. R., and Cunningham, D. (2011). Targeting angiogenesis in esophagogastric adenocarcinoma. *Oncologist* 16, 844–858. doi: 10.1634/theoncologist.2010-0387

Oliveira, M. J., Costa, A. M., Costa, A. C., Ferreira, R. M., Sampaio, P., Machado, J. C., et al. (2009). CagA associates with c-Met, E-cadherin, and p120-catenin in a multiproteic complex that suppresses *Helicobacter pylori*-induced cell-invasive phenotype. *J. Infect. Dis.* 200, 745–755. doi: 10.1086/604727

Ollauri-Ibanez, C., Lopez-Novoa, J. M., and Pericacho, M. (2017). Endoglin-based biological therapy in the treatment of angiogenesis-dependent pathologies. *Expert Opin. Biol. Ther.* 17, 1053–1063. doi: 10.1080/14712598.2017.1346607

Olofsson, A., Vallström, A., Petzold, K., Tegtmeyer, N., Schleucher, J., Carlsson, S., et al. (2010). Biochemical and functional characterization of *Helicobacter pylori* vesicles. *Mol. Microbiol.* 77, 1539–1555. doi: 10.1111/j.1365-2958.2010.07307.x

Palframan, S. L., Kwok, T., and Gabriel, K. (2012). Vacuolating cytotoxin A (VacA), a key toxin for *Helicobacter pylori* pathogenesis. *Front. Cell. Infect. Microbiol.* 2:92. doi: 10.3389/fcimb.2012.00092

Perrais, M., Rousseaux, C., Ducourouble, M. P., Courcol, R., Vincent, P., Jonckheere, N., et al. (2014). *Helicobacter pylori* urease and flagellin alter mucin gene expression in human gastric cancer cells. *Gastric Cancer* 17, 235–246. doi: 10.1007/s10120-013-0267-5

Pinto, M. P., Owen, G. I., Retamal, I., and Garrido, M. (2017). Angiogenesis inhibitors in early development for gastric cancer. *Expert Opin. Investig. Drugs* 26, 1007–1017. doi: 10.1080/13543784.2017.1361926

Plummer, M., de Martel, C., Vignat, J., Ferlay, J., Bray, F., and Franceschi, S. (2016). Global burden of cancers attributable to infections in 2012: a synthetic analysis. *Lancet Glob. Health* 4, e609–e616. doi: 10.1016/S2214-109X(16)30143-7

Sato, Y. (2013). The vasohibin family: a novel family for angiogenesis regulation. *J. Biochem.* 153, 5–11. doi: 10.1093/jb/mvs128

Schneider, C. A., Rasband, W. S., and Eliceiri, K. W. (2012). NIH Image to ImageJ: 25 years of image analysis. *Nat. Methods* 9, 671–675. doi: 10.1038/nmeth.2089

Schraw, W., Li, Y., McClain, M. S., van der Goot, F. G., and Cover, T. L. (2002). Association of *Helicobacter pylori* vacuolating toxin (VacA) with lipid rafts. *J. Biol. Chem.* 277, 34642–34650. doi: 10.1074/jbc.M203466200

Schwartz, J. T., and Allen, L. A. (2006). Role of urease in megasome formation and *Helicobacter pylori* survival in macrophages. *J. Leukoc. Biol.* 79, 1214–1225. doi: 10.1189/jlb.0106030

Stallone, G., Cormio, L., Netti, G. S., Infante, B., Selvaggio, O., Fino, G. D., et al. (2014). Pentraxin 3: a novel biomarker for predicting progression from prostatic inflammation to prostate cancer. *Cancer Res.* 74, 4230–4238. doi: 10.1158/0008-5472.CAN-14-0369

Strober, W. (2001). Trypan blue exclusion test of cell viability. *Curr. Protoc. Immunol.* 21, A.3B.1–A.3B.2. doi: 10.1002/0471142735.ima03bs21

Terebiznik, M. R., Raju, D., Vázquez, C. L., Torbricki, K., Kulkarni, R., Blanke, S. R., et al. (2009). Effect of *Helicobacter pylori's* vacuolating cytotoxin on the autophagy pathway in gastric epithelial cells. *Autophagy* 5, 370–379. doi: 10.4161/auto.5.3.7663

Teresa Pinto, A., Laranjeiro Pinto, M., Patricia Cardoso, A., Monteiro, C., Teixeira Pinto, M., Filipe Maia, A., et al. (2016). Ionizing radiation modulates human macrophages towards a pro-inflammatory phenotype preserving their pro-invasive and pro-angiogenic capacities. *Sci. Rep.* 6:18765. doi: 10.1038/srep18765

Tobin, N. P., Henehan, G. T., Murphy, R. P., Atherton, J. C., Guinan, A. F., Kerrigan, S. W., et al. (2008). *Helicobacter pylori*-induced inhibition of vascular endothelial cell functions: a role for VacA-dependent nitric oxide reduction. *Am. J. Physiol. Heart Circ. Physiol.* 295, H1403–H1413. doi: 10.1152/ajpheart.00240.2008

Uberti, A. F., Olivera-Severo, D., Wassermann, G. E., Scopel-Guerra, A., Moraes, J. A., Barcellos-de-Souza, P., et al. (2013). Pro-inflammatory properties and neutrophil activation by *Helicobacter pylori* urease. *Toxicon* 69, 240–249. doi: 10.1016/j.toxicon.2013.02.009

Vandercappellen, J., Van Damme, J., and Struyf, S. (2011). The role of the CXC chemokines platelet factor-4 (CXCL4/PF-4) and its variant (CXCL4L1/PF-4var) in inflammation, angiogenesis and cancer. *Cytokine Growth Factor Rev.* 22, 1–18. doi: 10.1016/j.cytogfr.2010.10.011

Wassermann, G. E., Olivera-Severo, D., Uberti, A. F., and Carlini, C. R. (2010). *Helicobacter pylori* urease activates blood platelets through a lipoxygenase-mediated pathway. *J. Cell. Mol. Med.* 14, 2025–2034. doi: 10.1111/j.1582-4934.2009.00901.x

Wroblewski, L. E., Shen, L., Ogden, S., Romero-Gallo, J., Lapierre, L. A., Israel, D. A., et al. (2009). *Helicobacter pylori* dysregulation of gastric epithelial tight junctions by urease-mediated myosin II activation. *Gastroenterology* 136, 236–246. doi: 10.1053/j.gastro.2008.10.011

Yeo, M., Kim, D. K., Han, S. U., Lee, J. E., Kim, Y. B., Cho, Y. K., et al. (2006). Novel action of gastric proton pump inhibitor on suppression of *Helicobacter pylori* induced angiogenesis. *Gut* 55, 26–33. doi: 10.1136/gut.2005.067454

Zhou, J., Goh, B. C., Albert, D. H., and Chen, C. S. (2009). ABT-869, a promising multi-targeted tyrosine kinase inhibitor: from bench to bedside. *J. Hematol. Oncol.* 2:33. doi: 10.1186/1756-8722-2-33

3

Intestinal Microbiota Influences Non-Intestinal Related Autoimmune Diseases

*Maria C. Opazo [1,2], Elizabeth M. Ortega-Rocha [3], Irenice Coronado-Arrázola [4], Laura C. Bonifaz [5], Helene Boudin [6], Michel Neunlist [6], Susan M. Bueno [4], Alexis M. Kalergis [4,7] and Claudia A. Riedel [1,2]**

[1] Laboratorio de Biología Celular y Farmacología, Departamento de Ciencias Biológicas, Facultad de Ciencias Biológicas, Millennium Institute on Immunology and Immunotherapy, Universidad Andres Bello, Santiago, Chile, [2] Facultad de Medicina, Millennium Institute on Immunology and Immunotherapy, Universidad Andres Bello, Santiago, Chile, [3] Laboratorio de Inmunobiología, Facultad de Medicina, Departamento de Biología Celular y Tisular, Universidad Nacional Autónoma de México, Mexico City, Mexico, [4] Departamento de Genética Molecular y Microbiología, Facultad de Ciencias Biológicas, Millennium Institute on Immunology and Immunotherapy, Pontificia Universidad Católica de Chile, Santiago, Chile, [5] Unidad de Investigación Médica en Inmunoquímica Hospital de Especialidades Centro Médico Nacional Siglo XXI, Instituto Mexicano del Seguro Social, Mexico City, Mexico, [6] Institut National de la Santé et de la Recherche Médicale U1235, Institut des Maladies de l'Appareil Digestif, Université de Nantes, Nantes, France, [7] Departamento de Endocrinología, Facultad de Medicina, Pontificia Universidad, Metropolitana, Chile

***Correspondence:**
Claudia A. Riedel
criedel99@yahoo.com;
claudia.riedel@unab.cl

The human body is colonized by millions of microorganisms named microbiota that interact with our tissues in a cooperative and non-pathogenic manner. These microorganisms are present in the skin, gut, nasal, oral cavities, and genital tract. In fact, it has been described that the microbiota contributes to balancing the immune system to maintain host homeostasis. The gut is a vital organ where microbiota can influence and determine the function of cells of the immune system and contributes to preserve the wellbeing of the individual. Several articles have emphasized the connection between intestinal autoimmune diseases, such as Crohn's disease with dysbiosis or an imbalance in the microbiota composition in the gut. However, little is known about the role of the microbiota in autoimmune pathologies affecting other tissues than the intestine. This article focuses on what is known about the role that gut microbiota can play in the pathogenesis of non-intestinal autoimmune diseases, such as Grave's diseases, multiple sclerosis, type-1 diabetes, systemic lupus erythematosus, psoriasis, schizophrenia, and autism spectrum disorders. Furthermore, we discuss as to how metabolites derived from bacteria could be used as potential therapies for non-intestinal autoimmune diseases.

Keywords: microbiota, autoimmune disease, gut, microbiome, skin, CNS

INTRODUCTION

Our body is colonized by millions of microorganisms that can survive in extreme environments surpassing difficult conditions, such as low pH or low oxygen (Peterson et al., 2015). The skin, gut, nasal, and oral cavities and genital tract are colonized by hundreds of different types of microorganisms and are known as "normal flora" or microbiota (Peterson et al., 2015). Lederberg defined the microbiota in 2001 as *"the ecological community of commensal, symbiotic, and pathogenic microorganisms that share our body space"* (Lederberg , 2001). For some authors the concept of microbiota comprehends mainly bacteria and while the concept of microbiota comprehends several different species among them are bacteria, archaea, fungi and viruses (Selber-Hnatiw et al., 2017). Recent scientific advances supported additionally by *"omics analyses"* have been crucial for the generation of a large amount of data relative to the composition of the microbiota (Almonacid et al., 2017). In fact, scientific progress has allowed the identification of the composition of the microbiota and the identification of specific microorganisms that live in the gut (Ferreira et al., 2017). The analysis of this information has contributed to revealing the complex relationship between the microbiota and the host. Evidence in the literature has shown that alterations in the proportion of these microorganisms can be associated to pathologies affecting humans (Aarts et al., 2017; Almonacid et al., 2017; Ferreira et al., 2017). Along these lines, in the past few years several scientific publications have shown a possible association between microbiota alterations and autoimmune diseases (Alkanani et al., 2015; Ma et al., 2015; Miyake et al., 2015; Breban et al., 2017; Kohling et al., 2017). These pathologies are characterized by an immune response against the body's own tissues causing inflammation and destruction of tissues and/or organs (Nagy et al., 2015). Autoimmune diseases are especially frequent in western countries, affecting majorly women (Davidson and Diamond, 2001). It has been proposed that lifestyle in this "modern era" can be affecting the microbiota composition causing a deregulation of the immune system (Berbers et al., 2017). Evidences in the literature have shown a strong link between microbiota composition and intestinal autoimmune diseases, such as Crohn's disease and inflammatory bowel disease (IBD) (Matsuoka and Kanai, 2015; Nishida et al., 2017; Powell and MacDonald, 2017). However, host gut microbiota seems also capable of influence autoimmune diseases that target tissues other than the intestine, including Type 1 diabetes (De Groot et al., 2017), multiple sclerosis (Hindson, 2017), arthritis (Felix et al., 2017), and psoriasis (Yan et al., 2017). Interestingly diseases like schizophrenia and autism are now considered to also have an inflammatory component suggesting that these ailments could also be associated to changes in intestinal microbiota (Dickerson et al., 2017; Vasquez, 2017; Wu, 2017; Yang et al., 2017; Cox and Weiner, 2018; Kopec et al., 2018). The aim of this review article is to analyze recent information supporting an association between gut microbiota composition and non-intestinal autoimmune diseases.

THE MICROBIOTA THROUGH HUMAN LIFE

An adult of 70 kg in average has around 39 trillion of bacteria and 30 trillion of human cells (Sender et al., 2016) and at least 20% of the metabolites in the blood are derived from commensal bacteria (Rook et al., 2017). The gut microbiota consists of about 2,000 different bacterial species (Llorente and Schnabl, 2015) and most of them reside at the distal intestine (Kamada et al., 2013b). In general, human gut microbiota is comprised by two main dominants phyla Firmicutes and Bacteroidetes, which are susceptible to alterations due to factors such as age, genetics, diet, environment, and infection (Gill et al., 2006). The neonatal microbiota is highly different compared to adult microbiota (Pickard et al., 2017). Neonatal microbiota is strongly influenced by type of delivery at birth. Thus, a vaginal delivery allows the colonization of the mother's gastrointestinal microorganisms to the neonate, meanwhile in a C-section delivery the infant will present more microorganisms related to mother's skin (Wampach et al., 2017).

Certain data support the notion that bacteria colonization in humans will begin in the gestation at the womb (Stinson et al., 2017). Consistently, several reports have detected the presence of bacterial DNA in the amniotic fluid, umbilical cord, placenta, meconium, and fetal membranes (Khan et al., 2016; Stinson et al., 2017; Tschoeke et al., 2017). This evidence is in contrast with the hypothesis of the sterile womb and that bacteria colonization in humans begins only at birth or at breastfeeding (Funkhouser and Bordenstein, 2013). The neonatal microbiota initially will resemble very much to individual maternal microbiota (Wampach et al., 2017). During the following years, the microbiota will be shaped and changed by nutritional, physiological, and/or pathological events occurring through life (Chu et al., 2016).

Evidence suggests that a proper microbiota homeostasis is required for the maturation of central nervous system (CNS), as well as the immune system during different developmental stages, such as infancy, adolescence, and adulthood (Rook et al., 2017). Certain microorganisms included in the microbiota will contribute to an appropriate development of various human tissues and organs. However, other microorganism could increase the susceptibility to suffering certain pathologies (Berbers et al., 2017). Therefore, the diet is an important factor that can lead to changes in the microbiota composition (Cui et al., 2017). It has been reported that only 24 h are sufficient to alter the composition of the microbiota after a change in the diet of an individual (Wu et al., 2011). For example, high fat diets increase the presence of enterotypes, such as *Bacteroides* meanwhile a fiber-rich diet increases the amount of the *Prevotella* genus (Wu et al., 2011). It has been shown that inappropriate changes in the microbiota composition, known as dysbiosis, could cause harmful consequences to the host (La Fata et al., 2017). For example dysbiosis has been reported for patients suffering from type I and type II diabetes, IBD and colorectal cancer (CRC) (Peterson et al., 2015). Because it would be of importance to understand how the microbiota composition can impair the wellness of the host, significant research efforts are currently in place to develop new treatments for these pathologies based on restoring a normal microbiota composition.

THE INTESTINAL BARRIERS FOR THE MICROBIOTA

The gut has developed different mechanisms to ensure a beneficial intestinal microbiota composition, as well as for regulating microbiota overgrowth and restricting pathogen colonization (Llorente and Schnabl, 2015; Gensollen et al., 2016). It is thought that the gut can produce an intestinal barrier by secreting mucus and pro-inflammatory molecules that contribute to the establishment of innate and adaptive immunity (Feng and Elson, 2011).

Intestinal epithelial cells are the first constituents of the gut barrier and they cover the intestinal lumen and separate the gut microbiota from the immune system (Farhadi et al., 2003; Feng and Elson, 2011). Epithelial cells are maintained together by tight junctions (TJs), adherents junctions (AJ), and desmosomes (Hartsock and Nelson, 2008). TJs are multiprotein complexes comprised of integral membrane proteins, such as claudins, occludins, and junctional adhesion molecules (Hartsock and Nelson, 2008). The TJs regulate the passing of solutes and fluids through the epithelial cells by passive paracellular diffusion (Choi et al., 2017). As part of the epithelial cell barrier are goblet cells, which secrete glycoproteins to the lumen forming an inner mucus layer that is closer to epithelium and an outer mucus layer that is in contact with bacteria (Hooper and Macpherson, 2010). Additionally, epithelial cells can secrete antimicrobial proteins, such as defensins, cathelicidins, and C-type lectins (Chairatana and Nolan, 2017). These molecules contribute at controlling bacterial growth by either enzymatically degrading their cell wall, disrupting the inner membrane or depriving bacteria from essential heavy metals (Mukherjee and Hooper, 2015). Additionally, enterocytes, enteroendocrine cells, globet cells, and Paneth cells can also produce antimicrobial proteins contributing to the antimicrobial activity (Chairatana and Nolan, 2017).

The three main lymphoid structures of gut immune system that locate at the mucosa are: (1) the Peyer's patches (PP), which is the mucosa-associated lymphoid tissue that can be found in clusters; (2) the lamina propria (LP) located as an isolated lymphoid tissue where effector lymphocytes secrete cytokines and immunoglobulins; and (3) the epithelium layer in which intraepithelial resident lymphocytes can be found (Richards et al., 2016; Shi et al., 2017). The secretion of IgA is considered to be an antimicrobial agent that is accomplished by the help of dendritic cells (DC) from the PP. IgA interacts with bacteria impeding their adhesion to epithelial cells and inhibiting bacterial motility (McGuckin et al., 2011).

The gut microbiota is tightly associated and has constant communication with the mucosal immune system. It is thought that the mucosal immune system limits the invasion of tissues by the normal flora, which entails a high microbial diversity as well as potential pathogens that could have been ingested with the diet (Hooper and Macpherson, 2010). Such a function is in part carried out by DCs located at the mucosal surface where they uptake antigens and prime lymphocytes. DCs can directly sample normal flora and pathogenic bacteria (Kelsall, 2008). Despite all of these barrier mechanisms, bacteria can find ways for trespassing them and go across the epithelial layer triggering bacteria killing mechanisms. Rapidly, trespassing bacteria suffer phagocytosis and elimination by the LP macrophages (Kelsall, 2008).

Activated DCs can promote the differentiation of T cells to regulate immune tolerance (Shi et al., 2017). In fact, there is a high content of T cells at the intestinal mucosa that can be divided in two major subpopulations known as type A or conventional (TCRαβ) located at the PPs and mesenteric lymph nodes and type B or non-conventional (TCRγδ) that can be found almost exclusively at the epithelium (Van Wijk and Cheroutre, 2010). Naïve T cells become activated into effector helper T cells (Th) by mainly differentiating into: (1) Th1 cells that contribute to the elimination of intracellular pathogens; (2) Th2 cells that protect against parasites and mediate allergic reactions; or (3) Th17 cells that contribute to the clearance of foreign pathogens (Geremia et al., 2014). Intestinal DCs can also regulate the differentiation of T cells to regulatory T cells (Tregs). The role of Tregs is to reduce and control the immune response in part by suppressing the activation and proliferation of T helper cells through the secretion of anti-inflammatory cytokines (O'garra and Vieira, 2004). Several studies support the notion that an alteration of the balance between T helper and Treg cells can be closely associated to intestinal autoimmune pathologies (Fasching et al., 2017; **Figure 1**).

MODULATION OF T CELL DIFFERENTIATION BY THE MICROBIOTA

Microbiota members can regulate the immune response through secretion of metabolites, such as short-chain fatty acids (SCFA). SCFAs are produced in the colon by the microbiota through fermentation of non-digestible carbohydrates including cellulose or inulin among others (Chen et al., 2015). The main products are acetate, propionate and butyrate, which are absorbed by the colon (Rios-Covian et al., 2016). While butyrate acts as an energy source for epithelial cells (Jung et al., 2015) and facilitates tight junction assembly (Peng et al., 2009), acetate and propionate are substrates for gluconeogenesis and lipogenesis in the liver and other peripheral organs (Rios-Covian et al., 2016).

SCFAs can modulate the intestinal immune response (Tremaroli and Backhed, 2012) by regulating T cell differentiation (Cavaglieri et al., 2003), epithelial barrier function, production of antimicrobial peptides, and the secretion of pro-inflammatory mediators (Johnson-Henry et al., 2014). Administration of butyrate in an animal model of colorectal colitis ameliorates the symptoms by increasing the percentage of Tregs and the production of IL-10 and IL-12 in peripheral blood, with an concomitant decrease of RORγt (a Th17 biomarker), IL-17 and IL-23 levels (Zhang et al., 2016). Furthermore, the addition *in vitro* of butyrate to human peripheral blood mononuclear cells (PBMCs) increased the differentiation of Tregs suggesting for this molecule a regulatory role in Treg/Th17 balance that influences the immune response (Zhang et al., 2016). Administration of SCFAs has been used in animal models of experimental autoimmune encephalomyelitis (EAE). It was observed that the oral administration of SCFAs butyrate, acetate, and propionate could significantly decrease EAE clinical score in mice (Mizuno et al., 2017). In these experiments, propionate showed the higher capacity to protect animals from the development of EAE (Mizuno et al., 2017) Interestingly, while treatment with propionate increased the frequency of Tregs in lymph nodes, treatment with butyrate did so in the spleens (Mizuno et al., 2017). These results reinforce the notion that

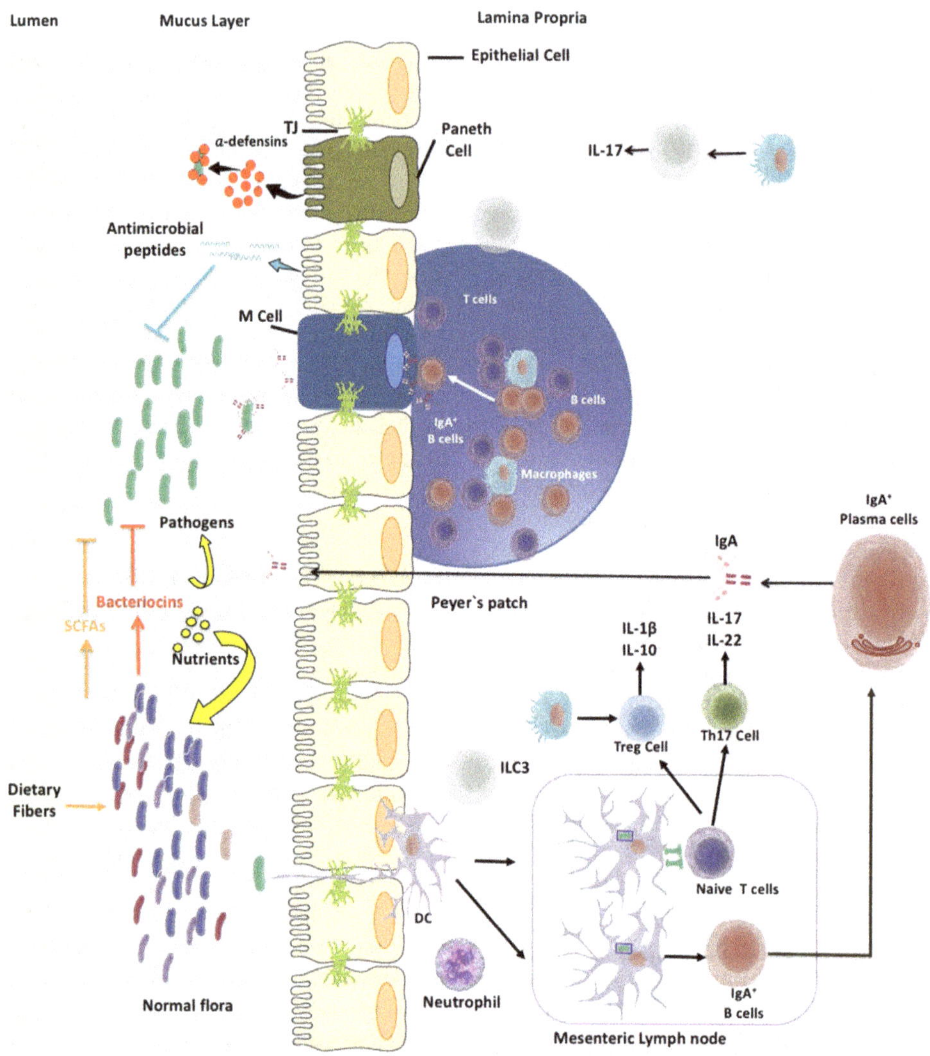

FIGURE 1 | Microbiota and pathogen control mechanisms of the gut immune system. The immune system of the gut has to deal with wide diversity of microbiota and pathogens. Thus, the immune system will help to establish a beneficial microbiota composition at the gut. Different mechanisms of the gut immune system have been discovered that control microbiota overgrowth and pathogens invasion. The gut immune system locates in the mucosa layer of the intestine mainly at the epithelium layer and Peyer's patches at the lamina propia. Enterocytes, enteroendocrine cells, globet cells, and Paneth cells, located in the intestinal epithelial layer, secrete antimicrobial peptides like defensins. It has been shown that defensins are produced in the course of innate immune defense to activate the adaptive immune response. Another mechanism to control microbiota is the secretion of IgA which is accomplished by dendritic cells (DC). IgGA by interacting with bacteria impedes their adhesion and inhibits bacteria motility. DCs are localized at mucosal surfaces in antigen uptake sites and at inductive lymphoid tissue; they can directly sampling the normal flora and pathogenic bacteria. In the mesenteric lymph node DCs can promote differentiation of T cells, to regulate immune tolerance. Once T cells are activated they differentiate to T helper cells (Th), like Th1, Th2, or Th17 cells. Intestinal DCs will also regulate the differentiation of T cells to T regulatory (Treg) cells. Treg cells have the capacity to suppress the activation and proliferation of Th cells by the secretion of anti-inflammatory cytokines.

SCFAs from the intestine can regulate systemic inflammation that is mediated by lymphocytes.

Hashimoto et al. by using *Ace2* knockout mice showed that a protein-free diet alters intestinal immunity (Hashimoto et al., 2012). Angiotensin converting enzyme-2 (ACE2) is a key regulatory enzyme of the renin-angiotensin system (RAS) as it catalyzes the conversion of angiotensin II (Ang II) to angiotensin 1-7 (Ang 1-7) the latter can bind the G-coupled protein Mas receptor inducing vasodilatation contrasting the effects of the binding of Ang II to its receptor AT-1 that promotes vasoconstriction and hypertension (Perlot and Penninger, 2013). ACE2 knockout male mice or $Ace2^{-/y}$ mice (Ace deficient at the × chromosome) induced with colitis and protein-deprived showed increased infiltration, ulceration, weight loss and higher diarrhea scores, as well as decreased serum levels of tryptophan (Trp) (Hashimoto et al., 2012). Trp is an essential amino acid for mammals and can only be obtained through the diet (Badawy, 2017). These knockout mice supplemented with Trp significantly improved colitis symptoms (Hashimoto et al., 2012). Additional analyses showed that these mice display an altered gut microbiota composition and an increase production of antimicrobial peptides, as compared to Trp-supplemented mice (Hashimoto et al., 2012).

Moreover, it has been observed that the microbiota produces catabolites from Trp or Trp-indole derivatives, such as Indole 3-acetamide, indole-3-acetic acid and indole-3-lactic acid and modulates the mucosal immune response through IL-22, which is produced by innate lymphoid cells 3 (ILC3) (Zelante et al., 2013). Consistently with these findings, Lamas et al. showed that the colitis associated knockout mice for *Card9* display a microbiota dysbiosis (Lamas et al., 2016). An adaptor protein involved in the immune response against fungi dysbiosis (Etienne-Mesmin et al., 2017). Authors showed that *Card9* knockout mice missed a Trp-metabolizing bacterium. Thus, the consequence is that these mice had low content of indole derivatives, which are important for the production of IL-22 by the ILC3 and T cells at the mucosa. Low levels of IL-22 generate a pro-inflammatory environment (Lamas et al., 2016), because this cytokine has anti-inflammatory properties and belongs to the IL-10 cytokine family (Parks et al., 2015). IL-22 participates in host defense against extracellular pathogens by eliciting innate defensive mechanisms that promote the expression of antimicrobial peptides at mucosal surfaces (Rutz et al., 2013) and is also involved in tissue repair by enhancing epithelial cell proliferation (Aujla and Kolls, 2009).

Additionally, IL-22 can influence intestinal epithelial cell glycosylation by inducing the expression of fucosyltransferase 2 (Fut2) that catalyzes the fucosylation of membrane proteins, a post translational modification needed for protection against enteric pathogens, such as *S. typhimurium* (Okumura and Takeda, 2017). Recent data support the notion that microbiota has immune-modulatory properties, however little is known about the identification of the specific bacteria genera responsible for the phenotype and also few is known at molecular level for which mechanisms these bacteria modulate the inflammatory state of the intestine. So far, it has been described that the presence of polysaccharide A (PSA) in the gut commensal *Bacteroides fragilis* induces the secretion of IL-10 by Tregs, which in turn decreases inflammation in the gut and in distant tissues, such as the brain (Ochoa-Reparaz et al., 2010; Dasgupta et al., 2014). These findings highlight the role of metabolites produced by the intestinal microbiota to modulate inflammation and their potential use as a therapeutic tool to treat inflammatory and autoimmune diseases.

WHAT DO WE KNOW ABOUT THE ROLE OF THE MICROBIOTA IN NON-INTESTINAL AUTOIMMUNE DISEASES?

Autoimmune Diseases

Autoimmune diseases are pathologies characterized by an inappropriate immune response against own tissues and molecules that results in tissue-specific or systemic inflammation that leads to organ damage and malfunction (Rose and Bona, 1993; Marmont, 1994). Causes for autoimmune disease are multifactorial and range from genetic predisposition to the exposition of environmental agents, such as infectious agents, xenobiotics, drugs, or stress (Davidson and Diamond, 2001). The disease progresses from initial naive lymphocyte activation to a chronic state characterized by an increase in the number of autoantigens targeted by T cells and antibodies. Activated autoreactive B cells can function as antigen presenting cells for novel peptides and express co-stimulatory molecules. Antigens are processed and presented to naive T cells leading to the activation of additional autoreactive B cells that present new epitopes up to a point in which there is autoreactivity to a large number of autoantigens (Lanzavecchia, 1995; Liang and Mamula, 2000). The production of autoantibodies induces damages to tissues by the formation of immune complexes, cytolysis, or phagocytosis of target self-cells and interfering with proper tissue and cellular functions (O'Garra et al., 1997). Although there are several autoimmune diseases, in this review we will focus on non-intestinal autoimmune disorders, for intestinal autoimmune diseases, please refer to other reports (Gallo et al., 2016; Blander et al., 2017; Passos and Moraes-Filho, 2017).

Graves's Disease and Hashimoto's Thyroiditis

The Grave's disease (GD) is an autoimmune disease characterized by the targeting of antigens derived from the thyroid gland. In GD there are autoantibodies against the thyroid stimulating hormone receptor (TSHR) (Kristensen, 2016). These autoantibodies activate the TSHR inducing the synthesis and secretion of thyroid hormones by the thyroid gland and causing hyperthyroidism. GD is the most common cause of hyperthyroidism and is more frequently observed in women than in men (Pokhrel and Bhusal, 2017). Shor et al. evaluated the prevalence of gastrointestinal auto antibodies in patients with Hashimoto's thyroiditis and Grave's disease (Shor et al., 2012). These are anti-gliadin antibodies (AGA), tissue transglutaminase (tTG) and anti *Saccharomyces cerevisiae* antibodies (ASCA). In particular ASCA have proven to be sensitive and highly specific for Crohn's disease. ASCA antibodies were highly prevalent in patients with GD (Shor et al., 2012). Analysis of fecal samples from GD patients showed an increased content of yeast supporting Schor's analyses (Covelli and Ludgate, 2017). It has also been observed the presence of antibodies against *Yersinia enterocolitica* and to *Helicobacter pylori,* but these responses vary among patients and are not observed in all the analyzed patients (Kohling et al., 2017). Next-generation sequencing projects intended to analyze and identify bacteria species in patients with GD. Using a TSHR immunized mouse model, it was observed an alteration of immunized animals when compared to controls. In humans, this modification is not fully observed, so far it has been observed in a small number of patients a significant decrease of the *Bacteroides* genus (Indigo, 2017). These are the first reports associating the gut microbiota and GD; therefore additional work must be accomplished to better understand the influence of the gut microbiota on the development of GD.

Hashimoto's thyroiditis (HT) is an autoimmune disease that is characterized by the infiltration of mononuclear cells in the thyroid, together with the production of autoantibodies against thyroglobulin and thyroid peroxidase (TPO) (Antonelli et al., 2015). It is thought that environmental factors, such as diets higher in iodide, contribute to the etiology of HT (Rose et al., 2002). Recently, research efforts have focused on the involvement of microbiota in the pathogenesis of autoimmune diseases. The transfer of microbiota from conventional rats to specific pathogen free (SPF) rats increased the susceptibility of the latter to experimental autoimmune thyroiditis (Penhale and Young, 1988), which provides further support for an influence of the microbiota during HT pathogenesis. The use of the probiotic mixture (VSL#3^{TM}) has been successful to reduce the susceptibility to developing autoimmune diseases, such as Type 1 diabetes and colitis by enhancing the production of IL-10 in Peyer's patches and the spleen (Calcinaro et al., 2005; Di Giacinto et al., 2005). Along these lines, it was important to explore whether probiotics could have a positive effect on HT. Contrarily to what was initially thought, the use probiotic strains of *Lactobacillus rhamnosus* HN001, *Bifidobacterium lactis* HN019, and *L. rhamnosus* GG failed to improve the disease outcome in a mouse model for autoimmune thyroiditis (Zhou and Gill, 2005). It has been demonstrated that a dysbiosis state can alter the epithelial barrier permeability leading to a condition known as "leaky gut" (Vaarala et al., 2008). At the histologic level, this is observed as morphological changes in epithelial cells and lymphocyte infiltration (Fritscher-Ravens et al., 2014). Interestingly, a similar observation has been made in patients with HT, in which both the space of two adjacent microvilli and the microvilli thickness are significantly increased. Furthermore, these patients were also evaluated for functional mucosal alterations using a lactulose/manitol test showing an increase in the recovery of lactulose/mannitol, which is consistent with the histological observations (Sasso et al., 2004). These data suggest that the microbiota and the epithelial barrier play an important role of during the pathogenesis of HT.

Type I Diabetes

Type 1 diabetes (T1D) is the most prevalent autoimmune disease in young people (<20 years), with a peak at 10–14 years old (Maahs et al., 2010) being more common in boys than in girls (Atkinson et al., 2014). The incidence of T1D is very variable worldwide, being higher in Europeans countries probably due to environmental factors (Xie et al., 2014) T1D is characterized by a T cell-mediated (CD4^{+} and CD8^{+}) destruction of β pancreatic cells (Atkinson et al., 2014). There are three major auto antigens associated to T1D, which are insulin, GAD65 (glutamic acid descarboxylase, 65 kDa isoform), and IA2 (Insulin autoantigen 2) (Ounissi-Benkalha and Polychronakos, 2008). The presence of antibodies specific for these antigens has been observed in the serum of T1D patients (Miao et al., 2007). A classical trio of symptoms characterizes T1D, which are polydipsia, polyphagia, and polyuria, accompanied by an overt hypoglycemia (Atkinson et al., 2014). All of them are used as hallmarks for T1D diagnosis in high-risk individuals, such as children and adolescents (Leslie, 2010).

The 60% of patients suffering from T1D has been attributed to a genetic cause (Ounissi-Benkalha and Polychronakos, 2008). The 50% of heritability of T1D is attributed to the human leukocyte antigen (HLA) alleles located in chromosome 6 and the rest is to non-HLA loci (Barrett et al., 2009; Redondo et al., 2017). It has been reported that are at least 40 non-HLA loci such *INS*, *CTLA4*, *PTPN22*, and *IL2RA* can contribute to disease susceptibility (Barrett et al., 2009). Moreover, T1D can also be triggered by environmental factors, such as cesarean or vaginal birth, diet, early infections in life etc. (Rewers and Ludvigsson, 2016). Experimental evidence has shown that the intestinal microbiota could induce T1D by priming the immune system at an early postnatal period (Endesfelder et al., 2016).

The first evidence linking the gut immune system and T1D derives from animal models. Non-obese diabetic (NOD) mice fed with regular commercial cereal-based chow and mice fed with a 10% casein-based diet presented the highest rates of T1D among the experimental groups (Elliott et al., 1988). These rates (26.9% cereal-based chow vs. 19.1% casein-rich diet) were significantly higher than the expected for this type of mice, which normally develop insulin-dependent diabetes at 200–250 days of age. Authors observed that the incidence of T1D in these mice was due to the 10% of casein in this diet, interestingly this percentage corresponds to the percentage of casein in cow milk (Elliott et al., 1988). Another important observation in children suffering T1D was the presence of antibodies against bovine serum albumin, a protein also contained in cow milk (Savilahti et al., 1988; Karjalainen et al., 1992; Saukkonen et al., 1996). These two observations support the notion that the diet could trigger the development of T1D, due that it contains potential antigens that will prime the immune system (Mejia-Leon and Barca, 2015; Rewers and Ludvigsson, 2016; Virtanen, 2016).

The notion that antigens derived from the diet can prime the immune system, suggests that the immune system is in contact with antigens and the intestinal permeability must be altered. In fact, there is evidence supporting a relationship between T1D and high intestinal permeability (Vaarala, 2008; Li and Atkinson, 2015; Maffeis et al., 2016). A study performed in 46 non-celiac T1D patients showed a significant increase of intestinal permeability as compared to healthy controls (Secondulfo et al., 2004). Authors performed electronic transmission microscopy (TEM) analyses over intestinal biopsies from non-celiac T1D patients. They observed a partial decrease in the microvilli together with morphological alterations at the tight junction domains (Secondulfo et al., 2004). Another study showed that T1D patients have high intestinal permeability measured as the urine levels of lactulose and mannitol 5 h after ingestion and high levels of zonulin in the serum (Sapone et al., 2006). Zonulin is a protein that can regulate intestinal permeability by disassembling tight junctions (Fasano et al., 2000). Studies performed in Biobreeding diabetes-prone (BBdp) rats, widely used as an animal model for studying human T1D (Bortell and Yang, 2012), showed increased intestinal permeability (Meddings et al., 1999). Using this animal model Neu et al. found in the small intestine of these animals a high number of globet cells and high intestinal mucus secretion before the onset of the disease, reflecting an inflammatory response at the intestine (Neu et al., 2005).

Other studies have found that intestinal microbiota could increase the probability to develop T1D. Studies performed in non-obese diabetic (NOD) mice at young age, when these animals are prediabetic, were infected by an oral gavage with wild type *C. rodentium* showed higher intestinal permeability, developed earlier insulitis (Lee et al., 2010) and showed an increased lymphocytic infiltration at the pancreas Langerhan's islets (In't Veld, 2011). These authors showed that the mutant strain of *C. rodentium* that lacks the ability to disrupt the intestinal barrier was unable to induce insulitis (Lee et al., 2010). Maffeis et al. observed in Italian T1D affected children an increased intestinal permeability that correlates with alterations in the microbiota composition (Maffeis et al., 2016). Interestingly, the authors found three microbial markers (*D. invisus, G. sanguinis,* and *B. longum*) highly represented in T1D affected children as compared to healthy controls (Maffeis et al., 2016). Furthermore, it has been observed that bio-breeding diabetes-resistant (BBDR) rats present more probiotic bacteria, such as *Bacterioides, Eubacterium,* and *Ruminococcus* (Roesch et al., 2009). It has also been observed in humans that the *Bacteroidaceae* family is over-represented in children with T1D together with a decrease of intestinal microbiota dominant species as *Bifidobacterium adolescentis* and *B. pseudocatenulatum* (De Goffau et al., 2013). Microbiota composition can be influenced by age, with major changes observed at early ages (Koenig et al., 2011; Arrieta et al., 2014; Rodriguez et al., 2015). Kostic et al. described that the microbiota of genetically-predisposed infants from 3 to 36 months old, based on HLA genotyping, has reduced alpha diversity and overabundance of *Blautia, Rikenellaceae, Ruminococcus,* and *Streptococcus* genera (Kostic et al., 2015). In contrast, Maffeis et al. (2016) showed that *D. invisus* was completely absent in this samples indicating that there is still contradictory data regarding the microbiota composition in T1D patients.

Multiple Sclerosis

Multiple sclerosis (MS) is the most common autoimmune disease that has the CNS as a target (Reich et al., 2018). The immune system in the MS patients reacts against proteins that are found in myelin and neurons inducing axonal damage and neuronal death (Lemus et al., 2018). The MS patient develops several symptoms that lead to chronic disability including cognition impairment, loss of motor control, and sensitivity (Yong et al., 2017). Several reports have shown that MS patients have dysbiosis at the intestinal microbiota and it has been proposed that MS patients could have a specific type of microbiome (Chen et al., 2016; Probstel and Baranzini, 2017; Shahi et al., 2017; Tremlett and Waubant, 2017). It was shown that MS patients have a relatively low abundance of the *Bacterioides, Parabacteroides, Prevotella,* and *Lactobacillus* genera and an increased abundance of *Akkermansia, Blautia, Ruminococcus,* and *Bifidobacterium* (Jangi et al., 2016; Freedman et al., 2017). Interestingly, *Akkermansia* is a mucin-degrading microorganism that transforms mucin into SCFAs, suggesting that this microorganism might be trying to compensate the inflammatory state of the MS patient (Derrien et al., 2004, 2011). Cekanaviciute et al. found that samples of gut microbiome from MS patients impaired the differentiation of T cells to $CD25^{+}FoxP3^{+}$ Treg cells (Cekanaviciute et al., 2017). These authors found that MS patients have a high presence of the *Akkermansia* genus, specifically *A. calcoaceticus* and *A. muciniphila* (Cekanaviciute et al., 2017). Further, it was observed that PBMCs from healthy donors showed an increased differentiation into effector T cells as compared to Treg cells, when exposed to *A. calcoaceticus* extracts from MS patients (Cekanaviciute et al., 2017). Once PBMCs are exposed to *A. muciniphila* extracts from MS patients the differentiation of T cells inclined toward to Th1 cells, suggesting that the microbiota of MS patients has a pro-inflammatory effect (Cekanaviciute et al., 2017).

There are several animal models to study MS, one of them is the experimental autoimmune encephalomyelitis (EAE) (Robinson et al., 2014). EAE has the advantage of reproducing most of the symptoms observed in humans and disease is mediated by T cells, as it is the case for MS patients (Stromnes and Goverman, 2006). The induction of EAE in rodents generates a T cell-mediated response, mainly of Th1 and Th17 types (Kleinewietfeld and Hafler, 2013). Interestingly, the function these cells is influenced by the composition microbiota (Wu and Wu, 2012). It has been shown that in normal conditions commensal microorganisms, such as segmented filamentous bacteria can activate these cells to keep a healthy immune response (Ivanov et al., 2009). Noteworthy, Lee et al. showed that the germ-free mice were more resistant to EAE (Lee et al., 2011). The authors observed that some of these mice did not develop symptoms, while and developed only mild symptoms and had a shorter period of EAE (Lee et al., 2011). Experiments of microbiota transfer from specific pathogen free mice (SPF) mice to germ-free mice enhanced the EAE symptoms in germ-free mice, supporting the notion that microbiota can influence the immune response during EAE (Lee et al., 2011).

Other studies have found that the microbiota can alter the ratio of cells that play important roles during autoimmune diseases, such as effector T cells vs. Tregs (Molloy et al., 2012; Kosiewicz et al., 2014). For example, *in vitro* re-stimulation with MOG_{35-55} of T cells from germ-free mice and SPF mice that have been previously immunized with MOG/CFA showed in SPF mice an increased secretion of IFNγ and IL-17, as compared to germ-free mice (Lee et al., 2011). Germ-free mice have increased frequencies of Tregs at day 8th before the onset of EAE and at day 15 at the peak of EAE symptoms (Lee et al., 2011). Recently, it was reported that EAE could be induced in mice that received microbiota from MS patients (Berer et al., 2017). By using next-generation sequencing analyses it was shown that the microbiota composition of MS patients has a low content of the *Sutterella* genus (Berer et al., 2017). It has been observed that this bacterium plays a beneficial role in patients that suffer from IBD (Morgan and Harris, 2015). There is evidence that Bacteroides can be beneficial for maintaining the homeostasis in models of intra-abdominal sepsis and experimental colitis (Tzianabos et al., 1995; Pagliuca et al., 2016). This seems to be the case for *B. fragilis*, as its polysaccharide (PSA) induces IL-10 secretion by Tregs (Ochoa-Reparaz et al., 2010). In fact, oral treatment with purified *Bacterioides fragilis* PSA has been shown to be beneficial because it reduces EAE scores, demyelination, IFNγ, and IL-17 and increases T cells conversion to Tregs and the content of IL-10 (Ochoa-Reparaz et al., 2010). Oral immunization with an oral vaccine of attenuated *Salmonella typhimurium* expressing the colonization factor antigen I (CFA/I) of Enterotoxigenic *Escherichia coli* (ETEC) to mice that suffer EAE decreased the EAE scores showing a decreased infiltration of $TCD4^{+}$ cells in the spinal cord (Jun et al., 2005). CFA/I plays an important role in the attachment of ETEC to the intestinal epithelia an important step for diarrhea pathogenesis (Li et al., 2009).

The question as to how the microbiota modulates de immune response in the MS and/or EAE remains to be addressed. Rumah et al. showed that bacteria metabolites could modulate the immune response (Rumah et al., 2013). These authors isolated a strain of *Costridium perfringens* type B bacillus from a woman that suffered MS and showed ovoid lesions at the *corpus callosum* (Rumah et al., 2013). By using a mouse model it was shown that protoxin (a protein secreted by this strain) caused BBB disruption (Finnie, 1984) and binds to myelin in the CNS inducing oligodedrocyte death, as observed in frozen sections of mouse retina (Rumah et al., 2013). Farrokhi et al. found that serum from MS patients has low levels of the lipid 654, this lipopeptide is secreted by commensal intestinal *Bacteroidetes* in healthy people (Farrokhi et al., 2013). It has been reported that the lipid 654 could work as a ligand for the human toll-like receptor 2 (TLR2), thus it could contribute at down-regulating innate immunity (Clark et al., 2013). The work of Farrokhi suggests that low levels of lipid 654 could be used as a biomarker of MS, however further research is required to demonstrate that this diagnostic approach would be accurate.

Evidence derived from the EAE model suggests that SCFAs can improve and balance the immune response. Mizuno et al. observed that the oral administration of propionate decreased EAE clinical scores and increased Tregs at the lymph nodes, thus it could favor the suppression effect of Tregs (Mizuno et al., 2017). Additional interesting work has provided evidence that supports the notion that the first symptoms of EAE begins at the intestine (Nouri et al., 2014). Nouri et al. in their article showed that there is an unbalance of Treg/Th17 toward Th17 pro-inflammatory response at the intestine (Nouri et al., 2014) Authors also showed an increased intestinal permeability, altered intestinal morphology across the small intestine characterized by depth crypt, gross mucosal thickness, and high expression of zonulin (Nouri et al., 2014). Summarizing, the evidence available in the literature suggests that intestinal microbiota could potentiate or modulate the immune response of MS or EAE specifically the ration or balance of Treg/Th17.

Systemic Lupus Erythematosus

Systemic Lupus Erythematosus (SLE) is a systemic autoimmune disease with unknown etiology that affects predominantly women. SLE is characterized by the presence of hyperactive and aberrant antibody response to nuclear and cytoplasmic antigens (La Paglia et al., 2017). Regarding the influence of microbiota over SLE development, microbiota composition analyses showed that SLE patients display intestinal dysbiosis. A decrease in the *Firmicutes* with an increase of the *Bacteroides* phyla was observed (Hevia et al., 2014). These bacteria are the most abundant components of the human microbiota and the same pattern has been observed in patients with Crohn's disease (Qin et al., 2010). Mouse models of lupus showed differences in microbiota composition, as compared to control mice. Females showed a more accelerated development of the disease that was associated with decreased levels of *Lactobacillaceae* and increased levels of *Lachnospiraceae* families (Zhang et al., 2014). Treatment with probiotics composed by *Lactobacillaceae* members has been used as anti-inflammatory therapies given its anti-inflammatory properties (Jirillo et al., 2012). Lopez et al. observed the influence of the microbiota over T cell differentiation in healthy and SLE patients (Lopez et al., 2016). These authors found an increase in lymphocyte activation and differentiation toward Th17 in SLE patients (Lopez et al., 2016). Even though, there is still no clarity about the role of microbiota in the development of SLE, the evidence suggests that the dysbiosis observed in the SLE patients could be related to this disease.

Psoriasis, Psoriasis Arthritis, and Other Skin Related Autoimmune Pathologies

The literature provides evidence for an association between intestinal microbiota with skin autoimmune diseases (Scher et al., 2015; Eppinga et al., 2016; Forbes et al., 2016; Zakostelska et al., 2016). Intestinal-related autoimmune diseases like Crohn's disease is a known comorbidity of psoriasis, patients with psoriasis have a 2.9-times higher risk of developing Crohn's disease as compared to the general population as well as Crohn's disease patients have a 7-times higher risk of developing psoriasis (Oliveira Mde et al., 2015). There is increasing evidence supporting a role of intestinal dysbiosis as a factor in the pathogenesis of Crohn's disease (Kaur et al., 2011) and this might as well be related to psoriasis pathology.

Another important comorbidity of psoriasis is psoriatic arthritis, which is a type of chronic spondyloarthritis with unknown etiology. A recent study characterized the composition of gut microbiota in patients with psoriatic arthritis, patients with psoriasis and healthy controls. The gut microbiota profile of both groups showed decreased bacterial diversity and a reduced relative abundance of some bacterial taxa as compared to healthy controls, such as *Akkermansia*, *Ruminococcus*, and *Pseudobutyrivibrio*. It is important to highlight that the microbiota profile of psoriatic arthritis resembled that published for patients with IBD, a finding that further supports a possible role for the gut microbiota in this skin disease (Scher et al., 2015). The directionality of this relationship remains poorly understood, but it opens a new and interesting research field.

Other skin diseases related to intestinal dysbiosis are scleroderma and vitiligo. In scleroderma (also known as systemic sclerosis) the majority of patients experience gastrointestinal tract dysfunction that might be related to gut microbiota composition. A study performed by Volkmann et al. (2017) shows a different microbial composition between two different cohorts of patients with systemic sclerosis and healthy controls. *Firmicutes* showed a significantly increased abundance in systemic sclerosis patients (63.5 and 42.8%) compared to healthy controls (33%). In contrast, *Bacteroidetes* decreased in one of the cohorts (21.3%) as compared to healthy controls (63.2%). This study also associated the presence of some genus with disease severity. In both systemic sclerosis cohorts, *Clostridium* was more abundant in patients with low gastrointestinal symptom severity, *Lactobacillus* was more abundant in patients with mild constipation and *Prevotella* was more abundant in patients with moderate to severe gastrointestinal symptom severity. Further research will elucidate the role and molecular pathways in which these genders contribute to disease pathogenesis (Volkmann et al., 2017).

Even though, there is information relative to the influence of intestinal microbiota over skin autoimmune diseases, there are data that make these pathologies more complex. Therefore, an influence of skin microbiota over the skin autoimmune diseases remains to be demonstrated (Sanford and Gallo, 2013; Statnikov et al., 2013; Tett et al., 2017). Briefly scientific work that relates skin microbiota with skin autoimmune diseases will be discussed due to the importance of the skin as a physical barrier that constantly interacts with factors from the environment, such as solar irradiation, grades of humidity or dryness and microorganisms. While a wide range of microbes inhabit the skin, the principal residents microbiota belong to one of these phyla: *Actinobacteria*, *Bacteroidetes*, *Firmicutes*, or *Proteobacteria*. Interactions between these microorganisms at the skin and the immune system have been suggested to influence tissue integrity and homeostasis (Sanford and Gallo, 2013). Similar to what happens in the gut, skin dysbiosis has been postulated to contribute to the pathology of diverse skin autoimmune diseases (Zeeuwen et al., 2013) like psoriasis, psoriasis arthritis and vitiligo (Gao et al., 2008; Castelino et al., 2014; Ganju et al., 2016). Studies related to chronic plaque psoriasis, the most common form of psoriasis, have shown that the composition of the microbiota both with skin lesions or not differed of healthy skin (Gao et al., 2008; Alekseyenko et al., 2013). Gao et al. showed that *Firmicutes* were the most abundant and diverse phylum present in the psoriatic patients with skin lesions (relative abundance of 46.2%) as compared to those that did not display lesions (39%) and with healthy subjects (24.4%) (Gao et al., 2008). In contrast, *Actinobacteria* has lower relative abundance in psoriatic patients with lesions (37.3%) compared to individuals with healthy skins (47.6%) (Gao et al., 2008). The phylum of *Proteobacteria* was less frequent in psoriatic patients (11.4%) as compared to subjects with healthy skin (21.9%). Alekseyenko et al. described three distinct types of bacteria from their data about the relative abundance of major phyla present in the skin, *Actinobacteria*, *Firmicutes*, and *Proteobacteria* (Alekseyenko et al., 2013). These results are consistent with some of the findings described above. Proteobacteria dominate the cutaneotype 1 they described, while the cutaneotype 2 has higher relative abundance of *Actinobacteria* and *Firmicutes*. These authors associated the cutaneotype 2 with psoriasis status in which the higher abundance of *Firmicutes* coincides with the results by Gao et al. (2008). The differences in the results could be attributed to as to where the sample was obtained from, as it has been demonstrated that skin microbial composition is dependent on the area of the body that is analyzed (Grice and Segre, 2011). Both studies provide evidence that skin microbiota composition is different in patients with psoriasis as compared to healthy controls. Nevertheless, the physiological meaning of these differences has yet to be defined.

The most recent study to date related to psoriasis is a metagenomic analysis that focused on the less explored diversity of the skin microbiota and provided evidence that these less characterized species inhabiting the skin might be relevant in disease pathogenesis. In this study, an increase in members of the genus *Staphylococcus* was associated to development of psoriasis (Tett et al., 2017).

The skin microbiota is not the only microbial compartment that has been associated to psoriasis pathogenesis. In a murine model of imiquimod-induced psoriasis-like skin inflammation, germ-free, and oral antibiotic-treated mice showed milder skin inflammation as compared to conventional reared mice, along with a decrease in $\gamma\delta$TCR and Th17 cells in draining lymph nodes and spleen. These cells are essential components of the IL-23/Th17 axis, which happens to be the main axis in psoriasis pathogenesis. These results suggest that the absence of microbiota or an alteration in their composition caused by antibiotic treatment can decrease the pro-inflammatory T cell response and thus diminish the severity of the imiquimod-induced skin inflammation (Zakostelska et al., 2016). Interestingly, in humans, a link between psoriasis and Crohn's disease has long been acknowledged (Hughes et al., 1983) and discussed extensively in previous articles (Najarian and Gottlieb, 2003). Finally, a recent study characterized for the first time the skin microbial composition of patients with the autoimmune disease vitiligo (Ganju et al., 2016). The data obtained were used to characterize a core skin microbiome for a lesional and non-lesional skin (Ganju et al., 2016). *Methylobacterium* constitutes a genus exclusive to lesional skin while *Anaerococcus*, *Microbacterium*, *Streptophyta*, and *Nocardiode* are exclusive to non-lesional skin (Ganju et al., 2016). It remains unclear whether the microbiota differences between groups are a cause or an effect of altered skin physiology of the depigmented patches. Therefore, further research is required to define the contribution of the bacterial component to the pathology of vitiligo (Ganju et al., 2016). Compared to the vast information about the role of microbiota in systemic autoimmune diseases, the contribution of intestinal microbiota to skin disease conditions has not been fully explored and requires further research.

AUTOIMMUNITY AND MICROBIOTA IN PSYCHIATRIC DISORDERS

Psychiatric disorders have complex etiologies likely resulting from environmental interactions with genetic factors (Tsuang, 2000; Chaste and Leboyer, 2012). Recently, comorbid immune system dysregulations have emerged as a relevant etiological agent in several psychiatric disorders, raising the concept that autoimmunity might be an important contributing factor (Severance et al., 2016). This notion is supported by occurrence of brain inflammation-induced psychosis and autoimmune encephalitis, such as the anti-NMDA receptor encephalitis. This latter disease is characterized by the presence of autoantibodies against the *N*-methyl-*D*-aspartate receptor

(NMDAR), a glutamatergic receptor in the brain involved in synaptic transmission (Guasp and Dalmau, 2017). Symptoms include a range of psychotic symptoms early in the course of the disease followed by neurologic deterioration and ultimately protracted cognitive and behavioral deficits (Dalmau et al., 2011). Remarkably, approximately 80% of patients recover with immunotherapy directed to remove the antibodies and antibody-producing plasma cells (Dalmau et al., 2017). Consistently with this notion, various autoantibodies have been detected in subgroups of schizophrenic patients (Pearlman and Najjar, 2014). In particular, meta-analyses have suggested that schizophrenic patients are three times more likely to have high levels of anti-NMDAR antibodies as compared to healthy controls (Pearlman and Najjar, 2014). Recently, Schwarz et al. analyzed fecal microbiota from a small cohort of patients with first-episode psychosis (FEP) (Schwarz et al., 2017). Interestingly, *Lactobacillus* and *Bifidobacterium* were increased in FEP patients and correlated with the psychotic symptoms severity (Schwarz et al., 2017). Although up to date this is the only report associating changes in the microbiota with psychotic severity in patients, it was also reported that autistic children show increased amounts of Lactobacillus in their intestinal microbiota (Adams et al., 2011; Schwarz et al., 2017). At family level, Schwarz et al. observed a decreased in the *Veillonellaceae* family an alteration of the microbiota composition that was also observed in depressive patients (Jiang et al., 2015).

As the largest organ of the immune system, the GI tract serves as an interface between the environment and the host. Therefore, alterations in gut cellular processes may influence immune homeostasis. Data generated to date suggest that increased intestinal permeability and alterations in the gut microbiota composition are strongly associated with psychiatric disorders and could represent potential sources of immune functional impairment (Fiorentino et al., 2016; Esnafoglu et al., 2017; Stevens et al., 2017). Gut microbiota seems to play a critical role in the bidirectional communication between the gastrointestinal tract and the CNS. In addition to regulating gastrointestinal functions, this microbiota-gut-brain axis has been shown to modulate brain functions, such as emotional behavior and stress-related responsiveness (Diaz Heijtz et al., 2011). The mechanisms implicated in these pathways, although not entirely characterized, involve humoral and/or neural route, such as the vagus nerve (De Palma et al., 2014). An involvement of the vagus nerve in the communication between the gut and the brain was supported by the observation that vagotomy abrogated the decrease of anxiety- and depression-related behavior induced by the probiotic *L. rhamnosus* in mice (Bravo et al., 2011). These observations suggest a close relationship between the different components of the gut-brain axis, several probiotics used in animal models have shown their efficacy with combined and correlated beneficial effects on the GI tract, such as intestinal barrier strengthening, HPA axis activation and behavior, including social interaction, anxiety, and exploratory behavior (Hsiao et al., 2013; Vanhaecke et al., 2017). On the other hand, mice exposed to antibiotics to alter the established microbiota, showed an increased in explorative behavior associated with an enhanced level of brain-derived neurotrophic factor (BDNF), an important growth factor for neuronal survival and synaptic plasticity (Bercik et al., 2011). However, another mouse strain exposed to a different antibiotic mixture induced a different behavioral phenotype consisting of an increased depressive-like behavior and altered social interaction, which was associated with reduced level of hippocampal BDNF activity. These data suggest that mouse strains or antimicrobial regimen can differently influence microbiota composition and in turn differently affect behavior (Guida et al., 2017). The use of the probiotic *Lactobacillus casei DG* in these animals was able to restore the behavioral phenotype and BDNF levels similar to controls (Guida et al., 2017). Interestingly, a decreased serum BDNF levels were observed in patients with major depressive disorders (Pedrotti Moreira et al., 2017) and pharmacological treatment that increases BDNF levels proved to be beneficial for depressive patients (Gupta et al., 2016). Along with the depressive-like behavior, mice exposed to antibiotics showed a marked dysbiosis characterized by a loss of bacterial diversity, an increase in *Protebacteria* and *Actinobacteria* and a decrease in *Bacteroidetes* and *Firmicutes*. The probiotic treatment was not able to restore this bacterial phenotype, but promoted the increase of *Lachnospiraceae*, a fiber-degrading and SCFA producer (Guida et al., 2017). In humans, either a decrease or an increase of *Lachnospiraceae* has been correlated with major depressive disorders (Naseribafrouei et al., 2014; Fung et al., 2017), indicating that there is still a controversy about microbiota composition in this pathology. Such a discrepancy could probably result from the influence of external factors (i.e., diet) between the patients cohorts used in these studies. The causal link of microbiota on GI and brain dysfunction has recently been shown for irritable bowel syndrome (IBS), a common intestinal disorder often accompanied by comorbid anxiety (De Palma et al., 2017). Colonization of germ-free mice with fecal microbiota from IBS patients induced altered GI transit, intestinal barrier dysfunctions, and anxiety-like behavior, suggesting a role for the gut microbiota in the expression of IBS (De Palma et al., 2017). The importance of microbiota has also been highlighted in neurodevelopmental disorders, such as autism spectrum disorder (ASD). In mice, pregnant animals exposition to poly(I:C) triggers a maternal immune activation that can cause in the offspring to atypical social and repetitive behavior reminiscent of ASD-related behavior. The mechanisms leading to behavioral abnormalities in the offspring required a particular type of maternal bacterium, the segmented filamentous bacteria (SFB), which induces intestinal T_H17 cells producing IL-17 (Kim et al., 2017). Interestingly, induction of T_H17 response by SFB has been shown to modulate gene expression of enteric neurons, which in turn influences microbiome/immune system crosstalk (Yissachar et al., 2017). Besides behavioral abnormalities, offspring from poly(I:C)-treated mice also develop GI symptoms, changes in gut bacterial population and intestinal barrier defects, as reported in some patients with ASD (Horvath and Perman, 2002). Treatment of the offspring with *B. fragilis* induced a remodeling of the microbiota composition ameliorated GI symptoms and reduced repetitive behavior. These preclinical results stimulated the development of pilot clinical studies using microbiome-driven therapies for ASD. Although not controlled and double-blinded, a clinical trial based on microbiota transfer of healthy donors in 7–16 years old children with ASD showed improvements in GI symptoms and in social and communication skills that are associated with bacterial community changes (Kang et al., 2017). Similarly, probiotic supplementation with *Bifidobacteria and Lactobacillus* species in 5–9 years ASD children modified the fecal microbiota composition and improved both GI symptoms and behavior (Shaaban et al., 2017). However, these studies were performed with a small number of patients, and wide-scale randomized controlled trials are needed to critically confirm the efficacy of probiotics in ASD. The use of probiotics or microbiota-derived metabolites that could selectively or simultaneously act on the different components of the microbiota-gut-brain axis raises alternative new treatments for CNS disorders. However, more information is still required to better understand the influence of the microbiota on CNS pathogenesis and to delineate the cellular and molecular mechanisms involved in the communication between microbiota, the gut, and the brain. Also, the implications of intestinal dysbiosis in the etiology and/or pathophysiology of brain diseases remain to be further defined and represent a major challenge for translational research.

EXTERNAL FACTORS THAT INFLUENCE THE MICROBIOTA

Microbiota is established by many factors that determine the characteristics for each individual, including genetic predisposition, an inheritance from the mother since the fetus is forming until breastfeeding and environmental factors, such as diet, culture, and geographic location (Yatsunenko et al., 2012). However, when there is an imbalance of microorganism's populations present in the gut, known as dysbiosis, many problems at the systemic level are triggered. This situation may cause an incorrect nutrient absorption, favor weight alterations and enhance some immune system diseases (Degruttola et al., 2016).

Diet is one of the important factors affecting the composition of microbiota in humans (Conlon and Bird, 2014; Sonnenburg and Backhed, 2016). The first major change in diet that humans experience is when the consumption of solid food begins. At this stage, microbiota composition and abundance suffer significant modifications, such as a decrease of *Bifidobacteria* and *Enterobacteria* (Fallani et al., 2011). This process occurs due to the new substrates that are available in the gut, leading to the proliferation of certain types of microbes (Fallani et al., 2011; Davis et al., 2017; Wampach et al., 2017). Later in life, each time that diet changes this phenomenon takes place, promoting the growth of some microorganisms more than others (Ottman et al., 2012; Odamaki et al., 2016; Sonnenburg and Backhed, 2016). In turn, this evolving microbiota will modulate the development and function of the immune system (Round and Mazmanian, 2009; Conlon and Bird, 2014; Kabat et al., 2014). However, microbiota analyses highlighted that although after a month of receiving a traditional diet, the composition of the microbiota took 1 year to change and be similar to the one found in other people with the same diet (Claesson et al., 2012).

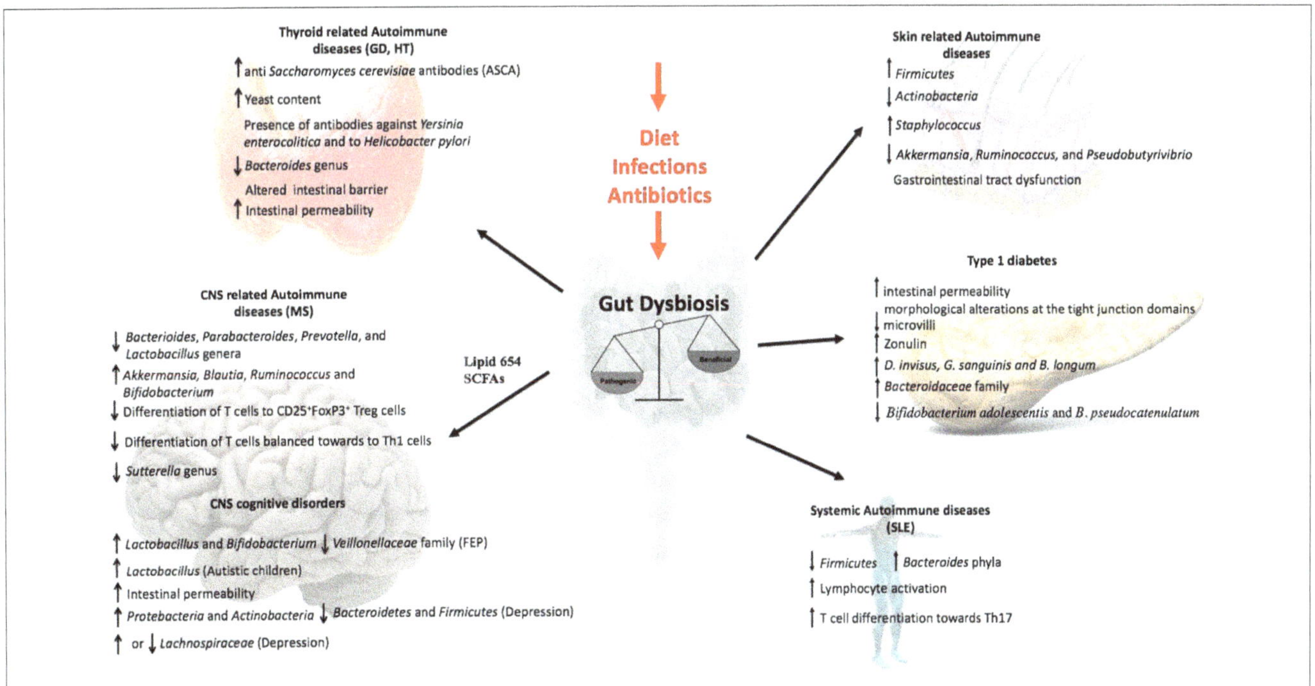

FIGURE 2 | Influence of the gut microbiota in non-intestinal diseases. Gut dysbiosis induced by external factors as diet, infections, or antibiotic overuse lead to an inflammatory response that influence the outcome of several autoimmune diseases as Grave's disease, Hashimoto's Thyroiditis, Multiple Sclerosis, SLE, and type1 diabetes. It has also been observed an important role in skin related autoimmune diseases as Psoriasis. Moreover, the evidences in the literature support that gut microbiota can influence CNS disorders like autism, depression, and schizophrenia.

Human studies have shown that there is a correlation in elderly between the microbiota location and diet, which can influence their health (Claesson et al., 2012). Additionally, analyses of microbiota composition had shown four different dietary groups and found that diet based on "low fat-high fiber" was associated with a more diverse microbiota. A study performed with C57BL/6 mice fed with high-fat diet was aimed at evaluating whether inflammation was due to microbiota changes or cytokines production. Results have shown that microbiota underwent changes 8 weeks after the treatment started, but increased IFNγ and TNF-α cytokines were only detected 16 weeks after administration of a high-fat diet (Guo et al., 2017). These observations underscore the importance of microbiota and corroborate the ability of diet to modulate microbiota composition.

Additionally, evaluation of the feces obtained from three different dietary groups ovo-lacto vegetarian, vegans, and omnivores, showed differences in microbiota composition (Ferrocino et al., 2015). Findings showed that *B. fragilis* group was diminished on ovo-lacto vegetarian and vegan volunteers, which is associated with low consumption of protein and animal fat (Wu et al., 2011). Also, a significant reduction for the loads for Lactic Acid Bacteria (LAB) was observed for the dietary groups ovo-lacto vegetarian and vegan, which may be due to the absence or low intake of some food such as cheese and yogurt (Zimmer et al., 2012).

Gluten-free diet is worldwide used for patients with celiac disease (CD), which is a chronic enteropathy caused mainly by gluten intolerance. It has been shown that the intestinal microbiota can be modified by a gluten-free diet: two of the groups that are reduced by such a diet are *Lactobacillus* and *Bifidobacterium,* which are considered as part of the group of healthy bacteria (De Palma et al., 2009; Lorenzo Pisarello et al., 2015). In contrast, some opportunistic bacteria from *Enterobacteriacea* family are increased as a result of gluten-free diets (De Palma et al., 2009; Lorenzo Pisarello et al., 2015). One possible explanation for these changes in the microbiota is the low carbohydrate intake due to the restrictions imposed by the gluten-free diet. Healthy bacteria usually use carbohydrates for their metabolism, which are needed for the colonization and fermentation inside the gastrointestinal tract (Sanz, 2010).

A diet that low in carbohydrates accessible for microbiota results in low levels of production of Short Chain Fatty Acids (SCFA) produced by bacteria from the microbiota. Butyrate, propionate, and acetate can modulate immune system by controlling inflammation and promoting an anti-inflammatory environment in the gut (Maslowski et al., 2009; Arpaia et al., 2013). However, when the diet undergoes a detrimental change, the abundance of these beneficial bacteria decreases and therefore SCFA production is reduced. Alteration of SCFA is common in obesity, celiac disease, and Type 2 Diabetes, because it is known that their action ameliorates the disease (Lin et al., 2012; Hong et al., 2016; Lerner et al., 2016).

Consistently with this notion, the Ma-Pi2 diet a diet rich in carbohydrates, whole grains and vegetables was shown to ameliorate dysbiosis and increment the diversity of microbiota

TABLE 1 | Alterations observed in the microbiota in non-intestinal autoimmune diseases.

Autoimmune disease	Observation	References
Grave's disease	↑ yeast Presence of antibodies against *Y. enterocolitica* and *H. pylori*. ↓ *Bacteroides*	Covelli and Ludgate, 2017 Kohling et al., 2017 Indigo, 2017
Hashimoto's thyroiditis (HT)	Dysbiosis Altered intestinal morphology ↑ intestinal permeability	Sasso et al., 2004
Multiple Sclerosis (MS) Murine EAE model Human	↓ *Sutterella* ↑ intestinal permeability ↑ Zonulin expression Th17 > Treg Dysbiosis ↓ *Bacteroides* ↓ Parbacteroides ↓ *Prevotella* ↓*Lactobacillus* ↑ *Akkermansia* ↓ *Blautia* ↓ *Ruminococcus* ↓ *Bifidiobacterium*	Berer et al., 2017 Nouri et al., 2014 Sturgeon and Fasano, 2016 Nouri et al., 2014 Chen et al., 2016 Jangi et al., 2016 Freedman et al., 2017
Systemic Lupus Erythematosus (SLE) Mouse model of SLE Human	↓ *La ctobacillus* ↑ *Lachnospiraceae* Dysbiosis ↓ *Firmicutes* ↓ *Bacteroides*	Hevia et al., 2014 Zhang et al., 2014
Psoriasis	↑ *Firmicutes* ↓ *Actinobacteria* ↑ *Proteobacteria* (Cutaneotype 1) ↑ *Actinobacteria* (Cutaneotype 2) ↑ *Firmicutes* (Cutaneotype 3) ↑ *Staphylococcus*	Gao et al., 2008 Alekseyenko et al., 2013 Tett et al., 2017
Psoriatic arthritis	↓ *Akkermansia* ↓ *Ruminococcus* ↓ *Pseudobutyrivibrio*	Scher et al., 2015
Scleroderma	↑ *Firmicutes* ↓ *Bacteroides* ↑ *Clostridium* ↑ *Lactobacillus* (mild gastrointestinal symptoms) ↑ *Prevotella* (moderate to severe gastrointestinal symptoms)	Volkmann et al., 2017
Vitiligo	*Methylobacterium* in lesional skin *Anaerococcus* in non-lesional skin *Microbacterium* in non-lesional skin *Streptophyta* (non-lesional skin) *Nocardiode* (non-lesional skin)	Ganju et al., 2016
Type 1 Diabetes	↑ intestinal permeability ↑ Zonulin ↑ *Bacteroideaceae* ↑ *Blautia* ↑ *Rikenellaceae* ↑ *Ruminococcus* ↑ *Sreptococcus*	Secondulfo et al., 2004; Sapone et al., 2006; Maffeis et al., 2016 Sapone et al., 2006 De Goffau et al., 2013 Kostic et al., 2015

in Type 2 Diabetes patients, as compared to untreated patients. Also, abundance of SCFA producers increased, such as *Bacteroides*, *Dorea*, and *Faecalibacterium*. Furthermore, the implementation of this diet has shown a potential role in the recovery of metabolic control in Type 2 Diabetes (Fallucca et al., 2014; Candela et al., 2016).

Overuse of Antibiotic Treatments

Overuse of antibiotics may cause a significant imbalance in microbiota and a disruption of the natural interaction between the microorganisms. One of the most important characteristics of a normal microbiota is the capacity to compete out infectious pathogens (Kamada et al., 2013a). Therefore, microbiota removal by antibiotics may allow the detrimental growth of pathogenic bacteria populations, increasing the probability of an infection. Additionally, antibiotics not only kill pathogens but also beneficial bacteria, eliminating as well the positive effect of the latter. Microbiota modulates the immune response through the molecules it produces, so if beneficial microorganisms decrease, a decrease in the modulation of the immune system can also be observed (Langdon et al., 2016).

In response to a constant exposure of an antibiotic, microorganisms can acquire genetic resistance, leading to an the increment of multi-drug resistance microorganisms (Jernberg et al., 2007), which can become a major public health problem due to the lack of new treatments capable of eliminating these bacteria. In the last years, many cases of infection caused by multi-drug resistant bacteria were reported and this number is expected to increase (Karam et al., 2016; Lee et al., 2016). The effects of overuse of antibiotics can be treated but not reversed. Restoration of the microbiota can take months or even years, but it will not be able to become the same as before (Jernberg et al., 2007, 2010). Importantly, it has also been described that newborns whose mothers have received antibiotics perinatally have a different microbiota composition, as compared to newborns whose mother have not been treated (Fallani et al., 2011). Due to the importance of first microorganisms in the gut of newborn, these changes in microbiota caused by excessive use of antibiotics may have long-term consequences (Langdon et al., 2016).

Interestingly, recent findings have highlighted the natural presence of antibiotic resistance genes in microbiota and their differential occurrence according to diet. Microbiota changes observed in ovo-lacto vegetarian and vegan diets, as compared to omnivores diet, are related to the presence of antibiotic resistance genes. A study performed with 144 volunteers found the presence of 12 antibiotic resistance genes in their microbiota. Among these genes, the occurrence of *erm*(A) (Erythromycin resistance methylase gene) has been exclusively detected in the feces of vegan subjects, which also show a low abundance of *tet*(K) (Tetracycline efflux protein), as compared to the genes present in the feces of omnivores. Interestingly, another antibiotic resistance gene with a higher occurrence observed in the feces of omnivores was *van*(B) (Vancomycin resistance gene; Milanovic et al., 2017).

CONCLUSIONS

This review article discusses data supporting the influence of the gut microbiota over non-intestinal autoimmune diseases. The central theme of this review is the intestine in which two important actors, microbiota and the immune system are controlling the response to non-intestinal autoimmune diseases (**Figure 2**, **Table 1**). Not much is known about the mechanisms of the interaction between microbiota and the immune system. However, today it is possible to identify certain members of the microbiota that regulate, balance or unbalance the immune response of the host. The current evidence supports the notion that changes or alterations of the microbial species that form part of the intestinal microbiota will affect the balance of Tregs and Th17 cells at the intestine, which could modify the immune response of non-intestinal autoimmune diseases. The experimental evidence suggesting that the cytokines secreted from Treg and Th17 will determine and influence non-intestinal autoimmune responses. It could also be possible that cells of the immune system located at the intestine could to move other organs to establish or modify an autoimmune response. The major message of this review is that the abundant data support the notion that the intestine is a critical organ the appropriate immune balance and for the prevention of non-intestinal autoimmune diseases. The key point is that by modifying the intestinal microbiota of a patient that suffers non-intestinal autoimmune disease it might be possible to improve the outcome of such illness. Interestingly, by modifying the diet it might be possible to improve the intestinal microbiota to promote an anti-inflammatory response of a patient suffering from autoimmunity. Thus, the scientific community has paid attention to the potential therapeutical benefits of manipulating the composition of the gut microbiota through oral administration of probiotic or modified organisms expressing selected self-antigens to treat these non-intestinal autoimmune diseases. Work remains to be done in order to fully understand the complex mechanisms of the intestinal microbiota that can impact non-intestinal autoimmune diseases.

AUTHOR CONTRIBUTIONS

MO, EO-R, and IC-A, have written the first draft of the manuscript. LB, CR, SB, HB, MN, and AK revised and improved the first draft. All authors have seen and agreed on the finally submitted version of the manuscript.

FUNDING

MO, IC-A, CR, SB, and AK: Millennium Institute on Immunology and Immunotherapy, IMII P09/16-F. IC-A: CONICYT 63140215. CR: Fondecyt 1161525, Nucleus project UNAB DI-471-15/N. SB: Fondecyt 1170964. AK: Fondecyt 1150862. HB and MN: Region Pays de la Loire (MIBIOGATE) and the Fondation pour la Recherche Medicale.

REFERENCES

Aarts, E., Ederveen, T. H. A., Naaijen, J., Zwiers, M. P., Boekhorst, J., Timmerman, H. M., et al. (2017). Gut microbiome in ADHD and its relation to neural reward anticipation. *PLoS ONE* 12:e0183509. doi: 10.1371/journal.pone.0183509

Adams, J. B., Johansen, L. J., Powell, L. D., Quig, D., and Rubin, R. A. (2011). Gastrointestinal flora and gastrointestinal status in children with autism–comparisons to typical children and correlation with autism severity. *BMC Gastroenterol.* 11:22. doi: 10.1186/1471-230X-11-22

Alekseyenko, A. V., Perez-Perez, G. I., De Souza, A., Strober, B., Gao, Z., Bihan, M., et al. (2013). Community differentiation of the cutaneous microbiota in psoriasis. *Microbiome* 1:31. doi: 10.1186/2049-2618-1-31

Alkanani, A. K., Hara, N., Gottlieb, P. A., Ir, D., Robertson, C. E., Wagner, B. D., et al. (2015). Alterations in intestinal microbiota correlate with susceptibility to type 1 diabetes. *Diabetes* 64, 3510–3520. doi: 10.2337/db14-1847

Almonacid, D. E., Kraal, L., Ossandon, F. J., Budovskaya, Y. V., Cardenas, J. P., Bik, E. M., et al. (2017). 16S rRNA gene sequencing and healthy reference ranges for 28 clinically relevant microbial taxa from the human gut microbiome. *PLoS ONE* 12:e0176555. doi: 10.1371/journal.pone.0176555

Antonelli, A., Ferrari, S. M., Corrado, A., Di Domenicantonio, A., and Fallahi, P. (2015). Autoimmune thyroid disorders. *Autoimmun. Rev.* 14, 174–180. doi: 10.1016/j.autrev.2014.10.016

Arpaia, N., Campbell, C., Fan, X., Dikiy, S., Van Der Veeken, J., Deroos, P., et al. (2013). Metabolites produced by commensal bacteria promote peripheral regulatory T-cell generation. *Nature* 504, 451–455. doi: 10.1038/nature12726

Arrieta, M. C., Stiemsma, L. T., Amenyogbe, N., Brown, E. M., and Finlay, B. (2014). The intestinal microbiome in early life: health and disease. *Front. Immunol.* 5:427. doi: 10.3389/fimmu.2014.00427

Atkinson, M. A., Eisenbarth, G. S., and Michels, A. W. (2014). Type 1 diabetes. *Lancet* 383, 69–82. doi: 10.1016/S0140-6736(13)60591-7

Aujla, S. J., and Kolls, J. K. (2009). IL-22: a critical mediator in mucosal host defense. *J. Mol. Med.* 87, 451–454. doi: 10.1007/s00109-009-0448-1

Badawy, A. A. (2017). Kynurenine pathway of tryptophan metabolism: regulatory and functional aspects. *Int. J. Tryptophan Res.* 10, 1–20. doi: 10.1177/1178646917691938

Barrett, J. C., Clayton, D. G., Concannon, P., Akolkar, B., Cooper, J. D., Erlich, H. A., et al. (2009). Genome-wide association study and meta-analysis find that over 40 loci affect risk of type 1 diabetes. *Nat. Genet.* 41, 703–707. doi: 10.1038/ng.381

Berbers, R. M., Nierkens, S., Van Laar, J. M., Bogaert, D., and Leavis, H. L. (2017). Microbial dysbiosis in common variable immune deficiencies: evidence, causes, and consequences. *Trends Immunol.* 38, 206–216. doi: 10.1016/j.it.2016.11.008

Bercik, P., Denou, E., Collins, J., Jackson, W., Lu, J., Jury, J., et al. (2011). The intestinal microbiota affect central levels of brain-derived neurotropic factor and behavior in mice. *Gastroenterology* 141, 599–609. doi: 10.1053/j.gastro.2011.04.052

Berer, K., Gerdes, L. A., Cekanaviciute, E., Jia, X., Xiao, L., Xia, Z., et al. (2017). Gut microbiota from multiple sclerosis patients enables spontaneous autoimmune encephalomyelitis in mice. *Proc. Natl. Acad. Sci. U.S.A.* 114, 10719–10724. doi: 10.1073/pnas.1711233114

Blander, J. M., Longman, R. S., Iliev, I. D., Sonnenberg, G. F., and Artis, D. (2017). Regulation of inflammation by microbiota interactions with the host. *Nat. Immunol.* 18, 851–860. doi: 10.1038/ni.3780

Bortell, R., and Yang, C. (2012). The BB rat as a model of human type 1 diabetes. *Methods Mol. Biol.* 933, 31–44. doi: 10.1007/978-1-62703-068-7_3

Bravo, J. A., Forsythe, P., Chew, M. V., Escaravage, E., Savignac, H. M., Dinan, T. G., et al. (2011). Ingestion of Lactobacillus strain regulates emotional behavior and central GABA receptor expression in a mouse via the vagus nerve. *Proc. Natl. Acad. Sci. U.S.A.* 108, 16050–16055. doi: 10.1073/pnas.1102999108

Breban, M., Tap, J., Leboime, A., Said-Nahal, R., Langella, P., Chiocchia, G., et al. (2017). Faecal microbiota study reveals specific dysbiosis in spondyloarthritis. *Ann. Rheum. Dis.* 76, 1614–1622. doi: 10.1136/annrheumdis-2016-211064

Calcinaro, F., Dionisi, S., Marinaro, M., Candeloro, P., Bonato, V., Marzotti, S., et al. (2005). Oral probiotic administration induces interleukin-10 production and prevents spontaneous autoimmune diabetes in the non-obese diabetic mouse. *Diabetologia* 48, 1565–1575. doi: 10.1007/s00125-005-1831-2

Candela, M., Biagi, E., Soverini, M., Consolandi, C., Quercia, S., Severgnini, M., et al. (2016). Modulation of gut microbiota dysbioses in type 2 diabetic patients by macrobiotic Ma-Pi 2 diet. *Br. J. Nutr.* 116, 80–93. doi: 10.1017/S0007114516001045

Castelino, M., Eyre, S., Upton, M., Ho, P., and Barton, A. (2014). The bacterial skin microbiome in psoriatic arthritis, an unexplored link in pathogenesis: challenges and opportunities offered by recent technological advances. *Rheumatology* 53, 777–784. doi: 10.1093/rheumatology/ket319

Cavaglieri, C. R., Nishiyama, A., Fernandes, L. C., Curi, R., Miles, E. A., and Calder, P. C. (2003). Differential effects of short-chain fatty acids on proliferation and production of pro- and anti-inflammatory cytokines by cultured lymphocytes. *Life Sci.* 73, 1683–1690. doi: 10.1016/S0024-3205(03)00490-9

Cekanaviciute, E., Yoo, B. B., Runia, T. F., Debelius, J. W., Singh, S., Nelson, C. A., et al. (2017). Gut bacteria from multiple sclerosis patients modulate human T cells and exacerbate symptoms in mouse models. *Proc. Natl. Acad. Sci. U.S.A.* 114, 10713–10718. doi: 10.1073/pnas.1711235114

Chairatana, P., and Nolan, E. M. (2017). Defensins, lectins, mucins, and secretory immunoglobulin A: microbe-binding biomolecules that contribute to mucosal immunity in the human gut. *Crit. Rev. Biochem. Mol. Biol.* 52, 45–56. doi: 10.1080/10409238.2016.1243654

Chaste, P., and Leboyer, M. (2012). Autism risk factors: genes, environment, and gene-environment interactions. *Dialogues Clin. Neurosci.* 14, 281–292.

Chen, J., Chia, N., Kalari, K. R., Yao, J. Z., Novotna, M., Soldan, M. M., et al. (2016). Multiple sclerosis patients have a distinct gut microbiota compared to healthy controls. *Sci. Rep.* 6:28484. doi: 10.1038/srep28484

Chen, J., Li, Y., Tian, Y., Huang, C., Li, D., Zhong, Q., et al. (2015). Interaction between microbes and host intestinal health: modulation by dietary nutrients and gut-brain-endocrine-immune axis. *Curr. Protein Pept. Sci.* 16, 592–603. doi: 10.2174/1389203716666150630135720

Choi, W., Yeruva, S., and Turner, J. R. (2017). Contributions of intestinal epithelial barriers to health and disease. *Exp. Cell Res.* 358, 71–77. doi: 10.1016/j.yexcr.2017.03.036

Chu, D. M., Antony, K. M., Ma, J., Prince, A. L., Showalter, L., Moller, M., et al. (2016). The early infant gut microbiome varies in association with a maternal high-fat diet. *Genome Med.* 8:77. doi: 10.1186/s13073-016-0330-z

Claesson, M. J., Jeffery, I. B., Conde, S., Power, S. E., O'connor, E. M., Cusack, S., et al. (2012). Gut microbiota composition correlates with diet and health in the elderly. *Nature* 488, 178–184. doi: 10.1038/nature11319

Clark, R. B., Cervantes, J. L., Maclejewski, M. W., Farrokhi, V., Nemati, R., Yao, X., et al. (2013). Serine lipids of Porphyromonas gingivalis are human and mouse Toll-like receptor 2 ligands. *Infect. Immun.* 81, 3479–3489. doi: 10.1128/IAI.00803-13

Conlon, M. A., and Bird, A. R. (2014). The impact of diet and lifestyle on gut microbiota and human health. *Nutrients* 7, 17–44. doi: 10.3390/nu7010017

Covelli, D., and Ludgate, M. (2017). The thyroid, the eyes and the gut: a possible connection. *J. Endocrinol. Invest.* 40, 567–576. doi: 10.1007/s40618-016-0594-6

Cox, L. M., and Weiner, H. L. (2018). Microbiota signaling pathways that influence neurologic disease. *Neurotherapeutics* 15, 135–145. doi: 10.1007/s13311-017-0598-8

Cui, C., Li, Y., Gao, H., Zhang, H., Han, J., Zhang, D., et al. (2017). Modulation of the gut microbiota by the mixture of fish oil and krill oil in high-fat diet-induced obesity mice. *PLoS ONE* 12:e0186216. doi: 10.1371/journal.pone.0186216

Dalmau, J., Geis, C., and Graus, F. (2017). Autoantibodies to synaptic receptors and neuronal cell surface proteins in autoimmune diseases of the central nervous system. *Physiol. Rev.* 97, 839–887. doi: 10.1152/physrev.00010.2016

Dalmau, J., Lancaster, E., Martinez-Hernandez, E., Rosenfeld, M. R., and Balice-Gordon, R. (2011). Clinical experience and laboratory investigations in patients with anti-NMDAR encephalitis. *Lancet Neurol.* 10, 63–74. doi: 10.1016/S1474-4422(10)70253-2

Dasgupta, S., Erturk-Hasdemir, D., Ochoa-Reparaz, J., Reinecker, H. C., and Kasper, D. L. (2014). Plasmacytoid dendritic cells mediate anti-inflammatory responses to a gut commensal molecule via both innate and adaptive mechanisms. *Cell Host Microbe* 15, 413–423. doi: 10.1016/j.chom.2014.03.006

Davidson, A., and Diamond, B. (2001). Autoimmune diseases. *N. Engl. J. Med.* 345, 340–350. doi: 10.1056/NEJM200108023450506

Davis, E. C., Wang, M., and Donovan, S. M. (2017). The role of early life nutrition in the establishment of gastrointestinal microbial composition and function. *Gut Microbes* 8, 143–171. doi: 10.1080/19490976.2016.1278104

De Goffau, M. C., Luopajarvi, K., Knip, M., Ilonen, J., Ruohtula, T., Harkonen, T., et al. (2013). Fecal microbiota composition differs between children with beta-cell autoimmunity and those without. *Diabetes* 62, 1238–1244. doi: 10.2337/db12-0526

De Groot, P. F., Belzer, C., Aydin, O., Levin, E., Levels, J. H., Aalvink, S., et al. (2017). Distinct fecal and oral microbiota composition in human type 1 diabetes, an observational study. *PLoS ONE* 12:e0188475. doi: 10.1371/journal.pone.0188475

De Palma, G., Collins, S. M., and Bercik, P. (2014). The microbiota-gut-brain axis in functional gastrointestinal disorders. *Gut Microbes* 5, 419–429. doi: 10.4161/gmic.29417

De Palma, G., Lynch, M. D., Lu, J., Dang, V. T., Deng, Y., Jury, J., et al. (2017). Transplantation of fecal microbiota from patients with irritable bowel syndrome alters gut function and behavior in recipient mice. *Sci. Transl. Med.* 9:eaaf6397. doi: 10.1126/scitranslmed.aaf6397

De Palma, G., Nadal, I., Collado, M. C., and Sanz, Y. (2009). Effects of a gluten-free diet on gut microbiota and immune function in healthy adult human subjects. *Br. J. Nutr.* 102, 1154–1160. doi: 10.1017/S0007114509371767

Degruttola, A. K., Low, D., Mizoguchi, A., and Mizoguchi, E. (2016). Current understanding of dysbiosis in disease in human and animal models. *Inflamm. Bowel Dis.* 22, 1137–1150. doi: 10.1097/MIB.0000000000000750

Derrien, M., Van Baarlen, P., Hooiveld, G., Norin, E., Muller, M., and De Vos, W. M. (2011). Modulation of mucosal immune response, tolerance, and proliferation in mice colonized by the mucin-degrader *Akkermansia muciniphila*. *Front. Microbiol.* 2:166. doi: 10.3389/fmicb.2011.00166

Derrien, M., Vaughan, E. E., Plugge, C. M., and De Vos, W. M. (2004). *Akkermansia muciniphila gen.* nov., sp. nov., a human intestinal mucin-degrading bacterium. *Int. J. Syst. Evol. Microbiol.* 54, 1469–1476. doi: 10.1099/ijs.0.02873-0

Di Giacinto, C., Marinaro, M., Sanchez, M., Strober, W., and Boirivant, M. (2005). Probiotics ameliorate recurrent Th1-mediated murine colitis by inducing IL-10 and IL-10-dependent TGF-beta-bearing regulatory cells. *J. Immunol.* 174, 3237–3246. doi: 10.4049/jimmunol.174.6.3237

Diaz Heijtz, R., Wang, S., Anuar, F., Qian, Y., Bjorkholm, B., Samuelsson, A., et al. (2011). Normal gut microbiota modulates brain development and behavior. *Proc. Natl. Acad. Sci. U.S.A.* 108, 3047–3052. doi: 10.1073/pnas.1010529108

Dickerson, F., Severance, E., and Yolken, R. (2017). The microbiome, immunity, and schizophrenia and bipolar disorder. *Brain Behav. Immun.* 62, 46–52. doi: 10.1016/j.bbi.2016.12.010

Elliott, R. B., Reddy, S. N., Bibby, N. J., and Kida, K. (1988). Dietary prevention of diabetes in the non-obese diabetic mouse. *Diabetologia* 31, 62–64.

Endesfelder, D., Engel, M., and Zu Castell, W. (2016). Gut immunity and type 1 diabetes: a melange of microbes, diet, and host interactions? *Curr. Diab. Rep.* 16:60. doi: 10.1007/s11892-016-0753-3

Eppinga, H., Sperna Weiland, C. J., Thio, H. B., Van Der Woude, C. J., Nijsten, T. E., Peppelenbosch, M. P., et al. (2016). Similar depletion of protective *Faecalibacterium prausnitzii* in psoriasis and inflammatory bowel disease, but not in hidradenitis suppurativa. *J. Crohns. Colitis* 10, 1067–1075. doi: 10.1093/ecco-jcc/jjw070

Esnafoglu, E., Cirrik, S., Ayyildiz, S. N., Erdil, A., Erturk, E. Y., Dagli, A., et al. (2017). Increased serum zonulin levels as an intestinal permeability marker in autistic subjects. *J. Pediatr.* 188, 240–244. doi: 10.1016/j.jpeds.2017.04.004

Etienne-Mesmin, L., Chassaing, B., and Gewirtz, A. T. (2017). Tryptophan: a gut microbiota-derived metabolites regulating inflammation. *World J. Gastrointest. Pharmacol. Ther.* 8, 7–9. doi: 10.4292/wjgpt.v8.i1.7

Fallani, M., Amarri, S., Uusijarvi, A., Adam, R., Khanna, S., Aguilera, M., et al. (2011). Determinants of the human infant intestinal microbiota after the introduction of first complementary foods in infant samples from five European centres. *Microbiology* 157, 1385–1392. doi: 10.1099/mic.0.042143-0

Fallucca, F., Porrata, C., Fallucca, S., and Pianesi, M. (2014). Influence of diet on gut microbiota, inflammation and type 2 diabetes mellitus. First experience with macrobiotic Ma-Pi 2 diet. *Diabetes Metab. Res. Rev.* 30(Suppl. 1), 48–54. doi: 10.1002/dmrr.2518

Farhadi, A., Banan, A., Fields, J., and Keshavarzian, A. (2003). Intestinal barrier: an interface between health and disease. *J. Gastroenterol. Hepatol.* 18, 479–497. doi: 10.1046/j.1440-1746.2003.03032.x

Farrokhi, V., Nemati, R., Nichols, F. C., Yao, X., Anstadt, E., Fujiwara, M., et al. (2013). Bacterial lipodipeptide, Lipid 654, is a microbiome-associated biomarker for multiple sclerosis. *Clin. Transl. Immunol.* 2:e8. doi: 10.1038/cti.2013.11

Fasano, A., Not, T., Wang, W., Uzzau, S., Berti, I., Tommasini, A., et al. (2000). Zonulin, a newly discovered modulator of intestinal permeability, and its expression in coeliac disease. *Lancet* 355, 1518–1519. doi: 10.1016/S0140-6736(00)02169-3

Fasching, P., Stradner, M., Graninger, W., Dejaco, C., and Fessler, J. (2017). Therapeutic potential of targeting the Th17/Treg axis in autoimmune disorders. *Molecules* 22:E134. doi: 10.3390/molecules22010134

Felix, K. M., Tahsin, S., and Wu, H. J. (2017). Host-microbiota interplay in mediating immune disorders. *Ann. N.Y. Acad. Sci.* doi: 10.1111/nyas.13508. [Epub ahead of print].

Feng, T., and Elson, C. O. (2011). Adaptive immunity in the host-microbiota dialog. *Mucosal Immunol.* 4, 15–21. doi: 10.1038/mi.2010.60

Ferreira, R. M., Pereira-Marques, J., Pinto-Ribeiro, I., Costa, J. L., Carneiro, F., MacHado, J. C., et al. (2017). Gastric microbial community profiling reveals a dysbiotic cancer-associated microbiota. *Gut* 67, 226–236. doi: 10.1136/gutjnl-2017-314205

Ferrocino, I., Di Cagno, R., De Angelis, M., Turroni, S., Vannini, L., Bancalari, E., et al. (2015). Fecal microbiota in healthy subjects following omnivore, vegetarian and vegan diets: culturable populations and rRNA DGGE profiling. *PLoS ONE* 10:e0128669. doi: 10.1371/journal.pone.0128669

Finnie, J. W. (1984). Ultrastructural changes in the brain of mice given *Clostridium perfringens* type D epsilon toxin. *J. Comp. Pathol.* 94, 445–452. doi: 10.1016/0021-9975(84)90031-8

Fiorentino, M., Sapone, A., Senger, S., Camhi, S. S., Kadzielski, S. M., Buie, T. M., et al. (2016). Blood-brain barrier and intestinal epithelial barrier alterations in autism spectrum disorders. *Mol. Autism* 7:49. doi: 10.1186/s13229-016-0110-z

Forbes, J. D., Van Domselaar, G., and Bernstein, C. N. (2016). The gut microbiota in immune-mediated inflammatory diseases. *Front. Microbiol.* 7:1081. doi: 10.3389/fmicb.2016.01081

Freedman, S. N., Shahi, S. K., and Mangalam, A. K. (2017). The "gut feeling": breaking down the role of gut microbiome in multiple sclerosis. *Neurotherapeutics* 15, 109–125. doi: 10.1007/s13311-017-0588-x

Fritscher-Ravens, A., Schuppan, D., Ellrichmann, M., Schoch, S., Rocken, C., Brasch, J., et al. (2014). Confocal endomicroscopy shows food-associated changes in the intestinal mucosa of patients with irritable bowel syndrome. *Gastroenterology* 147, 1012–1020. doi: 10.1053/j.gastro.2014.07.046

Fung, T. C., Olson, C. A., and Hsiao, E. Y. (2017). Interactions between the microbiota, immune and nervous systems in health and disease. *Nat. Neurosci.* 20, 145–155. doi: 10.1038/nn.4476

Funkhouser, L. J., and Bordenstein, S. R. (2013). Mom knows best: the universality of maternal microbial transmission. *PLoS Biol.* 11:e1001631. doi: 10.1371/journal.pbio.1001631

Gallo, A., Passaro, G., Gasbarrini, A., Landolfi, R., and Montalto, M. (2016). Modulation of microbiota as treatment for intestinal inflammatory disorders: an uptodate. *World J. Gastroenterol.* 22, 7186–7202. doi: 10.3748/wjg.v22.i32.7186

Ganju, P., Nagpal, S., Mohammed, M. H., Nishal Kumar, P., Pandey, R., Natarajan, V. T., et al. (2016). Microbial community profiling shows dysbiosis in the lesional skin of Vitiligo subjects. *Sci. Rep.* 6:18761. doi: 10.1038/srep18761

Gao, Z., Tseng, C. H., Strober, B. E., Pei, Z., and Blaser, M. J. (2008). Substantial alterations of the cutaneous bacterial biota in psoriatic lesions. *PLoS ONE* 3:e2719. doi: 10.1371/journal.pone.0002719

Gensollen, T., Iyer, S. S., Kasper, D. L., and Blumberg, R. S. (2016). How colonization by microbiota in early life shapes the immune system. *Science* 352, 539–544. doi: 10.1126/science.aad9378

Geremia, A., Biancheri, P., Allan, P., Corazza, G. R., and Di Sabatino, A. (2014). Innate and adaptive immunity in inflammatory bowel disease. *Autoimmun. Rev.* 13, 3–10. doi: 10.1016/j.autrev.2013.06.004

Gill, S. R., Pop, M., Deboy, R. T., Eckburg, P. B., Turnbaugh, P. J., Samuel, B. S., et al. (2006). Metagenomic analysis of the human distal gut microbiome. *Science* 312, 1355–1359. doi: 10.1126/science.1124234

Grice, E. A., and Segre, J. A. (2011). The skin microbiome. *Nat. Rev. Microbiol.* 9, 244–253. doi: 10.1038/nrmicro2537

Guasp, M., and Dalmau, J. (2017). Encephalitis associated with antibodies against the NMDA receptor. *Med. Clin.* doi: 10.1016/j.medcli.2017.10.015. [Epub ahead of print].

Guida, F., Turco, F., Iannotta, M., De Gregorio, D., Palumbo, I., Sarnelli, G., et al. (2017). Antibiotic-induced microbiota perturbation causes gut endocannabinoidome changes, hippocampal neuroglial reorganization and depression in mice. *Brain Behav. Immun.* 67, 230–245. doi: 10.1016/j.bbi.2017.09.001

Guo, X., Li, J., Tang, R., Zhang, G., Zeng, H., Wood, R. J., et al. (2017). High fat diet alters gut microbiota and the expression of paneth cell-antimicrobial peptides preceding changes of circulating inflammatory cytokines. *Mediators Inflamm.* 2017:9474896. doi: 10.1155/2017/9474896

Gupta, R., Gupta, K., Tripathi, A. K., Bhatia, M. S., and Gupta, L. K. (2016). Effect of mirtazapine treatment on serum levels of brain-derived neurotrophic factor and tumor necrosis factor-alpha in patients of major depressive disorder with severe depression. *Pharmacology* 97, 184–188. doi: 10.1159/000444220

Hartsock, A., and Nelson, W. J. (2008). Adherens and tight junctions: structure, function and connections to the actin cytoskeleton. *Biochim. Biophys. Acta* 1778, 660–669. doi: 10.1016/j.bbamem.2007.07.012

Hashimoto, T., Perlot, T., Rehman, A., Trichereau, J., Ishiguro, H., Paolino, M., et al. (2012). ACE2 links amino acid malnutrition to microbial ecology and intestinal inflammation. *Nature* 487, 477–481. doi: 10.1038/nature11228

Hevia, A., Milani, C., Lopez, P., Cuervo, A., Arboleya, S., Duranti, S., et al. (2014). Intestinal dysbiosis associated with systemic lupus erythematosus. *MBio* 5, e01548–e01514. doi: 10.1128/mBio.01548-14

Hindson, J. (2017). Multiple sclerosis: a possible link between multiple sclerosis and gut microbiota. *Nat. Rev. Neurol.* 13:705. doi: 10.1038/nrneurol.2017.142

Hong, J., Jia, Y., Pan, S., Jia, L., Li, H., Han, Z., et al. (2016). Butyrate alleviates high fat diet-induced obesity through activation of adiponectin-mediated pathway and stimulation of mitochondrial function in the skeletal muscle of mice. *Oncotarget* 7, 56071–56082. doi: 10.18632/oncotarget.11267

Hooper, L. V., and Macpherson, A. J. (2010). Immune adaptations that maintain homeostasis with the intestinal microbiota. *Nat. Rev. Immunol.* 10, 159–169. doi: 10.1038/nri2710

Horvath, K., and Perman, J. A. (2002). Autistic disorder and gastrointestinal disease. *Curr. Opin. Pediatr.* 14, 583–587. doi: 10.1097/00008480-200210000-00004

Hsiao, E. Y., McBride, S. W., Hsien, S., Sharon, G., Hyde, E. R., McCue, T., et al. (2013). Microbiota modulate behavioral and physiological abnormalities associated with neurodevelopmental disorders. *Cell* 155, 1451–1463. doi: 10.1016/j.cell.2013.11.024

Hughes, S., Williams, S. E., and Turnberg, L. A. (1983). Crohn's disease and psoriasis. *N. Engl. J. Med.* 308:101.

Indigo, P. (2017). *Investigation of Novel Biomarkers and Definition of the Role of the Microbiome in Graves' Orbitopathy*. Available online at: http://www.indigo-iapp.eu/publishable-summary/ (Accessed September 20, 2017).

In't Veld, P. (2011). Insulitis in human type 1 diabetes: the quest for an elusive lesion. *Islets* 3, 131–138. doi: 10.4161/isl.3.4.15728

Ivanov, I. I, Atarashi, K., Manel, N., Brodie, E. L., Shima, T., Karaoz, U., et al. (2009). Induction of intestinal Th17 cells by segmented filamentous bacteria. *Cell* 139, 485–498. doi: 10.1016/j.cell.2009.09.033

Jangi, S., Gandhi, R., Cox, L. M., Li, N., Von Glehn, F., Yan, R., et al. (2016). Alterations of the human gut microbiome in multiple sclerosis. *Nat. Commun.* 7:12015. doi: 10.1038/ncomms12015

Jernberg, C., Lofmark, S., Edlund, C., and Jansson, J. K. (2007). Long-term ecological impacts of antibiotic administration on the human intestinal microbiota. *ISME J.* 1, 56–66. doi: 10.1038/ismej.2007.3

Jernberg, C., Lofmark, S., Edlund, C., and Jansson, J. K. (2010). Long-term impacts of antibiotic exposure on the human intestinal microbiota. *Microbiology* 156, 3216–3223. doi: 10.1099/mic.0.040618-0

Jiang, H., Ling, Z., Zhang, Y., Mao, H., Ma, Z., Yin, Y., et al. (2015). Altered fecal microbiota composition in patients with major depressive disorder. *Brain Behav. Immun.* 48, 186–194. doi: 10.1016/j.bbi.2015.03.016

Jirillo, E., Jirillo, F., and Magrone, T. (2012). Healthy effects exerted by prebiotics, probiotics, and symbiotics with special reference to their impact on the immune system. *Int. J. Vitam. Nutr. Res.* 82, 200–208. doi: 10.1024/0300-9831/a000112

Johnson-Henry, K. C., Pinnell, L. J., Waskow, A. M., Irrazabal, T., Martin, A., Hausner, M., et al. (2014). Short-chain fructo-oligosaccharide and inulin modulate inflammatory responses and microbial communities in Caco2-bbe cells and in a mouse model of intestinal injury. *J. Nutr.* 144, 1725–1733. doi: 10.3945/jn.114.195081

Jun, S., Gilmore, W., Callis, G., Rynda, A., Haddad, A., and Pascual, D. W. (2005). A live diarrheal vaccine imprints a Th2 cell bias and acts as an anti-inflammatory vaccine. *J. Immunol.* 175, 6733–6740. doi: 10.4049/jimmunol.175.10.6733

Jung, T. H., Park, J. H., Jeon, W. M., and Han, K. S. (2015). Butyrate modulates bacterial adherence on LS174T human colorectal cells by stimulating mucin secretion and MAPK signaling pathway. *Nutr. Res. Pract.* 9, 343–349. doi: 10.4162/nrp.2015.9.4.343

Kabat, A. M., Srinivasan, N., and Maloy, K. J. (2014). Modulation of immune development and function by intestinal microbiota. *Trends Immunol.* 35, 507–517. doi: 10.1016/j.it.2014.07.010

Kamada, N., Chen, G. Y., Inohara, N., and Nunez, G. (2013a). Control of pathogens and pathobionts by the gut microbiota. *Nat. Immunol.* 14, 685–690. doi: 10.1038/ni.2608

Kamada, N., Seo, S. U., Chen, G. Y., and Nunez, G. (2013b). Role of the gut microbiota in immunity and inflammatory disease. *Nat. Rev. Immunol.* 13, 321–335. doi: 10.1038/nri3430

Kang, D. W., Adams, J. B., Gregory, A. C., Borody, T., Chittick, L., Fasano, A., et al. (2017). Microbiota Transfer Therapy alters gut ecosystem and improves gastrointestinal and autism symptoms: an open-label study. *Microbiome* 5:10. doi: 10.1186/s40168-016-0225-7

Karam, G., Chastre, J., Wilcox, M. H., and Vincent, J. L. (2016). Antibiotic strategies in the era of multidrug resistance. *Crit. Care* 20:136. doi: 10.1186/s13054-016-1320-7

Karjalainen, J., Martin, J. M., Knip, M., Ilonen, J., Robinson, B. H., Savilahti, E., et al. (1992). A bovine albumin peptide as a possible trigger of insulin-dependent diabetes mellitus. *N. Engl. J. Med.* 327, 302–307. doi: 10.1056/NEJM199207303270502

Kaur, N., Chen, C. C., Luther, J., and Kao, J. Y. (2011). Intestinal dysbiosis in inflammatory bowel disease. *Gut Microbes* 2, 211–216. doi: 10.4161/gmic.2.4.17863

Kelsall, B. (2008). Recent progress in understanding the phenotype and function of intestinal dendritic cells and macrophages. *Mucosal Immunol.* 1, 460–469. doi: 10.1038/mi.2008.61

Khan, K. N., Fujishita, A., Masumoto, H., Muto, H., Kitajima, M., Masuzaki, H., et al. (2016). Molecular detection of intrauterine microbial colonization in women with endometriosis. *Eur. J. Obstet. Gynecol. Reprod. Biol.* 199, 69–75. doi: 10.1016/j.ejogrb.2016.01.040

Kim, S., Covington, A., and Pamer, E. G. (2017). The intestinal microbiota: antibiotics, colonization resistance, and enteric pathogens. *Immunol. Rev.* 279, 90–105. doi: 10.1111/imr.12563

Kleinewietfeld, M., and Hafler, D. A. (2013). The plasticity of human Treg and Th17 cells and its role in autoimmunity. *Semin. Immunol.* 25, 305–312. doi: 10.1016/j.smim.2013.10.009

Koenig, J. E., Spor, A., Scalfone, N., Fricker, A. D., Stombaugh, J., Knight, R., et al. (2011). Succession of microbial consortia in the developing infant gut microbiome. *Proc. Natl. Acad. Sci. U.S.A.* 108(Suppl. 1), 4578–4585. doi: 10.1073/pnas.1000081107

Kohling, H. L., Plummer, S. F., Marchesi, J. R., Davidge, K. S., and Ludgate, M. (2017). The microbiota and autoimmunity: their role in thyroid autoimmune diseases. *Clin. Immunol.* 183, 63–74. doi: 10.1016/j.clim.2017.07.001

Kopec, A. M., Fiorentino, M. R., and Bilbo, S. D. (2018). Gut-immune-brain dysfunction in Autism: importance of sex. *Brain Res.* doi: 10.1016/j.brainres.2018.01.009

Kosiewicz, M. M., Dryden, G. W., Chhabra, A., and Alard, P. (2014). Relationship between gut microbiota and development of T cell associated disease. *FEBS Lett.* 588, 4195–4206. doi: 10.1016/j.febslet.2014.03.019

Kostic, A. D., Gevers, D., Siljander, H., Vatanen, T., Hyotylainen, T., Hamalainen, A. M., et al. (2015). The dynamics of the human infant gut microbiome in development and in progression toward type 1 diabetes. *Cell Host Microbe* 17, 260–273. doi: 10.1016/j.chom.2015.01.001

Kristensen, B. (2016). Regulatory B and T cell responses in patients with autoimmune thyroid disease and healthy controls. *Dan. Med. J.* 63:B5177.

La Fata, G., Weber, P., and Mohajeri, M. H. (2017). Probiotics and the gut immune system: indirect regulation. *Probiotics Antimicrob. Proteins* 10, 11–21. doi: 10.1007/s12602-017-9322-6

La Paglia, G. M. C., Leone, M. C., Lepri, G., Vagelli, R., Valentini, E., Alunno, A., et al. (2017). One year in review 2017: systemic lupus erythematosus. *Clin. Exp. Rheumatol.* 35, 551–561.

Lamas, B., Richard, M. L., Leducq, V., Pham, H. P., Michel, M. L., Da Costa, G., et al. (2016). CARD9 impacts colitis by altering gut microbiota metabolism of tryptophan into aryl hydrocarbon receptor ligands. *Nat. Med.* 22, 598–605. doi: 10.1038/nm.4102

Langdon, A., Crook, N., and Dantas, G. (2016). The effects of antibiotics on the microbiome throughout development and alternative approaches for therapeutic modulation. *Genome Med.* 8:39. doi: 10.1186/s13073-016-0294-z

Lanzavecchia, A. (1995). How can cryptic epitopes trigger autoimmunity? *J. Exp. Med.* 181, 1945–1948.

Lederberg, J., M. A. (2001). 'Ome sweet' omics - a genealogical treasury of words. *Scientist* 15:8.

Lee, A. S., Gibson, D. L., Zhang, Y., Sham, H. P., Vallance, B. A., and Dutz, J. P. (2010). Gut barrier disruption by an enteric bacterial pathogen accelerates insulitis in NOD mice. *Diabetologia* 53, 741–748. doi: 10.1007/s00125-009-1626-y

Lee, J. H., Kim, S. K., Kim, S. K., Han, S. B., Lee, J. W., Lee, D. G., et al. (2016). Increase in antibiotic-resistant gram-negative bacterial infections in febrile neutropenic children. *Infect. Chemother.* 48, 181–189. doi: 10.3947/ic.2016.48.3.181

Lee, Y. K., Menezes, J. S., Umesaki, Y., and Mazmanian, S. K. (2011). Proinflammatory T-cell responses to gut microbiota promote experimental autoimmune encephalomyelitis. *Proc. Natl. Acad. Sci. U.S. A.* 108(Suppl. 1), 4615–4622. doi: 10.1073/pnas.1000082107

Lemus, H. N., Warrington, A. E., and Rodriguez, M. (2018). Multiple sclerosis: mechanisms of disease and strategies for myelin and axonal repair. *Neurol. Clin.* 36, 1–11. doi: 10.1016/j.ncl.2017.08.002

Lerner, A., Patricia, J., and Matthias, T. (2016). Nutrients, bugs and us: the short-chain fatty acids story in celiac disease. *Int. J. Celiac Dis.* 4, 92–94. doi: 10.12691/ijcd-4-3-12

Leslie, R. D. (2010). Predicting adult-onset autoimmune diabetes: clarity from complexity. *Diabetes* 59, 330–331. doi: 10.2337/db09-1620

Li, X., and Atkinson, M. A. (2015). The role for gut permeability in the pathogenesis of type 1 diabetes–a solid or leaky concept? *Pediatr. Diabetes* 16, 485–492. doi: 10.1111/pedi.12305

Li, Y. F., Poole, S., Nishio, K., Jang, K., Rasulova, F., McVeigh, A., et al. (2009). Structure of CFA/I fimbriae from enterotoxigenic *Escherichia coli*. *Proc. Natl. Acad. Sci. U.S.A.* 106, 10793–10798. doi: 10.1073/pnas.0812843106

Liang, B., and Mamula, M. J. (2000). Molecular mimicry and the role of B lymphocytes in the processing of autoantigens. *Cell. Mol. Life Sci.* 57, 561–568. doi: 10.1007/PL00000718

Lin, H. V., Frassetto, A., Kowalik, E. J. Jr., Nawrocki, A. R., Lu, M. M., Kosinski, J. R., et al. (2012). Butyrate and propionate protect against diet-induced obesity and regulate gut hormones via free fatty acid receptor 3-independent mechanisms. *PLoS ONE* 7:e35240. doi: 10.1371/journal.pone.0035240

Llorente, C., and Schnabl, B. (2015). The gut microbiota and liver disease. *Cell. Mol. Gastroenterol. Hepatol.* 1, 275–284. doi: 10.1016/j.jcmgh.2015.04.003

Lopez, P., De Paz, B., Rodriguez-Carrio, J., Hevia, A., Sanchez, B., Margolles, A., et al. (2016). Th17 responses and natural IgM antibodies are related to gut microbiota composition in systemic lupus erythematosus patients. *Sci. Rep.* 6:24072. doi: 10.1038/srep24072

Lorenzo Pisarello, M. J., Vintini, E. O., Gonzalez, S. N., Pagani, F., and Medina, M. S. (2015). Decrease in lactobacilli in the intestinal microbiota of celiac children with a gluten-free diet, and selection of potentially probiotic strains. *Can. J. Microbiol.* 61, 32–37. doi: 10.1139/cjm-2014-0472

Ma, Y., Shi, N., Li, M., Chen, F., and Niu, H. (2015). Applications of next-generation sequencing in systemic autoimmune diseases. *Genomics Proteomics Bioinformatics* 13, 242–249. doi: 10.1016/j.gpb.2015.09.004

Maahs, D. M., West, N. A., Lawrence, J. M., and Mayer-Davis, E. J. (2010). Epidemiology of type 1 diabetes. *Endocrinol. Metab. Clin. North Am.* 39, 481–497. doi: 10.1016/j.ecl.2010.05.011

Maffeis, C., Martina, A., Corradi, M., Quarella, S., Nori, N., Torriani, S., et al. (2016). Association between intestinal permeability and faecal microbiota composition in Italian children with beta cell autoimmunity at risk for type 1 diabetes. *Diabetes Metab. Res. Rev.* 32, 700–709. doi: 10.1002/dmrr.2790

Marmont, A. M. (1994). Defining criteria for autoimmune diseases. *Immunol. Today* 15:388. doi: 10.1016/0167-5699(94)90178-3

Maslowski, K. M., Vieira, A. T., Ng, A., Kranich, J., Sierro, F., Yu, D., et al. (2009). Regulation of inflammatory responses by gut microbiota and chemoattractant receptor GPR43. *Nature* 461, 1282–1286. doi: 10.1038/nature08530

Matsuoka, K., and Kanai, T. (2015). The gut microbiota and inflammatory bowel disease. *Semin. Immunopathol.* 37, 47–55. doi: 10.1007/s00281-014-0454-4

McGuckin, M. A., Linden, S. K., Sutton, P., and Florin, T. H. (2011). Mucin dynamics and enteric pathogens. *Nat. Rev. Microbiol.* 9, 265–278. doi: 10.1038/nrmicro2538

Meddings, J. B., Jarand, J., Urbanski, S. J., Hardin, J., and Gall, D. G. (1999). Increased gastrointestinal permeability is an early lesion in the spontaneously diabetic BB rat. *Am. J. Physiol.* 276, G951–G957. doi: 10.1152/ajpgi.1999.276.4.G951

Mejia-Leon, M. E., and Barca, A. M. (2015). Diet, microbiota and immune system in type 1 diabetes development and evolution. *Nutrients* 7, 9171–9184. doi: 10.3390/nu7115461

Miao, D., Yu, L., and Eisenbarth, G. S. (2007). Role of autoantibodies in type 1 diabetes. *Front. Biosci.* 12, 1889–1898. doi: 10.2741/2195

Milanovic, V., Osimani, A., Aquilanti, L., Tavoletti, S., Garofalo, C., Polverigiani, S., et al. (2017). Occurrence of antibiotic resistance genes in the fecal DNA of healthy omnivores, ovo-lacto vegetarians and vegans. *Mol. Nutr. Food Res.* 61, 61:1601098. doi: 10.1002/mnfr.201601098

Miyake, S., Kim, S., Suda, W., Oshima, K., Nakamura, M., Matsuoka, T., et al. (2015). Dysbiosis in the gut microbiota of patients with multiple sclerosis, with a striking depletion of species belonging to clostridia XIVa and IV clusters. *PLoS ONE* 10:e0137429. doi: 10.1371/journal.pone.0137429

Mizuno, M., Noto, D., Kaga, N., Chiba, A., and Miyake, S. (2017). The dual role of short fatty acid chains in the pathogenesis of autoimmune disease models. *PLoS ONE* 12:e0173032. doi: 10.1371/journal.pone.0173032

Molloy, M. J., Bouladoux, N., and Belkaid, Y. (2012). Intestinal microbiota: shaping local and systemic immune responses. *Semin. Immunol.* 24, 58–66. doi: 10.1016/j.smim.2011.11.008

Morgan, B. P., and Harris, C. L. (2015). Complement, a target for therapy in inflammatory and degenerative diseases. *Nat. Rev. Drug Discov.* 14, 857–877. doi: 10.1038/nrd4657

Mukherjee, S., and Hooper, L. V. (2015). Antimicrobial defense of the intestine. *Immunity* 42, 28–39. doi: 10.1016/j.immuni.2014.12.028

Nagy, G., Huszthy, P. C., Fossum, E., Konttinen, Y., Nakken, B., and Szodoray, P. (2015). Selected aspects in the pathogenesis of autoimmune diseases. *Mediators Inflamm.* 2015:351732. doi: 10.1155/2015/351732

Najarian, D. J., and Gottlieb, A. B. (2003). Connections between psoriasis and Crohn's disease. *J. Am. Acad. Dermatol.* 48, 805–821. quiz: 822–804. doi: 10.1067/mjd.2003.540

Naseribafrouei, A., Hestad, K., Avershina, E., Sekelja, M., Linlokken, A., Wilson, R., et al. (2014). Correlation between the human fecal microbiota and depression. *Neurogastroenterol. Motil.* 26, 1155–1162. doi: 10.1111/nmo.12378

Neu, J., Reverte, C. M., MacKey, A. D., Liboni, K., Tuhacek-Tenace, L. M., Hatch, M., et al. (2005). Changes in intestinal morphology and permeability in the biobreeding rat before the onset of type 1 diabetes. *J. Pediatr. Gastroenterol. Nutr.* 40, 589–595. doi: 10.1097/01.MPG.0000159636.19346.C1

Nishida, A., Inoue, R., Inatomi, O., Bamba, S., Naito, Y., and Andoh, A. (2017). Gut microbiota in the pathogenesis of inflammatory bowel disease. *Clin. J. Gastroenterol.* 11, 1–10. doi: 10.1007/s12328-017-0813-5

Nouri, M., Bredberg, A., Westrom, B., and Lavasani, S. (2014). Intestinal barrier dysfunction develops at the onset of experimental autoimmune encephalomyelitis, and can be induced by adoptive transfer of auto-reactive T cells. *PLoS ONE* 9:e106335. doi: 10.1371/journal.pone.0106335

Ochoa-Reparaz, J., Mielcarz, D. W., Wang, Y., Begum-Haque, S., Dasgupta, S., Kasper, D. L., et al. (2010). A polysaccharide from the human commensal *Bacteroides fragilis* protects against CNS demyelinating disease. *Mucosal Immunol.* 3, 487–495. doi: 10.1038/mi.2010.29

Odamaki, T., Kato, K., Sugahara, H., Hashikura, N., Takahashi, S., Xiao, J. Z., et al. (2016). Age-related changes in gut microbiota composition from newborn to centenarian: a cross-sectional study. *BMC Microbiol.* 16:90. doi: 10.1186/s12866-016-0708-5

O'Garra, A., Steinman, L., and Gijbels, K. (1997). CD4+ T-cell subsets in autoimmunity. *Curr. Opin. Immunol.* 9, 872–883. doi: 10.1016/S0952-7915(97)80192-6

O'garra, A., and Vieira, P. (2004). Regulatory T cells and mechanisms of immune system control. *Nat. Med.* 10, 801–805. doi: 10.1038/nm0804-801

Okumura, R., and Takeda, K. (2017). Roles of intestinal epithelial cells in the maintenance of gut homeostasis. *Exp. Mol. Med.* 49:e338. doi: 10.1038/emm.2017.20

Oliveira Mde, F., Rocha Bde, O., and Duarte, G. V. (2015). Psoriasis: classical and emerging comorbidities. *An. Bras. Dermatol.* 90, 9–20. doi: 10.1590/abd1806-4841.20153038

Ottman, N., Smidt, H., De Vos, W. M., and Belzer, C. (2012). The function of our microbiota: who is out there and what do they do? *Front. Cell. Infect. Microbiol.* 2:104. doi: 10.3389/fcimb.2012.00104

Ounissi-Benkalha, H., and Polychronakos, C. (2008). The molecular genetics of type 1 diabetes: new genes and emerging mechanisms. *Trends Mol. Med.* 14, 268–275. doi: 10.1016/j.molmed.2008.04.002

Pagliuca, C., Cicatiello, A. G., Colicchio, R., Greco, A., Cerciello, R., Auletta, L., et al. (2016). Novel approach for evaluation of *Bacteroides fragilis* protective role against *Bartonella henselae* liver damage in immunocompromised murine model. *Front. Microbiol.* 7:1750. doi: 10.3389/fmicb.2016.01750

Parks, O. B., Pociask, D. A., Hodzic, Z., Kolls, J. K., and Good, M. (2015). Interleukin-22 signaling in the regulation of intestinal health and disease. *Front. Cell. Dev. Biol.* 3:85. doi: 10.3389/fcell.2015.00085

Passos, M., and Moraes-Filho, J. P. (2017). Intestinal microbiota in digestive diseases. *Arq. Gastroenterol.* 54, 255–262. doi: 10.1590/s0004-2803.201700000-31

Pearlman, D. M., and Najjar, S. (2014). Meta-analysis of the association between N-methyl-d-aspartate receptor antibodies and schizophrenia, schizoaffective disorder, bipolar disorder, and major depressive disorder. *Schizophr. Res.* 157, 249–258. doi: 10.1016/j.schres.2014.05.001

Pedrotti Moreira, F., Borges, C. J., Wiener, C. D., Da Silva, P. M., Portela, L. V., Lara, D. R., et al. (2017). Serum brain-derived neurotrophic factor levels in subjects with major depressive disorder with previous suicide attempt: a population-based study. *Psychiatry Res.* doi: 10.1016/j.psychres.2017.09.033

Peng, L., Li, Z. R., Green, R. S., Holzman, I. R., and Lin, J. (2009). Butyrate enhances the intestinal barrier by facilitating tight junction assembly via activation of AMP-activated protein kinase in Caco-2 cell monolayers. *J. Nutr.* 139, 1619–1625. doi: 10.3945/jn.109.104638

Penhale, W. J., and Young, P. R. (1988). The influence of the normal microbial flora on the susceptibility of rats to experimental autoimmune thyroiditis. *Clin. Exp. Immunol.* 72, 288–292.

Perlot, T., and Penninger, J. M. (2013). ACE2 - from the renin-angiotensin system to gut microbiota and malnutrition. *Microbes Infect.* 15, 866–873. doi: 10.1016/j.micinf.2013.08.003

Peterson, C. T., Sharma, V., Elmen, L., and Peterson, S. N. (2015). Immune homeostasis, dysbiosis and therapeutic modulation of the gut microbiota. *Clin. Exp. Immunol.* 179, 363–377. doi: 10.1111/cei.12474

Pickard, J. M., Zeng, M. Y., Caruso, R., and Nunez, G. (2017). Gut microbiota: role in pathogen colonization, immune responses, and inflammatory disease. *Immunol. Rev.* 279, 70–89. doi: 10.1111/imr.12567

Pokhrel, B., and Bhusal, K. (2017). *Graves Disease.* Treasure Island, FL: StatPearls.

Powell, N., and MacDonald, T. T. (2017). Recent advances in gut immunology. *Parasite Immunol.* 39, 1–11. doi: 10.1111/pim.12430

Probstel, A. K., and Baranzini, S. E. (2017). The role of the gut microbiome in multiple sclerosis risk and progression: towards characterization of the "MS microbiome". *Neurotherapeutics* 15, 126–134. doi: 10.1007/s13311-017-0587-y

Qin, J., Li, R., Raes, J., Arumugam, M., Burgdorf, K. S., Manichanh, C., et al. (2010). A human gut microbial gene catalogue established by metagenomic sequencing. *Nature* 464, 59–65. doi: 10.1038/nature08821

Redondo, M. J., Oram, R. A., and Steck, A. K. (2017). Genetic risk scores for type 1 diabetes prediction and diagnosis. *Curr. Diab. Rep.* 17:129. doi: 10.1007/s11892-017-0961-5

Reich, D. S., Lucchinetti, C. F., and Calabresi, P. A. (2018). Multiple sclerosis. *N. Engl. J. Med.* 378, 169–180. doi: 10.1056/NEJMra1401483

Rewers, M., and Ludvigsson, J. (2016). Environmental risk factors for type 1 diabetes. *Lancet* 387, 2340–2348. doi: 10.1016/S0140-6736(16)30507-4

Richards, J. L., Yap, Y. A., McLeod, K. H., MacKay, C. R., and Marino, E. (2016). Dietary metabolites and the gut microbiota: an alternative approach to control inflammatory and autoimmune diseases. *Clin. Transl. Immunol.* 5:e82. doi: 10.1038/cti.2016.29

Rios-Covian, D., Ruas-Madiedo, P., Margolles, A., Gueimonde, M., De Los Reyes-Gavilan, C. G., and Salazar, N. (2016). Intestinal short chain fatty acids and their link with diet and human health. *Front. Microbiol.* 7:185. doi: 10.3389/fmicb.2016.00185

Robinson, A. P., Harp, C. T., Noronha, A., and Miller, S. D. (2014). The experimental autoimmune encephalomyelitis (EAE) model of MS: utility for understanding disease pathophysiology and treatment. *Handb. Clin. Neurol.* 122, 173–189. doi: 10.1016/B978-0-444-52001-2.00008-X

Rodriguez, J. M., Murphy, K., Stanton, C., Ross, R. P., Kober, O. I., Juge, N., et al. (2015). The composition of the gut microbiota throughout life, with an emphasis on early life. *Microb. Ecol. Health Dis.* 26:26050. doi: 10.3402/mehd.v26.26050

Roesch, L. F., Lorca, G. L., Casella, G., Giongo, A., Naranjo, A., Pionzio, A. M., et al. (2009). Culture-independent identification of gut bacteria correlated with the onset of diabetes in a rat model. *ISME J.* 3, 536–548. doi: 10.1038/ismej.2009.5

Rook, G., Backhed, F., Levin, B. R., McFall-Ngai, M. J., and McLean, A. R. (2017). Evolution, human-microbe interactions, and life history plasticity. *Lancet* 390, 521–530. doi: 10.1016/S0140-6736(17)30566-4

Rose, N. R., and Bona, C. (1993). Defining criteria for autoimmune diseases (Witebsky's postulates revisited). *Immunol. Today* 14, 426–430. doi: 10.1016/0167-5699(93)90244-F

Rose, N. R., Bonita, R., and Burek, C. L. (2002). Iodine: an environmental trigger of thyroiditis. *Autoimmun. Rev.* 1, 97–103. doi: 10.1016/S1568-9972(01)00016-7

Round, J. L., and Mazmanian, S. K. (2009). The gut microbiota shapes intestinal immune responses during health and disease. *Nat. Rev. Immunol.* 9, 313–323. doi: 10.1038/nri2515

Rumah, K. R., Linden, J., Fischetti, V. A., and Vartanian, T. (2013). Isolation of *Clostridium perfringens* type B in an individual at first clinical presentation of multiple sclerosis provides clues for environmental triggers of the disease. *PLoS ONE* 8:e76359. doi: 10.1371/journal.pone.0076359

Rutz, S., Eidenschenk, C., and Ouyang, W. (2013). IL-22, not simply a Th17 cytokine. *Immunol. Rev.* 252, 116–132. doi: 10.1111/imr.12027

Sanford, J. A., and Gallo, R. L. (2013). Functions of the skin microbiota in health and disease. *Semin. Immunol.* 25, 370–377. doi: 10.1016/j.smim.2013.09.005

Sanz, Y. (2010). Effects of a gluten-free diet on gut microbiota and immune function in healthy adult humans. *Gut Microbes* 1, 135–137. doi: 10.4161/gmic.1.3.11868

Sapone, A., De Magistris, L., Pietzak, M., Clemente, M. G., Tripathi, A., Cucca, F., et al. (2006). Zonulin upregulation is associated with increased gut permeability in subjects with type 1 diabetes and their relatives. *Diabetes* 55, 1443–1449. doi: 10.2337/db05-1593

Sasso, F. C., Carbonara, O., Torella, R., Mezzogiorno, A., Esposito, V., Demagistris, L., et al. (2004). Ultrastructural changes in enterocytes in subjects with Hashimoto's thyroiditis. *Gut* 53, 1878–1880. doi: 10.1136/gut.2004.047498

Saukkonen, T., Savilahti, E., Madacsy, L., Arato, A., Korner, A., Barkai, L., et al. (1996). Increased frequency of IgM antibodies to cow's milk proteins in Hungarian children with newly diagnosed insulin-dependent diabetes mellitus. *Eur. J. Pediatr.* 155, 885–889. doi: 10.1007/BF02282839

Savilahti, E., Akerblom, H. K., Tainio, V. M., and Koskimies, S. (1988). Children with newly diagnosed insulin dependent diabetes mellitus have increased levels of cow's milk antibodies. *Diabetes Res.* 7, 137–140.

Scher, J. U., Ubeda, C., Artacho, A., Attur, M., Isaac, S., Reddy, S. M., et al. (2015). Decreased bacterial diversity characterizes the altered gut microbiota in patients with psoriatic arthritis, resembling dysbiosis in inflammatory bowel disease. *Arthritis Rheumatol.* 67, 128–139. doi: 10.1002/art.38892

Schwarz, E., Maukonen, J., Hyytiainen, T., Kieseppa, T., Oresic, M., Sabunciyan, S., et al. (2017). Analysis of microbiota in first episode psychosis identifies preliminary associations with symptom severity and treatment response. *Schizophr. Res.* 192, 398–403. doi: 10.1016/j.schres.2017.04.017

Secondulfo, M., Iafusco, D., Carratu, R., Demagistris, L., Sapone, A., Generoso, M., et al. (2004). Ultrastructural mucosal alterations and increased intestinal permeability in non-celiac, type I diabetic patients. *Dig. Liver Dis.* 36, 35–45. doi: 10.1016/j.dld.2003.09.016

Selber-Hnatiw, S., Rukundo, B., Ahmadi, M., Akoubi, H., Al-Bizri, H., Aliu, A. F., et al. (2017). Human gut microbiota: toward an ecology of disease. *Front. Microbiol.* 8:1265. doi: 10.3389/fmicb.2017.01265

Sender, R., Fuchs, S., and Milo, R. (2016). Revised estimates for the number of human and bacteria cells in the body. *PLoS Biol.* 14:e1002533. doi: 10.1371/journal.pbio.1002533

Severance, E. G., Tveiten, D., Lindstrom, L. H., Yolken, R. H., and Reichelt, K. L. (2016). The gut microbiota and the emergence of autoimmunity: relevance to major psychiatric disorders. *Curr. Pharm. Des.* 22, 6076–6086. doi: 10.2174/1381612822666160914183804

Shaaban, S. Y., El Gendy, Y. G., Mehanna, N. S., El-Senousy, W. M., El-Feki, H. S. A., Saad, K., et al. (2017). The role of probiotics in children with autism spectrum disorder: a prospective, open-label study. *Nutr. Neurosci.* doi: 10.1080/1028415X.2017.1347746. [Epub ahead of print].

Shahi, S. K., Freedman, S. N., and Mangalam, A. K. (2017). Gut microbiome in multiple sclerosis: the players involved and the roles they play. *Gut Microbes* 8, 607–615. doi: 10.1080/19490976.2017.1349041

Shi, N., Li, N., Duan, X., and Niu, H. (2017). Interaction between the gut microbiome and mucosal immune system. *Mil. Med. Res.* 4:14. doi: 10.1186/s40779-017-0122-9

Shor, D. B., Orbach, H., Boaz, M., Altman, A., Anaya, J. M., Bizzaro, N., et al. (2012). Gastrointestinal-associated autoantibodies in different autoimmune diseases. *Am. J. Clin. Exp. Immunol.* 1, 49–55.

Sonnenburg, J. L., and Backhed, F. (2016). Diet-microbiota interactions as moderators of human metabolism. *Nature* 535, 56–64. doi: 10.1038/nature18846

Statnikov, A., Alekseyenko, A. V., Li, Z., Henaff, M., Perez-Perez, G. I., Blaser, M. J., et al. (2013). Microbiomic signatures of psoriasis: feasibility and methodology comparison. *Sci. Rep.* 3:2620. doi: 10.1038/srep02620

Stevens, B. R., Goel, R., Seungbum, K., Richards, E. M., Holbert, R. C., Pepine, C. J., et al. (2017). Increased human intestinal barrier permeability plasma biomarkers zonulin and FABP2 correlated with plasma LPS and altered gut microbiome in anxiety or depression. *Gut.* doi: 10.1136/gutjnl-2017-314759

Stinson, L. F., Payne, M. S., and Keelan, J. A. (2017). Planting the seed: origins, composition, and postnatal health significance of the fetal gastrointestinal microbiota. *Crit. Rev. Microbiol.* 43, 352–369. doi: 10.1080/1040841X.2016.1211088

Stromnes, I. M., and Goverman, J. M. (2006). Active induction of experimental allergic encephalomyelitis. *Nat. Protoc.* 1, 1810–1819. doi: 10.1038/nprot.2006.285

Sturgeon, C., and Fasano, A. (2016). Zonulin, a regulator of epithelial and endothelial barrier functions, and its involvement in chronic inflammatory diseases. *Tissue Barriers* 4:e1251384. doi: 10.1080/21688370.2016.1251384

Tett, A., Pasolli, E., Farina, S., Truong, D. T., Asnicar, F., Zolfo, M., et al. (2017). Unexplored diversity and strain-level structure of the skin microbiome associated with psoriasis. *NPJ Biofilms Microbiomes* 3:14. doi: 10.1038/s41522-017-0022-5

Tremaroli, V., and Backhed, F. (2012). Functional interactions between the gut microbiota and host metabolism. *Nature* 489, 242–249. doi: 10.1038/nature11552

Tremlett, H., and Waubant, E. (2017). The multiple sclerosis microbiome? *Ann. Transl. Med.* 5:53. doi: 10.21037/atm.2017.01.63

Tschoeke, D. A., De Oliveira, L. S., Leomil, L., Tanuri, A., and Thompson, F. L. (2017). Pregnant women carrying microcephaly foetuses and Zika virus contain potentially pathogenic microbes and parasites in their amniotic fluid. *BMC Med. Genomics* 10:5. doi: 10.1186/s12920-016-0242-1

Tsuang, M. (2000). Schizophrenia: genes and environment. *Biol. Psychiatry* 47, 210–220. doi: 10.1016/S0006-3223(99)00289-9

Tzianabos, A. O., Kasper, D. L., Cisneros, R. L., Smith, R. S., and Onderdonk, A. B. (1995). Polysaccharide-mediated protection against abscess formation in experimental intra-abdominal sepsis. *J. Clin. Invest.* 96, 2727–2731. doi: 10.1172/JCI118340

Vaarala, O. (2008). Leaking gut in type 1 diabetes. *Curr. Opin. Gastroenterol.* 24, 701–706. doi: 10.1097/MOG.0b013e32830e6d98

Vaarala, O., Atkinson, M. A., and Neu, J. (2008). The "perfect storm" for type 1 diabetes: the complex interplay between intestinal microbiota, gut permeability, and mucosal immunity. *Diabetes* 57, 2555–2562. doi: 10.2337/db08-0331

Van Wijk, F., and Cheroutre, H. (2010). Mucosal T cells in gut homeostasis and inflammation. *Expert Rev. Clin. Immunol.* 6, 559–566. doi: 10.1586/eci.10.34

Vanhaecke, T., Aubert, P., Grohard, P. A., Durand, T., Hulin, P., Paul-Gilloteaux, P., et al. (2017). *L. fermentum* CECT 5716 prevents stress-induced intestinal barrier dysfunction in newborn rats. *Neurogastroenterol. Motil.* 29:e13069. doi: 10.1111/nmo.13069

Vasquez, A. (2017). Biological plausibility of the gut-brain axis in autism. *Ann. N.Y. Acad. Sci.* 1408, 5–6. doi: 10.1111/nyas.13516

Virtanen, S. M. (2016). Dietary factors in the development of type 1 diabetes. *Pediatr. Diabetes* 17(Suppl. 22), 49–55. doi: 10.1111/pedi.12341

Volkmann, E. R., Hoffmann-Vold, A. M., Chang, Y. L., Jacobs, J. P., Tillisch, K., Mayer, E. A., et al. (2017). Systemic sclerosis is associated with specific alterations in gastrointestinal microbiota in two independent cohorts. *BMJ Open Gastroenterol.* 4:e000134. doi: 10.1136/bmjgast-2017-000134

Wampach, L., Heintz-Buschart, A., Hogan, A., Muller, E. E. L., Narayanasamy, S., Laczny, C. C., et al. (2017). Colonization and succession within the human gut microbiome by archaea, bacteria, and microeukaryotes during the first year of life. *Front. Microbiol.* 8:738. doi: 10.3389/fmicb.2017.00738

Wu, G. D., Chen, J., Hoffmann, C., Bittinger, K., Chen, Y. Y., Keilbaugh, S. A., et al. (2011). Linking long-term dietary patterns with gut microbial enterotypes. *Science* 334, 105–108. doi: 10.1126/science.1208344

Wu, H. J., and Wu, E. (2012). The role of gut microbiota in immune homeostasis and autoimmunity. *Gut Microbes* 3, 4–14. doi: 10.4161/gmic.19320

Wu, W. L. (2017). Association among gut microbes, intestinal physiology, and autism. *EBioMedicine* 25, 11–12. doi: 10.1016/j.ebiom.2017.10.013

Xie, Z., Chang, C., and Zhou, Z. (2014). Molecular mechanisms in autoimmune type 1 diabetes: a critical review. *Clin. Rev. Allergy Immunol.* 47, 174–192. doi: 10.1007/s12016-014-8422-2

Yan, D., Issa, N., Afifi, L., Jeon, C., Chang, H. W., and Liao, W. (2017). The role of the skin and gut microbiome in psoriatic disease. *Curr. Dermatol. Rep.* 6, 94–103. doi: 10.1007/s13671-017-0178-5

Yang, Y., Tian, J., and Yang, B. (2017). Targeting gut microbiome: a novel and potential therapy for autism. *Life Sci.* 194, 111–119. doi: 10.1016/j.lfs.2017.12.027

Yatsunenko, T., Rey, F. E., Manary, M. J., Trehan, I., Dominguez-Bello, M. G., Contreras, M., et al. (2012). Human gut microbiome viewed across age and geography. *Nature* 486, 222–227. doi: 10.1038/nature11053

Yissachar, N., Zhou, Y., Ung, L., Lai, N. Y., Mohan, J. F., Ehrlicher, A., et al. (2017). An intestinal organ culture system uncovers a role for the nervous system in microbe-immune crosstalk. *Cell* 168, 1135–1148.e1112. doi: 10.1016/j.cell.2017.02.009

Yong, H., Chartier, G., and Quandt, J. (2017). Modulating inflammation and neuroprotection in multiple sclerosis. *J. Neurosci. Res.* doi: 10.1002/jnr.24090. [Epub ahead of print].

Zakostelska, Z., Malkova, J., Klimesova, K., Rossmann, P., Hornova, M., Novosadova, I., et al. (2016). Intestinal microbiota promotes psoriasis-like skin inflammation by enhancing Th17 response. *PLoS ONE* 11:e0159539. doi: 10.1371/journal.pone.0159539

Zeeuwen, P. L., Kleerebezem, M., Timmerman, H. M., and Schalkwijk, J. (2013). Microbiome and skin diseases. *Curr. Opin. Allergy Clin. Immunol.* 13, 514–520. doi: 10.1097/ACI.0b013e328364ebeb

Zelante, T., Iannitti, R. G., Cunha, C., De Luca, A., Giovannini, G., Pieraccini, G., et al. (2013). Tryptophan catabolites from microbiota engage aryl hydrocarbon receptor and balance mucosal reactivity via interleukin-22. *Immunity* 39, 372–385. doi: 10.1016/j.immuni.2013.08.003

Zhang, H., Liao, X., Sparks, J. B., and Luo, X. M. (2014). Dynamics of gut microbiota in autoimmune lupus. *Appl. Environ. Microbiol.* 80, 7551–7560. doi: 10.1128/AEM.02676-14

Zhang, M., Zhou, Q., Dorfman, R. G., Huang, X., Fan, T., Zhang, H., et al. (2016). Butyrate inhibits interleukin-17 and generates Tregs to ameliorate colorectal colitis in rats. *BMC Gastroenterol.* 16:84. doi: 10.1186/s12876-016-0500-x

Zhou, J. S., and Gill, H. S. (2005). Immunostimulatory probiotic *Lactobacillus rhamnosus* HN001 and *Bifidobacterium lactis* HN019 do not induce pathological inflammation in mouse model of experimental autoimmune thyroiditis. *Int. J. Food Microbiol.* 103, 97–104. doi: 10.1016/j.ijfoodmicro.2004.11.031

Zimmer, J., Lange, B., Frick, J. S., Sauer, H., Zimmermann, K., Schwiertz, A., et al. (2012). A vegan or vegetarian diet substantially alters the human colonic faecal microbiota. *Eur. J. Clin. Nutr.* 66, 53–60. doi: 10.1038/ejcn.2011.141

4

The Role of Type 2 Diabetes for the Development of Pathogen-Associated Cancers in the Face of the HIV/AIDS Epidemic

Melissa J. Blumenthal†, Sylvia Ujma†, Arieh A. Katz and Georgia Schäfer*

Receptor Biology Research Unit, Division of Medical Biochemistry and Structural Biology, Institute of Infectious Disease and Molecular Medicine, Department of Integrative Biomedical Sciences, Faculty of Health Sciences, SA-MRC Gynecology Cancer Research Centre, University of Cape Town, Cape Town, South Africa

***Correspondence:**
Georgia Schäfer
georgia.schafer@uct.ac.za

†These authors have contributed equally to this work.

The contribution of HIV to the development of pathogen-associated cancers has long been recognized, as has the contribution of type 2 diabetes for the development of several types of cancer. While HIV/AIDS-associated immunosuppression reduces immunosurveillance and indirectly contributes favorably to cancerogenesis, diabetes directly increases cancer development due to chronic low-grade inflammation, dysregulated glucose metabolism, hyperactivation of insulin-responsive pathways, and anti-apoptotic signaling. Pathogen-associated cancers contribute significantly to the cancer burden particularly in low- and middle-income countries. In those countries, the incidence of type 2 diabetes has increased alarmingly over the last decades, in part due to rapid changes in diet, lifestyle, and urbanization. It is likely that the HIV/AIDS epidemic and the steadily increasing rate of type 2 diabetes display synergistic effects on oncogenesis. Although this possible link has not been extensively investigated, it might become more important in the years to come not least due to the stimulating effects of antiretroviral therapy on the development of type 2 diabetes. This review provides an overview of the current understanding of pathogen- and diabetes- associated cancers with focus on geographical regions additionally burdened by the HIV/AIDS epidemic. As both HIV and carcinogenic infections as well as the onset of type 2 diabetes involve environmental factors that can be avoided to a certain extent, this review will support the hypothesis that certain malignancies are potentially preventable. Deploying effective infection control strategies together with educational policies on diet and lifestyle may in the long term reduce the burden of preventable cancers which is of particular relevance in low-resource settings.

Keywords: type 2 diabetes, pathogen-associated cancers, HIV/AIDS, HPV, KSHV, low- and middle-income countries, sub-Saharan Africa

INTRODUCTION

The development of cancer is a complex multistep process. It is well-understood that the lack of responsiveness to signals from the microenvironment together with the accumulation of aberrations in multiple cellular regulatory systems can eventually lead to the characteristic loss of growth control displayed by cancer cells (Hanahan and Weinberg, 2011). Oncogenesis is typically initiated by a non-lethal genetic or epigenetic alteration leading to abnormal proliferation of a single cell. Apart from the genetic constitution of an individual, this can be caused by multiple agents including radiation, chemicals and persistent infection with oncogenic microbes, the latter causing about 15–20% of all human cancers (Plummer et al., 2016).

Although necessary, initiation alone is not sufficient for tumor formation. In addition, tumor promoters are needed to induce the initiated cells to transform and become malignant. Tumor promoters are generally non-tumorigenic by themselves but rather reversibly stimulate cell proliferation and/or provide a tumor-friendly environment (e.g., hormones, chronic inflammation, and immunosuppression). The combined action of initiators and promoters can then eventually give rise to cells that become gradually and irreversibly malignant through a progressive series of alterations (Vincent and Gatenby, 2008).

Smoking and alcohol consumption, obesity and physical inactivity are the worldwide leading risk factors for cancer death, with oncogenic pathogens significantly contributing to cancer incidence in low-and middle-income countries which are often additionally burdened by the HIV/AIDS epidemic (Danaei et al., 2005). The leading types of cancer-causing infections worldwide are *Helicobacter pylori*, human papillomavirus (HPV), hepatitis B virus (HBV) and hepatitis C virus (HCV), while Kaposi's sarcoma-associated herpesvirus (KSHV) is particularly important in the sub-Saharan African context. Co-infection with human immunodeficiency virus (HIV) substantially enhances the incidence of pathogen-associated cancers (Working Group on the Evaluation of Carcinogenic Risks to Humans [IARC], 2012). Although HIV is not considered an oncogenic virus, it indirectly impacts on cancerogenesis through immune deficiency and impaired immune surveillance, thereby increasing the effects of oncogenic infections (Working Group on the Evaluation of Carcinogenic Risks to Humans [IARC], 2012). Cancer-promoting effects have also been ascribed to the chronic metabolic and hormonal disturbances as seen in type 2 diabetes (Giovannucci et al., 2010), a condition that is no longer considered a disease primarily affecting the industrialized world but has become increasingly common in low-resource settings (Hu, 2011).

All three conditions, namely type 2 diabetes, HIV-associated immunosuppression and oncogenic pathogen infections, not only contribute to cancer development, they are also largely preventable. Fundamental changes in public policies with regard to diet and lifestyle modifications, education and training on infection prevention as well as nation-wide prophylactic vaccination programs against HBV and HPV are predicted to have a significant impact on the cancer burden in low- and middle- income countries (Sylla and Wild, 2012).

PATHOGEN-ASSOCIATED CANCER DEVELOPMENT IN THE CONTEXT OF HIV/AIDS

Cancers attributable to infectious agents are an important component of the global cancer burden. Assessments dating from 1990 to 2012 have attributed 1/6th of global cancer cases to infectious etiologies and in sub-Saharan Africa, which is heavily burdened with HIV/AIDS, this is greater than 30% (Pisani et al., 1997; Parkin, 2006; de Martel et al., 2012; Plummer et al., 2016). Oncogenic infectious agents include viruses: HCV, HBV, high-risk HPV, KSHV, Epstein–Barr virus (EBV), human T-cell lymphotrophic virus type-1 (HTLV-1) and Merkel cell polyomavirus (MCPyV) (Houben et al., 2010; Working Group on the Evaluation of Carcinogenic Risks to Humans [IARC], 2012; Schäfer et al., 2015); bacteria: *Helicobacter pylori* (Forman et al., 1991; Nomura et al., 1991; Parsonnet et al., 1991); and parasites: *Opisthorchis viverrini*, *Clonorchis sinensis*, and *Schistosoma haematobium* (International Agency for Research on Cancer Working Group, 1994; Honjo et al., 2005; Bouvard et al., 2009). Additionally, HIV is classified as carcinogenic, although its mechanism is indirect via cell-mediated immune deficiency and needs to be in conjunction with another infectious agent (Working Group on the Evaluation of Carcinogenic Risks to Humans [IARC], 2012). Not surprisingly, the exceptional elevation of pathogen-associated cancers in the developing world is, not least, exacerbated in the high HIV/AIDS context (Parkin et al., 2005; Grulich et al., 2007).

The introduction of the highly active antiretroviral therapy (HAART) strategy has substantially reduced the number of AIDS-related deaths and extended the lifespans of HIV infected individuals (Palmisano and Vella, 2011). This extended lifespan has led to the emergence of a range of HIV-associated malignancies, again particularly burdening sub-Saharan Africa, that were not often seen preceding the introduction of HAART when average lifespan following HIV infection was significantly less (Frisch et al., 2001; Grulich et al., 2007; Coghill et al., 2013; Antiretroviral Therapy Cohort Collaboration, 2017). In contrast, HAART also had a profound preventative effect on some, but not all, HIV-associated malignancies. Kaposi's sarcoma (KS) incidence in Western countries was reported to decrease by greater than 90% from 1994 to 2003, spanning the introduction of HAART in 1996 (Mocroft et al., 2004). Similarly, incidence of EBV-associated non-Hodgkin lymphoma decreased by greater than 40% after the introduction of HAART in Western countries (International Collaboration on HIV and Cancer, 2000). However, incidences of HPV-associated cervical cancer and non-AIDS defining cancers have not yet been seen to be reduced (International Collaboration on HIV and Cancer, 2000). Although promising, the reductions of incidences of particularly KS and non-Hodgkin lymphoma in Western countries, has not been mirrored in resource-limited, developing countries. In fact, GLOBOCAN age standardized incidence rates reported in 2002 and 2012, indicate an increase in incidence of non-Hodgkin lymphoma in males and females in Southern and Northern Africa (Parkin et al., 2005; Torre et al., 2015). This is corroborated in a Ugandan study over the period 1991–1995 to 2002–2006, which reports an annual increase in incidence of non-Hodgkin lymphoma by 6.7 and 11.0% in men and women, respectively (Parkin et al., 2010). Similarly, KS incidence in Ugandan women has increased (1.4% annually, 10% over the period), while in men incidence has slightly decreased (2.8% annually, 30% over the period); this in contrast to the large (>90%) reductions in

KS incidence in Western countries over a similar period, and concomitant with the large scale roll-out of HAART (Mocroft et al., 2004; Parkin et al., 2010; Casper, 2011). This disparity has been attributed to a delayed and stilted availability of HAART in low-resource settings; indeed, it has been noted that even in sub-Saharan countries with relatively well-established antiretroviral therapy (ART) programs, KS incidence has not decreased as expected (Casper, 2011). Further, Nguyen et al. (2008) found that up to half of AIDS-related KS patients treated with HAART and chemotherapy never achieved total remission, which was in concordance with other studies (Dupin et al., 1999; Dupont et al., 2000; Bihl et al., 2007; Nguyen et al., 2008). It is therefore predicted that cancers caused by infectious agents will become a burgeoning complication of long-term HIV infection (Grulich et al., 2007; Sasco et al., 2010; Casper, 2011).

Oncogenic organisms infect, but do not kill their target cells, leading to persistent infection. This is facilitated by various immune evasion strategies driven by the expression of pathogen-encoded proteins and subversion of cellular regulation of proliferation and apoptosis (McLaughlin-Drubin and Munger, 2008; Mesri et al., 2014). Perhaps the best example of this is oncogenic HPV infection of basal cells of the cervical epithelium, which precedes development of virtually all cases of cervical cancer by decades (Woodman et al., 2007; Castellsague, 2008). HPV oncogenes E6 and E7 mitigate host innate immune responses through inhibition of the interferon pathway (Ronco et al., 1998; Park et al., 2000) and similarly, E5 oncoprotein causes downregulation of MHC class I (Campo et al., 2010). Likewise, HBV and HCV infection, which together account for approximately 80% of hepatocellular carcinoma cases, promote cirrhosis through non-cytocidal chronic infection of hepatocytes (Parkin et al., 2005; El-Serag, 2012). HBV-encoded X antigen (HBx) and HCV-encoded core, non-structural protein 5A (NS5A) and NS3 antigens inhibit innate antiviral signaling pathways as well as apoptosis, conferring a survival advantage to infected hepatocytes (Mesri et al., 2014). Persistent infection through immune evasion is further facilitated in an immunosuppressive environment, such as in HIV infection, where host-mediated anti-tumor responses are extinguished.

Persistent infection can be accompanied by chronic inflammation. Persistent HBV and HCV infection lead to chronic inflammation of the liver (hepatitis) which promotes cancer development (Mesri et al., 2014). Similarly, key to the oncogenic potential of *Helicobacter pylori,* to which approximately 90% of new stomach cancer cases are attributed, is its ability to persist in the gastric mucosa for decades, eliciting chronic inflammation through the expression of virulence factors *CagA* (cytotoxin-associated gene A) and *VacA* (vacuolating cytotoxin A) (Wang et al., 2014; Plummer et al., 2015, 2016). Chronic low-grade inflammation is also present in HIV infected individuals on ART treatment and is associated with cancer development (Marks et al., 2013; Maartens et al., 2014).

Persistent oncogenic infection is necessary but often not sufficient to trigger carcinogenesis, but rather requires precipitating co-factors for the development of malignancy (McLaughlin-Drubin and Munger, 2008; Mesri et al., 2010). Often, immunosuppression plays this role, made evident by the enhanced incidence of infection-related cancers and cancers suspected to have infectious etiology seen in both HIV-positive patients and immunosuppressed post-transplant cohorts (Grulich et al., 2007). Of those, KS is the most common AIDS-related malignancy and a significant public health burden in sub-Saharan Africa, where KSHV seroprevalence rates as high as 50% have been reported (Mesri et al., 2010). While KSHV infection accounts for 100% of KS cases, alone it is asymptomatic and not sufficient for tumorigenesis, requiring HIV-related or another form of immunosuppression [e.g., standardized incidence ratio (SIR) for KS in HIV/AIDS cohort versus transplant cohort is 3640.0 (3326–3976) versus 208.0 (114–349), respectively] amongst other potential co-factors, to trigger KS development (Grulich et al., 2007; Mesri et al., 2010; Plummer et al., 2016). Moreover, due to shared routes of transmission, HPV and HIV coinfection is common and HIV infection increases the probability of HPV persistent infection resulting in increased relative risk [5.8 (3.0–11.3)] of cervical cancer development compared to HPV infection in the absence of HIV (Strickler et al., 2005; Grulich et al., 2007; Working Group on the Evaluation of Carcinogenic Risks to Humans [IARC], 2012). Similarly, HIV co-infection with either HBV or HCV increases the rate of progression of HBV- or HCV-mediated liver damage and the SIR of HBV/HCV-mediated liver cancer [5.22 (3.32–8.20)] (Graham et al., 2001; Grulich et al., 2007; Chen et al., 2009; Nikolopoulos et al., 2009).

Furthermore, a number of infectious cancers show distinct geographical distributions or population-specific prevalence. Before the HIV epidemic, KS was considered rare except for hotspots in the Mediterranean and Eastern Europe (Classic KS) and Central and Eastern Africa (Endemic KS). Now, AIDS-related KS is prevalent across sub-Saharan Africa, but its peculiar geographical epidemiology has led to speculation that host genetic factors may influence seroconversion after exposure to KSHV and/or subsequent KS development (Mesri et al., 2010; Cavallin et al., 2014). Interestingly, while HCV is an important risk factor for the development of hepatocellular carcinoma in the United States, Europe and Japan, HBV contributes more substantially to the development of liver cancer globally and particularly in countries with low human development index (Barth et al., 2010; Chung et al., 2010; Plummer et al., 2016).

Besides HIV immunosuppression as outlined above, environmental factors such as host diet, physical inactivity, behaviors such as smoking, reproductive factors, and co-factors leading to smoldering chronic inflammation are thought to further influence the natural history of oncogenic infections and as a consequence of globalization, these are thought to become more important in the developing world (Parkin et al., 2005; Ajuwon et al., 2009; Plummer et al., 2016).

DIABETES-ASSOCIATED CANCER DEVELOPMENT IN THE CONTEXT OF HIV/AIDS

Type 2 diabetes is a non-communicable disease, characterized by insulin resistance and hyperglycemia (Zaccardi et al., 2016).

Globally, type 2 diabetes is a major problem, but prevalence of the disease is particularly rapidly increasing in low- and middle-income countries (Guariguata et al., 2014). This is largely due to the changes in lifestyle and diet brought about by rapid urbanization, such as decreased physical activity as well as increased consumption of refined carbohydrates and sugar sweetened beverages (Hu, 2011). On that note, it was shown that only 1–2 servings of sugar-sweetened beverages per day increase diabetes risk by 26% (Malik et al., 2010). In 2013, low- and middle-income countries had the highest prevalence of type 2 diabetes and it is projected that Africa will experience a 109% increase in cases over the next 22 years (Guariguata et al., 2014). The most undiagnosed cases of type 2 diabetes occur in low- and middle-income countries due to a lack of resources necessary for diagnosis, meaning that often the disease is only detected after complications have already developed (Beagley et al., 2014). The Lancet Diabetes & Endocrinology Commission on diabetes in sub-Saharan Africa provides a comprehensive and up-to-date analysis of the vast economic burden that diabetes places on the resource-constrained health systems found in those regions (Atun et al., 2017).

As outlined above, low- and middle-income countries are also highly burdened by the HIV/AIDS epidemic, and 2–4 fold higher prevalence of dysglycemia in HIV-infected individuals in South Africa has been reported (Dave et al., 2011; Levitt et al., 2016). Although the mechanisms are not well-understood, the presence of HIV infection itself may contribute to diabetogenesis, both directly through inflammation and immune activation, and indirectly through immunodeficiency (Kalra and Agrawal, 2013; Lake and Currier, 2013; Levitt et al., 2016). Moreover, treatment by HAART may be directly or indirectly linked to the development of type 2 diabetes in HIV-infected patients (Hadigan and Kattakuzhy, 2014). The increased life expectancy of HIV-infected patients on HAART treatment has dramatically changed the natural history of HIV infection (Samaras, 2009), resulting in the emergence of more chronic illnesses, including type 2 diabetes (Hasse et al., 2011). Moreover, certain nucleoside reverse transcriptase inhibitors (NRTIs) and protease inhibitors (PIs) have been associated with the development of insulin resistance and an increased incidence of type 2 diabetes in HIV-infected individuals, though the literature has been contentious about whether PIs do indeed play a role (Behrens et al., 1999; Brown et al., 2005; Tien et al., 2007; De Wit et al., 2008; Capeau et al., 2012). A large cross-sectional study recently published reported a significantly higher odds ratio (OR) of diabetes and metabolic syndrome (OR 3.85 and 1.45, respectively, 95% CI) among ART-exposed patients compared to their naïve counterparts, although the association between ART and diabetes was not interpreted as cause and effect (Nduka et al., 2017). HAART is also known to cause lipodystrophy and hyperlipidemia, conditions common to insulin resistance and type 2 diabetes, therefore indirectly increasing the risk of development of type 2 diabetes in HIV-infected individuals who are on HAART (Samaras, 2009). The high prevalence of HIV/AIDS in today's era of HAART may therefore further substantially contribute to the increase in type 2 diabetes predicted for low- and middle-income countries.

Of the various complications associated with type 2 diabetes, cancer development, incidence, prognosis, and mortality have been linked to the long-term effects of the disease (Giovannucci et al., 2010). For example, a meta-analysis of 23 studies reported increased mortality across all cancer types in diabetes patients (HR 1.41; 95% CI, 1.28–1.55) (Barone et al., 2008). Specifically, an increased risk of colon cancer has been associated with type 2 diabetes [summary relative risk (SRR) = 1.30] (Larsson et al., 2005), and a cohort study showed that diabetic patients with stages 2 and 3 colon cancer had higher mortality rates and cancer recurrence as compared to non-diabetic patients (Meyerhardt et al., 2003). Individuals with type 2 diabetes had a SRR of 1.94 for the development of pancreatic cancer (Ben et al., 2011) and a SRR of 2.01 for hepatocellular carcinoma development (Wang et al., 2012). Another study described synergistic interactions between diabetes mellitus and hepatocellular carcinoma (OR, 9.9; 95% CI, 2.5–39.3) which was further found to be strikingly associated with heavy alcohol consumption and chronic hepatitis virus infection (OR, 53.9; 95% CI, 7.0–415.7) (Hassan et al., 2002). Type 2 diabetes has also been associated with a 42% increase in kidney cancer risk (Larsson and Wolk, 2011) as well as a 20% increase in risk of developing breast cancer (Larsson et al., 2007). Overall, type 2 diabetes is associated with increased mortality in cancer patients and an overall poor prognosis of cancer (Barone et al., 2008).

Both type 2 diabetes and cancer are highly complex diseases affecting many cellular processes. However, they share several risk factors, such as alcohol consumption, smoking, obesity, diet and physical inactivity, but the possible biological links between the two diseases are not yet completely understood. Possible mechanisms for a direct link between cancer and type 2 diabetes include hyperglycemia, hyperinsulinemia, and inflammation. Firstly, hyperglycemia has been suggested to be one of the possible influences of type 2 diabetes on cancer, mainly due to the Warburg effect: a well-known observation that cancer cells tend to undergo aerobic glycolysis and therefore consume more glucose than normal cells in order to accumulate precursor molecules for biomass rather than energy production (Vander Heiden et al., 2009). Additionally, high levels of glucose are linked to increases in WNT signaling, which enhances proliferation (Garcia-Jimenez et al., 2014), as well as upregulation of the oxidative response genes, leading to increased reactive oxygen species and mutations (Turturro et al., 2007). Secondly, hyperinsulinemia may also be a potential link between type 2 diabetes and cancer, as insulin is not only a metabolic hormone but also a growth factor that has anti-apoptotic and mitogenic effects via activation of the insulin receptor (Vigneri et al., 2016). Of the different insulin receptor isoforms the A isoform, which has predominant mitogenic activity, is often overexpressed in cancer cells, providing a selective growth advantage to malignant cells when exposed to insulin (Vigneri et al., 2016). High levels of circulating insulin due to insulin resistance or insulin treatment also result in reduced insulin-like growth factor binding protein (IGFBP), leading to increased insulin-like growth factor 1 (IGF-1), which has more potent anti-apoptotic and mitogenic effects than insulin (Giovannucci et al., 2010). However, high levels of insulin can also spill over to IGF-1 receptors, and indeed it was shown that both the insulin receptor and the IGF-1 receptor can act as identical portals to the regulation of gene expression with differences between insulin and IGF-1 effects due to a modulation of the amplitude of the signal created by the specific ligand-receptor interaction (Boucher et al., 2010). Hyperinsulinemia also indirectly leads to increased levels of estrogen and androgens by reducing the hepatic synthesis of sex hormone-binding globulin (Calle and Kaaks, 2004); aberrant steroid hormone metabolism is associated with a higher risk of certain cancers, including breast and endometrial cancer. Lastly, excessive caloric intake often associated with urbanization and an increasing Westernized lifestyle leads to obesity which is not only a well-known risk factor for the development of type 2 diabetes but is also linked to cancer development (Hjartaker et al., 2008). In South Africa, 68% of women and 31% of men are overweight or obese (Department of Health, 2016). Additionally, consumption of sugar sweetened beverages has approximately doubled in rural areas since 2005, with 56% of women and 63% of men consuming these beverages, which further contributes to the increasing prevalence of obesity here (Vorster et al., 2014). Chronic low-grade adipose tissue inflammation is not only a symptom of obesity but is also known to be a recognizable feature of the metabolic syndrome and a major cause of the decreased insulin sensitivity seen in type 2 diabetes (van Kruijsdijk et al., 2009; Shu et al., 2012). Moreover, obesity can induce sustained systemic production of reactive oxygen species which can eventually lead to somatic mutations and neoplastic transformation (Manna and Jain, 2015). As an endocrine organ, excess adipose tissue secretes elevated levels of various cytokines, hormones and growth factors including interleukin-6 (IL-6), tumor necrosis factor alpha (TNF-α), plasminogen activator inhibitor-1 (PAI-1) and leptin that can alter the body's ability to appropriately respond to insulin (van Kruijsdijk et al., 2009). TNF-α has been shown to promote cell survival through the NF-κB pathway, and IL-6 mediates cell proliferation and survival through the JAK/STAT pathway (van Kruijsdijk et al., 2009). Type 2 diabetes is therefore associated with a general dysregulated innate immune response (Paich et al., 2013). Together with metabolic disruptions in insulin signaling, this manifestation of immune dysfunction common to obesity and type 2 diabetes present a favorable environment for cancer cell proliferation, invasion, and survival (Allavena et al., 2008; van Kruijsdijk et al., 2009).

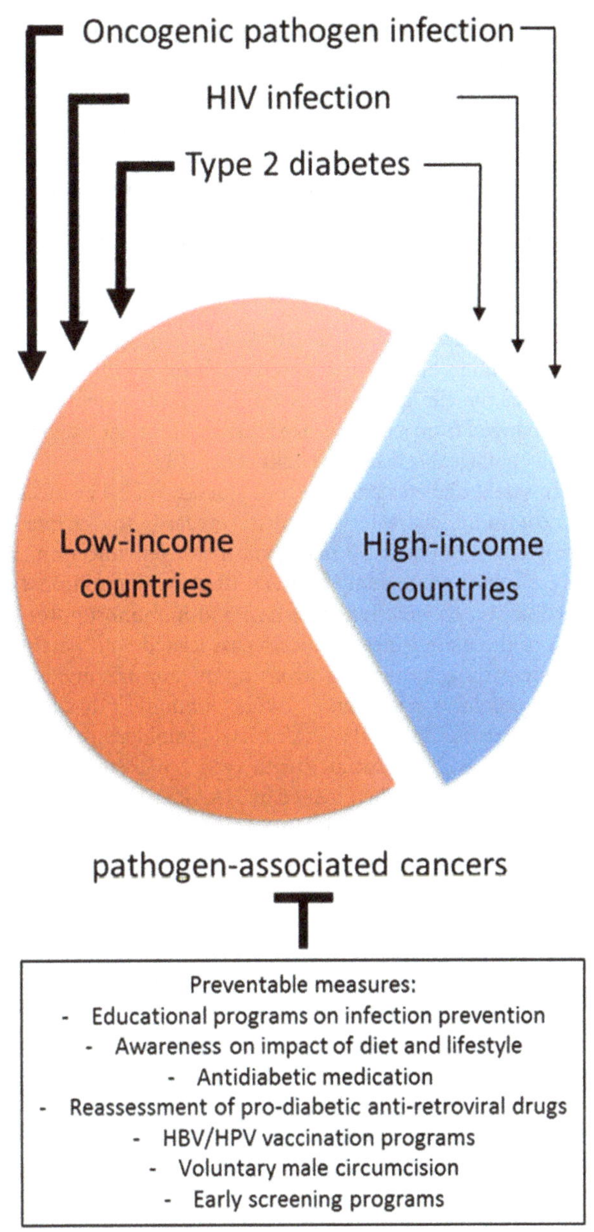

FIGURE 1 | The relative contribution of oncogenic pathogen infection, HIV infection and type 2 diabetes for pathogen-associated cancers in low-income versus high-income countries and the potential prevention of these malignancies.

THE LINK BETWEEN TYPE 2 DIABETES AND PATHOGEN-ASSOCIATED CANCERS IN THE CONTEXT OF HIV/AIDS

Low- and middle-income countries are projected to carry the majority of the world-wide cancer burden over the next decades, highlighting the emergence of cancer as a major public health problem (Sylla and Wild, 2012). While chronic infection with oncogenic pathogens has long been identified as a main contributor, the impact of HIV infection, particularly in the HAART era, as well as the ever-increasing incidence of type 2 diabetes represent emerging risk factors for morbidity and mortality in those regions of the world. Indeed, patients living with HIV/AIDS have an increased burden of non-communicable diseases relative to HIV-uninfected individuals, with more than 25% predicted to develop three or more non-communicable diseases by 2030 (Smit et al., 2015).

Globally, two-thirds of infection-attributable cancers occur in less developed countries (Plummer et al., 2016) (**Figure 1**), although the true incidence rates within the African continent are very uncertain due to underreporting and the data from GLOBOCAN often not being comprehensive. Nevertheless, low-resource settings also carry by far the largest burden of the HIV epidemic: in 2015, an estimated 36.7 million people were living with HIV globally of whom approximately 19.0 million (i.e., more than 50%) live in Southern Africa (Global AIDS, 2016). These numbers have been increasing over the years (from 31.0 million in 2002 to 36.7 million in 2016) due to the life-extending effects of HAART (Zaidi et al., 2013). Moreover, two-thirds of all diabetes cases as a consequence of rapid changes in lifestyle, urbanization and population aging are reported to occur in low- and middle-income countries (Wild et al., 2004; Hu, 2011), representing a growing public health issue in the HIV-infected population, especially as the clinical course of HIV infection in the HAART era has changed from a progressive illness with a fatal outcome to a chronic manageable disease (Deeks et al., 2013).

Both type 2 diabetes and the consequences of HIV infection share common characteristics with regard to facilitating cancerogenesis initiated by oncogenic pathogen infection, but is there a causal relationship between these two conditions? As outlined above, chronic inflammation and immunosuppression are two of the main cancer hallmarks associated with persistent oncogenic pathogen infection adverting the normal functioning of the cellular machinery. While immune dysfunction is characteristic for HIV infection, smoldering chronic inflammation is also associated with type 2 diabetes and HIV infection (particularly when treated by HAART), highlighting the importance of these two conditions as promoting environments for the development of pathogen-associated cancers. Although type 2 diabetes and HIV infection might constitute independent risk factors for pathogen-associated cancers in general, some striking synergism has been described for hepatitis virus-associated hepatocellular carcinoma. Indeed, overwhelming evidence in the literature points toward an association between co-infection of HIV and HBV/HCV together with insulin resistance and/or diabetes and a significantly enhanced risk of liver disease (Merchante et al., 2009; DallaPiazza et al., 2010; Howard et al., 2010; Salmon et al., 2012; Elkrief et al., 2014; Hadigan and Kattakuzhy, 2014; Lo Re et al., 2014; Oliver et al., 2016). This was found to be further exacerbated by certain antiretroviral drugs such as didanosine and/or stavudine (Blanco et al., 2011).

This well-documented link of HIV infection, type 2 diabetes and liver cancer is less evident for other pathogen-associated malignancies. For example, only case reports on HIV-related KS in the presence of type 2 diabetes are currently available, calling attention to the risk of delayed diagnosis of KS in patients on ART with a relatively high CD4 count (Chan and Pakianathan, 2011). Although no such case report on the link between HIV, type 2 diabetes and cervical cancer exists, an interesting recent study describes the combination of metformin, the worldwide most widely prescribed first-line therapeutic drug for type 2 diabetes and known for its antitumor properties (Kasznicki et al., 2014), together with nelfinavir, an HIV protease inhibitor. This drug combination showed promising effects on HPV-associated cervical cancer cell growth *in vitro* and *in vivo* (Xia et al., 2017). It is highly likely that other pathogen-associated cancers also benefit from the underlying cancer-friendly environment in the presence of both HIV infection and type 2 diabetes. Their cancer-promoting contributions are unlikely to be separate entities but rather present complex interactions facilitating cancerogenesis especially in a setting where these risk factors predominate.

In light of the low resources and the often deficient health care infrastructure in less developed countries, concerted efforts on cancer prevention rather than cancer treatment will likely have a sustainable effect on the reduction of cancer. The first step to prevention is the identification of risk factors and/or the etiological agent. Indeed, infections have been suggested to be one of the most important preventable causes of cancer in general, not least reflected by the significantly disparate incidence rates of pathogen-associated malignancies in industrialized versus low- and middle-income countries (**Figure 1** and Kuper et al., 2000). Highly effective prophylactic vaccines exist for some of the most common etiological agents of pathogen-associated cancers, namely HBV and HPV types 16 and 18, causing liver and cervical cancer, respectively, the two most common causes of cancer death in Africa (Sylla and Wild, 2012). Although the HBV vaccine is relatively inexpensive, national HBV infant immunization programs as seen in many African countries account only for 10% coverage in Africa (Plummer et al., 2016). The HPV vaccines are still rather expensive to produce, limiting efficient coverage of the population in the most affected areas (Hanson et al., 2015). Moreover, of the 13 HPV genotypes classified as carcinogenic (Working Group on the Evaluation of Carcinogenic Risks to Humans [IARC], 2012), the HPV vaccines currently available in low-resource settings only target the most common oncogenic genotypes 16 and 18 which account for approximately 70% of invasive cervical cancers globally. In sub-Saharan Africa however, other carcinogenic HPV types, such as HPV45 and 35, occur relatively more frequently than in other world regions as they seem to be more affected by changes in immunodeficiency levels (De Vuyst et al., 2013; Clifford et al., 2016). Therefore, even if there was saturation coverage of vaccinated populations in those regions of the world, the reduction in cervical cancer will fall well short of 100%. In this regard, voluntary medical male circumcision has a significant protective effect not only against HIV but also high-risk HPV, HBV and other sexually transmitted infections (Castellsague et al., 2002; Tobian et al., 2014; Wahome et al., 2017). Although highly cost-effective, implementation of the WHO recommended goal of 80% circumcision coverage among men aged 15–49 years in 13 countries in Eastern and Southern Africa with high HIV prevalence has been very slow and is far from being reached (Tobian et al., 2014). To reduce pathogen-associated cancers in low-resource settings both HPV/HBV vaccination and male circumcision should be advocated. Even so, efforts in the reduction of infection-related cancers are often offset by an increasing number of new cases that are associated with (among others) dietary and lifestyle factors (Bray et al., 2012). This is further exacerbated by the adverse effects of HAART on the development of type 2 diabetes and low-grade chronic inflammation seen in HIV/AIDS patients (Maartens et al., 2014). Therefore, programs to implement nation-wide prophylactic vaccination against HBV and HPV together with concerted efforts to reduce type 2 diabetes risk and the risk of acquiring sexually transmitted infections such as HIV, HBV/HCV and HPV, would have a significant impact on cancer incidence and mortality (**Figure 1**). Indeed, several randomized clinical trials have demonstrated that diet and lifestyle modifications are highly effective in preventing type 2 diabetes in different ethnic and racial groups (Knowler et al., 2002; Lindstrom et al., 2006; Ramachandran et al., 2006; Li et al., 2008).

CONCLUSION

It has become evident over the last decades that the nature of comorbidities in HIV-infected individuals has changed substantially, particularly with regards to tumorigenesis and oncogenic disease progression. Although the descriptive data presented here may not lead to a definitive scientific interpretation, they clearly support the hypothesis that some of the highest cancer risk factors that predominate in resource-limited settings (such as oncogenic pathogen infection, HIV infection and type 2 diabetes) are potentially avoidable. It is suspected that there might be a link between these risk factors, particularly between HIV infection, its treatment and the onset of non-communicable diseases such as type 2 diabetes. Effective interventions including population-based vaccination against HBV and HPV together with HIV prevention and cervical cancer screening programs as well as awareness, counseling and educational programs on changes in diet and physical activity would lead to significant reductions of the cancer burden in those areas of the world. Early intervention programs not only prevent disease onset and complications but are clearly much simpler and cheaper than treating later stage disease. Research activities to understand the synergistic effects between the risk factors discussed in this review are needed and should be a focus of future scientific efforts.

AUTHOR CONTRIBUTIONS

GS led the conception and design of this article, drafted, revised and approved its final version. MB and SU equally contributed to drafting individual sections, while AK critically revised the article.

ACKNOWLEDGMENT

This work was supported by funding from the Poliomyelitis Research Foundation (PRF), the Cancer Association of South Africa (CANSA), and the National Research Foundation (NRF) of South Africa.

REFERENCES

Ajuwon, K. M., Banz, W., and Winters, T. A. (2009). Stimulation with Peptidoglycan induces interleukin 6 and TLR2 expression and a concomitant downregulation of expression of adiponectin receptors 1 and 2 in 3T3-L1 adipocytes. *J. Inflamm.* 6:8. doi: 10.1186/1476-9255-6-8

Allavena, P., Garlanda, C., Borrello, M. G., Sica, A., and Mantovani, A. (2008). Pathways connecting inflammation and cancer. *Curr. Opin. Genet. Dev.* 18, 3–10. doi: 10.1016/j.gde.2008.01.003

Antiretroviral Therapy Cohort Collaboration (2017). Survival of HIV-positive patients starting antiretroviral therapy between 1996 and 2013: a collaborative analysis of cohort studies. *Lancet HIV* 4, e349–e356. doi: 10.1016/S2352-3018(17)30066-8

Atun, R., Davies, J. I., Gale, E. A. M., Barnighausen, T., Beran, D., Kengne, A. P., et al. (2017). Diabetes in sub-Saharan Africa: from clinical care to health policy. *Lancet Diabetes Endocrinol.* 5, 622–667. doi: 10.1016/S2213-8587(17)30181-X

Barone, B. B., Yeh, H. C., Snyder, C. F., Peairs, K. S., Stein, K. B., Derr, R. L., et al. (2008). Long-term all-cause mortality in cancer patients with preexisting diabetes mellitus: a systematic review and meta-analysis. *JAMA* 300, 2754–2764. doi: 10.1001/jama.2008.824

Barth, R. E., Huijgen, Q., Taljaard, J., and Hoepelman, A. I. (2010). Hepatitis B/C and HIV in sub-Saharan Africa: an association between highly prevalent infectious diseases. A systematic review and meta-analysis. *Int. J. Infect. Dis.* 14, e1024–e1031. doi: 10.1016/j.ijid.2010.06.013

Beagley, J., Guariguata, L., Weil, C., and Motala, A. A. (2014). Global estimates of undiagnosed diabetes in adults. *Diabetes. Res. Clin. Pract.* 103, 150–160. doi: 10.1016/j.diabres.2013.11.001

Behrens, G., Dejam, A., Schmidt, H., Balks, H. J., Brabant, G., Korner, T., et al. (1999). Impaired glucose tolerance, beta cell function and lipid metabolism in HIV patients under treatment with protease inhibitors. *AIDS* 13, F63–F70. doi: 10.1097/00002030-199907090-00001

Ben, Q., Xu, M., Ning, X., Liu, J., Hong, S., Huang, W., et al. (2011). Diabetes mellitus and risk of pancreatic cancer: a meta-analysis of cohort studies. *Eur. J. Cancer* 47, 1928–1937. doi: 10.1016/j.ejca.2011.03.003

Bihl, F., Mosam, A., Henry, L. N., Chisholm, J. V. III, Dollard, S., Gumbi, P., et al. (2007). Kaposi's sarcoma-associated herpesvirus-specific immune reconstitution and antiviral effect of combined HAART/chemotherapy in HIV clade C-infected individuals with Kaposi's sarcoma. *AIDS* 21, 1245–1252. doi: 10.1097/QAD.0b013e328182df03

Blanco, F., Barreiro, P., Ryan, P., Vispo, E., Martin-Carbonero, L., Tuma, P., et al. (2011). Risk factors for advanced liver fibrosis in HIV-infected individuals: role of antiretroviral drugs and insulin resistance. *J. Viral. Hepat.* 18, 11–16. doi: 10.1111/j.1365-2893.2009.01261.x

Boucher, J., Tseng, Y. H., and Kahn, C. R. (2010). Insulin and insulin-like growth factor-1 receptors act as ligand-specific amplitude modulators of a common pathway regulating gene transcription. *J. Biol. Chem.* 285, 17235–17245. doi: 10.1074/jbc.M110.118620

Bouvard, V., Baan, R., Straif, K., Grosse, Y., Secretan, B., El Ghissassi, F., et al. (2009). A review of human carcinogens–Part B: biological agents. *Lancet Oncol.* 10, 321–322. doi: 10.1016/S1470-2045(09)70096-8

Bray, F., Jemal, A., Grey, N., Ferlay, J., and Forman, D. (2012). Global cancer transitions according to the human development index (2008-2030): a population-based study. *Lancet Oncol.* 13, 790–801. doi: 10.1016/S1470-2045(12)70211-5

Brown, T. T., Li, X., Cole, S. R., Kingsley, L. A., Palella, F. J., Riddler, S. A., et al. (2005). Cumulative exposure to nucleoside analogue reverse transcriptase inhibitors is associated with insulin resistance markers in the Multicenter AIDS cohort study. *AIDS* 19, 1375–1383. doi: 10.1097/01.aids.0000181011.62385.91

Calle, E. E., and Kaaks, R. (2004). Overweight, obesity and cancer: epidemiological evidence and proposed mechanisms. *Nat. Rev. Cancer* 4, 579–591. doi: 10.1038/nrc1408

Campo, M. S., Graham, S. V., Cortese, M. S., Ashrafi, G. H., Araibi, E. H., Dornan, E. S., et al. (2010). HPV-16 E5 down-regulates expression of surface HLA class I and reduces recognition by CD8 T cells. *Virology* 407, 137–142. doi: 10.1016/j.virol.2010.07.044

Capeau, J., Bouteloup, V., Katlama, C., Bastard, J. P., Guiyedi, V., Salmon-Ceron, D., et al. (2012). Ten-year diabetes incidence in 1046 HIV-infected patients started on a combination antiretroviral treatment. *AIDS* 26, 303–314. doi: 10.1097/QAD.0b013e32834e8776

Casper, C. (2011). The increasing burden of HIV-associated malignancies in resource-limited regions. *Annu. Rev. Med.* 62, 157–170. doi: 10.1146/annurev-med-050409-103711

Castellsague, X. (2008). Natural history and epidemiology of HPV infection and cervical cancer. *Gynecol. Oncol.* 110(3 Suppl. 2), S4–S7. doi: 10.1016/j.ygyno.2008.07.045

Castellsague, X., Bosch, F. X., Munoz, N., Meijer, C. J., Shah, K. V., de Sanjose, S., et al. (2002). Male circumcision, penile human papillomavirus infection, and cervical cancer in female partners. *N. Engl. J. Med.* 346, 1105–1112. doi: 10.1056/NEJMoa011688

Cavallin, L. E., Goldschmidt-Clermont, P., and Mesri, E. A. (2014). Molecular and cellular mechanisms of KSHV oncogenesis of Kaposi's sarcoma associated with HIV/AIDS. *PLOS Pathog.* 10:e1004154. doi: 10.1371/journal.ppat.1004154

Chan, S. Y., and Pakianathan, M. (2011). Delayed diagnosis of Kaposi's sarcoma in a HIV positive man with a high CD4 count and suppressed viral load. *Sex Transm. Infect.* 87, 609–610. doi: 10.1136/sextrans-2011-050189

Chen, T. Y., Ding, E. L., Seage Iii, G. R., and Kim, A. Y. (2009). Meta-analysis: increased mortality associated with hepatitis C in HIV-infected persons is unrelated to HIV disease progression. *Clin. Infect. Dis.* 49, 1605–1615. doi: 10.1086/644771

Chung, H., Ueda, T., and Kudo, M. (2010). Changing trends in hepatitis C infection over the past 50 years in Japan. *Intervirology* 53, 39–43. doi: 10.1159/000252782

Clifford, G. M., de Vuyst, H., Tenet, V., Plummer, M., Tully, S., and Franceschi, S. (2016). Effect of HIV infection on human papillomavirus types causing invasive cervical cancer in Africa. *J. Acquir. Immune Defic. Syndr.* 73, 332–339. doi: 10.1097/QAI.0000000000001113

Coghill, A. E., Newcomb, P. A., Madeleine, M. M., Richardson, B. A., Mutyaba, I., Okuku, F., et al. (2013). Contribution of HIV infection to mortality among cancer patients in Uganda. *AIDS* 27, 2933–2942. doi: 10.1097/01.aids.0000433236.55937.cb

DallaPiazza, M., Amorosa, V. K., Localio, R., Kostman, J. R., and Lo Re, V. (2010). Prevalence and risk factors for significant liver fibrosis among HIV-monoinfected patients. *BMC Infect. Dis.* 10:116. doi: 10.1186/1471-2334-10-116

Danaei, G., Vander Hoorn, S., Lopez, A. D., Murray, C. J., Ezzati, M., and Comparative Risk Assessment collaborating group. (2005). Causes of cancer in the world: comparative risk assessment of nine behavioural and environmental risk factors. *Lancet* 366, 1784–1793. doi: 10.1016/S0140-6736(05)67725-2

Dave, J. A., Lambert, E. V., Badri, M., West, S., Maartens, G., and Levitt, N. S. (2011). Effect of nonnucleoside reverse transcriptase inhibitor-based antiretroviral therapy on dysglycemia and insulin sensitivity in South African HIV-infected patients. *J. Acquir. Immune Defic. Syndr.* 57, 284–289. doi: 10.1097/QAI.0b013e318221863f

de Martel, C., Ferlay, J., Franceschi, S., Vignat, J., Bray, F., Forman, D., et al. (2012). Global burden of cancers attributable to infections in 2008: a review and synthetic analysis. *Lancet Oncol.* 13, 607–615. doi: 10.1016/s1470-2045(12)70137-7

De Vuyst, H., Alemany, L., Lacey, C., Chibwesha, C. J., Sahasrabuddhe, V., Banura, C., et al. (2013). The burden of human papillomavirus infections and related diseases in sub-saharan Africa. *Vaccine* 31(Suppl. 5), F32–F46. doi: 10.1016/j.vaccine.2012.07.092

De Wit, S., Sabin, C. A., Weber, R., Worm, S. W., Reiss, P., Cazanave, C., et al. (2008). Incidence and risk factors for new-onset diabetes in HIV-infected patients: the data collection on adverse events of anti-HIV drugs (D:A:D) study. *Diabetes Care* 31, 1224–1229. doi: 10.2337/dc07-2013

Deeks, S. G., Lewin, S. R., and Havlir, D. V. (2013). The end of AIDS: HIV infection as a chronic disease. *Lancet* 382, 1525–1533. doi: 10.1016/S0140-6736(13)61809-7

Department of Health (2016). *South Africa Demographic and Health Survey.* Available at: http://www.statssa.gov.za/publications/Report%2003-00-09/Report%2003-00-092016.pdf [accessed June 23, 2017].

Dupin, N., Rubin De Cervens, V., Gorin, I., Calvez, V., Pessis, E., Grandadam, M., et al. (1999). The influence of highly active antiretroviral therapy on AIDS-associated Kaposi's sarcoma. *Br. J. Dermatol.* 140, 875–881. doi: 10.1046/j.1365-2133.1999.02818.x

Dupont, C., Vasseur, E., Beauchet, A., Aegerter, P., Berthe, H., de Truchis, P., et al. (2000). Long-term efficacy on Kaposi's sarcoma of highly active antiretroviral therapy in a cohort of HIV-positive patients. CISIH 92. Centre d'information et de soins de l'immunodeficience humaine. *AIDS* 14, 987–993. doi: 10.1097/00002030-200005260-00010

Elkrief, L., Chouinard, P., Bendersky, N., Hajage, D., Larroque, B., Babany, G., et al. (2014). Diabetes mellitus is an independent prognostic factor for major liver-related outcomes in patients with cirrhosis and chronic hepatitis C. *Hepatology* 60, 823–831. doi: 10.1002/hep.27228

El-Serag, H. B. (2012). Epidemiology of viral hepatitis and hepatocellular carcinoma. *Gastroenterology* 142, 1264–1273e1261. doi: 10.1053/j.gastro.2011.12.061

Forman, D., Newell, D. G., Fullerton, F., Yarnell, J. W., Stacey, A. R., Wald, N., et al. (1991). Association between infection with *Helicobacter pylori* and risk of gastric cancer: evidence from a prospective investigation. *BMJ* 302, 1302–1305. doi: 10.1136/bmj.302.6788.1302

Frisch, M., Biggar, R. J., Engels, E. A., and Goedert, J. J. (2001). Association of cancer with AIDS-related immunosuppression in adults. *JAMA* 285, 1736–1745. doi: 10.1001/jama.285.13.1736

Garcia-Jimenez, C., Garcia-Martinez, J. M., Chocarro-Calvo, A., and De la Vieja, A. (2014). A new link between diabetes and cancer: enhanced WNT/beta-catenin signaling by high glucose. *J. Mol. Endocrinol.* 52, R51–R66. doi: 10.1530/jme-13-0152

Giovannucci, E., Harlan, D. M., Archer, M. C., Bergenstal, R. M., Gapstur, S. M., Habel, L. A., et al. (2010). Diabetes and cancer: a consensus report. *CA Cancer J. Clin.* 60, 207–221. doi: 10.3322/caac.20078

Global AIDS (2016). *Report on the Global AIDS Epidemic 2016.* Available at: http://www.unaids.org/sites/default/files/media_asset/2016-AIDS-data_en.pdf [accessed June 22, 2017].

Graham, C. S., Baden, L. R., Yu, E., Mrus, J. M., Carnie, J., Heeren, T., et al. (2001). Influence of human immunodeficiency virus infection on the course of hepatitis C virus infection: a meta-analysis. *Clin. Infect. Dis.* 33, 562–569. doi: 10.1086/321909

Grulich, A. E., van Leeuwen, M. T., Falster, M. O., and Vajdic, C. M. (2007). Incidence of cancers in people with HIV/AIDS compared with immunosuppressed transplant recipients: a meta-analysis. *Lancet* 370, 59–67. doi: 10.1016/S0140-6736(07)61050-2

Guariguata, L., Whiting, D. R., Hambleton, I., Beagley, J., Linnenkamp, U., and Shaw, J. E. (2014). Global estimates of diabetes prevalence for 2013 and projections for 2035. *Diabetes Res. Clin. Pract.* 103, 137–149. doi: 10.1016/j.diabres.2013.11.002

Hadigan, C., and Kattakuzhy, S. (2014). Diabetes mellitus type 2 and abnormal glucose metabolism in the setting of human immunodeficiency virus. *Endocrinol. Metab. Clin. North Am.* 43, 685–696. doi: 10.1016/j.ecl.2014.05.003

Hanahan, D., and Weinberg, R. A. (2011). Hallmarks of cancer: the next generation. *Cell* 144, 646–674. doi: 10.1016/j.cell.2011.02.013

Hanson, C. M., Eckert, L., Bloem, P., and Cernuschi, T. (2015). Gavi HPV programs: application to implementation. *Vaccines* 3, 408–419. doi: 10.3390/vaccines3020408

Hassan, M. M., Hwang, L. Y., Hatten, C. J., Swaim, M., Li, D., Abbruzzese, J. L., et al. (2002). Risk factors for hepatocellular carcinoma: synergism of alcohol with viral hepatitis and diabetes mellitus. *Hepatology* 36, 1206–1213. doi: 10.1053/jhep.2002.36780

Hasse, B., Ledergerber, B., Furrer, H., Battegay, M., Hirschel, B., Cavassini, M., et al. (2011). Morbidity and aging in HIV-infected persons: the Swiss HIV cohort study. *Clin. Infect. Dis.* 53, 1130–1139. doi: 10.1093/cid/cir626

Hjartaker, A., Langseth, H., and Weiderpass, E. (2008). Obesity and diabetes epidemics: cancer repercussions. *Adv. Exp. Med. Biol.* 630, 72–93. doi: 10.1007/978-0-387-78818-0_6

Honjo, S., Srivatanakul, P., Sriplung, H., Kikukawa, H., Hanai, S., Uchida, K., et al. (2005). Genetic and environmental determinants of risk for cholangiocarcinoma via *Opisthorchis viverrini* in a densely infested area in Nakhon Phanom, northeast Thailand. *Int. J. Cancer* 117, 854–860. doi: 10.1002/ijc.21146

Houben, R., Shuda, M., Weinkam, R., Schrama, D., Feng, H., Chang, Y., et al. (2010). Merkel cell polyomavirus-infected Merkel cell carcinoma cells require expression of viral T antigens. *J. Virol.* 84, 7064–7072. doi: 10.1128/JVI.02400-09

Howard, A. A., Hoover, D. R., Anastos, K., Wu, X., Shi, Q., Strickler, H. D., et al. (2010). The effects of opiate use and hepatitis C virus infection on risk of diabetes mellitus in the Women's Interagency HIV Study. *J. Acquir. Immune Defic. Syndr.* 54, 152–159. doi: 10.1097/QAI.0b013e3181d0c911

Hu, F. B. (2011). Globalization of diabetes: the role of diet, lifestyle, and genes. *Diabetes Care* 34, 1249–1257. doi: 10.2337/dc11-0442

International Agency for Research on Cancer Working Group (1994). Infection with liver flukes (*Opisthorchis viverrini, Opisthorchis felineus* and *Clonorchis sinensis*). *IARC Monogr. Eval. Carcinog. Risks Hum.* 61, 121–175.

International Collaboration on HIV and Cancer (2000). Highly active antiretroviral therapy and incidence of cancer in human immunodeficiency virus-infected adults. *J. Natl. Cancer Inst.* 92, 1823–1830. doi: 10.1093/jnci/92.22.1823

Kalra, S., and Agrawal, N. (2013). Diabetes and HIV: current understanding and future perspectives. *Curr. Diab. Rep.* 13, 419–427. doi: 10.1007/s11892-013-0369-9

Kasznicki, J., Sliwinska, A., and Drzewoski, J. (2014). Metformin in cancer prevention and therapy. *Ann. Trans. Med.* 2, 57. doi: 10.3978/j.issn.2305-5839.2014.06.01

Knowler, W. C., Barrett-Connor, E., Fowler, S. E., Hamman, R. F., Lachin, J. M., Walker, E. A., et al. (2002). Reduction in the incidence of type 2 diabetes with lifestyle intervention or metformin. *N. Engl. J. Med.* 346, 393–403. doi: 10.1056/NEJMoa012512

Kuper, H., Adami, H. O., and Trichopoulos, D. (2000). Infections as a major preventable cause of human cancer. *J. Intern. Med.* 248, 171–183. doi: 10.1046/j.1365-2796.2000.00742.x

Lake, J. E., and Currier, J. S. (2013). Metabolic disease in HIV infection. *Lancet Infect. Dis.* 13, 964–975. doi: 10.1016/S1473-3099(13)70271-8

Larsson, S. C., Mantzoros, C. S., and Wolk, A. (2007). Diabetes mellitus and risk of breast cancer: a meta-analysis. *Int. J. Cancer* 121, 856–862. doi: 10.1002/ijc.22717

Larsson, S. C., Orsini, N., and Wolk, A. (2005). Diabetes mellitus and risk of colorectal cancer: a meta-analysis. *J. Natl. Cancer Inst.* 97, 1679–1687. doi: 10.1093/jnci/dji375

Larsson, S. C., and Wolk, A. (2011). Diabetes mellitus and incidence of kidney cancer: a meta-analysis of cohort studies. *Diabetologia* 54, 1013–1018. doi: 10.1007/s00125-011-2051-6

Levitt, N. S., Peer, N., Steyn, K., Lombard, C., Maartens, G., Lambert, E. V., et al. (2016). Increased risk of dysglycaemia in South Africans with HIV; especially those on protease inhibitors. *Diabetes Res. Clin. Pract.* 119, 41–47. doi: 10.1016/j.diabres.2016.03.012

Li, G., Zhang, P., Wang, J., Gregg, E. W., Yang, W., Gong, Q., et al. (2008). The long-term effect of lifestyle interventions to prevent diabetes in the China Da Qing Diabetes Prevention Study: a 20-year follow-up study. *Lancet* 371, 1783–1789. doi: 10.1016/S0140-6736(08)60766-7

Lindstrom, J., Ilanne-Parikka, P., Peltonen, M., Aunola, S., Eriksson, J. G., Hemio, K., et al. (2006). Sustained reduction in the incidence of type 2 diabetes by lifestyle intervention: follow-up of the finnish diabetes prevention study. *Lancet* 368, 1673–1679. doi: 10.1016/S0140-6736(06)69701-8

Lo Re, V. III., Kallan, M. J., Tate, J. P., Localio, A. R., Lim, J. K., Goetz, M. B., et al. (2014). Hepatic decompensation in antiretroviral-treated patients co-infected with HIV and hepatitis C virus compared with hepatitis C virus-monoinfected patients: a cohort study. *Ann. Intern. Med.* 160, 369–379. doi: 10.7326/m13-1829

Maartens, G., Celum, C., and Lewin, S. R. (2014). HIV infection: epidemiology, pathogenesis, treatment, and prevention. *Lancet* 384, 258–271. doi: 10.1016/S0140-6736(14)60164-1

Malik, V. S., Popkin, B. M., Bray, G. A., Despres, J. P., Willett, W. C., and Hu, F. B. (2010). Sugar-sweetened beverages and risk of metabolic syndrome and type 2 diabetes: a meta-analysis. *Diabetes Care* 33, 2477–2483. doi: 10.2337/dc10-1079

Manna, P., and Jain, S. K. (2015). Obesity, oxidative stress, adipose tissue dysfunction, and the associated health risks: causes and therapeutic strategies. *Metab. Syndr. Relat. Disord.* 13, 423–444. doi: 10.1089/met.2015.0095

Marks, M. A., Rabkin, C. S., Engels, E. A., Busch, E., Kopp, W., Rager, H., et al. (2013). Markers of microbial translocation and risk of AIDS-related lymphoma. *AIDS* 27, 469–474. doi: 10.1097/QAD.0b013e32835c1333

McLaughlin-Drubin, M. E., and Munger, K. (2008). Viruses associated with human cancer. *Biochim. Biophys. Acta* 1782, 127–150. doi: 10.1016/j.bbadis.2007.12.005

Merchante, N., Rivero, A., de Los Santos-Gil, I., Merino, D., Marquez, M., Lopez-Ruz, M. A., et al. (2009). Insulin resistance is associated with liver stiffness in HIV/HCV co-infected patients. *Gut* 58, 1654–1660. doi: 10.1136/gut.2009.179085

Mesri, E. A., Cesarman, E., and Boshoff, C. (2010). Kaposi's sarcoma and its associated herpesvirus. *Nat. Rev. Cancer* 10, 707–719. doi: 10.1038/nrc2888

Mesri, E. A., Feitelson, M. A., and Munger, K. (2014). Human viral oncogenesis: a cancer hallmarks analysis. *Cell Host Microbe* 15, 266–282. doi: 10.1016/j.chom.2014.02.011

Meyerhardt, J. A., Catalano, P. J., Haller, D. G., Mayer, R. J., Macdonald, J. S., Benson, A. B., et al. (2003). Impact of diabetes mellitus on outcomes in patients with colon cancer. *J. Clin. Oncol.* 21, 433–440. doi: 10.1200/jco.2003.07.125

Mocroft, A., Kirk, O., Clumeck, N., Gargalianos-Kakolyris, P., Trocha, H., Chentsova, N., et al. (2004). The changing pattern of Kaposi sarcoma in patients with HIV, 1994-2003: the EuroSIDA Study. *Cancer* 100, 2644–2654. doi: 10.1002/cncr.20309

Nduka, C. U., Stranges, S., Kimani, P. K., Sarki, A. M., and Uthman, O. A. (2017). Is there sufficient evidence for a causal association between antiretroviral therapy and diabetes in HIV-infected patients? A meta-analysis. *Diabetes Metab. Res. Rev.* 33:e2902. doi: 10.1002/dmrr.2902

Nguyen, H. Q., Magaret, A. S., Kitahata, M. M., Van Rompaey, S. E., Wald, A., and Casper, C. (2008). Persistent Kaposi sarcoma in the era of highly active antiretroviral therapy: characterizing the predictors of clinical response. *AIDS* 22, 937–945. doi: 10.1097/QAD.0b013e3282ff6275

Nikolopoulos, G. K., Paraskevis, D., Hatzitheodorou, E., Moschidis, Z., Sypsa, V., Zavitsanos, X., et al. (2009). Impact of hepatitis B virus infection on the progression of AIDS and mortality in HIV-infected individuals: a cohort study and meta-analysis. *Clin. Infect. Dis.* 48, 1763–1771. doi: 10.1086/599110

Nomura, A., Stemmermann, G. N., Chyou, P. H., Kato, I., Perez-Perez, G. I., and Blaser, M. J. (1991). *Helicobacter* pylori infection and gastric carcinoma among Japanese Americans in Hawaii. *N. Engl. J. Med.* 325, 1132–1136. doi: 10.1056/nejm199110173251604

Oliver, N. T., Hartman, C. M., Kramer, J. R., and Chiao, E. Y. (2016). Statin drugs decrease progression to cirrhosis in HIV/hepatitis C virus coinfected individuals. *AIDS* 30, 2469–2476. doi: 10.1097/qad.0000000000001219

Paich, H. A., Sheridan, P. A., Handy, J., Karlsson, E. A., Schultz-Cherry, S., Hudgens, M. G., et al. (2013). Overweight and obese adult humans have a defective cellular immune response to pandemic H1N1 influenza A virus. *Obesity* 21, 2377–2386. doi: 10.1002/oby.20383

Palmisano, L., and Vella, S. (2011). A brief history of antiretroviral therapy of HIV infection: success and challenges. *Ann. Ist. Super. Sanita* 47, 44–48. doi: 10.4415/ANN_11_01_10

Park, J. S., Kim, E. J., Kwon, H. J., Hwang, E. S., Namkoong, S. E., and Um, S. J. (2000). Inactivation of interferon regulatory factor-1 tumor suppressor protein by HPV E7 oncoprotein. Implication for the E7-mediated immune evasion mechanism in cervical carcinogenesis. *J. Biol. Chem.* 275, 6764–6769. doi: 10.1074/jbc.275.10.6764

Parkin, D. M. (2006). The global health burden of infection-associated cancers in the year 2002. *Int. J. Cancer* 118, 3030–3044. doi: 10.1002/ijc.21731

Parkin, D. M., Bray, F., Ferlay, J., and Pisani, P. (2005). Global cancer statistics, 2002. *CA Cancer J. Clin.* 55, 74–108. doi: 10.3322/canjclin.55.2.74

Parkin, D. M., Nambooze, S., Wabwire-Mangen, F., and Wabinga, H. R. (2010). Changing cancer incidence in Kampala, Uganda, 1991-2006. *Int. J. Cancer* 126, 1187–1195. doi: 10.1002/ijc.24838

Parsonnet, J., Friedman, G. D., Vandersteen, D. P., Chang, Y., Vogelman, J. H., Orentreich, N., et al. (1991). *Helicobacter pylori* infection and the risk of gastric carcinoma. *N. Engl. J. Med.* 325, 1127–1131. doi: 10.1056/nejm199110173251603

Pisani, P., Parkin, D. M., Munoz, N., and Ferlay, J. (1997). Cancer and infection: estimates of the attributable fraction in 1990. *Cancer Epidemiol. Biomarkers Prev.* 6, 387–400.

Plummer, M., de Martel, C., Vignat, J., Ferlay, J., Bray, F., and Franceschi, S. (2016). Global burden of cancers attributable to infections in 2012: a synthetic analysis. *Lancet Glob. Health* 4, e609–e616. doi: 10.1016/S2214-109X(16)30143-7

Plummer, M., Franceschi, S., Vignat, J., Forman, D., and de Martel, C. (2015). Global burden of gastric cancer attributable to *Helicobacter pylori*. *Int. J. Cancer* 136, 487–490. doi: 10.1002/ijc.28999

Ramachandran, A., Snehalatha, C., Mary, S., Mukesh, B., Bhaskar, A. D., Vijay, V., et al. (2006). The Indian diabetes prevention programme shows that lifestyle modification and metformin prevent type 2 diabetes in Asian Indian subjects with impaired glucose tolerance (IDPP-1). *Diabetologia* 49, 289–297. doi: 10.1007/s00125-005-0097-z

Ronco, L. V., Karpova, A. Y., Vidal, M., and Howley, P. M. (1998). Human papillomavirus 16 E6 oncoprotein binds to interferon regulatory factor-3 and inhibits its transcriptional activity. *Genes Dev.* 12, 2061–2072. doi: 10.1101/gad.12.13.2061

Salmon, D., Bani-Sadr, F., Loko, M. A., Stitou, H., Gervais, A., Durant, J., et al. (2012). Insulin resistance is associated with a higher risk of hepatocellular carcinoma in cirrhotic HIV/HCV-co-infected patients: results from ANRS CO13 HEPAVIH. *J. Hepatol.* 56, 862–868. doi: 10.1016/j.jhep.2011.11.009

Samaras, K. (2009). Prevalence and pathogenesis of diabetes mellitus in HIV-1 infection treated with combined antiretroviral therapy. *J. Acquir. Immune Defic. Syndr.* 50, 499–505. doi: 10.1097/QAI.0b013e31819c291b

Sasco, A. J., Jaquet, A., Boidin, E., Ekouevi, D. K., Thouillot, F., Lemabec, T., et al. (2010). The challenge of AIDS-related malignancies in sub-Saharan Africa. *PLOS ONE* 5:e8621. doi: 10.1371/journal.pone.0008621

Schäfer, G., Blumenthal, M. J., and Katz, A. A. (2015). Interaction of human tumor viruses with host cell surface receptors and cell entry. *Viruses* 7, 2592–2617. doi: 10.3390/v7052592

Shu, C. J., Benoist, C., and Mathis, D. (2012). The immune system's involvement in obesity-driven type 2 diabetes. *Semin. Immunol.* 24, 436–442. doi: 10.1016/j.smim.2012.12.001

Smit, M., Brinkman, K., Geerlings, S., Smit, C., Thyagarajan, K., Sighem, A., et al. (2015). Future challenges for clinical care of an ageing population infected with HIV: a modelling study. *Lancet Infect. Dis.* 15, 810–818. doi: 10.1016/S1473-3099(15)00056-0

Strickler, H. D., Burk, R. D., Fazzari, M., Anastos, K., Minkoff, H., Massad, L. S., et al. (2005). Natural history and possible reactivation of human papillomavirus in human immunodeficiency virus-positive women. *J. Natl. Cancer Inst.* 97, 577–586. doi: 10.1093/jnci/dji073

Sylla, B. S., and Wild, C. P. (2012). A million africans a year dying from cancer by 2030: what can cancer research and control offer to the continent? *Int. J. Cancer* 130, 245–250. doi: 10.1002/ijc.26333

Tien, P. C., Schneider, M. F., Cole, S. R., Levine, A. M., Cohen, M., DeHovitz, J., et al. (2007). Antiretroviral therapy exposure and incidence of diabetes mellitus in the Women's interagency HIV study. *AIDS* 21, 1739–1745. doi: 10.1097/QAD.0b013e32827038d0

Tobian, A. A., Kacker, S., and Quinn, T. C. (2014). Male circumcision: a globally relevant but under-utilized method for the prevention of HIV and other sexually transmitted infections. *Annu. Rev. Med.* 65, 293–306. doi: 10.1146/annurev-med-092412-090539

Torre, L. A., Bray, F., Siegel, R. L., Ferlay, J., Lortet-Tieulent, J., and Jemal, A. (2015). Global cancer statistics, 2012. *CA Cancer J. Clin.* 65, 87–108. doi: 10.3322/caac.21262

Turturro, F., Friday, E., and Welbourne, T. (2007). Hyperglycemia regulates thioredoxin-ROS activity through induction of thioredoxin-interacting protein (TXNIP) in metastatic breast cancer-derived cells MDA-MB-231. *BMC Cancer* 7:96. doi: 10.1186/1471-2407-7-96

van Kruijsdijk, R. C., van der Wall, E., and Visseren, F. L. (2009). Obesity and cancer: the role of dysfunctional adipose tissue. *Cancer Epidemiol. Biomarkers Prev.* 18, 2569–2578. doi: 10.1158/1055-9965.epi-09-0372

Vander Heiden, M. G., Cantley, L. C., and Thompson, C. B. (2009). Understanding the Warburg effect: the metabolic requirements of cell proliferation. *Science* 324, 1029–1033. doi: 10.1126/science.1160809

Vigneri, R., Goldfine, I. D., and Frittitta, L. (2016). Insulin, insulin receptors, and cancer. *J. Endocrinol. Invest.* 39, 1365–1376. doi: 10.1007/s40618-016-0508-7

Vincent, T. L., and Gatenby, R. A. (2008). An evolutionary model for initiation, promotion, and progression in carcinogenesis. *Int. J. Oncol.* 32, 729–737.

Vorster, H. H., Kruger, A., Wentzel-Viljoen, E., Kruger, H. S., and Margetts, B. M. (2014). Added sugar intake in South Africa: findings from the adult prospective Urban and rural epidemiology cohort study. *Am. J. Clin. Nutr.* 99, 1479–1486. doi: 10.3945/ajcn.113.069005

Wahome, E., Ngetsa, C., Mwambi, J., Gelderblom, H. C., Manyonyi, G. O., Micheni, M., et al. (2017). Hepatitis B virus incidence and risk factors among human immunodeficiency virus-1 negative men who have sex with men in Kenya. *Open Forum Infect. Dis.* 4:ofw253. doi: 10.1093/ofid/ofw253

Wang, C., Wang, X., Gong, G., Ben, Q., Qiu, W., Chen, Y., et al. (2012). Increased risk of hepatocellular carcinoma in patients with diabetes mellitus: a systematic review and meta-analysis of cohort studies. *Int. J. Cancer* 130, 1639–1648. doi: 10.1002/ijc.26165

Wang, F., Meng, W., Wang, B., and Qiao, L. (2014). *Helicobacter pylori*-induced gastric inflammation and gastric cancer. *Cancer Lett.* 345, 196–202. doi: 10.1016/j.canlet.2013.08.016

Wild, S., Roglic, G., Green, A., Sicree, R., and King, H. (2004). Global prevalence of diabetes: estimates for the year 2000 and projections for 2030. *Diabetes Care* 27, 1047–1053. doi: 10.2337/diacare.27.5.1047

Woodman, C. B., Collins, S. I., and Young, L. S. (2007). The natural history of cervical HPV infection: unresolved issues. *Nat. Rev. Cancer* 7, 11–22. doi: 10.1038/nrc2050

Working Group on the Evaluation of Carcinogenic Risks to Humans [IARC] (2012). Biological agents. Volume 100 B. A review of human carcinogens. *IARC Monogr. Eval. Carcinog Risks Hum.* 100(Pt B), 1–441.

Xia, C., Chen, R., Chen, J., Qi, Q., Pan, Y., Du, L., et al. (2017). Combining metformin and nelfinavir exhibits synergistic effects against the growth of human cervical cancer cells and xenograft in nude mice. *Sci. Rep.* 7:43373. doi: 10.1038/srep43373

Zaccardi, F., Webb, D. R., Yates, T., and Davies, M. J. (2016). Pathophysiology of type 1 and type 2 diabetes mellitus: a 90-year perspective. *Postgrad. Med. J.* 92, 63–69. doi: 10.1136/postgradmedj-2015-133281

Zaidi, J., Grapsa, E., Tanser, F., Newell, M. L., and Barnighausen, T. (2013). Dramatic increase in HIV prevalence after scale-up of antiretroviral treatment. *AIDS* 27, 2301–2305. doi: 10.1097/QAD.0b013e328362e832

5

Case of Meningitis in a Neonate Caused by an Extended-Spectrum-Beta-Lactamase-Producing Strain of Hypervirulent *Klebsiella pneumoniae*

Khalit S. Khaertynov[1]*, Vladimir A. Anokhin[1], Yuri N. Davidyuk[2], Irina V. Nicolaeva[1], Svetlana V. Khalioullina[1], Dina R. Semyenova[1], Evgeny Y. Alatyrev[3], Natalia N. Skvortsova[3] and Levon G. Abrahamyan[4]*

[1] Department of Children Infectious Diseases, Kazan State Medical University, Kazan, Russia, [2] Institute of Fundamental Medicine and Biology, Kazan Federal University, Kazan, Russia, [3] Intensive Care Unit No 2, Republican Clinical Infectious Diseases Hospital, Kazan, Russia, [4] Laboratory for Animal Molecular Virology, Research Group on Infectious Diseases in Production Animals and Swine and Poultry Infectious Diseases Research Center, Faculty of Veterinary Medicine, Université de Montréal, Saint-Hyacinthe, QC, Canada

Correspondence:
Khalit S. Khaertynov
khalit65@rambler.ru
Levon G. Abrahamyan
levon.abrahamyan@umontreal.ca

Klebsiella pneumoniae is one of the most important infectious agents among neonates. This pathogen has a potential to develop an increased antimicrobial resistance and virulence. The classic non-virulent strain of *K. pneumoniae*, producing an extended-spectrum beta-lactamases (ESBL), is associated with nosocomial infection mainly in preterm neonates. Hypervirulent *K. pneumoniae* strains are associated with invasive infection among previously healthy ambulatory patients, and most of them exhibit antimicrobial susceptibility. During the last few years, several cases of diseases caused by hypervirulent *K. pneumoniae* producing ESBL have been registered in different geographical regions of the world. However, reports of such cases in neonates are rare. Here, we reported that this pathogen can cause pyogenic meningitis in full-term neonate with poor prognosis. A previously healthy, full-term, 12-day-old neonate was admitted to the infectious diseases hospital with suspected meningitis. The clinical symptoms included loss of appetite, irritability, fever, seizures, and a bulging anterior fontanelle. The analysis of the cerebrospinal fluid confirmed the diagnosis of meningitis. Blood and cerebrospinal fluid cultures were positive for *K. pneumoniae*, producing ESBL. *K. pneumoniae* isolates were resistant to aminopenicillins, 3rd generation cephalosporins but were sensitive to imipenem and meropenem. The "string test" was positive. The study of the virulence factors of *K. pneumoniae* by PCR revealed the presence of the *rmpA* gene. A combination of *K. pneumoniae* virulence and drug resistance complicated by cerebral oedema led to the death of the neonate. We concluded that both the risk of developing severe forms of infection and the outcome of the disease due to *K. pneumonia* are associated with the phenotypic features of the pathogen such as its antibiotic susceptibility and virulence factors. Emergence of the ESBL-producing strain of hypervirulent *K. pneumoniae* could represent a new serious threat to public health, suggesting an urgent need to enhance clinical awareness and epidemiological surveillance.

Keywords: *Klebsiella pneumoniae*, extended-spectrum β-lactamases, hypervirulent, meningitis, neonate

INTRODUCTION

Subject

Here, we report a case of neonatal meningitis caused by an ESBL-producing hypervirulent *Klebsiella pneumoniae* strain in a 12-day-old, male neonate. A 40-week-gestation male, with a birth weight of 3400 grams was born by cesarean delivery to a 24-year-old woman. The infant's Apgar scores were 8 and 9 at delivery, and he was discharged on the 5th day after delivery. The mother gave no history of infections before delivery and no complications during pregnancy. Blood and cerebrospinal fluid cultures (CSF) of the infant patient were positive for *K. pneumoniae*.

The aim of this study was to determine the antibiotic susceptibility and virulence factors of *K. pneumoniae* isolated from a neonate with purulent meningitis. We investigated the antibiotic susceptibility of *K. pneumoniae*, the ability of the microorganism for production of extended-spectrum β-lactamases (ESBL), and its virulent factors: the *rmpA* gene and the hypermucoviscosity phenotype identified by a positive string test.

The Institutional Review Board of the Republican Clinical Infectious Diseases Hospital approved this study and written informed consent was obtained from a subject's parents, according to the guidelines approved under this protocol (Federal Law "Protection of Health Right of Citizens of Russian Federation" N323- FL, 11.21.2011).

Bacterial Isolates

One milliliter of blood sample was collected by a sterile syringe and mixed with 20 ml of Brain-Heart Infusion broth (Conda Pronadisa, Spain). This mixture was incubated at 37°C for 7 days, streaked onto the surface of blood agar and MacConkey agar (Oxoid, United Kingdom), and incubated at 37°C for 24 h (Collee et al., 1996). In order to isolate *K. pneumoniae* from CSF, a chocolate agar and blood medium were used (Oxoid, United Kingdom). Bacterial isolates were identified according to morphological and biochemical tests (Gram stain, capsule stain, motility test, indole production test, urease production test, Methyl Red test, Voges–Proskauer test) (MacFaddin, 2000) and confirmed by matrix-assisted laser desorption-ionization time-of-flight mass spectrometry (Microflex, Bruker Daltonics, Bremen, Germany).

Gram Stain

Bacterial isolates were resuspended in normal saline for Gram stain. Smear was prepared on a glass slide, air dried and fixed by gentle heating. The slide was flooded with crystal violet for 1 min. The stain was washed off with excess of tap water. Gram's iodine was poured over the slide for 1 min. The slide was washed and destained with ethyl alcohol. Finally, counter staining was done with safranin for 30 s. Slides were washed again, dried and examined under the microscope.

For Capsule Staining

India Ink method was used. We placed a single drop of India ink on a clean microscope slide. Then, we removed some colonies from culture plate with a flamed loop and mixed them in the drop of India ink. Then, we placed the end of another clean microscope slide at an angle on the original slide containing the microorganisms. Next, we spread drop out so that it formed a thin film. After 5 min, we saturated the slide with crystal violet for 1 min and carefully rinsed it with water. The slide was air-dried for 5 min. Then, the slide was examined under the microscope using an oil immersion objective lens and looked for purple cells surrounded by a clear halo on a dark background.

Motility Test

Colonies of isolated microorganisms from an 18–24 h culture were inoculated into the medium by stabbing the center of the medium (HiMedia, India) to a depth of 1,5 cm. The inoculated medium was incubated at 37°C for 18 h. A positive motility test was indicated by a diffuse zone of growth flaring from the line of inoculation.

For the Indole Production Test

Conventional tube method was used. Colonies of microorganism were inoculated in tryptophan broth and were incubated at 37°C for 24 h in ambient air. Then, 0,5 ml of Kovac's reagent was added to the broth culture. The test was considered positive if a pink colored ring appeared after the addition of reagent. Negative test is indicated if no color change occurred after the addition of reagent.

Urease Production Test

Colonies of isolated microorganism from an overnight Brain-Heart Infusion broth were streaked onto the surface of a urea agar slant. The tube of medium was incubated at 37°C in ambient air for 7 days. The test was positive if a pink color appeared.

Methyl Red and Voges–Proskauer Tests

Colonies of isolated microorganism were inoculated into Methyl Red/Voges–Proskauer broth tube. The tube of medium was incubated at 37°C for 24 h. After incubation, we removed two – 1 mL aliquots and placed them into two small tubes: one tube was for the methyl red test and the other for the Voges–Proskauer test. For the *Methyl Rose test,* we added five drops of methyl red to one tube. A red color at the surface was considered a positive result. For the *Voges–Proskauer test,* we added 0.6mL of 5% alpha naphthol, followed by 0.2 mL of 40% potassium hydroxide and shook the tube gently. A positive test was represented by the development of a red color 15 min after the addition of the reagents.

Antibiotic Susceptibility Testing

The antibiotic susceptibility of *K. pneumoniae* isolates was determined by the Kirby-Bauer disk diffusion method according to Clinical Laboratory Standards Institute guidelines (CLSI) (Patel et al., 2015). Suspension of *K. pneumoniae* isolate was spread by sterile glass rods on the surface of *Mueller Hinton agar* (Oxoid, United Kingdom). Then antibiotic disks (Bio-Rad, France) were placed onto the surface of the inoculated *Mueller Hinton agar* plate. The plate was then incubated at 37°C for 18 h. Antimicrobial susceptibility was determined by measuring the diameter of the inhibition zone according to CLSI (2015). All antibiotics used for this test are listed in **Table 1**.

TABLE 1 | The susceptibility of *K. pneumoniae* to antibiotics.

Antibiotic	Concentration (mg)	Values of diameter of inhibition zones (mm)	Susceptibility
Ampicillin	25	0	R
Ampicillin/clavulanate	30	0	R
Ceftriaxone	30	0	R
Ceftazidime	30	0	R
Cefotaxime	30	0	R
Ciprofloxacin	5	13	I
Co-trimoxazole	25	0	R
Imipenem	10	25	S
Meropenem	10	24	S
Amikacin	30	16	I
Gentamicin	10	0	R

S, susceptible; I, intermediate; R, resistant.

Test for Production of Extended-Spectrum β-Lactamases (ESBL)

The *K. pneumoniae* isolates were tested for ESBL by using the double-disk method according CLSI (Patel et al., 2015).

Amoxicillin/clavulanate disks were placed in the center of *Mueller Hinton* agar plate (Oxoid, United Kingdom). The disk of ceftazidime and cefotaxime were placed at the distance of 20 mm from the amoxicillin/clavulanic acid disk. The plates were incubated aerobically at 37°C for 18 h before the zone size recorded. A positive result was indicated when the inhibition zones around any of the cephalosporin disks was augmented in the direction of the disk containing clavulanic acid.

Hypermucoviscosity Testing

Single colonies, cultured on Brain Heart infusion agar plates (Conda Pronadisa, Spain), were obtained and tested for their ability to form viscous strings. The hypermucoviscosity was defined by the formation of viscous strings > 5 mm length (Yu et al., 2007; Shon et al., 2013).

DNA Extraction

Some colonies from the surface of MacConkey agar were suspended in 50 μl of sterile water. Total DNA was extracted from suspended cells using an extraction kit ("Litech," Russia) according to the manufacturer's recommendations.

PCR Detection of Virulence-Associated Genes

DNA samples were analyzed using polymerase chain reaction (PCR) with primer pair for the *rmpA* (5′-ACGACTTTCAAGAGAAATGA-3′ forward and 5′-CATAGATGTCATAATCACAC-3′ reverse). Amplification was performed using C1000 Thermo Cycler ("Bio-Rad Laboratories," United States) applying the following program: (1) DNA denaturation at 94°C, 3 min; (2) 35 cycles at 94°C, 30 s; 45°C, 30 s; 72°C, 35 s; (3) final extension at 72°C, 5 min; (4) reaction termination at 4°C. The amplicons were separated in 1% agarose gel and purified by using GeneJET Gel Extraction Kit (Thermo Scientific, United States) according to the manufacturer's recommendations. The PCR-products were sequenced using the 3730 DNA Analyzer (Life Technologies, United States) to confirm the presence of the *rmpA* gene.

Case

A full-term, 12-day-old, male neonate was admitted to the infectious diseases hospital with suspected meningitis on the 3rd day of illness. During the first 2 days, irritability and a loss of appetite were observed. On admission day, the infant had a temperature of 39°C and seizures. He looked noticeably ill and sleepy. On physical examination, his anterior fontanelle was bulging. The skin was pale, without rash. Chest, abdomen, and heart examinations did not show any abnormalities. The heart rate was 156 beats per minute, respiratory rate – 40 per minute. The liver and spleen were not enlarged. Chest X-ray was normal. The initial blood analysis revealed increased C-reactive protein (100 mg/L), presepsin (2932 pg/mL) and procalcitonin (more than 10 ng/mL). The initial complete blood cell count (CBC) analysis did not reveal any changes. CBC showed a erythrocytes count of 5,4 × 10^{12}/L, a white blood cell (WBC) count of 6,4 × 10^9/L, with 22% segmented neutrophils, 62% lymphocytes, 15% monocytes, 1% eosinophils, and 235 × 10^9/L platelets. A lumbar puncture was performed: CSF was turbid, physico-chemical examination showed 21 000 WBC/mm^3 with 90% neutrophils, 10% lymphocytes. CSF protein was 290 mg/dL, glucose – 0,3 mmol/L. Serum glucose was 8 mmol/L. The latex antigen test was negative for *Haemophilus influenzae B*, *Neisseria meningitides*, *Escherichia coli*, and *Streptococcus* group B. The cranial ultrasonography was performed and demonstrated thickening of the ventricular walls. The course of disease was complicated by the development of cerebral edema. The Pediatric Glasgow Coma Scale Score was 5. Changes in WBCs were found only on the 3rd day after hospitalization (**Table 2**). WBC examination showed 28.3 × 10^9/L leukocytes with 77% neutrophils. The duration of leukocytosis and neutrophilia were 15 and 23 days, respectively. From the 2nd day of the hospitalization, the platelet count dropped to 25 × 10^9/L. The duration of thrombocytopenia was 8 days. Blood and CSFs were positive for *K. pneumoniae* producing ESBL. Colonies of

TABLE 2 | Complete blood cells counts during hospitalization.

Days of hospitalization	1	3	8	15	23
Erythrocytes, × 10^{12}/L	5,4	3,3	3,4	3,5	3,6
Hb, g/dl	142	133	135	137	132
WBC, × 10^9/L	6,4	28,3	59,3	25,1	6,4
Banded, %	0	1	8	3	1
Segmented, %	22	76	62	70	74
Eosinophils, %	1	2	4	1	0
Lymphocytes, %	62	18	21	24	20
Monocytes, %	15	3	5	2	5
Platelets, × 10^9/L	235	31	105	410	238

Hb, hemoglobin; WBC, white blood cells.

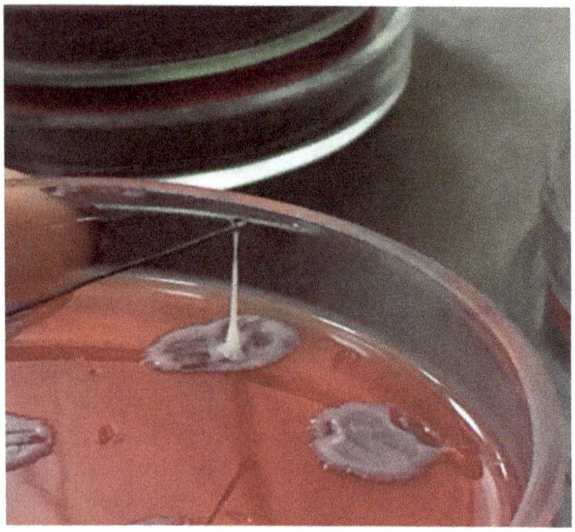

FIGURE 1 | Hypermucoviscosity phenotype of *Klebsiella pneumoniae.* When the colonies were touched with a loop and the loop lifted vertically from the surface of the blood agar plate, the mucoid isolates adhered to the loop.

bacteria isolated on media were gray, mucoid, with diameters up to 2–4 mm, gram-negative, contained a thick capsule, and were non-motile (motility test was negative). Colonies of bacteria were positive for urease and *Voges–Proskauer* tests, and were itive negative for indole and Methyl Red tests. CSF culture for other bacteria was negative. The "string test" was positive (**Figure 1**). The study of the virulence factors by PCR revealed the presence of the *rmpA* (regulator of the mucoid phenotype) gene. The treatment of the patient included comprehensive antibiotics (ampicillin, amikacin, meropenem, cefoperazone), dexamethasone, IgM-enriched intravenous immunoglobulin, infusion therapy and mechanical ventilation. On admission day, a neonate was started on ampicillin (200 mg/kg/day) and amikacin (10 mg/kg/day). Both antibiotics a neonate received within 3 days, but did not show any clinical improvement. Following the isolation of *K. pneumoniae* (after 3 days), meropenem (120mg/kg/day) was administered, which a neonate received for 15 days. From the 19th day after hospitalization until the death, the patient received cefoperazone (100mg/kg/day). Despite the therapy, the patient died on the 35th day of the disease. The post-mortem examination revealed purulent meningoencephalitis, ventriculitis with the outcome of total cerebral leukomalacia, scattered pulmonary atelectasis, bilateral pneumonia, and the depletion of the thymus and spleen.

BACKGROUND

Klebsiella pneumoniae is one of the leading causes of hospital-acquired infection and neonatal sepsis (Janda and Abbott, 2006; Jones, 2010; Camacho-Gonzalez et al., 2013). The risk of severe bacterial infections such as sepsis and meningitis in neonates is associated mainly with neonatal factors: prematurity, low birth weight, and immaturity of innate and adaptive immunity (Cuenca et al., 2013; Cortese et al., 2016). Additionally, pathogenic features of the *K. pneumoniae* such as virulence and antibiotic resistance can define the course and outcome of the infection (Al-Hasan et al., 2011; Jacob et al., 2013). *K. pneumoniae* is an opportunistic pathogen often resistant to multiple antibiotics. During the last few decades, ESBL positive *K. pneumoniae* isolates have been recovered worldwide, especially in intensive care units (ICU) (Canton et al., 2008; Gelband et al., 2015). ESBLs can inactivate all penicillins and cephalosporins, including 3rd generation cephalosporins (Gelband et al., 2015). In neonates, *K. pneumoniae* median resistance to ampicillin was 94% and cephalosporins 84% in Asia; 100% and 50% in Africa (Le Doare et al., 2015). The prevalence of ESBL-producing strains of *K. pneumoniae* in the United States is 23%, in some countries of Europe up to 85–100% (Gelband et al., 2015). These microorganisms can cause outbreaks of neonatal sepsis in hospitals and neonatal ICU (Haller et al., 2015; Khaertynov et al., 2016). Virulence factors of *K. pneumoniae* play an important role in the development of infection. The factors that are implicated in the virulence of *K. pneumoniae* strains include the capsular polysaccharide, lipopolysaccharide, fimbrial adhesins, and siderophores (Broberg et al., 2014; Li et al., 2014). In the mid-1980s and 1990s, reports from Taiwan described cases of disease caused by hypervirulent strains of *K. pneumoniae* (hv-KP) (Liu et al., 1986; Cheng et al., 1991; Wang et al., 1998). A combination of clinical and bacterial phenotypic features of the hv-KP distinguishes it from the "classic" *K. pneumoniae* strains (Shon et al., 2013). One of these features is its ability to cause severe invasive infection (liver abscesses, meningitis, endophthalmitis) in previously healthy ambulatory patients. The second distinctive characteristic is the hypermucoviscous phenotype, which results in mucoid colonies on agar plates. This phenotype is defined by a positive "string test." A positive string test is indicated by a microbiological inoculation loop able to generate a viscous string > 5 mm the length by stretching bacterial colonies on an agar plate (Yu et al., 2007; Shon et al., 2013). The hypermucoviscous phenotype of *K. pneumoniae* is associated with the presence of *rmpA* and *rmpA2* genes (Decré et al., 2011; Bialek-Davenet et al., 2014). The hypervirulent strains of *K. pneumoniae* currently spread throughout the world (Decré et al., 2011; Bialek-Davenet et al., 2014). Until recently, it was believed that the classic, non-virulent strains of *K. pneumoniae* producing ESBL and the hv-KP strains evolved separately, and have been considered as independent of each other. However, in 2014 an hv-KP able to produce ESBL (Zhang et al., 2015) was found in China, and in 2015 a clinical case caused by hv-KP producing ESBL was reported in France (Surgers et al., 2016). It is likely the frequency of these cases will grow worldwide. These cases were mainly observed in adult patients. The reports of such cases in neonates are extremely rare (Shankar et al., 2016).

DISCUSSION

Neonatal infection can occur in term infants because of birth risk factors and exposure to pathogens in the community as well. Neonatal sepsis and meningitis are more common in preterm newborns with low gestational age and low birthweight (Kavuncuoğlu et al., 2013; Samuelsson et al., 2014). *K. pneumoniae* infection is a typical nosocomial infection in neonates with the combination of these factors. However, in the case reported here, the disease occurred in a full-term baby. The mother of the baby did not have clinical signs of infectious disease. The neonatal meningitis ensues when pathogenic virulence factors overcome host defense mechanisms. For instance, the presence of a capsule at cell surface protects *K. pneumoniae* from opsonization and phagocytosis by macrophages and neutrophils (Li et al., 2014). On the other hand, capsular polysaccharide of *K. pneumoniae* suppress the early inflammatory response by inhibition of IL-8 expression through the inhibition of TLR4 signaling (Li et al., 2014). Thus, the pathogenic potential of the microorganism plays an important role in the disease outcome. In the reported case, the *K. pneumoniae* isolates produced ESBL and were absolutely resistant to aminopenicillins, 3rd generation cephalosporins and gentamicin, with diameters of inhibition zones of 0 mm for each of them. *K. pneumoniae* isolates were sensitive only to imipenem and meropenem with diameters of inhibition zones of 25 and 24 mm, respectively. Intermediate sensitivity was observed for amikacin and co-trimoxazole with diameters of inhibition zones of 16 mm and 13 mm, respectively. Additionally, these isolates were hypervirulent (i.e., positive "string test" and presence of *rmpA*). In this case, neonatal meningitis was caused by ESBL-producing strain of hv-KP. An unfavorable outcome has been associated with the inefficiency and late onset of antibacterial therapy, as well as the formation of a severe inflammatory reaction from the membranes and brain matter. Bacterial meningitis in neonates is an independent risk factor for mortality: mortality rates of meningitis caused by *K. pneumoniae* reaching 17.1% (Watson et al., 2003). We noted the absence of changes in WBC on admission day despite the massive pyogenic process in the cerebrospinal fluid. Given the fact of bacteremia, this unusual situation with the redistribution of neutrophils in newborn fluids cannot be explained only by the biological characteristics of the microorganism. Likely, the nature of the immune response to a severe invasive infection in a newborn patient takes place. The primary reaction of the newborn child in the tissues of the central nervous system is associated with the redistribution of neutrophil chemoattractants: with an increase in their concentration in the cerebrospinal fluid, their level in the blood should be reduced. We regret that we were unable to confirm this assumption. For example, simultaneous assessment of interleukin-8 in the blood and cerebrospinal fluid could have provided confirmation. However, we do not rule out that such changes are associated with specific biological characteristics of the microorganism. Meningitis caused by hypervirulent *K. pneumoniae* is associated with potential mortality. Emergence of hypervirulent strains of *K. pneumoniae* producing EXBL can represent a major challenge for patient treatment. In our study, the most sensitive antibiotics to hypervirulent ESBL-producing *K. pneumoniae* strains were meropenem and imipenem. In cases of neonatal sepsis or neonatal meningitis caused by hypervirulent strains of *K. pneumoniae* producing EXBL, these two carbapenems should be considered as first-line therapy and should be administered as soon as possible.

CONCLUDING REMARKS

The risk of developing severe forms of infection due to *K. pneumonia* and the outcome of the disease are associated not only with neonatal factors (low gestational age, very low birth weight), but also with the features of the microorganism: its antibiotic susceptibility and virulence. ESBL-producing strain of hypervirulent *K. pneumoniae* causes invasive infection (pyogenic meningitis) in full-term neonate with poor prognosis.

AUTHOR CONTRIBUTIONS

KK design of the study and wrote the paper. Discussed the results and implications, wrote the manuscript. VA design of the study and wrote the paper. YD DNA extraction of *K. pneumoniae* strains with subsequent genotyping by PCR method to determine virulence factors. IN design of the study. SK wrote the paper. DS collection of clinical data. EA collection and interpretation of clinical data. NS isolation of *K. pneumoniae* colonies, determination of their antibiotic resistance and ability to produce of extended spectrum β-lactamase. LA wrote the paper. Discussed the results and implications, wrote the manuscript.

ACKNOWLEDGMENTS

This study was performed according to the Russian Government Program of Competitive Growth of Kazan Federal University and subsidy allocated to Kazan Federal University for the state assignment in the sphere of scientific activities. Some of the experiments were conducted using the equipment of Interdisciplinary center for collective use and Pharmaceutical Research and Education Center, Kazan (Volga Region) Federal University, Kazan, Russia. Authors would like to thank Mackenzie Waltke for proofreading.

REFERENCES

Al-Hasan, M. N., Huskins, W. C., Lahr, B. D., Eckel-Passow, J. E., and Baddour, L. M. (2011). Epidemiology and outcome of Gram-negative bloodstream infection in children: a population-based study. *Epidemiol. Infect.* 139, 791–796. doi: 10.1017/S0950268810001640 1640

Bialek-Davenet, S., Criscuolo, A., Ailloud, F., Passet, V., Jones, L., Delannoy-Vieillard, A. S., et al. (2014). Genomic definition of hypervirulent and multidrug-resistant *Klebsiella pneumoniae* clonal groups. *Emerg. Infect. Dis.* 20, 1812–1820. doi: 10.3201/eid2011.14020622

Broberg, C. A., Palacios, M., and Miller, V. L. (2014). *Klebsiella*: a long way to go towards understanding this enigmatic jet-setter. *F1000Prime Rep.* 6:64. doi: 10.12703/P6-64

Camacho-Gonzalez, A., Spearman, P. W., and Stoll, B. J. (2013). Neonatal infectious diseases: evaluation of neonatal sepsis. *Pediatr. Clin. North Am.* 60, 367–389. doi: 10.1016/j.pcl.2012.12.003

Canton, R., Novais, A., Valverde, A., Machado, E., Peixe, L., Baquero, F., et al. (2008). Prevalence and spread of extended-spectrum b-lactamase-producing *Enterobacteriaceae* in Europe. *Clin. Microbiol. Infect.* 14, 144–153. doi: 10.1111/j.1469-0691.2007.01850

Cheng, D. L., Liu, Y. C., Yen, M. Y., Liu, C. Y., and Wang, R. S. (1991). Septic metastatic lesions of pyogenic liver abscess. Their association with *Klebsiella pneumoniae* bacteremia in diabetic patients. *Arch. Intern. Med.* 151, 1557–1559. doi: 10.1001/archinte.1991.00400080059010

CLSI (2015). *Performance Standards for Antimicrobial Susceptibility Testing; Twenty-Fifth Informational Supplement.* CLSI Document M100-S25. Wayne, PA: Clinical and Laboratory Standards Institute.

Collee, J. G., Mackie, T. J., and McCartney, J. E. (1996). *Practical Medical Microbiology.* New York, NY: Churchill Livingstone.

Cortese, F., Scicchitano, P., Gesualdo, M., Filaninno, A., De Giorgi, E., Schettini, F., et al. (2016). Early and late infections in newborns: where do we stand? A review. *Pediatr. Neonatol.* 57, 265–273. doi: 10.1016/j.pedneo.2015.09.007

Cuenca, A. G., Wynn, J. L., Moldawer, L. L., and Levy, O. (2013). Role of innate immunity in neonatal infection. *Am. J. Perinatol.* 30, 105–112. doi: 10.1055/s-0032-1333412

Decré, D., Verdet, C., Emirian, A., Le Gourrierec, T., Petit, J. C., Offenstadt, G., et al. (2011). Emerging severe and fatal infections due to *Klebsiella pneumoniae* in two university hospitals in France. *J. Clin. Microbiol.* 49, 3012–3014. doi: 10.1128/JCM.00676-11

Gelband, H., Miller-Petrie, M., Pant, S., Gandra, S., Levinson, J., Barter, D., et al. (2015). *The State of the World's Antibiotics.* Washington, DC: Center for Disease Dynamics, Economics, Policy.

Haller, S., Eller, C., Hermes, J., Kaase, M., Steglich, M., Radonic, A., et al. (2015). What caused the outbreak of ESBL-producing *Klebsiella pneumoniae* in a neonatal intensive care unit, Germany 2009 to 2012? Reconstructing transmission with epidemiological analysis and whole-genome sequencing. *BMJ* 5:e007397. doi: 10.1136/bmjopen-2014-007397

Jacob, J. T., Klein, E., Laxminarayan, R., Beldavs, Z., Lynfield, R., Kallen, A., et al. (2013). Vital signs: carbapenem resistant *Enterobacteriaceae. Morb. Mortal. Wkly Rep.* 62, 165–170.

Janda, J. M., and Abbott, S. L. (eds). (2006). "The genera *Klebsiella* and *Raoultella*," in *The Enterobacteria*, 2nd Edn (Washington, DC: ASM Press), 115–129.

Jones, R. N. (2010). Microbial etiologies of hospital-acquired bacterial pneumonia and ventilator-associated bacterial pneumonia. *Clin. Infect. Dis.* 51, 81–87. doi: 10.1086/653053

Kavuncuoğlu, S., Gürsoy, S., Türel, Ö., Aldemir, E. Y., and Hoşaf, E. (2013). Neonatal bacterial meningitis in Turkey: epidemiology, risk factors, and prognosis. *J. Infect. Dev. Ctries.* 7, 73–81. doi: 10.3855/jidc.2652

Khaertynov, K. S., Anohin, V. A., Nikolaeva, I. V., Semenova, D. R., Lyubin, S. A., and Agapova, I. V. (2016). Neonatal sepsis caused by *Klebsiella. Med. News North Caucasus* 11, 82–86.

Le Doare, K., Bielicki, J., Heath, P. T., and Sharland, M. (2015). Systematic review of antibiotic resistance rates among gram-negative bacteria in children with sepsis in resource-limited countries. *J. Pediatr. Infect. Dis. Soc.* 4, 11–20. doi: 10.1093/jpids/piu014

Li, B., Zhao, Y., Liu, C., and Zhou, D. (2014). Molecular pathogenesis of *Klebsiella pneumonia. Future Microbiol.* 9, 1071–1081. doi: 10.2217/fmb.14.48

Liu, Y. C., Cheng, D. L., and Lin, C. L. (1986). *Klebsiella pneumoniae* liver abscess associated with septic endophthalmitis. *Arch. Intern. Med.* 146, 1913–1916. doi: 10.1001/archinte.1986.00360220057011

MacFaddin, J. F. (2000). *Biochemical Tests for Identification of Medical Bacteria*, 3rd Edn. Philadelphia, PA: Lippincott Williams & Wilkins.

Patel, J. B., Cockerill, F. R., Bradford, P. A., Eliopoulos, G. M., Hindler, J. A., Jenkins, S. J., et al. (2015). *Performance Standards for Antimicrobial Susceptibility testing*, 25th Edn. Wayne, PA: Clinical and Laboratory Standards Institute.

Samuelsson, A., Isaksson, B., Hanberger, H., and Olhager, E. (2014). Late-onset neonatal sepsis, risk factors and interventions: an analysis of recurrent outbreaks of *Serratia marcescens*, 2006–2011. *J. Hosp. Infect.* 86, 57–63. doi: 10.1016/j.jhin.2013.09.017

Shankar, C., Santhanam, S., Kumar, M., Gupta, V., Ragupathi, N. K. D., and Veeraraghavan, B. (2016). Draft genome sequence of an extended-spectrum—lactamase-positive hypervirulent *Klebsiella pneumoniae* strain with novel sequence type 2318 isolated from a neonate. *Genome Announc.* 4:e01273-16. doi: 10.1128/genomeA.01273-16

Shon, A. S., Bajwa, R. P., and Russo, T. A. (2013). Hypervirulent (hypermucoviscous) *Klebsiella pneumoniae*: a new and dangerous breed. *Virulence* 4, 107–118. doi: 10.4161/viru.22718

Surgers, L., Boyd, A., Girard, P. M., Arlet, G., and Decré, D. (2016). ESBL-producing strain of hypervirulent *Klebsiella pneumoniae* K2, France. *Emerg. Infect. Dis.* 22, 1687–1688. doi: 10.3201/eid2209.160681

Wang, J. H., Liu, Y. C., Lee, S. S., Yen, M. Y., Chen, Y. S., Wang, J. H., et al. (1998). Primary liver abscess due to *Klebsiella pneumoniae* in Taiwan. *Clin. Infect. Dis.* 26, 1434–1438. doi: 10.1086/516369

Watson, R. S., Carcillo, J. A., Linde-Zwirble, W. T., Clermont, G., Lidicker, J., and Angus, D. C. (2003). The epidemiology of severe sepsis in children in the United States. *Am. J. Respir. Crit. Care Med.* 167, 695–701. doi: 10.1164/rccm.200207-682OC

Yu, V. L., Hansen, D. S., and Ko, W. C. (2007). Virulence characteristics of *Klebsiella* and clinical manifestations of *K. pneumoniae* bloodstream infections. *Emerg. Infect. Dis.* 13, 986–993. doi: 10.3201/eid1307.070187

Zhang, R., Lin, D., Chan, E. W., Gu, D., Chen, G. X., and Chen, S. (2015). Emergence of carbapenem-resistant serotype K1 hypervirulent *Klebsiella pneumoniae* strains in China. *Antimicrob. Agents Chemother.* 60, 709–711. doi: 10.1128/AAC.02173-15

6

Microbes and Viruses are Bugging the Gut in Celiac Disease: Are They Friends or Foes?

Aaron Lerner [1,2], Marina Arleevskaya [3], Andreas Schmiedl [2] and Torsten Matthias [2]*

[1] The Ruth and Bruce Rappaport Faculty of Medicine, Technion Israel Institute of Technology, Haifa, Israel, [2] Department of Research, AESKU.KIPP Institute, Wendelsheim, Germany, [3] Central Research Laboratory, Kazan State Medical Academy Kazan, Kazan, Russia

***Correspondence:**
Aaron Lerner
aaronlerner1948@gmail.com

The links between microorganisms/viruses and autoimmunity are complex and multidirectional. A huge number of studies demonstrated the triggering impact of microbes and viruses as the major environmental factors on the autoimmune and inflammatory diseases. However, growing evidences suggest that infectious agents can also play a protective role or even abrogate these processes. This protective crosstalk between microbes/viruses and us might represent a mutual beneficial equilibrium relationship between two cohabiting ecosystems. The protective pathways might involve post-translational modification of proteins, decreased intestinal permeability, Th1 to Th2 immune shift, induction of apoptosis, auto-aggressive cells relocation from the target organ, immunosuppressive extracellular vesicles and down regulation of auto-reactive cells by the microbial derived proteins. Our analysis demonstrates that the interaction of the microorganisms/viruses and celiac disease (CD) is always a set of multidirectional processes. A deeper inquiry into the CD interplay with Herpes viruses and *Helicobacter pylori* demonstrates that the role of these infections, suggested to be potential CD protectors, is not as controversial as for the other infectious agents. The outcome of these interactions might be due to a balance between these multidirectional processes.

Keywords: celiac disease, bacteria, viruses, gut, microbiome, environmental inducer, environmental protectors

INTRODUCTION

Infection and Autoimmunity

The relationship between infections and autoimmunity is complex. Microbial and viral infections might act as environmental triggers inducing or propagating autoimmune and inflammatory processes, resulting in symptomatic presentation of a disease in genetically high risk individuals (Lerner, 2015; Arleevskaya et al., 2017). An autoimmune disease onset following an infectious agent exposure has been well-documented (Pordeus et al., 2008; Bogdanos et al., 2015; Sakkas and Bogdanos, 2016). At least, for CD, the following infections were suggested to be associated with the disease: viruses: enterovirus, Epstein-Barr virus (EBV), Cytomegalovirus (CMV), hepatitis C virus (HCV), hepatitis B virus (HBV), and rotavirus, microbes: Bacteroides species, *Campylobacter jejuni*, Pneumococcus, *Mycobacterium tuberculosis*, and *Helicobacter pylori* (Lerner, 2015). However, recent serological evidence suggests the opposite outcome, which is the protection against autoimmune conditions following bacterial/viral exposure (Christen and von Herrath, 2005). At least the suggestive protector agents for CD were CMV, EBV, Rubella, and Herpes simplex type 1 virus (HSV1) when compared to healthy people (Plot and Amital, 2009; Jansen et al., 2016). According to the "hygiene hypothesis," the excessively sterile environment leads to the enhanced incidence of autoimmune disorders, asthma, and allergies, thus, associating surge of CD incidence with decreased infectious environment (Lerner et al., 2015b,e; Bloomfield et al., 2016).

Celiac Disease

Celiac disease is a life-long autoimmune disease (Lerner et al., 1996) mainly of the proximal intestine, affecting genetically predisposed individuals. Gluten, the storage protein of wheat, is the environmental inducer of the disease in addition to other structurally related molecules found in barley, rye, and oat (Lerner, 2014). Many environmental factors were suggested to induce or enhance the disease: multiple infections (Lerner and Reif, 2015), early infections (Myléus et al., 2012), early gastrointestinal infections (Beyerlein et al., 2017), lack of breast feeding (Lerner and Matthias, 2016c), time and amount of gluten consumption (Chmielewska et al., 2015), microbiome/dysbiome repertoire (Lerner et al., 2015a; Lerner and Matthias, 2017a,b), mode of delivery (Decker et al., 2011), early vaccination (Kemppainen et al., 2017) or early consumption of antibiotics (Canova et al., 2014) and geo-epidemiological influences (Lerner, 1994, 2015; Reif and Lerner, 2004b; Lerner and Matthias, 2015a). The abnormal immune response is directed, in particular, against tissue transglutaminase (tTG), representing the autoantigen, (Reif and Lerner, 2004a; Lerner et al., 2015c) and the two main autoantibodies, anti-endomysium and anti-tTG antibodies, are the most prevalent serological markers used to screen for the condition (Shamir et al., 2002; Lerner and Matthias, 2015d). Recently, the list of CD serological markers was expanded by two additional autoantibodies: anti-deamidated gliadin peptide and anti- tTG neo-epitope antibodies, found to be reliable for CD diagnosis (Rozenberg et al., 2012; Lerner and Blank, 2014; Lerner et al., 2015e). As yet, HLA-DQ2 and HLA-DQ8 are known predisposing genetic factors. The sequential events in disease progression were unraveled in the last years and gave rise to multiple future therapeutic strategies (Lerner, 2010). Notably, its epidemiological, incidental, and clinical presentation are changing continuously, and new clinical pictures are reported and expand the abundance of clinical variance of the disease (Lerner et al., 2015d). In fact, age of disease onset increases and the traditional enteric presentation is more and more replaced by extraintestinal manifestations. Skin (Lerner et al., 2015d), endocrine (Lerner and Matthias, 2016d; Lerner et al., 2017), hepatic (Anania et al., 2015), metabolic (Eliyah Livshits et al., 2017), skeletal (Lerner and Matthias, 2016a), rheumatic (Lerner and Matthias, 2015b), geriatric (Lerner and Matthias, 2015c), hematological (Branski et al., 1992), neurological (Zelnik et al., 2004; Lerner et al., 2012), gynecological and infertility (Mårild et al., 2012; Casella et al., 2016), oral and dental (Cantekin et al., 2015), hypercoagulability (Lerner and Blank, 2014), cardiac (Lerner et al., 2015d), and behavioral abnormalities (Zelnik et al., 2004) are often described. Those epidemiological and clinical changes can explain why the disease is diagnosed during the whole human life-span including in the elderly (Lerner and Matthias, 2015c). There is no doubt that in the last decades its incidence is constantly increasing, ranging between 1 and 3% nowadays (Lerner, 2014; Lerner et al., 2015b). The present review will concentrate, expand and update on the multiple faces of the inductive/protective roles that infectious agents might play in CD pathogenesis. This aspect is further interesting since pathogens are the major drivers of human selective genetic adaptation during evolution (Vatsiou et al., 2016), and the question of microbes that are bugging the celiac patient "are they friends or foes?" is the subject of the current review.

Infections and CD

It should be clarified that, although the trigger role of microorganisms and viruses in the CD development was undoubtedly traced in numerous investigations, it substantially differs from other immune pathogenesis like rheumatoid arthritis (as a classic model of an autoimmune disease; Arleevskaya et al., 2016; Kemppainen et al., 2017).

The induction of rheumatoid arthritis most likely occurs under the influence of the burden of many trivial infections, influencing the patient's immune system due to the frequent and prolonged infectious episodes (Arleevskaya et al., 2014). Individuals at CD risk apparently do not have such features in their mucosal immunity, nor significant defects in systemic anti-infective protection, impacting infection susceptibility. Since all the CD studies are focused only on the disease link with various gastrointestinal infections, such association is different from what was shown in rheumatoid arthritis (Riddle et al., 2012).

The number of infectious agents related to CD is continuously increasing (**Figure 1**). Examples for viruses enterovirus, EBV, Cytomegalovirus (CMV), HCV, HBV, and rotavirus And for

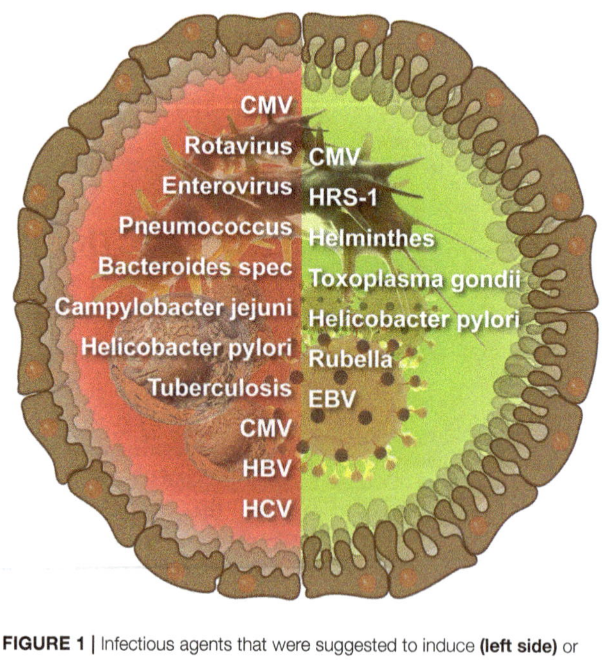

FIGURE 1 | Infectious agents that were suggested to induce **(left side)** or protect against **(right side)** intestinal celiac disease.

microbes *Bacteroides* species, *C. jejuni*, *Pneumococcus*, *M. tuberculosis*, and *H. pylori* (Lerner, 2015). However, links between CD and infections were more associative and less causative, thus, far from being elucidated. Moreover, the mutually exclusive hypotheses about the provocative and protective role of a particular microorganism/virus in CD pathogenesis were suggested and discussed in various publications.

It appears that the essential condition for the CD induction is a gastrointestinal infection (Kemppainen et al., 2017). Apparently, the other major condition is an early childhood—namely immature gastrointestinal tract, immature immune system, and gastrointestinal microbiome at the early phase of formation. The beginning of gut colonization by microorganisms set the stage for the cross talks between the epithelium, enteric lymphoid tissue, and microflora, all together establishing the intestinal barrier and as a consequence, a strictly dosed delivery of macromolecules into the internal environment and shaping of mucosal tolerance to food antigens and normal flora (Makarova et al., 2014).

So, in the vulnerable infant period any gastrointestinal infection, even a transitory one, is potentially able to disturb these processes of gut microbiome maturation and the establishment of local immunity and immune tolerance, including that against food and microbial antigens. Apparently, deleterious coincidence of these circumstances leads to an error in the negative selection of gluten-reactive lymphocyte clones.

Thus, the community of microorganisms, being extremely vulnerable during the ripening period, appears to be an inert system in adults. For example, in adults it needs no more than 30–60 days to restore gut microflora after the exposure to antibiotics (Spanhaak et al., 1998; Tannock et al., 2000). At the same time, a weekly clindamycin treatment of a newborn reduces Bacteroides diversity for the next 2 years (Jernberg et al., 2007). The same infections, capable of altering the fate of a sick infant, are merely a light ripples on the ocean surface for an adult microbiome.

In conclusion, there is an undoubted link between CD development and microorganisms, and this link looks to be rather specific. Gastrointestinal infections in predisposed infants with an immature gastrointestinal tract and immune system might shape gut microbiome in the immature and therefore labile circumstances. Such an unfortunate combination could trigger early CD development or becomes a ticking time bomb, represented by the structural features of the gut microbiome and persistence of gluten-reactive lymphocyte clones with latent basal cell proliferation without overt disruptive inflammatory activation.

GUT MICROBIOME SIGNATURE IN CELIAC DISEASE

Gut microbiome analysis in the healthy adult human populations revealed about 1150 bacterial species, the majority (50–75%) being represented by Firmicutes, and then Bacteroidetes (10–50%), Actinobacteria (1–10%), with fewer than 1% being Proteobacteria (Manichanh et al., 2012). Apparently, the HLA system, to a certain extent, shapes microbiome structure. Besides, polymorphisms of some other non-HLA genes were found to correlate with a certain microbiome structure (Spor et al., 2011). Interestingly, in addition to the HLA system, microbiome composition may be due to CD-associated polymorphisms of defensin, some molecules of Toll-like receptor signaling pathways and vitamin D receptor genes (San-Pedro et al., 2005; Fernandez-Jimenez et al., 2010; Wang et al., 2016). Whole genome study of 93 individuals and 16S rRNA gene pyrosequencing of their body microflora revealed 83 alliances between genetic variance in host sequence and plethora of specific microbial taxa (Blekhman et al., 2015). In particular, the links with CD-associated host genes were revealed. In addition to the host genes related to immunity, a link was found between the microbiome composition and SNP of the genes not related to immunity. For example, the authors revealed an interesting correlation between the abundance of Bifidobacterium in the gastrointestinal tract and host genetic variation in LCT gene, encoding the lactase enzyme hydrolyzing dietary lactose. This gene SNPs are known to be associated with lactose intolerance, which is frequently associated with celiac disease (Ojetti et al., 2005). Bifidobacterium is able to metabolize lactose, and there are some strains preferring lactose instead of glucose. The authors suggested that the problems with individual's consumption of milk products might impact the richness of Bifidobacterium in the gastrointestinal tract.

The results of gut microbiome structure investigations in the infants at CD risk as well as in the therapy-naïve patients at the disease onset are somewhat contradictory. Besides the bulk of the results was obtained by study of feces, while the principal for CD microbe community in the small intestine boundary layers has its own peculiarities, although in a certain extent it is associated with fecal microbes. However, a certain tendency can be traced. A single and rather limited study of mucosa-associated microbiota in the proximal gut—using enteric samples from 45 children with CD and 18 clinical controls born during the "Swedish CD epidemic"—demonstrated only marginally differences between the groups. Enrichment with Clostridium, Prevotella, and Actinomyces was revealed in the most of the CD samples (Ou et al., 2009). Feces studies demonstrated, that infants genetically predisposed to CD, had significantly higher abundance of Firmicutes (Clostridium) and Proteobacteria (Escherichia/Shigella) and desreased proportions of Actinobacteria (Bifidobacterium) and Bacteroidetes compared to low-risk infants (Sellitto et al., 2012; Olivares et al., 2015). In a proof of concept study, Sellitto and co-workers have traced the longitudinal changes in the microbial populations colonizing from birth to 24 months in 30 genetically predisposed infants. They demonstrated that even at 2 years of age their microbiota do not resemble that of adults, while in not at-risk infants the maturation was complete at 1 year of age. The group was divided into an early and a late gluten exposure groups (17 and 13 infants, respectively). The authors showed that genetically susceptible infants may benefit from delayed gluten exposure not before 12 months of age. A hypothesis was forwarded that lack of maturity of the enteric microbiota faced with early gluten consumption can induce or accelerate the autoimmunogenetic process. Not less interesting was the infant's metabolome. When solid food was introduced at 6 months of age, succinate, acetate, propionate, and butyrate accumulated in their stools. However, by 2 years of age, butyrate, and acetate were the dominant short-chain fatty acids (SCFA). Since bacteroidetes are associated most strongly with propionate, while Firmicuters are negatively correlated to SCFAs production (Koenig et al., 2011), Sellitto's group envisioned that the high Firmicutes and low Bactriodetes abundance in CD infants results in down production of those protective SCFAs, thereby abrogating enteric health and predisposing them to autoimmune diseases. The decrease in *Lactobacillus* spp. associated with lower lactate production, observed in between 6 and 12 months of age, accompanied by decreased SCFAs' feces repertoire, during a vulnerable time of mucosal immune maturation and microbiome compositional changes might lead to loss of tolerance to non-self-antigens like gluten in those CD genetically predisposed infants (Sellitto et al., 2012). Once again it points to the important relations connecting nutrition to microbiome composition and diversity, its metabolome and the local maturation and functioning of the immune system.

From this perspective, it is interesting to compare the composition of the gut flora in infants at CD risk and premature babies with a priori immature gut. Arboleya and coauthors compared the gradual establishment of the intestinal microbiome in very-low birth-weight preterm infants with that of healthy full-term, vaginally born, breast-fed neonates using 16S rRNA gene profiling and quantitative PCR for the various microbial taxa. It was demonstrated that preterm neonates sheltered a higher relative proportion of Firmicutes at 2 days of age, and of Proteobacteria in the later sampling times, compared to control babies. Prematurity reflected reduced levels of Bacteroidetes at day 2 and as well as in later sampling times together with Actinobacteria (Arboleya et al., 2016). In addition, very-low birth-weight preterm infants frequently displayed a lag in establishing an adult microbiota compared to full-term children (Weng and Walker, 2013). So, the parallels to the peculiarities of the gut flora in CD prone individuals seem to be obvious. Combining the results of Arboleya et al. and Sellitto et al. about the enteric mucosal immaturity and the unbalanced microbiome found early in life and in CD high-risk infants, it can be suggested that by ingesting gluten peptides, the disease will progress in these individuals, unlike in non-CD high-risk premature infants, that will never develop CD. The features of CD gut microbiome, incorporated in early childhood seem to persist in the adulthood even despite gluten withdrawal (Nistal et al., 2012; Wacklin et al., 2014).

Caminero and co-workers demonstrated that gluten amounts in feces of healthy volunteers, CD patients and individuals under risk receiving gluten-free or normal diet depended on gluten intake. The greatest amount of gluten was found in fecal samples from healthy volunteers being on normal diet, with a significant decrease in the untreated CD patients and the individuals under risk. It is noteworthy that in all the groups fecal peptidase activity against the gluten-derived peptide 33-mer inversely correlated with gluten amount in the samples (Caminero et al., 2015). It looks like the increased functional proteolytic activity of gut microflora in CD patients can affect gluten excretion. The same research group isolated 144 strains belonging to 35 microbial species that might be involved in gluten digestion in the human intestine. Most of the strains were part of the phyla Firmicutes and Actinobacteria, mainly from the genera Lactobacillus, Streptococcus, Staphylococcus, Clostridium and Bifidobacterium (Caminero et al., 2014). Ninety-four of these strains were capable to metabolize gluten, 61 of them showed an extracellular proteolytic activity of gluten proteins, and several strains showed a peptidase activity toward the "supra-molecule" 33-mer peptide, the luminal immunogenic molecule in CD patients (Caminero et al., 2014). At the end of the day, there is a certain difference in gluten proteolysis by various bacteria, and the immunogenicity of the generated peptide fragments might be different. It should be noted that these studies were carried out in cultures, in which the glutenase activity of aggregate microbial community as a whole (biofilm) in the gut boundary layer might significantly differ from the isolated activity of the individual members of this community.

It is known that the microbiome impact gastrointestinal and systemic functions by its metabolome, the most studied one being the short chain fatty acids (SCFA). Most recently, the topic of nutrition, microbiome, and SCFA associations in CD was updated (Lerner et al., 2016). Multiple beneficial effects to the host were attributed to them. Changes in microbiota and their SCFA production is clearly related to the pathogenesis of CD. Interestingly, peculiar dysbiosis and significant changes in stool SCFA profile were described in several autoimmune diseases, one of those is in Behcet's disease where decreased butyrate production was suggested to play a role in its pathogenesis (Consolandi et al., 2015).

Taken together, the microbiota/dysbiota disbalance may present a risk factor for CD either directly by influencing the mucosal immune responses or by intensifying inflammatory responses to gluten. In contrary, several microbial species are capable to break down gliadin and perhaps therefore decrease the immunopathogenicity of consumed gliadin (Sjöberg et al., 2013; Carding et al., 2015; Lerner and Matthias, 2015a; Rostami-Nejad et al., 2015).

COEXISTENCE OF CERTAIN INFECTIONS AND CD: A CRITICAL LOOK AT THE ISSUE

It is of interest how CD affected individuals survived in the presence of harmful conditions (increased gluten content and toxicity in wheat, increased gluten consumption worldwide; Lerner et al., 2017) and despite them, thrived and expanded? (Lerner, 2011; Lerner et al., 2015b). Despite being underprivileged with nutritional deficiencies, failure to thrive and high morbidity and mortality, a substantial increase in the disease incidence is observed in the last decades. There are several theories explaining this paradox. One is positive evolutionary selection, in which the celiac patient accumulates protective genes (Lerner, 2011). The other is due to some pathogens which are the major drivers of human selective genetic adaptation (Vatsiou et al., 2016) that could have been beneficial environmental factors, protecting the CD populations. Indeed, in contrast to the observations that infections may induce CD, some infection agents were assumed to have a protective impact (Christen and von Herrath, 2005; Gaisford and Cooke, 2009; Kivity et al., 2009; Plot et al., 2009).

This assumption was based in particular on a lower incidence of the serum antibodies against Cytomegalovirus (CMV), EBV, and Rubella in CD patients when compared to healthy people (Plot and Amital, 2009). Another argument for the protective effect is the inverse correlation between serum anti-CMV, -EBV, and/or -Herpes simplex type 1 virus (HSV1) IgG levels and anti-tTG antibodies (Jansen et al., 2016).

Viruses

It should be specified that Jansen and coauthors determined the antiviral antibody levels in the sera samples of 6-year old children (Jansen et al., 2016). CMV single infection and combined CMV, EBV, and/or herpes simplex virus type 1 infection antibodies were inversely associated with strongly tTg-IgA positivity. The authors suggested that the serological profile may indicate a protective effect of herpesvirus infections in the pathogenesis of celiac disease autoimmunity. It is accepted that by this age IgG and IgM production is close to that of the adults. However, the immune system is still immature and its reaction is not fully functional at this age even in healthy children, whereas the immune system of CD prone children, at least, the local immune defense, is somewhat delayed in the maturation. Thus, Jansen et al. suggested explanation should be taken with a grain of salt.

In Plot's publication, the age profile of the studied cohorts was not presented (Plot and Amital, 2009). There are some curious details in this publication which need to be interpreted. First, while the prevalence of the anti-EBV capsid antigen and anti-EBV nuclear antigen IgG in the CD patients was significantly lower than that in the controls, the prevalence of the anti-EBV early antigen IgG was comparable in the two groups and the prevalence of anti-EBV capsid antigen IgM, though unreliably, was more than twice higher in the CD group. In general, the anti-EBV capsid antigen IgMs are known to be produced during the acute phase (the first days—6 months from the onset of the disease) or during acute exacerbation of chronic EBV infection (http://www.tiensmed.ru/news/epstein-barr-bc1.html#nov1). In addition, if the anti-EBV early antigen IgG is not concurrently revealed, it may indicate incubation period or the very beginning of the infection (up to 1 week of symptoms). So, either in the CD patients this generally latent infection is apt to more frequent exacerbations, or, given the reduced frequency of the studied IgG antiviral antibodies, the existence of some features of the antiviral antibody production in CD can be assumed. Secondly, revealed by PCR, CMV DNA presence in the samples is not always accompanied by the presence of serum specific antibodies. This situation is typical in particular for the infants with immature immune system (Dong et al., 2004, 2005).

A number of publications on the HBV vaccine non-responsiveness in CD might attest for possible unique features of the antiviral antibody response formation (Noh et al., 2003; Park et al., 2007; Urganci and Kalyoncu, 2013), further criticizing the assumption that decrease antibodies activities in CD patients represent a protective effect.

As for the inverse correlation of the antiviral and anti-tTG antibodies demonstrated by Jansen et al. (2016), similar patterns are not uncommon in autoimmune diseases, and this fact by no means demonstrates a lesser exposure to the infections. For example, high levels of autoantibodies against double-stranded DNA, reflecting the activity and severity of systemic lupus erythematosus, are quite often combined with lower levels of antibodies to particular bacterial DNA (Pisetsky and Drayton, 1997). The inverse correlation of those indexes is usually explained by a distorted immune humoral response.

Additionally, it should be specified that, in general, in Herpesvirus infections and viral hepatitis the specific antibodies are not the principal players in the antiviral defense but are accepted to be the reliable serological markers for an infection (Grinde, 2013). It is advisable to note that caution should be used for the interpretation of the protective role of these infections in CD, relying only on data on the incidence of the corresponding antibodies.

As for Rubella infection, the specific antibodies are the major antiviral response players. However, the incidence of CD in children vaccinated with inactivated rubella virus as part of polio vaccine was close to that in the unvaccinated children (Myléus et al., 2012). Thus, a reduced incidence of the anti-rubella IgG antibodies demonstrated by Plot and co-workers can mean an equally probable lower exposure of CD patients to Rubella and the above-discussed features of the specific IgG antibody production. Moreover, since the antiviral immune response is always multi-componental, the disturbed antibody formation, although being a weak link of an antiviral defense, does not necessarily entail an increased susceptibility to Rubella.

The data which might testify for the direct and reverse links of CD to Herpes virus infection are summarized in **Table 1**. The analysis of the data demonstrates that the links of CD and herpes infections are multi-directional. On one hand there are some peculiarities, which can promote the viral infecting: (1) CD-associated DQA1*0501/DQB1*0201 genotype, which is also due to the imperfect response against Herpes viral infection; (2) the typical CD immature gastro—intestinal tract and the delayed process of microbiome maturation, which might be risk factors for the virus infecting; (3) the typical CD mucosal overexpression of epidermal growth factor receptors, by which Herpes viruses enter the cells; (4) increased expression of IL-33, suppressing local antiviral immunity in CD patients. On the other hand, the increased levels of several humoral factors with the antiviral activity; increased expression of some cytokines, which promote mucosa maturation and thus increase its' resistance to the viruses; as well as some potential features of CD microbiome that might indicate a backward link between CD and Herpes viral infection. The protective effect of the infection on atopic manifestations was demonstrated in the case of the early (infancy or early childhood) EBV exposure, while the later infection predisposes to the atopic disease (Nilsson et al., 2005, 2009). So, if to extrapolate the data on the links of herpes and atopic diseases to CD, it is likely that the early (infancy or early childhood) EBV exposure might play a protective role, while the later infection might trigger CD or have no impact on it at all.

TABLE 1 | Direct (⇑⇑) and reverse (⇑⇓) links of CD and Herpes virus infections.

⇑⇑	⇑⇓
Markedly impaired binding and presentation of some herpes antigens to the TCRs in CD-associated DQA1*0501/DQB1*0201 carriers (Koelle et al., 1997; Reichstetter et al., 1999) might be due to the imperfect antiviral immune response as well as to the peculiarities of antibody production.	–
Increased HSV2, CMV and EBV DNA levels in the stool samples were observed among premature neonates with intrauterine growth restriction compared with those infants born appropriate for gestational age (Naing et al., 2013). The immature gastro–intestinal tract and the delayed process of microbiome maturation might be the typical signs of CD (Sellitto et al., 2012), that might be risk factors for the virus infecting in infancy as well as for the higher rates of the clinical manifestations of the infection.	Virus-shaped cytokine levels might to some extent promote the maturation of the local immune system and intestinal tissues, lagging behind in the CD-prone individuals: IL-6 promotes enterocyte differentiation and inhibits enterocyte apoptosis, TNF-alpha promotes intestinal growth (Rollwagen et al., 1998; Maheshwari, 2004), IFN-gamma increases macromolecular transport in the immature gut particularly across Peyer's patches. This Peyer's patch-targeted effect can be important for setting mucosal immune responses against dietary antigens early in life and aiding their immune exclusion (Sütas et al., 1997).
Herpes viruses were revealed in the inflamed gastrointestinal tract mucosa, but never in the endoscopically healthy tissue (Ramanathan et al., 2000; Roblin et al., 2011). It is unclear whether the inflamed mucosa is a consequence of the viral infection or the inflamed tissues "draw" viruses, due to the expressing of the corresponding receptors. Epidermal growth factor receptors, by which Herpes viruses enter the cells are overexpressed in CD gut mucosa, that being due to gliadin stimulatory effect (Barone et al., 2007; Juuti-Uusitalo et al., 2009).	In CD the level of various humoral factors with a pronounced diverse direct and indirect antiviral activity in the inflamed intestinal tissues are increased (defensins, IFN-gamma, IFN-alpha, TNF-alpha, IL-6, IL-15 the latter being necessary for the development and function of NK/NKT cells and maintenance of naive and memory CD8(+) T cells; (Forsberg et al., 2004; Hazrati et al., 2006; Di Sabatino et al., 2007; Brottveit et al., 2013; Meresse et al., 2015)), that might have a protective effect on the infection.
Microbiome features might impact antiviral immunity via stimulation of IL-33 (alarmin) released by mucosal epithelium, which suppresses local antiviral immunity by blocking the migration of effector T cells to mucosa, thereby inhibiting the production of IFN-γ, a critical cytokine for antiviral defense, at local infection sites (Oh et al., 2016). Serum levels and intestinal tissue expression of IL-33 and its receptor in CD patients were found to be increased (López-Casado et al., 2015).	Pre-treatment of HeLa monolayer with inactivated *Staphylococcus aureus* cells before HSV infection increases expression of TNF-a, IL-6, and IL-8 genes, that being due to the protection from the occurrence of virus mediated cytopathic effect and to decrease of viral multiplication rate (Bleotu et al., 2015). Vaginal Lactobacillus strains neutralize lactic acid and thus, acidic pH values needed for the viral replication, as well as to macrophage activation (Conti et al., 2009; Khani et al., 2012). Microbiota might impact the antiviral defense via regulation of the natural killer T cells at the frontiers of the mucosal immune system (Zeissig and Blumberg, 2014). So, certain shifts in the structure of the microbiome mighty inhibit viral infection.

Helicobacter pylori (Hp)

The permanent interest in CD and Hp infection coexistence is quite natural, due to the gut-stomach axis (Lerner and Matthias, 2016b). The infectious inflammatory process directly in the gastrointestinal tract—CD epicenter, which might shape the local immune system and microbiota, might obviously play a role in CD pathogenesis. In addition, both CD and Hp infection in a number of cases are associated with the diffuse lymphocytic gastroenteropathy (Lynch et al., 1995; Broide et al., 2007; Pai, 2014). However, diffuse lymphocytic gastroenteropathy is far from being obligatory attributed only to both entities (Wu and Hamilton, 1999; Nielsen et al., 2014). Besides, lymphocytic gastritis and a subsequently villous atrophy are accepted to be a non-specific manifestation of many pathological conditions in the gastrointestinal tract, due to a wide variety of infectious, immunologic or any inflammatory stimuli raising intraepithelial lymphocyte numbers. Lymphocytic duodenitis and increased intraepithelial lymphocytosis are known to be associated with diseases that are completely different in their pathogenesis, such as autoimmune disorders like CD (Broide et al., 2007; Rostami et al., 2010), tropical sprue, food protein intolerance, Hp-induced duodenitis, peptic duodenitis, parasitic, and viral infections, intestinal lymphoma (Chang et al., 2005; Brown et al., 2006; Pallav et al., 2012; Rosinach et al., 2012; Shmidt et al., 2014) drugs' induced duodenitis (non-steroidal anti-inflammatory drug; Shmidt et al., 2014) and small-intestine bacterial overgrowth (Lappinga et al., 2010). The differential diagnosis of lymphocytic gastritis is not less restricted. CD and HP are not the only ones. Various non-HP infections, inflammatory conditions and several non-celiac autoimmune diseases were described (Broide et al., 2007; Polydorides, 2014).

The interest in the CD—HP infection link is fueled by the well-known data, indicating that childhood infection with HP could protect against the development of Crohn's disease, severe gastric-reflux disease, Barrett's esophagus and esophagus adenocarcinoma (Chen and Blaser, 2008). Yet, as for the protective role of Hp in CD, the available data are limited and quite contradictory. The prevalence of CD among Hp-positive adults was 0.05% compared with 0.09% among Hp-negative individuals (statistically non-significant) while the prevalence of Crohn's disease among Hp-positive patients was 0.07% compared with 0.24% among Hp-negative patients (Bartels et al., 2016). Based on these data, at least in adults, the protective effect of Hp on CD is minimal, if at all existing. However, given the fact that in childhood gastrointestinal infection appears to be a more important condition for CD triggering than in adults, this conclusion is not necessarily true in the case of early exposure to Hp (Kemppainen et al., 2017). Unfortunately, we failed to find the similar data on the CD frequency in children infected with Hp early in life.

The incidences of Hp and CD worldwide vary enormously (9–100%, 0.3–3.9%, respectively; Rostami-Nejad et al., 2016). Most of the studies aimed to determine the ratio of Hp infected individuals in CD and non-CD control groups. In our opinion, this study design gives less information about the inductive/protective effect of Hp infection on the CD development as on the susceptibility of the CD patients for the infection. The results of various studies on Hp both in children and adults are contradictory (**Table 2**). The spread in the ratios of both Hp infected CD patients and non-CD controls in these publications might be due to the national and age-related characteristics of the studied cohorts (Eusebi et al., 2014). As for the diametrically opposed regularities of HP incidence in CD and non-CD groups, a meticulously analysis of these publications, did not lead us to any reason for the conflicting results, but to the possible differences in the poorly described clinical characteristics of the controls. In these studies, the authors examined the collections of endoscopically obtained biopsies and sera allocating the cases into CD and non-CD (control) groups. It is obvious that the persons accepted as controls underwent the relevant examination because they had any gastroenterological problems associated or not associated with HP infection.

The analysis of the literature data which might testify the direct and reverse links of CD and Hp infection (**Table 3**) shows that the interaction of the two diseases represents an interweaving of differently directed processes. Perhaps the end result might depend on the balance of these processes, being deeply individual in each specific case. Important is the assumption that the direct or reverse CD/HP link may depend on the age at which the encounter with the bacterium occurred. At least, it is important for allergies–Hp links. Our attempt to test this hypothesis failed, because the literary data accumulated to the present moment are largely insufficient.

POTENTIAL MECHANISMS FOR BENEFICIAL BUGS' EFFECTS IN CELIAC GUT

Multiple potential pathophysiological avenues were suggested to understand the microbial-gut cross-talks in CD.

Post-translational Modification of Protein (PTMP) from Non-self- to Self-proteins

Endogenous and microbial enzymes are capable to generate intestinal enzymatic neo-antigens via PTMP. The modifications taking place in the intestinal lumen include peptides crosslinking, de/amination/deamidation by the transglutaminases, de/phosphorylation, a/deacetylation, de/tyrosination, and many other enzymatic modifications exist (Lerner et al., 2016). Related to the present topic, the human endogenous intestinal enzymes, tTG and its family member, the exogenous microbial transglutaminases, induce multiple neo-epitopes on the TG-gliadin cross-linked complex resulting in the formation of antibodies against the complexes in CD. CD is a classical disease where luminal PTMP is driving the disease. It seems logical that a microbial agent might modify non-self-peptide to self-one—reducing its immunogenicity. Additionally, in CD, some microbe strains might modify gluten in the lumen, thus preventing or aggravating the inflammatory cascade and the intestinal damage progression via PTMP (Caminero et al., 2016).

Horizontal Gene Transfer in the Human Gut Lumen

Given the extensive influence of the microbiota on human health, the gut-microbiome integrity is of prime importance for host health and survival. In this regards, our bodies' "second genome" cohabit with the human one to form a stable equilibrium for the two kingdom's long term survival. As opposed to long-term evolutionary events, newer genetic manipulations with microorganisms, plants, animals, or nutrients, applying new food technologies and/or microbial engineered delivery systems or novel mode of therapies are rapidly evolving.

Due to the close relationship and intimate cross-talks between the human and the gut's biospheres, consumption of the modified genetic cargo into the human intestinal ecosystem might occur. It was hypothesized that modern probiotic ingestion, genetically manipulated food consumption and genetically manipulated microorganism usage are potential genetic driving forces for changing the evolutionary equilibrium established during the last millions of years (Cho and Blaser, 2012). Horizontal gene exchange is the ability to transfer genetic material between contacting biological domains, including eukaryote (plants, animals, and man), prokaryote (microbes), and viruses (Aminov, 2011; Ruggiero et al., 2015). Despite not being investigated in CD, various virulent genes, the most studied one is the antibiotic resistance gene, were described to be laterally transferred. It is hypothesized that the opposite might occur. This infectious genetic cargo might include anti-inflammatory/pro-apoptotic/Treg or other immune-modulatory genes, attenuating or abrogating autoimmunity.

Infections as Tight Junction Closure Enhancers

The tight junction protein, Zonulin, is involved in the regulation of the intestinal permeability between gut epithelial cells. Several clinical trials with Zonulin antagonist (Larazotide acetate, AT-1001, Alba Therapeutics, USA) demonstrated the promising therapeutic effect in CD (Lerner, 2010; Khaleghi et al., 2016). Larazotide acetate—an octa-peptide derived from a cholera toxin ZO, antagonizing zonulin via receptor blockade—is aimed to decrease the paracellular transport caused by gluten and thus to suppress the activation of the pathological immune cascade. In addition to the above mentioned cholera toxin derivative, many other factors produced by microorganisms can improve tight junction performance, modulating intestinal permeability. *Salmonella enterica serovar*, *Escherichia coli*, and *C. jejuni* modulated enteric epithelial barrier functions in chickens (Awad et al., 2012, 2014, 2015), and the probiotics *Lactobacillus casei* DN-114001 and *E. coli* strain Nissle 1917 decreased intestinal epithelium permeability in human intestinal originated cell lines (Parassol et al., 2005; Zyrek et al., 2007; Trebichavsky et al., 2010).

TABLE 2 | The incidence of *Helicobacter pylori* infection (Hp-positive, %) in CD patients and non-CD controls.

Age characteristics of groups	Hp-positive CD patients, %	Hp-positive non-CD controls, %	References
Adults	36%	41%	Simondi et al., 2015
	86% (82% untreated, 95% treated)	97%	Diamanti et al., 1999
	20.7% (Untreated) 32.4% (treated)	55.3%	Ciacci et al., 2000
	Frequency increased with age in groups.		
	12.5%	30%	Lasa et al., 2015
Children (age, years)	21.8% (Median 8.2 years)	23.8% (Median 8.9 years)	Aydogdu et al., 2008
	18.5% (Median6.8 years)	17.3% (Median6.8 years)	Luzza et al., 1999
	5.4% (3–12 years)	6.8% (3–12 years)	Jozefczuk et al., 2015
	30.6 (<18 years)	33.8% (<18 years)	Guz-Mark et al., 2014
	2.7% (Median5.7 years)	15.6% (Median7.4 years)	Nenna et al., 2012
	11.4% (1–18 years)	50% (1–18 years)	Narang et al., 2016

Taken together, modulation of gut permeability by infectious agent, counteracting the breached tight junction integrity in CD, might represent a protective pathway.

Molecular Mimicry between Infectious Agents and Self-antigens

Generally, molecular mimicry between foreign (infectious/environmental) and self-antigens is a well-described pathway of autoimmune disease induction. Recently, it was suggested that antigen mimicry between foreign and self-antigens might be due to the long-term regulation of inflammation (Pontes-de-Carvalho et al., 2013). In a cohort of African patients, infected with *Schistosoma* it was found that the parasite inhibited production of anti-nuclear antibodies (Mutapi et al., 2011). More recently, apparent effectiveness of rotavirus vaccination was found to prevent the onset of CD autoimmunity (Silvester and Leffler, 2016). This finding gives indirect evidence for the persistence of regulatory cells in the lack of stimulation of the immune system by pathogen-derived processes. The strength of the immune adjustment, however, may increase with the uninterrupted presence of the pathogen or its antigens. Thus, molecular mimicry can represent a protective mechanism of autoimmunity.

Th2 to Th1 Shift

Inflammation, given rise by microbes, viruses and especially by parasites such as helminths, can shift the Th1 pathway to Th2 one, resulting in a more immunosuppressive state where regulatory T cells might be induced or be activated (Shor et al., 2013). Recent studies have supplied such an evidence for pathogen-specific regulatory cells in *Leishmania major*, Herpes simplex virus, and Friend retrovirus (murine leukemia virus) infections (Christen and von Herrath, 2005). During the acute phase of the infection this Th2 profile counter-regulates Th1-driven autoimmune pathologies. Along the chronic stage of infection, immune-regulatory networks arise, mainly led by regulatory T cells. These cells produce IL-10 and TGFβ, which has observative effect on Th1-related autoimmune diseases, such type 1 diabetes mellitus or CD. In fact, several helminths were tried in CD patients with encouraging results (Croese et al., 2015). Treatment with helminthes or helminthes ova ameliorated the clinical pictures of several autoimmune conditions in patients as well as in animal models (Smallwood et al., 2017). A major recent contribution to the field is the helminth phosphorylcholine proved to be an immunemodulatory molecule. Most recently, tuftsin-phosphorylcholine, a novel helminth-based compound was shown to reduce pro-inflammatory cytokine production and induced anti-inflammatory cytokine expression and Treg and Breg cell expansion in mouse models of rheumatoid arthritis, lupus nephritis, and colitis (Bashi et al., 2015b, 2016; Shor et al., 2015).

It is conceivable, that the ability of helminthic parasites to attenuate host immune responses into an anti-inflammatory/regulatory phenotype is attributed to the endogenous component that the parasites secrete and/or excrete interacting with immune effector cells to regulate their function (Lund et al., 2014; Selmi, 2016).

An additional mechanism was suggested for the helminth's immunomodulation of autoimmunity, in addition to the Th1 to Th2 shift. Accelerated T and B regulatory phenotypes, decreased levels of the inflammatory cytokines like IFNγ and Il-17 or vice versa, promoting IL-4, IL-10, and TGF-β release (Bashi et al., 2015a). Since CD is a Th1 profile disease, shifting the immune pathway to Th2 profile might reduce the intestinal damage (Lerner, 2010).

Immune Activation Induced Cell Death

Inflammation can cause a substantial hyperactivation of auto-aggressive lymphocytes, leading to activation-induced cell death and attenuate the systemic load of aggressive T cells. It seems that repeated encounter with powerful antigenic stimuli leading to restriction of an immune response is well-established in viral infections, where the primary response undergoes a major restriction after antigen elimination. EBV, HBV, and CMV infections are some of the examples. Similarly, administration of mycobacterial products, such as bacilli *Calmette-Guérin*, prevented the onset and recurrence of type 1 diabetes mellitus in NOD mice by inducing apoptosis

TABLE 3 | Direct (⇑⇑), reverse (⇑⇓) or no (⊗) links of CD and Hp infection.

	⇑⇑	⇑⇓ or ⊗
Clinic	The cases of fresh HP infection in the CD patients and the reports of CD onset right after the carried *H. pylori* infection both in children and adults were described (Cârdei et al., 2003; Villanacci et al., 2006).	The milder CD forms were found to be more prevalent in HP-positive adults (Villanacci et al., 2006). The data, received in children are contradictory (Guz-Mark et al., 2014; Narang et al., 2016). On a gluten free diet the normalization of the duodenal mucosa was independent of presence/absence of HP both in adults and children (Bardella et al., 2007; Aydogdu et al., 2008).
Genetic	DQA1*03:01 was found to be often in both CD and HP-positive duodenal ulcer patients (Azuma et al., 1995; Mubarak et al., 2013). TNF-308 (G > A) SNP increases risk of CD and persistent HPinfection (Khan et al., 2016). The−336G CD209 allele[#] associated with a higher HP infection severity/susceptibility might be involved in CD susceptibility in HLA-DQ2 negative patients. (Núñez et al., 2006).	DQA1*0201 allele associated with the high CD risk was significantly rarer in the HP-positive duodenal ulcer patients than in the HP-negative controls (Azuma et al., 1995; Lionetti et al., 2014). HLA-DRB1*0301 and DRB1*07 associated with high CD risk in some ethnic groups are involved in the of some HPproteins recognition and in subsequent activation of gastric T cells within the framework of antiinfective immune response (Bilbao et al., 2002; talová et al., 2002; Bergman et al., 2005).
Gastrointestinal functions	Hp infection leads to the abnormal gut permeability, due to increased production of pro-inflammatory cytokines (Caron et al., 2015). At that the subjects with latent CD have an abnormal permeability (Peña and Crusius, 1998; Sapone et al., 2011) The abnormal mucosal permeability increases the gluten availability for the gluten-specific lymphocyte clones in the Peyer's Plaques.	CD patients were found to have high basal and stimulated acid-forming function, while a comfortable microenvironment for HPincludeыhypochlorhydria (Il'chenko et al., 1991; Savarino et al., 1999; Krums et al., 2011; Harris et al., 2013). Indeed, HPcan only survive for minutes in the stomach lumen (pH of 1–2) and must quickly migrate to the gastric epithelial surface (Schreiber et al., 2005).
Innate immune	–	Hpcolonizes the gastric mucosa by adhering to the mucous epithelial cells via the fucosylated blood group antigens H-type 1 and Leb (Magalhães and Reis, 2010). In principle, the typical for CD immaturity of the gastrointestinal tractincludes weak functions of the mucosal barrier and a lack of bacteria colonization (Forchielli and Walker, 2005). However, single publications indicated no features of the glycocalyx/mucous layer carbohydrate structures in CD (Toft-Hansen et al., 2013).
	The inflammatory cells in the Hpinfection in epithelium and lamina propria express inducible NO-synthase with excess free radicals due to the alterations and exacerbation of inflammation with impaired regeneration processes (Cherdantseva et al., 2014). The similar events occur after gluten exposure in the gastrointestinal mucosa of gluten-sensitive patients, being due to the in injury of the small-intestinal tissue (Holmgren Peterson et al., 1998; Niveloni et al., 2000).	Increased tissues concentration of nitric oxide metabolites in CD might have a protective effect against Hp (Gobert and Wilson, 2016). At the same time Hp uses diverse strategies to promote its survival. All Hpstrains encode proteins important for detoxifying reactive oxygen species and its arginase limits NO production by macrophage-, neutrophil- and epithelial cell-derived nitric oxide synthase (Salama et al., 2013). So, the passing suppression of CD- caused inflammation by Hp is quite possible. Defensins' levels are increased in CD mucosa (Vordenbäumen et al., 2010). During Hp infections, these cationic peptides with antimicrobial properties play a pivotal role in the innate immune responses and are able to eradicate the bacteria (Pero et al., 2017). It should be noted that according to some data, HP strains were resistant to these factors (Nuding et al., 2013).
	Hp induces apoptosis of gastric epithelial cells directly and via modulation TRAIL-mediated apoptosis signaling (Tsai and Hsu, 2010). This effect might contribute to epithelial apoptosis and villous atrophy—CD hallmark (Shalimar et al., 2013).	In Hp positive CD patients a significantly lower prevalence of atrophic gastritis was observed when compared with Hp negative ones (Santarelli et al., 2006). That might be due to the expression of several DNA repair proteins in the inflamed tissue accumulating damaged host DNA (Salama et al., 2013). On the other hand, Hp can gain a foothold in gastrointestinal tract only in the mild CD cases. It is in line with the data, demonstrating the higher inflammation in correlation with lower bacterial upload (Salama et al., 2013).
	Proinflammatory cytokine production in the framework of anti Hp immune reaction might be due to CD triggering (Crabtree, 1996).	Increased local levels of proinflammatory cytokines in CD might have a protective effect against the fresh Hp infection (Eiró et al., 2012; Di Sabatino et al., 2016).
	Gastroduodenal response to chronic Hp infection include IL-8secretion, that being due to neutrophil migration and activation (Crabtree, 1996). These events might trigger CD, as the cells play important role in CD pathogenesis (Lammers et al., 2015).	The increased infiltration by activated neutrophil was demonstrated in CD mucosa (Hällgren et al., 1989). That might have a protective effect while HPexposure.

(Continued)

TABLE 3 | Continued

	⇑⇑	⇑⇓ or ⊗
Adaptive immunity	After the challenge of 4-weeks aged (infants) and 6-weeks aged (adults) mice with HP strain T-cell activation in the gastric samples was demonstrated including the pathways for pro-inflammatory molecules (nitric oxide, iNOS), this effect increased over time (Kienesberger et al., 2016).	Hp re-programs dendritic cells playing a crucial role in Hp recognition toward a tolerance-promoting phenotype; HP-exposed DCs fail to induce effector T-cell responses of the Th1 and Th17 type *in vitro* and *in vivo*; instead, they preferentially induce the expression of the Treg-specific transcription factor FoxP3, the surface marker CD25 and the anti-inflammatory cytokine IL-10 in naive T-cells (Salama et al., 2013). The role of this effect in protection from protection against allergies, asthma and inflammatory bowel diseases, was demonstrated (Oertli and Müller, 2012). Besides, at least two virulence factors are known to inhibit human T-cells. VacAvia β2 integrin reception inhibits T-cell proliferation and prevents nuclear translocation of the T-cell transcription factor NF-AT and its subsequent transactivation of T-cell-specific immune response genes. The other virulence determinant—γ-glutamyl-transpeptidase blocks proliferation of T-cells (Salama et al., 2013). As the interaction of the virulent molecules with T-cells is non-specific, a bystander gluten-specific T-cell repression is quite possible. It's a purely speculativehypothesis. No one research was published on this issue.
Microbiome	Lactobacillus species (*Lactobacillus johnsonii*, Lactobacillus murinus, *Lactobacillus reuteri*) were able to inhibit Hpgrowth *in vitro* (Zaman et al., 2014; Delgado et al., 2015). *Streptococcus mitis*, a commensal microorganism of the human stomach, was found to inhibit Hpgrowth and to drive its conversion from a spiral to a coccoidal form (Khosravi et al., 2014). Just the same Lactobacillus and Streptococcus species appeared to be ability to degrade and remove gluten derivatives (Fernandez-Feo et al., 2013; Duar et al., 2015). The impact of these coincidences on both CD and Hp infection remain unclear because (1) the studies of activities were carried using cultivated and then isolated microbes, whereas the glutenase activity of aggregate microbial community as a whole (biofilm) in gut boundary layer may significantly differ from the isolated activity of the individual members of this community; (2) the immunogenicity of the generated peptide fragments might be different that might be due to the opposite effect on CD.	

#CD209 is a dendritic and macrophage surface molecule involved in pathogen recognition and immune activation, Hp infection in particular (Bergman et al., 2006; Núñez et al., 2006). It was found to be overexpressed in the Hp infected gastric epithelial cells and to mediate Th1 differentiation, which may be involved in gastric mucosal injury (Wu et al., 2014).

of autoreactive T cells (Christen and von Herrath, 2005). In view of the fact that viruses are inducers of immune cells apoptosis while sparing the Treg cells (Che et al., 2015) and apoptosis is enhanced in CD (Shalimar et al., 2013), it is suggested that viruses, by abrogating immune activation, might attenuate intestinal autoimmune progression in CD.

Infection at Another Location might Keep Auto-Aggressive Cells from Reaching the Site of Autoimmune Destruction

As suggested by Christen (Christen and von Herrath, 2005), an infectious inflammation elsewhere in the body might keep auto-aggressive cells from arriving into the sites of autoimmune destruction, that might be due to the abrogation of type 1 diabetes in NOD mice after LCMV infection. The authors suggested that this occurred because the "abrogative" virus grew predominantly in peripheral lymphoid organs and other sites rather than the pancreas or its islets themselves. Thus, the sites of severe inflammation might act as a filter for auto-aggressive T cells removing them from the circuit and depriving them from homing the pancreatic islets. Similar scenarios might operate where infection with B. coxsackievirus or *Salmomella typhi murium* protected against autoimmunity (Tracy et al., 2002; Raine et al., 2006).

Immunosuppression by Extracellular Vesicles

Release of extracellular vesicles is a natural phenomenon of almost all cell types. They derive either from multivesicular bodies or from the cellular plasma membrane. Those vesicles contain a subset of cell derived proteins, lipids, including nucleic acids. Extracellular vesicles regulate immune responses against pathogens, as well as autoimmunity. It is suggested that these suppressive vesicles would prevent peripheral self-antigens and commonly encountered foreign antigens from causing chronic inflammation and autoimmunity. Following this lines, it is hypothesized that various infectious agents can induce those regulatory extracellular vesicles, counteracting autoimmune pathways, playing a protective anti-autoimmune role (Robbins and Morelli, 2014; Robbins et al., 2016).

Infectious Agents' Secretion of Anti-Autoreactive T Cells Proteins

Infections with helminths can prevent or attenuate auto-inflammatory/immune diseases. In addition to their Th1 to Th2 shift, most recently, Helminth secreted proteins were shown to prevent autoimmunity. The excretory/secretory products of Fasciola hepatica contain immune-modulatory molecules that arbitrate protection from autoimmune diabetes via the activation and provision of a regulatory immune environment (Lund et al., 2014). Such a mechanism was not studied in CD, but might explain the new potential therapeutic strategy to treat CD with *Necator Americanus* larvae (Croese et al., 2015; Giacomin et al., 2015).

CONCLUSIONS

The cross-talks between infections and autoimmunity are complex (**Figure 1**). Most of the data indicate that microbes and viruses are major environmental factors in autoimmunity induction. However, growing evidences conversely suggest that infectious agent can abrogate or protect against autoimmunity. This protective evolutionary cross-talks between microbes/viruses and us might represent a mutual beneficial equilibrium relationship between two cohabiting ecosystems. The protective pathways might involve PTMP, decreased intestinal permeability, Th1 to Th2 immune shift, induction of inflammatory immune cell apoptosis, auto-aggressive cells relocation from the target organ, immunosuppressive extracellular vesicles and anti-autoreactive cell immune-regulatory proteins.

Yet, our analysis demonstrates that the interaction of the microorganisms /viruses and CD is always a set of multi-directional processes. With a detailed consideration of possible mechanisms of CD and CMV, EBV, Herpes simplex type 1, Rubella, *H. pylori*, it can be assumed that the role of these infections suggested to be potential CD protectors infections, is not so unambiguous positive and the outcome of this interactions might be due to a balance between these multi-directional processes. In summary, there are more publications on the inducer role of infections in CD, and the few ones advocating the protective role should be further explored. The present review expend on several avenues that can be studied to understand the protective cross-talks between infectious agents and CD. Apprehending them can potentially suggest new therapeutic strategies for CD.

AUTHOR CONTRIBUTIONS

AL: designed, wrote, edited, submitted, MA: designed, wrote, AS: literature search, revised, reviewed, TM: literature search, edited, and revised.

ACKNOWLEDGMENTS

The authors thank Mr. Alf Neu for the artistic design of the figure.

REFERENCES

Aminov, R. (2011). Horizontal gene exchange in environmental microbiota. *Front. Microbiol.* 2:158. doi: 10.3389/fmicb.2011.00158

Anania, C., De Luca, E., De Castro, G., Chiesa, C., and Pacifico, L. (2015). Liver involvement in pediatric celiac disease. *World J. Gastroenterol.* 21, 5813–5822. doi: 10.3748/wjg.v21.i19.5813

Arboleya, S., Sánchez, B., Solís, G., Fernández, N., Suárez, M., Hernández-Barranco, A. M., et al. (2016). Impact of prematurity and perinatal antibiotics on the developing intestinal microbiota: a functional inference study. *Int. J. Mol. Sci.* 17:E649. doi: 10.3390/ijms17050649

Arleevskaya, M. I., Gabdoulkhakova, A. G., Filina, Y. V., Miftakhova, R. R., Bredberg, A., and Tsybulkin, A. P. (2014). A transient peak of infections during onset of rheumatoid arthritis: a 10-year prospective cohort study. *BMJ Open* 4:e005254. doi: 10.1136/bmjopen-2014-005254

Arleevskaya, M. I., Kravtsova, O. A., Lemerle, J., Renaudineau, Y., and Tsibulkin, A. P. (2016). How rheumatoid arthritis can result from provocation of the immune system by microorganisms and viruses. *Front. Microbiol.* 7:1296. doi: 10.3389/fmicb.2016.01296

Arleevskaya, M. I., Manukyan, G., Inoue, R., and Aminov, R. (2017). Editorial: Microbial and environmental factors in autoimmune and inflammatory diseases. *Front. Immunol.* 8:243. doi: 10.3389/fimmu.2017.00243

Awad, W. A., Aschenbach, J. R., Khayal, B., Hess, C., and Hess, M. (2012). Intestinal epithelial responses to *Salmonella enterica serovar Enteritidis*: effects on intestinal permeability and ion transport. *Poult Sci.* 91, 2949–2957. doi: 10.3382/ps.2012-02448

Awad, W. A., Hess, C., Khayal, B., Aschenbach, J. R., and Hess, M. (2014). *In vitro* exposure to *Escherichia coli* decreases ion conductance in the jejunal epithelium of broiler chickens. *PLoS ONE* 9:e92156. doi: 10.1371/journal.pone.0092156

Awad, W. A., Molnár, A., Aschenbach, J. R., Ghareeb, K., Khayal, B., Hess, C., et al. (2015). Campylobacter infection in chickens modulates the intestinal epithelial barrier function. *Innate Immun.* 21, 151–160. doi: 10.1177/1753425914521648

Aydogdu, S., Cakir, M., Yuksekkaya, H. A., Tumgor, G., Baran, M., and Arikan, C. (2008). *Helicobacter pylori* infection in children with celiac disease. *Scand. J. Gastroenterol.* 43, 1088–1093. doi: 10.1080/00365520802101846

Azuma, T., Ito, Y., Miyaji, H., Dojyo, M., Tanaka, Y., Hirai, M., et al. (1995). Immunogenetic analysis of the human leukocyte antigen DQA1 locus in patients with duodenal ulcer or chronic atrophic gastritis harbouring *Helicobacter pylori*. *Eur. J. Gastroenterol. Hepatol.* 7(Suppl. 1), S71–S73.

Bardella, M. T., Velio, P., Cesana, B. M., Prampolini, L., Casella, G., Di Bella, C., et al. (2007). Coeliac disease: a histological follow-up study. *Histopathology* 50, 465–471. doi: 10.1111/j.1365-2559.2007.02621.x

Barone, M. V., Gimigliano, A., Castoria, G., Paolella, G., Maurano, F., Paparo, F., et al. (2007). Growth factor-like activity of gliadin, an alimentary protein: implications for coeliac disease. *Gut* 56, 480–488. doi: 10.1136/gut.2005.086637

Bartels, L. E., Jepsen, P., Christensen, L. A., Gerdes, L. U., Vilstrup, H., and Dahlerup, J. F. (2016). Diagnosis of *Helicobacter Pylori* infection is associated with lower prevalence and subsequent incidence of Crohn's Disease. *J. Crohns Colitis* 10, 443–448. doi: 10.1093/ecco-jcc/jjv229

Bashi, T., Bizzaro, G., Ben-Ami Shor, D., and Blank, M., Shoenfeld, Y. (2015a). The mechanisms behind helminth's immunomodulation in autoimmunity. *Autoimmun. Rev.* 14, 98–104. doi: 10.1016/j.autrev.2014.10.004

Bashi, T., Blank, M., Ben-Ami Shor, B. A., Fridkin, M., Gendelman, O., Versini, M., et al. (2015b). Successful modulation of murine lupus nephritis with tuftsin-phosphorylcholine. *J. Autoimmun.* 59, 1–7. doi: 10.1016/j.jaut.2015.3.001

Bashi, T., Shovman, O., Fridkin, M., Volkov, A., Barshack, I., Blank, M., et al. (2016). Novel therapeutic compound tuftsin-phosphorylcholine attenuates collagen-induced arthritis. *Clin. Exp. Immunol.* 184, 19–28. doi: 10.1111/cei.12745

Bergman, M. P., Vandenbroucke-Grauls, C. M., Appelmelk, B. J., D'Elios, M. M., Amedei, A., Azzurri, A., et al. (2005). The story so far: *Helicobacter pylori* and gastric autoimmunity. *Int. Rev. Immunol.* 24, 63–91. doi: 10.1080/08830180590884648

Bergman, M., Del Prete, G., van Kooyk, Y., and Appelmelk, B. (2006). *Helicobacter pylori* phase variation, immune modulation and gastric autoimmunity. *Nat. Rev. Microbiol.* 4, 151–159. doi: 10.1038/nrmicro1344

Beyerlein, A., Donnachie, E., and Ziegler, A. -G. (2017). Infections in early life and development of celiac disease. *Am. J. Epidemiol.* doi: 10.1093/aje/kwx190. [Epub ahead of print].

Bilbao, J. R., Martín-Pagola, A., Vitoria, J. C., Zubillaga, P., Ortiz, L., and Castaño, L. (2002). HLA-DRB1 and MHC class 1 chain-related A haplotypes in Basque families with celiac disease. *Tissue Antigens* 60, 71–76. doi: 10.1034/j.1399-0039.2002.600109.x

Blekhman, R., Goodrich, J. K., Huang, K., Sun, Q., Bukowski, R., Bell, J. T., et al. (2015). Host genetic variation impacts microbiome composition across human body sites. *Genome Biol.* 16:191. doi: 10.1186/s13059-015-0759-1

Bleotu, C., Chifiriuc, M. C., Lazăr, V., Drăguşel, R., and Matei, L., Aldea, I. M., et al. (2015). Influence of *Staphylococcus aureus* attachment to the herpes simplex virus infected cells. *Rom. J. Morphol. Embryol.* 56, 433–437.

Bloomfield, S. F., Rook, G. A., Scott, E. A., Shanahan, F., Stanwell-Smith, R., and Turner, P. (2016). Time to abandon the hygiene hypothesis: new perspectives on allergic disease, the human microbiome, infectious disease prevention and the role of targeted hygiene. *Perspect. Public Health.* 136, 213–224. doi: 10.1177/1757913916650225

Bogdanos, D. P., Smyk, D. S., Rigopoulou, E. I., Sakkas, L. I., and Shoenfeld, Y. (2015). Infectomics and autoinfectomics: a tool to study infectious-induced autoimmunity. *Lupus* 24, 364–373. doi: 10.1177/0961203314559088

Branski, D., Ashkenazy, A., Frier, S., and Lerner, A. (1992). "Extra intestinal manifestation and associated disorders of celiac disease," in *Gluten-Sensitive Enteropathy, Front Gastrointest Res*, eds D. Branski, P. Rozen, and M. F. Kaganoff (Basel: Karger), 164–175.

Broide, E., Sandbank, J., Habler, L., Scapa, E., Kimchi, N. A., Shapiro, M., et al. (2007). The immunohistochemistry profile of lymphocytic gastritis in celiac disease and *Helicobacter pylori* infection- Interplay between infection and inflammation. *Mediators Inflamm.* 2007:81838. doi: 10.1155/2007/81838

Brottveit, M., Beitnes, A. C., Tollefsen, S., Bratlie, J. E., Jahnsen, F. L., Johansen, F. E., et al. (2013). Mucosal cytokine response after short-term gluten challenge in celiac disease and non-celiac gluten sensitivity. *Am. J. Gastroenterol.* 108, 842–850. doi: 10.1038/ajg.2013.91

Brown, I., Mino-Kenudson, M., Deshpande, V., and Lauwers, G. Y. (2006). Intraepithelial lymphocytosis in architecturally preserved proximal small intestinal mucosa: an increasing diagnostic problem with a wide differential diagnosis. *Arch. Pathol. Lab. Med.* 130, 1020–1025. doi: 10.1043/1543-2165(2006)130[1020:]ILIAPP2.0.CO;2

Caminero, A., Galipeau, H. J., McCarville, J. L., Johnston, C. W., Bernier, S. P., Russell, A. K., et al. (2016). Duodenal bacteria from patients with celiac disease and healthy subjects distinctly affect gluten breakdown and immunogenicity. *Gastroenterology* 151, 670–683. doi: 10.1053/j.gastro.2016.06.041

Caminero, A., Herrán, A. R., Nistal, E., Pérez-Andrés, J., Vaquero, L., Vivas, S., et al. (2014). Diversity of the cultivable human gut microbiome involved in gluten metabolism: isolation of microorganisms with potential interest for coeliac disease. *FEMS Microbiol. Ecol.* 88, 309–319. doi: 10.1111/1574-6941.12295

Caminero, A., Nistal, E., Herrán, A. R., Pérez-Andrés, J., Ferrero, M. A., Vaquero Ayala, L., et al. (2015). Differences in gluten metabolism among healthy volunteers, coeliac disease patients and first-degree relatives. *Br. J. Nutr.* 114, 1157–1167. doi: 10.1017/S0007114515002767

Canova, C., Zabeo, V., Pitter, G., Romor, P., Baldovin, T., Zanotti, R., et al. (2014). Association of maternal education, early infections, and antibiotic use with celiac disease: a population-based birth cohort study in northeastern Italy. *Am. J. Epidemiol.* 180, 76–85. doi: 10.1093/aje/kwu101

Cantekin, K., Arslan, D., and Delikan, E. (2015). Presence and distribution of dental enamel defects, recurrent aphthous lesions and dental caries in children with celiac disease. *Pak. J. Med. Sci.* 31, 606–609. doi: 10.12669/pjms.313.6960

Cârdei, E., Moraru, D., Trandafir, L., Bozomitu, L., and Mihăilă, D. (2003). Celiac disease associated with *Helicobacter pylori* infection. *Rev. Med. Chir. Soc. Med. Nat. Iasi.* 107, 633–635.

Carding, S., Verbeke, K., Vipond, D. T., Corfe, B. M., and Owen, L. J. (2015). Dysbiosis of the gut microbiota in disease. *Microb. Ecol. Health Dis.* 26:26191. doi: 10.3402/mehd.v26.26191

Caron, T. J., Scott, K. E., Fox, J. G., and Hagen, S. J. (2015). Tight junction disruption: *Helicobacter pylori* and dysregulation of the gastric mucosal barrier. *World, J. Gastroenterol.* 21, 11411–11427. doi: 10.3748/wjg.v21.i40.11411

Casella, G., Orfanotti, G., Giacomantonio, L., Bella, C. D., Crisafulli, V., Villanacci, V., et al. (2016). Celiac disease and obstetrical-gynecological contribution. *Gastroenterol. Hepatol. Bed Bench.* 9, 241–249.

Chang, F., Mahadeva, U., and Deere, H. (2005). Pathological and clinical significance of increased intraepithelial lymphocytes (IELs) in small bowel mucosa. *APMIS* 113, 385–399. doi: 10.1111/j.1600-0463.2005.apm_204.x

Che, J. W., Kraft, A. R., Selin, L. K., and Welsh, R. M. (2015). Regulatory T cells resist virus infection-induced apoptosis. *J. Virol.* 89, 2112–2120. doi: 10.1128/JVI.02245-14

Chen, Y., and Blaser, M. J. (2008). *Helicobacter pylori* colonization is inversely associated with childhood asthma. *J. Infect. Dis.* 198, 553–560. doi: 10.1086/590158

Cherdantseva, L. A., Potapova, O. V., Sharkova, T. V., Belyaeva, Y. Y., and Shkurupiy, V. A. (2014). Association of *Helicobacter pylori* and iNOS production by macrophages and lymphocytes in the gastric mucosa in chronic gastritis. *J. Immunol. Res.* 2014:762514. doi: 10.1155/2014/762514

Chmielewska, A., Pieścik-Lech, M., Szajewska, H., and Shamir, R. (2015). Primary prevention of celiac disease: environmental factors with a focus on early nutrition. *Ann. Nutr. Metab.* 67, 43–50. doi: 10.1159/000440992

Cho, I., and Blaser, M. J. (2012). The human microbiome: at the interface of health and disease. *Nat. Rev. Genet.* 13, 260–270. doi: 10.1038/nrg3182

Christen, U., and von Herrath, M. G. (2005). Infections and autoimmunity—good or bad? *J. Immunol.* 174, 7481–7486. doi: 10.4049/jimmunol.174.12.7481

Ciacci, C., Squillante, A., Rendina, D., Limauro, S., Bencivenga, C., Labanca, F., et al. (2000). *Helicobacter pylori* infection and peptic disease in coeliac disease. *Eur. J. Gastroenterol. Hepatol.* 12, 1283–1287. doi: 10.1097/00042737-200012120-00004

Consolandi, C., Turroni, S., Emmi, G., Severgnini, M., Fiori, J., Peano, C., et al. (2015). Behçet's syndrome patients exhibit specific microbiome signature. *Autoimmun. Rev.* 14, 269–276. doi: 10.1016/j.autrev.2014.11.009

Conti, C., Malacrino, C., and Mastromarino, P. (2009). Inhibition of herpes simplex virus type 2 by vaginal lactobacilli. *J. Physiol. Pharmacol.* 60(Suppl. 6), 19–26.

Crabtree, J. E. (1996). Immune and inflammatory responses to *Helicobacter pylori* infection. *Scand. J. Gastroenterol. Suppl.* 215, 3–10. doi: 10.3109/00365529609094526

Croese, J., Giacomin, P., Navarro, S., Clouston, A., McCann, L., Dougall, A., et al. (2015). Experimental hookworm infection and gluten microchallenge promote tolerance in celiac disease. *J. Allergy Clin. Immunol.* 135, 508–516. doi: 10.1016/j.jaci.2014.07.022

Decker, E., Hornef, M., and Stockinger, S. (2011). Cesarean delivery is associated with celiac disease but not inflammatory bowel disease in children. *Gut Microbes.* 2:91–98. doi: 10.4161/gmic.2.2.15414

Delgado, S., Leite, A. M., Ruas-Madiedo, P., and Mayo, B. (2015). Probiotic and technological properties of *Lactobacillus* spp. strains from the human stomach in the search for potential candidates against gastric microbial dysbiosis. *Front. Microbiol.* 5:766. doi: 10.3389/fmicb.2014.00766

Di Sabatino, A., Giuffrida, P., Fornasa, G., Salvatore, C., Vanoli, A., Naviglio, S., et al. (2016). Innate and adaptive immunity in self-reported nonceliac gluten sensitivity versus celiac disease. *Dig. Liver Dis.* 48, 745–752. doi: 10.1016/j.dld.2016.03.024

Di Sabatino, A., Pickard, K. M., Gordon, J. N., Salvati, V., Mazzarella, G., Beattie, R. M., et al. (2007). Evidence for the role of interferon-alfa production by dendritic cells in the Th1 response in celiac disease. *Gastroenterology* 133, 1175–1187. doi: 10.1053/j.gastro.2007.08.018

Diamanti, A., Maino, C., Niveloni, S., Pedreira, S., Vazquez, H., Smecuol, E., et al. (1999). Characterization of gastric mucosal lesions in patients with celiac disease: a prospective controlled study. *Am. J. Gastroenterol.* 94, 1313–1319. doi: 10.1111/j.1572-0241.1999.01082.x

Dong, G. P., Shang, S. Q., Du, L. Z., Yu, X. L., Xu, Y. P., and Wu, X. J. (2004). Detection of four human herpesviruses DNA and virus-specific IgM antibody in blood specimens of infants. *Zhonghua Er Ke Za Zhi* 42, 367–370.

Dong, G., Shang, S., Liang, L., and Yu, X. (2005). Determination of the six major human herpesviruses in cerebrospinal fluid and blood specimens of children. *Acta Paediatr.* 94, 38–43. doi: 10.1080/08035250410022477

Duar, R. M., Clark, K. J., Patil, P. B., Hernández, C., Brüning, S., Burkey, T. E., et al. (2015). Identification and characterization of intestinal lactobacilli strains capable of degrading immunotoxic peptides present in gluten. *Appl. Microbiol.* 118, 515–527. doi: 10.1111/jam.12687

Eiró, N., González-Reyes, S., González, L., González, L. O., Altadill, A., Andicoechea, A., et al. (2012). Duodenal expression of Toll-like receptors and interleukins are increased in both children and adultceliac patients. *Dig. Dis. Sci.* 57, 2278–2285. doi: 10.1007/s10620-012-2184-6

Eliyah Livshits, O., Shaoul, R., Reifen, R., Matthias, T., and Lerner, A. (2017). Can celiac disease present along with childhood obesity? *Int. J. Celiac Dis.* 5, 19–23. doi: 10.12691/ijcd-5-1-7

Eusebi, L. H., Zagari, R. M., and Bazzoli, F. (2014). Epidemiology of *Helicobacter pylori* infection. *Helicobacter* 19(Suppl. 1), 1–5. doi: 10.1111/hel.12165

Fernandez-Feo, M., Wei, G., Blumenkranz, G., Dewhirst, F. E., Schuppan, D., Oppenheim, F. G., et al. (2013). The cultivable human oral gluten-degrading microbiome and its potential implications in coeliac disease and gluten sensitivity. *Clin. Microbiol. Infect.* 19, E386–E394. doi: 10.1111/1469-0691.12249

Fernandez-Jimenez, N., Castellanos-Rubio, A., Plaza-Izurieta, L., Gutierrez, G., Castaño, L., Vitoria, J. C., et al. (2010). Analysis of beta-defensin and Toll-like receptor gene copy number variation in celiac disease. *Hum. Immunol.* 71, 833–836. doi: 10.1016/j.humimm.2010.05.012

Forchielli, M. L., and Walker, W. A. (2005). The effect of protective nutrients on mucosal defense in the immature intestine. *Acta Paediatr. Suppl.* 94, 74–83. doi: 10.1080/08035320510043592

Forsberg, G., Fahlgren, A., Hörstedt, P., Hammarström, S., Hernell, O., and Hammarström, M. L. (2004). Presence of bacteria and innate immunity of intestinal epithelium in childhood celiac disease. *Am. J. Gastroenterol.* 99, 894–904. doi: 10.1111/j.1572-0241.2004.04157.x

Gaisford, W., and Cooke, A. (2009). Can infections protect against autoimmunity? *Curr. Opin. Rheumatol.* 21, 391–396. doi: 10.1097/BOR.0b013e32832c2dee

Giacomin, P., Zakrzewski, M., Croese, J., Su, X., Sotillo, J., McCann, L., et al. (2015). Experimental hookworm infection and escalating gluten challenges are associated with increased microbial richness in celiac subjects. *Sci. Rep.* 5:13797. doi: 10.1038/srep13797

Gobert, A. P., and Wilson, K. T. (2016). The immune battle against *Helicobacter pylori* infection: NO offense. *Trends Microbiol.* 24, 366–376. doi: 10.1016/j.tim.2016.02.005

Grinde, B. (2013). Latency and reactivation - viral strategies and host response. *J. Oral. Microbiol.* 5, 1–9. doi: 10.3402/jom.v5i0.22766

Guz-Mark, A., Zevit, N., Morgenstern, S., and Shamir, R. (2014). Duodenal intraepithelial lymphocytosis is common in children without coeliac disease, and is not meaningfully influenced by *Helicobacter pylori* infection. *Aliment. Pharmacol. Ther.* 39, 1314–1320. doi: 10.1111/apt.12739

Hällgren, R., Colombel, J. F., Dahl, R., Fredens, K., Kruse, A., Jacobsen, N. O., et al. (1989). Neutrophil and eosinophil involvement of the small bowel in patients with celiac disease and Crohn's disease: studies on the secretion rate and immunohistochemical localization of granulocyte granule constituents. *Am. J. Med.* 86, 56–64. doi: 10.1016/0002-9343(89)90230-1

Harris, P. R., Serrano, C. A., Villagrán, A., Walker, M. M., Thomson, M., Duarte, I., et al. (2013). *Helicobacter pylori*-associated hypochlorhydria in children, and development of iron deficiency. *J. Clin. Pathol.* 66, 343–347. doi: 10.1136/jclinpath-2012-201243

Hazrati, E., Galen, B., Lu, W., Wang, W., Ouyang, Y., Keller, M. J., et al. (2006). Human alpha- and beta-defensins block multiple steps in herpes simplex virus infection. *J. Immunol.* 177, 8658–8666. doi: 10.4049/jimmunol.177.12.8658

Holmgren Peterson, K., Fälth-Magnusson, K., Magnusson, K. E., Stenhammar, L., and Sundqvist, T. (1998). Children with celiac disease express inducible nitric oxide synthase in the small intestine during gluten challenge. *Scand. J. Gastroenterol.* 33, 939–943. doi: 10.1080/003655298750026958

Il'chenko, A. A., Korshunova, V. M., Aruin, L. I., Zhukhovitskiĭ, V. G., Dugasheva, L. G., and Radakova, E. D. (1991). The intestinal microflora and acid-forming function of the stomach in peptic ulcer patients with *Helicobacter pylori* bacteriosis. *Z. Mikrobiol. Epidemiol. Immunobiol.* 10, 17–19.

Jansen, M. A., van den Heuvel, D., van der Zwet, K. V., Jaddoe, V. W., Hofman, A., Escher, J. C., et al. (2016). Herpesvirus infections and transglutaminase type 2 antibody positivity in childhood: the generation R study. *J. Pediatr. Gastroenterol. Nutr.* 63, 423–430. doi: 10.1097/MPG.0000000000001163

Jernberg, C., Lofmark, S., and Edlund, C., Jansson, J. K. (2007). Long-term ecological impacts of antibiotic administration on the human Intestinal microbiota. *ISME J.* 1, 56–66. doi: 10.1038/ismej.2007.3

Jozefczuk, J., Bancerz, B., Walkowiak, M., Glapa, A., Nowak, J., Piescikowska, J., et al. (2015). Prevalence of Helicobacter pylori infection in pediatric celiac disease. *Eur. Rev. Med. Pharmacol. Sci.* 19, 2031–2035.

Juuti-Uusitalo, K., Lindfors, K., Mäki, M., Patrikainen, M., Isola, J., and Kaukinen, K. (2009). Inhibition of epithelial growth factor receptor signalling does not preserve epithelial barrier function after *in vitro* gliadin insult. *Scand. J. Gastroenterol.* 44, 820–825. doi: 10.1080/00365520902898119

Kemppainen, K. M., Lynch, K. F., Liu, E., Lönnrot, M., Simell, V., Briese, T., et al. (2017). Factors that increase risk of celiac disease autoimmunity after a gastrointestinal infection in early life. *Clin. Gastroenterol. Hepatol.* 15, 694.e5–702.e5. doi: 10.1016/j.cgh.2016.10.033

Khaleghi, S., Ju, J. M., Lamba, A., and Murray, J. A. (2016). The potential utility of tight junction regulation in celiac disease: focus on larazotide acetate. *Ther. Adv. Gastroenterol.* 9, 37–49. doi: 10.1177/1756283X15616576

Khan, S., Mandal, R. K., Jawed, A., Wahid, M., Panda, A. K., Areeshi, M. Y., et al. (2016). TNF-α−308 G > A (rs1800629) Polymorphism is associated with celiac disease: a meta-analysis of 11 case-control studies. *Sci. Rep.* 6:32677. doi: 10.1038/srep32677

Khani, S., Motamedifar, M., Golmoghaddam, H., Hosseini, H. M., and Hashemizadeh, Z. (2012). *In vitro* study of the effect of a probiotic bacterium *Lactobacillus rhamnosus* against herpes simplex virus type 1. *Braz. J. Infect. Dis.* 16, 129–135. doi: 10.1016/S1413-8670(12)70293-3

Khosravi, Y., Dieye, Y., Loke, M. F., Goh, K. L., and Vadivelu, J. (2014). *Streptococcus mitis* induces conversion of *Helicobacter pylori* to coccoid cells during co-culture *in vitro*. *PLoS ONE* 9:e112214. doi: 10.1371/journal.pone.0112214

Kienesberger, S., Cox, L. M., Livanos, A., Zhang, X. S., Chung, J., Perez-Perez, G. I., et al. (2016). Gastric *Helicobacter pylori* infection affects local and distant microbial populations and host responses. *Cell. Rep.* 14, 1395–1407. doi: 10.1016/j.celrep.2016.01.017

Kivity, S., Agmon-Levin, N., Blank, M., and Shoenfeld, Y. (2009). Infections and autoimmunity–friends or foes? *Trends Immunol.* 30, 409–414. doi: 10.1016/j.it.2009.05.005

Koelle, D. M., Johnson, M. L., Ekstrom, A. N., Byers, P., and Kwok, W. W. (1997). Preferential presentation of herpes simplex virus T-cell antigen by HLA DQA1*0501/DQB1*0201 in comparison to HLA DQA1*0201/DQB1*0201. *Hum. Immunol.* 53, 195–205. doi: 10.1016/S0198-8859(97)00034-7

Koenig, J. E., Spor, A., Scalfone, N., Fricker, A. D., Stombaugh, J., Knight, R., et al. (2011). Succession of microbial consortia in the developing infant gut microbiome. *Proc. Natl. Acad. Sci. U.S.A.* 108 (Suppl. 1), 4578–4585. doi: 10.1073/pnas.1000081107

Kotalová, R., Vraná, M., Dobrovolná, M., Nevoral, J., and Loudová, M. (2002). [HLA-DRB1/DQA1/DQB1 alleles and haplotypes in Czech children with celiac sprue]. *Cas. Lek. Cesk.* 141, 518–522.

Krums, L. M., Sabel'nikova, E. A., and Parfenov, A. I. (2011). Functional condition of the stomach, pancreas, liver and gallbladder in celiac disease. *Ter. Arkh.* 83, 20–24.

Lammers, K. M., Chieppa, M., Liu, L., Liu, S., Omatsu, T., Janka-Junttila, M., et al. (2015). Gliadin induces neutrophil migration via engagement of the formyl peptide receptor, FPR1. *PLoS ONE* 10:e0138338. doi: 10.1371/journal.pone.0138338

Lappinga, P. J., Abraham, S. C., Murray, J. A., Vetter, E. A., Patel, R., and Wu, T. T. (2010). Small intestinal bacterial overgrowth: histopathologic features and clinical correlates in an underrecognized entity. *Arch Pathol. Lab Med.* 134, 264–270.

Lasa, J., Zubiaurre, I., Dima, G., Peralta, D., and Soifer, L. (2015). *HELICOBACTER PYLORI* PREVALENCE IN PATIENTS WITH CELIAC DISEASE: results from a cross-sectional study. *Arq. Gastroenterol.* 52, 139–142. doi: 10.1590/s0004-28032015000200012

Lerner, A. (1994). Factors affecting the clinical presentation and time diagnosis of celiac disease: The Jerusalem and the West Bank-Gaza experience (editorial). *Isr. J. Med. Sci.* 30, 294–295.

Lerner, A. (2010). New therapeutic strategies for celiac disease. *Autoimmun. Rev.* 9, 144–147. doi: 10.1016/j.autrev.2009.05.002

Lerner, A. (2011). The last two millennias eco-catastrophes are the driving forces for thepotential genetic advantage mechanisms in celiac disease. *Med. Hypotheses* 77, 773–776. doi: 10.1016/j.mehy.2011.07.034

Lerner, A. (2014). Serological diagnosis of celiac disease –moving beyond the tip of the iceberg. *Int. J. Celiac Dis.* 2, 64–66. doi: 10.12691/ijcd-2-2-8

Lerner, A. (2015). "Non nutritional environmental factors associated with celiac disease: infections and vaccinations," in *Vaccines and Autoimmunity*, eds Y. Shoenfeld, N. Agmon-Levin, and L. Tomljenovic (Hoboken, NJ: Wiley Blackwell), 301–306.

Lerner, A., Aminov, R., and Matthias, T. (2016). Dysbiosis may trigger autoimmune diseases via inappropriate posttranslational modification of host proteins. *Front. Microbiol.* 7:84. doi: 10.3389/fmicb.2016.00084

Lerner, A., and Blank, M. (2014). Hypercoagulability in celiac disease-an update. *Autoimmun. Rev.* 13, 1138–1141. doi: 10.1016/j.autrev.2014.07.004

Lerner, A., and Matthias, T. (2015a). Changes in intestinal tight junction permeability associated with industrial food additives explain the rising incidence of autoimmune disease. *Autoimmun. Rev.* 14, 479–489. doi: 10.1016/j.autrev.2015.01.009

Lerner, A., and Matthias, T. (2015b). Rheumatoid arthritis-celiac disease relationship: joints get that gut feeling. *Autoimmun. Rev.* 14, 1038–1047. doi: 10.1016/j.autrev.2015.07.007

Lerner, A., and Matthias, T. (2015c). Increased knowledge and awareness of celiac disease will benefit the elderly. *Int. J. Celiac Dis.* 3, 112–114. doi: 10.12691/ijcd-3-3-6

Lerner, A., and Matthias, T. (2015d). Editorial: Celiac disease: intestinal, heart and skin inter-connections. *Int. J. Celiac Dis.* 3, 28–30. doi: 10.12691/ijcd-3-1-6

Lerner, A., and Matthias, T. (2016a). Gut- bone cross talks and implications in celiac disease. *Int. J. Celiac Dis.* 4, 19–23. doi: 10.12691/ijcd-4-1-4

Lerner, A., and Matthias, T. (2016b). The gut-stomach axis: *Helicobacter pylori* and celiac disease. *Int. J. Celiac Dis.* 4, 77–79.

Lerner, A., and Matthias, T. (2016c). The jigsaw of breast feeding and celiac disease. *Int. J Celiac Dis.* 4, 87–89. doi: 10.12691/ijcd-3-3-4

Lerner, A., and Matthias, T. (2016d). Autoimmune thyroid diseases in celiac disease: if and when to screen? *Int. J Celiac Dis.* 4, 124–126. doi: 10.12691/ijcd-4-4-10

Lerner, A., and Matthias, T. (2017a). Extraintestinal manifestations of CD: common pathways in the gut-remote organs' axes. *Int. J. Celiac Dis.* 5, 24–27. doi: 10.12691/ijcd-5-1-5

Lerner, A., and Matthias, T. (2017b). Gluten free diet- tough alley in torrid time. *Int. J. Celiac Dis.* 5, 50–55. doi: 10.12691/ijcd-5-2-4

Lerner, A., and Reif, S. (2015). "Chapter 50: Nonnutritional environmental factors associated with Celiac disease: the infectome," in *Infections and Autoimmunity, 2nd Edn.*, eds Y. Shoenfeld, N. Agmon-Levine, and N. R. Rose (Amsterdam: Elsevier), 829–837.

Lerner, A., Blank, M., and Shoenfeld, Y. (1996). Celiac disease and autoimmunity. *Isr. J. Med. Sci.* 32, 33–36.

Lerner, A., Jeremias, P., and Matthias, T. (2015a). The world incidence and prevalence of autoimmune diseases is increasing: a review. *Int. J. Celiac Dis.* 3, 151–155. doi: 10.12691/ijcd-3-4-8

Lerner, A., Jeremias, P., and Matthias, T. (2017). The gut-thyroid axis: beyond the thyroid: what's happening in the gut. *Endocrinol. Cennections* 6, R52–R58. doi: 10.1530/EC-17-0021

Lerner, A., Jermias, P., and Matthias, T. (2015b). The world incidence of celiac disease is increasing: a review. *Int. J. Recent Sci. Res.* 7, 5491–5496.

Lerner, A., Makhoul, B., and Eliakim, R. (2012). Neurological manifestations of celiac disease in children and adults. *Eur. Neurolog. J.* 4, 15–20. doi: 10.1016/j.autrev.2014.11.009

Lerner, A., Neidhöfer, S., and Matthias, T. (2015c). Transglutaminase 2 and anti transglutaminase 2 autoantibodies in celiac disease and beyond: Part A: TG2 double-edged sword: gut and extraintestinal involvement. *Immunome Res.* 11, 101–105. doi: 10.4172/1745-7580.10000101

Lerner, A., Neidhöfer, S., and Matthias, T. (2015d). Transglutaminase 2 and anti transglutaminase 2 autoantibodies in celiac disease and beyond. Part B: Anti-Transglutaminase 2 autoantibodies: friends or enemies. *Immunome Res.* 11, 3–7.

Lerner, A., Neidhöfer, S., and Matthias, T. (2015e). Serological markers and/or intestinal biopsies in the case-finding of celiac disease. *Int. J. Celiac Dis.* 3, 53–55.

Lionetti, E., Castellaneta, S., Francavilla, R., Pulvirenti, A., Tonutti, E., Amarri, S., et al. (2014). SIGENP (Italian Society of Pediatric Gastroenterology, Hepatology, and Nutrition) Working Group on Weaning and CD Risk. Introduction of gluten, HLA status, and the risk of celiac disease in children. *N. Engl. J. Med.* 371, 1295–1303. doi: 10.1056/NEJMoa1400697

López-Casado, M. A., Lorite, P., and Palomeque, T., Torres, M. I. (2015). Potential role of the IL-33/ST2 axis in celiac disease. *Cell. Mol. Immunol.* 14, 285–292. doi: 10.1038/cmi.2015.85

Lund, M. E., O'Brien, B. A., Hutchinson, A. T., Robinson, M. W., Simpson, A. M., Dalton, J. P., et al. (2014). Secreted proteins from the helminth Fasciola hepatica inhibit the initiation of autoreactive T cell responses and prevent diabetes in the NOD mouse. *PLoS ONE* 9:e86289. doi: 10.1371/journal.pone.0086289

Luzza, F., Mancuso, M., Imeneo, M., Mesuraca, L., Contaldo, A., Giancotti, L., et al. (1999). *Helicobacter pylori* infection in children with celiac disease: prevalence and clinicopathologic features. *J. Pediatr. Gastroenterol. Nutr.* 28, 143–146. doi: 10.1097/00005176-199902000-00009

Lynch, D. A., Sobala, G. M., Dixon, M. F., Gledhill, A., Jackson, P., Crabtree, J. E., et al. (1995). Lymphocytic gastritis and associated small bowel disease: a diffuse lymphocytic gastroenteropathy? *J. Clin. Pathol.* 48, 939–945. doi: 10.1136/jcp.48.10.939

Magalhães, A., and Reis, C. A. (2010). *Helicobacter pylori* adhesion to gastric epithelial cells is mediated by glycan receptors. *Braz. J. Med. Biol. Res.* 43, 611–618. doi: 10.1590/S0100-879X2010007500049

Maheshwari, A. (2004). Role of cytokines in human intestinal villous development. *Clin. Perinatol.* 31, 143–155. doi: 10.1016/j.clp.2004.03.003

Makarova, S. G., Boldyreva, M. N., Lavrova, T., and Ye., Petrovskaya, M. I. (2014). Intestinal Microbiocenosis, Food Tolerance and Food Allergy. Current State of a Problem. *Voprosy Sovremennoj Pediatrii* 13, 21–29. doi: 10.15690/vsp.v13i3.1024

Manichanh, C., Borruel, N., Casellas, F., and Guarner, F. (2012). The gut microbiota in IBD. *Nat. Rev. Gastroenterol. Hepatol.* 9, 599–608. doi: 10.1038/nrgastro.2012.152

Mårild, K., Stephansson, O., Montgomery, S., Murray, J. A., and Ludvigsson, J. F. (2012). Pregnancy outcome and risk of celiac disease in offspring: a nationwide case-control study. *Gastroenterology.* 142, 39.e3–45.e3. doi: 10.1053/j.gastro.2011.09.047

Meresse, B., Korneychuk, N., Malamut, G., and Cerf-Bensussan, N. (2015). Interleukin-15, a master piece in the immunological jigsaw of celiac disease. *Dig. Dis.* 33, 122–130. doi: 10.1159/000369521

Mubarak, A., Spierings, E., Wolters, V., van Hoogstraten, I., Kneepkens, C. M., and Houwen, R. (2013). Human leukocyte antigen DQ2.2 and celiac disease. *J. Pediatr. Gastroenterol. Nutr.* 56, 428–430. doi: 10.1097/MPG.0b013e31827913f9

Mutapi, F., Imai, N., Nausch, N., Bourke, C. D., Rujeni, N., Mitchell, K. M., et al. (2011). Schistosome infection intensity is inversely related to auto-reactive antibody levels. *PLoS ONE.* 6:e19149. doi: 10.1371/journal.pone.0019149

Myléus, A., Stenlund, H., Hernell, O., Gothefors, L., Hammarström, M. L., Persson, L. Å., et al. (2012). Early vaccinations are not risk factors for celiac disease. *Pediatrics* 130, e63–e70. doi: 10.1542/peds.2011-2806

Naing, Z., Rayner, B., Killikulangara, A., Vunnam, K., Leach, S., McIver, C. J., et al. (2013). Prevalence of viruses in stool of premature neonates at a neonatal intensive care unit. *J. Paediatr. Child Health* 49, E221–E226. doi: 10.1111/jpc.12113

Narang, M., Puri, A. S., Sachdeva, S., Singh, J., Kumar, A., and Saran, R. K. (2016). Celiac disease and *H. Pylori* infection in children: is there any association? *J. Gastroenterol. Hepatol. J Gastroenterol. Hepatol.* 32, 1178–1182. doi: 10.1111/jgh.13654

Nenna, R., Magliocca, F. M., Tiberti, C., Mastrogiorgio, G., Petrarca, L., Mennini, M., et al. (2012). Endoscopic and histological gastric lesions in children with celiac disease: mucosal involvement is not only confined to the duodenum. *J. Pediatr. Gastroenterol. Nutr.* 55, 728–732. doi: 10.1097/MPG.0b013e318266aa9e

Nielsen, J. A., Roberts, C. A., Lager, D. J., Putcha, R. V., Jain, R., and Lewin, M. (2014). Lymphocytic gastritis is not associated with active *Helicobacter pylori* infection. *Helicobacter* 19, 349–355. doi: 10.1111/hel.12139

Nilsson, C., Larsson Sigfrinius, A. K., Montgomery, S. M., Sverremark-Ekström, E., Linde, A., Lilja, G., et al. (2009). Epstein-Barr virus and cytomegalovirus are differentially associated with numbers of cytokine-producing cells and early atopy. *Clin. Exp. Allergy* 39, 509–517. doi: 10.1111/j.1365-2222.2008.03147.x

Nilsson, C., Linde, A., Montgomery, S. M., Gustafsson, L., Näsman, P., Blomberg, M. T., et al. (2005). Does early EBV infection protect against IgE sensitization? *J. Allergy Clin. Immunol.* 116, 438–444. doi: 10.1016/j.jaci.2005.04.027

Nistal, E., Caminero, A., Vivas, S., Ruiz de Morales, J. M., Sáenz de Miera, L. E., Rodríguez-Aparicio, L. B., et al. (2012). Differences in faecal bacteria populations and faecal bacteria metabolism in healthy adults and celiac disease patients. *Biochimie* 94, 1724–1729. doi: 10.1016/j.biochi.2012.03.025

Niveloni, S., Weksler-Zangen, S., Pedreira, S., Dezi, R., Granot, E., Doldan, I., et al. (2000). Time course of nitric oxide synthase generation after gluten exposure in the rectal mucosa of gluten-sensitive patients. *Scand. J. Gastroenterol.* 35, 1150–1156. doi: 10.1080/003655200750056619

Noh, K. W., Poland, G. A., and Murray, J. A. (2003). Hepatitis B vaccine nonresponse and celiac disease. *Am. J. Gastroenterol.* 98, 2289–2292. doi: 10.1111/j.1572-0241.2003.07701.x

Nuding, S., Gersemann, M., Hosaka, Y., Konietzny, S., Schaefer, C., Beisner, J., et al. (2013). Gastric antimicrobial peptides fail to eradicate *Helicobacter pylori* infection due to selective induction and resistance. *PLoS ONE* 8:e73867. doi: 10.1371/journal.pone.0073867

Núñez, C., Rueda, B., Martínez, A., Maluenda, C., Polanco, I., López-Nevot, M. A., et al. (2006). A functional variant in the CD209 promoter is associated with

DQ2-negative celiac disease in the Spanish population. *World J. Gastroenterol.* 12, 4397–4400. doi: 10.3748/wjg.v12.i27.4397

Oertli, M., and Müller, A. (2012). *Helicobacter pylori* targets dendritic cells to induce immune tolerance, promote persistence and confer protection against allergic asthma. *Gut Microbes* 3, 566–571. doi: 10.4161/gmic.21750

Oh, J. E., Kim, B. C., Chang, D. H., Kwon, M., Lee, S. Y., Kang, D., et al. (2016). Dysbiosis-induced IL-33 contributes to impaired antiviral immunity in the genital mucosa. *Proc. Natl. Acad. Sci. U.S.A.* 113, E762–E771. doi: 10.1073/pnas.1518589113

Ojetti, V., Nucera, G., Migneco, A., Gabrielli, M., Lauritano, C., Danese, S., et al. (2005). High prevalence of celiac disease in patients with lactose intolerance. *Digestion* 71, 106–110. doi: 10.1159/000084526

Olivares, M., Neef, A., Castillejo, G., Palma, G. D., Varea, V., Capilla, A., et al. (2015). The HLA-DQ2 genotype selects for early intestinal microbiota composition in infants at high risk of developing coeliac disease. *Gut* 64, 406–417. doi: 10.1136/gutjnl-2014-306931

Ou, G., Hedberg, M., Hörstedt, P., Baranov, V., Forsberg, G., Drobni, M., et al. (2009). Proximal small intestinal microbiota and identification of rod-shaped bacteria associated with childhood celiac disease. *Am. J. Gastroenterol.* 104, 3058–3067. doi: 10.1038/ajg.2009.524

Pai, R. K. A. (2014). Practical approach to small bowel biopsy interpretation: celiac disease and its mimics. *Semin. Diagn. Pathol.* 31, 124–136. doi: 10.1053/j.semdp.2014.02.006

Pallav, K., Leffler, D. A., Tariq, S., Kabbani, T., Hansen, J., Peer, A., et al. (2012). Noncoeliac enteropathy: the differential diagnosis of villous atrophy in contemporary clinical practice. *Aliment. Pharmacol. Ther.* 35, 380–390. doi: 10.1111/j.1365-2036.2011.04938.x

Parassol, N., Freitas, M., Thoreux, K., Dalmasso, G., Bourdet-Sicard, R., and Rampal, P. (2005). *Lactobacillus casei* DN-114 001 inhibits the increase in paracellular permeability of enteropathogenic *Escherichia coli*-infected T84 cells. *Res. Microbiol.* 156, 256–262. doi: 10.1016/j.resmic.2004.09.013

Park, S. D., Markowitz, J., Pettei, M., Weinstein, T., Sison, C. P., Swiss, S. R., et al. (2007). Failure to respond to hepatitis B vaccine in children with celiac disease. *J. Pediatr. Gastroenterol. Nutr.* 44, 431–435. doi: 10.1097/MPG.0b013e3180320654

Peña, A. S., and Crusius, J. B. (1998). Food allergy, coeliac disease and chronic inflammatory bowel disease in man. *Vet. Q.* 20 (Suppl. 3), S49–S52.

Pero, R., Coretti, L., Nigro E., Lembo, F., Laneri, S., Lombardo, B., et al. (2017). β-defensins in the fight against *Helicobacter pylori*. *Molecules* 22:424. doi: 10.3390/molecules22030424

Pisetsky, D. S., and Drayton, D. M. (1997). Deficient expression of antibodies specific for bacterial DNA by patients with systemic lupus erythematosus. *Proc. Assoc. Am. Phys.* 109, 237–244.

Plot, L., Amital, H., Barzilai, O., Ram, M., Bizzaro, N., and Shoenfeld, Y. (2009). Infections may have a protective role in the etiopathogenesis of celiac disease. *Ann. N. Y. Acad. Sci.* 1173, 670–674. doi: 10.1111/j.1749-6632.2009.04814.x

Plot, L., and Amital, H. (2009). Infectious associations of Celiac disease. *Autoimmun Rev.* 8, 316–319. doi: 10.1016/j.autrev.2008.10.001

Polydorides, A. D. (2014). Pathology and differential diagnosis of chronic, noninfectious gastritis. *Semin. Diagn. Pathol.* 31, 114–123. doi: 10.1053/j.semdp.2014.02.008

Pontes-de-Carvalho, L., Mengel, J., Figueiredo, C. A., Social Changes, Asthma and Allergy in Latin America (SCAALA)'s Study Group, and Alcântara-Neves, N. M. (2013). Antigen mimicry between infectious agents and self or environmental antigens may lead to long-term regulation of inflammation. *Front. Immunol.* 4:314. doi: 10.3389/fimmu.2013.00314

Pordeus, V., Szyper-Kravitz, M., Levy, R. A., Vaz, N. M., and Shoenfeld, Y. (2008). Infections and autoimmunity: a panorama. *Clin. Rev. Allergy Immunol.* 34, 283–99. doi: 10.1007/s12016-007-8048-8

Raine, T., Zaccone, P., Mastroeni, P., and Cooke, A. (2006). Salmonella typhimurium infection in nonobese diabetic mice generates immunomodulatory dendritic cells able to prevent type 1 diabetes. *J. Immunol.* 177, 2224–2233. doi: 10.4049/jimmunol.177.4.2224

Ramanathan, J., Rammouni, M., Baran, J. Jr., and Khatib, R. (2000). Herpes simplex virus esophagitis in the immunocompetent host: an overview. *Am. J. Gastroenterol.* 95, 2171–2176. doi: 10.1111/j.1572-0241.2000.02299.x

Reichstetter, S., Kwok, W. W., and Nepom, G. T. (1999). Impaired binding of a DQ2 and DQ8-binding HSV VP16 peptide to a DQA1*0501/DQB1*0302 trans class II heterodimer. *Tissue Antigens* 53, 101–105. doi: 10.1034/j.1399-0039.1999.530111.x

Reif, S., and Lerner, A. (2004b). "Celiac disease and infection," in *Infections and Autoimmunity*, eds Y. Shoenfeld and N. Rose (Amsterdam: Elsevier), 689–692.

Reif, S., and Lerner, A. (2004a). Tissue transglutaminase—the key player in celiac disease: a review. *Autoimmun. Rev.* 3, 40–45. doi: 10.1016/S1568-9972(03)00065-X

Riddle, M. S., Murray, J. A., and Porter, C. K. (2012). The incidence and risk of celiac disease in a healthy US adult population. *Am. J. Gastroenterol.* 107, 1248–1255. doi: 10.1038/ajg.2012.130

Robbins, P. D., Dorronsoro, A., and Booker, C. N. (2016). Regulation of chronic inflammatory and immune processes by extracellular vesicles. *J. Clin. Invest.* 126, 1173–1180. doi: 10.1172/JCI81131

Robbins, P. D., and Morelli, A. E. (2014). Regulation of immune responses by extracellular vesicles. *Nat. Rev. Immunol.* 14, 195–208. doi: 10.1038/nri3622

Roblin, X., Pillet, S., Oussalah, A., Berthelot, P., Del Tedesco, E., Phelip, J. M., et al. (2011). Cytomegalovirus load in inflamed intestinal tissue is predictive of resistance to immunosuppressive therapy in ulcerative colitis. *Am. J. Gastroenterol.* 106, 2001–2008. doi: 10.1038/ajg.2011.202

Rollwagen, F. M., Yu, Z. Y., Li, Y. Y., and Pacheco, N. D. (1998). IL-6 rescues enterocytes from hemorrhage induced apoptosis *in vivo* and *in vitro* by abcl-2 mediated mechanism. *Clin. Immunol. Immunopathol.* 89, 205–213. doi: 10.1006/clin.1998.4600

Rosinach, M., Esteve, M., González, C., Temiño, R., Mariné, M., Monzón, H., et al. (2012). Lymphocytic duodenosis: aetiology and long-term response to specific treatment. *Dig. Liver Dis.* 44, 643–648. doi: 10.1016/j.dld.2012.03.006

Rostami, K. A., Al Dulaimi, D., Rostami Nejad, M., Villanacci, V., and Danciu, M. (2010). Microscopic enteritis and pathomechanism of malabsorption. *Auto Immun. Highlights* 1, 37–38. doi: 10.1007/s13317-010-0006-4

Rostami-Nejad, M., Ishaq, S., Al Dulaimi, D., Zali, M. R., and Rostami, K. (2015). The role of infectiousmediators and gut microbiome in the pathogenesis of celiac disease. *Arch. Iran Med.* 18, 244–249.

Rostami Nejad, M., Javad Ehsani-Ardakani, M., Assadzadeh, H., Shahbazkhani, B., Ierardi, E., Losurdo, G., et al. (2016). Pathological and clinical correlation between celiac disease and *Helicobacter pylori* infection; a review of controversial reports. *Middle East J. Dig. Dis.* 8, 85–92. doi: 10.15171/mejdd.2016.12

Rozenberg, O., Lerner, A., Pacht, A., Grinberg, M., Reginashvili, D., Henig, C., et al. (2012). Novel algorithm for childhood celiac disease serological diagnosis based upon intestinal biopsies. *Crit. Rev. Allerg. Immunol.* 42, 331–341. doi: 10.1007/s12016-010-8250-y

Ruggiero, M. A., Gordon, D. P., Orrell, T. M., Bailly, N., et al. (2015). A higher level classification of all living organisms. *PLoS ONE* 10:e0119248. doi: 10.1371/journal.pone.0119248

Sakkas, L. I., and Bogdanos, D. P. (2016). Infections as a cause of autoimmune rheumatic diseases. *Autoimmun. Highlights* 7, 13. doi: 10.1007/s13317-016-0086-x

Salama, N. R., Hartung, M. L., and Müller, A. (2013). Life in the human stomach: persistence strategies of the bacterial pathogen *Helicobacter pylori*. *Nat. Rev. Microbiol.* 11, 385–399. doi: 10.1038/nrmicro3016

San-Pedro, J. I., Bilbao, J. R., Perez de Nanclares, G., Vitoria, J. C., Martul, P., and Castaño, L. (2005). Heterogeneity of vitamin D receptor gene association with celiac disease and type 1 diabetes mellitus. *Autoimmunity* 38, 439–444. doi: 10.1080/08916930500288455

Santarelli, L., Gabrielli, M., Santoliquido, A., Cuoco, L., Cazzato, A., Candelli, M., et al. (2006). Interaction between *Helicobacter pylori* infection and untreated coeliac disease on gastric histological pattern. *Scand. J. Gastroenterol.* 41, 532–535. doi: 10.1080/00365520500349549

Sapone, A., Lammers, K. M., Casolaro, V., Cammarota, M., Giuliano, M. T., De Rosa, M., et al. (2011). Divergence of gut permeability and mucosal immune gene expression in two gluten-associated conditions: celiac disease and gluten sensitivity. *BMC. Med.* 9:23. doi: 10.1186/1741-7015-9-23

Savarino, V., Mela, G. S., Zentilin, P., Lapertosa, G., Bisso, G., Mele, M. R., et al. (1999). Histological and functional recovery in patients with multifocal atrophic gastritis after eradication of *Helicobacter pylori* infection. *Ital. J. Gastroenterol. Hepatol.* 31, 4–8.

Schreiber, S., Bücker, R., Groll, C., Azevedo-Vethacke, M., Garten, D., Scheid, P., et al. (2005). Rapid loss of motility of *Helicobacter pylori* in the gastric lumen *in vivo*. *Infect. Immun.* 73, 1584–1589. doi: 10.1128/IAI.73.3.1584-1589.2005

Sellitto, M., Bai, G., Serena, G., Fricke, W. F., Sturgeon, C., Gajer, P., et al. (2012). Proof of concept of microbiome-metabolome analysis and delayed gluten exposure on celiac disease autoimmunity in genetically at-risk infants. *PLoS ONE* 7:e33387. doi: 10.1371/journal.pone.0033387

Selmi, C. (2016). Are helminths to be trusted as allies in the war against autoimmunity and chronic inflammation? *Isr. Med. Assoc. J.* 18, 139–140.

Shalimar, D. M., Das, P., Sreenivas, V., Gupta, S. D., Panda, S. K., and Makharia, G. K. (2013). Mechanism of villous atrophy in celiac disease: role of apoptosis and epithelial regeneration. *Arch. Pathol. Lab. Med.* 13, 1262–1269. doi: 10.5858/arpa.2012-0354-OA

Shamir, R., Eliakim, R., Lahat, N., Sobel, E., and Lerner, A. (2002). ELISA assay of anti endomysial antibodies in the diagnosis of celiac disease: comparison with immunofluorescence assay of anti endomysial antibodies and tissue transglutaminase antibodies. *Isr. Med. Assoc. J.* 4, 594–596.

Shmidt, E., Smyrk, T. C., Boswell, C. L., Enders, F. T., and Oxentenko, A. S. (2014). Increasing duodenal intraepithelial lymphocytosis found at upper endoscopy: time trends and associations. *Gastrointest. Endosc.* 80, 105–111. doi: 10.1016/j.gie.2014.01.008

Shor, B.-A. D., Bashi, T., Lachnish, J., Fridkin, M., Bizzaro, G., Barshak, I., et al. (2015). Phosphorylcholine-tuftsin compound prevents development of dextransulfate-sodium-salt induced murine colitis: implications for the treatment of human inflammatory bowel disease. *J. Autoimmun.* 56, 111–117. doi: 10.1016/j.jaut.2014.11.001

Shor, B.-A. D., Harel, M., Eliakim, R., and Shoenfeld, Y. (2013). The hygiene theory harnessing helminths and their ova to treat autoimmunity. *Clin. Rev. Allergy Immunol.* 45, 211–216. doi: 10.1007/s12016-012-8352-9

Silvester, J. A., and Leffler, D. A. (2016). Is autoimmunity infectious? the effect of gastrointestinal viral infections and vaccination on risk of celiac disease autoimmunity. *Clin. Gastroenterol. Hepatol.* 15, 703–705. doi: 10.1016/j.cgh.2016.12.014

Simondi, D., Ribaldone, D. G., Bonagura, G. A., Foi, S., Sapone, N., Garavagno, M., et al. (2015). *Helicobacter pylori* in celiac disease and in duodenal intraepithelial lymphocytosis: active protagonist or innocent bystander? *Clin. Res. Hepatol. Gastroenterol.* 39, 740–745. doi: 10.1016/j.clinre.2015.03.005

Sjöberg, V., Sandström, O., Hedberg, M., Hammarström, S., Hernell, O., and Hammarström, M. L. (2013). Intestinal T-cell responses in celiac disease — impact of celiac disease associated bacteria. *PLoS ONE* 8:e53414. doi: 10.1371/journal.pone.0053414

Smallwood, T. B., Giacomin, P. R., Loukas, A., Mulvenna, J. P., Clark, R. J., and Miles, J. J. (2017). Helminth Immunomodulation in Autoimmune Disease. *Front Immunol.* 8:453. doi: 10.3389/fimmu.2017.00453

Spanhaak, S., Havenaar, R., and Schaafsma, G. (1998). The effect of consumption of milk fermented by *Lactobacillus casei* strain Shirota on the intestinal microflora and immune parameters in humans. *Eur. J. Clin. Nutr.* 52, 899–907. doi: 10.1038/sj.ejcn.1600663

Spor, A., Koren, O., and Ley, R. (2011). Unravelling the effects of the environment and host genotype on the gut microbiome. *Nat. Rev. Microbiol.* 9, 279–290. doi: 10.1038/nrmicro2540

Sütas, Y., Autio, S., Rantala, I., and Isolauri, E. (1997). IFN-gamma enhances macromolecular transport across Peyer's patches in suckling rats: implications for natural immune responses to dietary antigens early in life. *J. Pediatr. Gastroenterol. Nutr.* 24, 162–169. doi: 10.1097/00005176-199702000-00009

Tannock, G. W., Munro, K., Harmsen, H. J., et al. (2000). Analysis of the fecal microflora of human subjects consuming a probiotic product containing *Lactobacillus rhamnosus* DR20. *Appl. Environ. Microbiol.* 66, 2578–2588. doi: 10.1128/AEM.66.6.2578-2588.2000

Toft-Hansen, H., Nielsen, C., Biagini, M., Husby, S., and Lillevang, S. T. (2013). Lectin staining shows no evidence of involvement of glycocalyx/mucous layer carbohydrate structures in development of celiac disease. *Nutrients* 5, 4540–4552. doi: 10.3390/nu5114540

Tracy, S., Drescher, K. M., Chapman, N. M., Kim, K. S., Carson, S. D., Pirruccello, S., et al. (2002). Toward testing the hypothesis that group B coxsackieviruses (CVB) trigger insulin-dependent diabetes: inoculating nonobese diabetic mice with CVB markedly lowers diabetes incidence. *J. Virol.* 76, 12097–12111. doi: 10.1128/JVI.76.23.12097-12111.2002

Trebichavsky, I., Splichal, I., Rada, V., and Splichalova, A. (2010). Modulation of natural immunity in the gut by *Escherichia coli* strain Nissle 1917. *Nutr. Rev.* 68, 459–464. doi: 10.1111/j.1753-4887.2010.00305.x

Tsai, H. F., and Hsu, P. N. (2010). Interplay between*Helicobacter pylori* and immune cells in immunepathogenesis of gastric inflammation and mucosal pathology. *Cell Mol. Immunol.* 7, 255–259. doi: 10.1038/cmi.2010.2

Urganci, N., and Kalyoncu, D. (2013). Response to hepatitis A and B vaccination in pediatric patients with celiac disease. *J. Pediatr. Gastroenterol. Nutr.* 56, 408–411. doi: 10.1097/MPG.0b013e31827af200

Vatsiou, A. I., Bazin, E., and Gaggiotti, O. E. (2016). Changes in selective pressures associated with human population expansion may explain metabolic and immune related pathways enriched for signatures of positive selection. *BMC. Genomics.* 17:504. doi: 10.1186/s12864-016-2783-2

Villanacci, V., Bassotti, G., Liserre, B., Lanzini, A., Lanzarotto, F., and Genta, R. M. (2006). *Helicobacter pylori* infection in patients with celiac disease. *Amer. J. Gastroenterol.* 101, 1880–1885. doi: 10.1111/j.1572-0241.2006.00621.x

Vordenbäumen, S., Pilic, D., Otte, J. M., Schmitz, F., and Schmidt-Choudhury, A. (2010). Defensin-mRNA expression in the upper gastrointestinal tract is modulated in children with celiac disease and *Helicobacter pylori*-positive gastritis. *J. Pediatr. Gastroenterol. Nutr.* 50, 596–600. doi: 10.1097/MPG.0b013e3181cd26cd

Wacklin, P., Laurikka, P., Lindfors, K., Collin, P., Salmi, T., Lähdeaho, M. L., et al. (2014). Altered duodenal microbiota composition in celiac disease patients suffering from persistent symptoms on a long-term gluten-free diet. *Am. J. Gastroenterol.* 109, 1933–1941. doi: 10.1038/ajg.2014.355

Wang, J., Thingholm, L. B., Skiecevičienė, J., Rausch, P., Kummen, M., Hov, J. R., et al. (2016). Genome-wide association analysis identifies variation in vitamin D receptor and other host factors influencing the gut microbiota. *Nat. Genet.* 48, 1396–1406. doi: 10.1038/ng.3695

Weng, M., and Walker, W. A. (2013). The role of gut microbiota in programming the immune phenotype. *J. Dev. Orig. Health Dis.* 4, 203–214. doi: 10.1017/S2040174412000712

Wu, J., Lin, K., Zeng, J., Liu, W., Yang, F., Wang, X., et al. (2014). Role of DC-SIGN in *Helicobacter pylori* infection of gastrointestinal cells. *Front. Biosci.* 19, 825–834. doi: 10.2741/4250

Wu, T. T., and Hamilton, S. R. (1999). Lymphocytic gastritis: association with etiology and topology. *Am. J. Surg. Pathol.* 23, 153–158. doi: 10.1097/00000478-199902000-00003

Zaman, C., Osaki, T., Hanawa, T., Yonezawa, H., Kurata, S., and Kamiya, S. (2014). Analysis of the microbial ecology between *Helicobacter pylori* and the gastric microbiota of Mongolian gerbils. *J. Med. Microbiol.* 63, 129–137. doi: 10.1099/jmm.0.061135-0

Zeissig, S., and Blumberg, R. S. (2014). Commensal microbial regulation of natural killer T cells at the frontiers of the mucosal immune system. *FEBS Lett.* 588, 4188–4194. doi: 10.1016/j.febslet.2014.06.042

Zelnik, N., Pacht, A., Obeid, R., and Lerner, A. (2004). Range of neurological disorders in patients with celiac disease. *Pediatrics* 113, 1672–1676. doi: 10.1542/peds.113.6.1672

Zyrek, A. A., Cichon, C., Helms, S., Enders, C., Sonnenborn, U., and Schmidt, M. A. (2007). Molecular mechanisms underlying the probiotic effects of *Escherichia coli* Nissle 1917 involve ZO-2 and PKCzeta redistribution resulting in tight junction and epithelial barrier repair. *Cell. Microbiol.* 9, 804–816. doi: 10.1111/j.1462-5822.2006.00836.x

7

Human Endogenous Retrovirus-K and TDP-43 Expression Bridges ALS and HIV Neuropathology

Renée N. Douville[1,2] and Avindra Nath[3]*

[1] Department of Biology, University of Winnipeg, Winnipeg, MB, Canada, [2] Department of Immunology, University of Manitoba, Winnipeg, MB, Canada, [3] Section of Infections of the Nervous System, National Institute of Neurological Diseases and Stroke, National Institutes of Health, Bethesda, MD, United States

***Correspondence:**
Renée N. Douville
r.douville@uwinnipeg.ca

Despite the repetitive association of endogenous retroviruses in human disease, the mechanisms behind their pathological contributions remain to be resolved. Here we discuss how neuronal human endogenous retrovirus-K (HERV-K) expression in human immunodeficiency virus (HIV)-infected individuals is a distinct pathological aspect of HIV-associated neurological conditions, such as HIV encephalitis and HIV-associated neurocognitive disorders. Enhanced neuronal HERV-K levels were observed in the majority of HIV-infected individuals, and to a higher degree in brain tissue marked by HIV replication. Moreover, we highlight an important neuropathological overlap between amyotrophic lateral sclerosis and HIV encephalitis, that being the formation of neurotoxic TDP-43 deposits in neurons. Herein, we argue for enhanced transdisciplinary research in the field of ERV biology, using an example of how HERV-K expression has novel mechanistic and therapeutic implications for HIV neuropathology.

Keywords: human immunodeficiency virus (HIV), human endogenous retrovirus-K (HERV-K), TDP-43, NeuroAIDS, amyotrophic lateral sclerosis (ALS)

INTRODUCTION

Originating from ancient retroviruses that overcame host defense mechanisms and permanently integrated into the DNA of our hominid ancestors, endogenous retroviruses (ERVs) occupy over 8% of the human genome. The process of retroviral endogenation has resulted in at least 31 independently acquired ERV genera in the human genome (Belshaw et al., 2005; Blikstad et al., 2008; Subramanian et al., 2011). Despite roles in homeostasis (Brattas et al., 2017; Meyer et al., 2017), ERVs are increasingly being recognized as integral players in the pathogenesis of many human diseases [reviewed in Ruprecht et al. (2008), Balada et al. (2009), Manghera et al. (2014), Christensen (2016)]. Furthermore, concrete examples in other species indicate how ERVs may drive pathogenic mechanisms such as cellular transformation and immune dysregulation [reviewed in Kassiotis (2014), Mager and Stoye (2015)]. This is illustrated by mice deficient in select TLRs (−3, −7, −9), which exhibit endogenously derived MuLV viremia and development of acute T cell lymphoblastic leukemia (Yu et al., 2012). It also highlights the fact that both innate and adaptive immune responses are essential for control of ERV expression (Stetson et al., 2008; Hurst and Magiorkinis, 2015); conversely, ERVs also regulate immunity genes (Hurst and Magiorkinis, 2015; Chuong et al., 2016). Neurological effects caused by ERVs are also documented. Neurovirulent strains of MuLV such as Cas-Br-E cause infection of microglial cells with neurodegeneration in the brain and spinal cord which resembles amyotrophic lateral sclerosis

(ALS) and is mediated by the envelope protein of the virus (Lynch and Sharpe, 2000; Jolicoeur et al., 2003).

Ongoing clinical trials seek to determine the value of ERVs as biomarkers and therapeutic targets (clinicaltrials.gov NCT02437110 and NCT02782858) (Alfahad and Nath, 2013). Breakthroughs in one specialty are likely to translate into other disease contexts, due to the overlap of ERV expression patterns in multiple conditions (Brutting et al., 2017). Herein, we argue for enhanced transdisciplinary research in the field of ERV biology, using an example of how endogenous retrovirus-K (HERV-K) expression has novel implications for human immunodeficiency virus (HIV) neuropathology.

HIV INFECTION: MORE THAN ONE RETROVIRUS AT PLAY?

Even with antiretroviral therapy, the clinical treatment of HIV infection is often complicated by neurocognitive disorders (Robertson et al., 2007). The occurrence of mild neurocognitive deficits, such as those impacting daily living activities, have notably increased among HIV^{+} populations - despite a decline in the more severe forms of HIV-associated neurocognitive disorders (HAND) with the advent of antiretroviral therapy (McArthur et al., 2010). Even worse, there is currently no targeted treatment to prevent the onset or progression of HAND. Clinical trials with a wide variety of neuroprotective drugs, anti-inflammatory agents, and antioxidants have failed or shown only minor effects. Risk factors for the progression to HAND include genetic, viral, and co-morbid factors, such as drug use and increasing age (Saylor et al., 2016).

Human immunodeficiency virus enters the central nervous system (CNS) soon after initial infection. Whether HIV drives neurodegeneration by slow and progressive pathological changes or sudden alterations caused by systemic immunosuppression is unclear. In the CNS, productive HIV infection is supported by cell types such as astrocytes, microglia, and macrophages which subsequently elicit chronic pro-inflammatory responses [reviewed in Kraft-Terry et al. (2010)]. Both HIV infection and inflammatory signals mediated by cytokines such as IL-6, IL-1β, TNFα, and IFNγ, can trigger the expression of ERVs (Serra et al., 2003; Contreras-Galindo et al., 2007b), and specifically HERV-K (Manghera et al., 2016b).

Human immunodeficiency virus infection can promote ERV expression in proliferating peripheral blood mononuclear cells (PBMC) (Contreras-Galindo et al., 2007b). Longitudinal analysis of PBMC from HIV-infected patients shows that increased HERV-K expression precedes spikes of HIV replication in select individuals (Contreras-Galindo et al., 2007a). Enhanced HERV-K levels were observed in patients treated sub-optimal therapeutic doses of antiretrovirals, or those who outright failed to respond to HAART therapy (Contreras-Galindo et al., 2006, 2007a). Further evidence for a dynamically intertwined relationship between HERV-K and HIV replication stems form the observation that HIV elite controllers have robust cellular and antibody responses against the HERV-K (HML-2) capsid protein (de Mulder et al., 2017).

Until recently, it was unclear if HERV-K re-activation stays limited to peripheral tissues or is a feature of HIV neuroinvasion. Independent groups have now shown that HERV-K proteins accumulate in cortical neurons of patients with HIV infection (Bhat et al., 2014). Specifically, here we sought to determine if HIV infection in the brain is associated with the up-regulation of HERV-K expression, and additional markers of neuronal dysfunction.

AN EXPLORATION OF HERV-K EXPRESSION IN HIV^{+} BRAIN TISSUE

We have previously demonstrated enhanced HERV-K expression in cortical and spinal neurons of patients with ALS (Douville et al., 2011; Li et al., 2015). Therefore, we examined the extent of cortical HERV-K expression in HIV patients with encephalitis and/or HIV-associated neurocognitive disorder (HIV-E/HAND, $n = 6$,), HIV patients without encephalitis (HIV, $n = 9$), and individuals with chronic systemic illness (controls, $n = 7$), through detection and localization of the viral reverse transcriptase (RT) protein within autopsy tissues (**Table 1** and **Figure 1**).

In both HIV-infected groups, increased HERV-K RT protein was detectable (using AbNova #H00002087-A01 antibody), but surprisingly expressed at similar levels (**Figure 1A**). Based on the findings of Contreras-Galindo et al. (2007a), we expected HERV-K induction to occur immediately preceding or during HIV replication in the brain. HIV-E is a multifocal disease; therefore, varying levels of HIV replication occurs within the many regions of the brain. This leads to an intrinsic sampling bias when examining excised brain specimens, as select tissue samples may not be representative of the global pattern of HIV-associated pathology. Future studies would benefit from larger sample sizes and from sampling multiple brain regions per individual to improve the chances of identifying focal lesions. Considering these caveats, we evaluated the degree of HIV replication in each tissue specimen based on the presence or absence of HIV p24 positive cells as determined by immunohistochemistry, and stratified the tissues from HIV-infected individuals accordingly. HERV-K RT expression was significantly elevated in brain tissue with p24 reactivity (**Figure 1B**). This finding is consistent with the observation that productive HIV infection in PBMC triggers HERV-K expression (Contreras-Galindo et al., 2007b; Laderoute et al., 2007). Since HIV^{+} patients who fail to respond to HAART therapy exhibit elevated HERV-K levels in PBMC (Contreras-Galindo et al., 2007a), our results suggest that HERV-K expression in the brain may reflect inadequate drug penetration into the CNS or an unsuccessful response to antiretroviral treatment. Moreover, plasma HIV loads were associated with HERV-K RT measurements in cortical tissue (Spearman's correlation $p = 0.052$), supportive of the idea that systemic HIV replication favors HERV-K re-activation in both the CNS and peripheral compartment. Productive HIV infection in neocortical tissues is characteristic of HIV-E/HAND (McArthur et al., 2010), and could also play a significant role in milder neurocognitive disorders. Moreover, robust HERV-K expression

TABLE 1 | Cortical brain tissue specimens.

Case	Brain bank	Diagnosis	Tissue	Age (years)	Gender	PMI	CD4	Plasma viral load	CSF viral load
CB164	CNTC	HIV+	Parietal lobe	35	M	5	211	2827	78
CC128	CNTC	HIV+	Parietal lobe	47	M	12	306	4953	ND
CE132	CNTC	HIV+/HIV-E	Parietal lobe	39	M	7	26	ND	0
7101868276	TRANR	HIV+/HIV-E	Parietal cortex	41	M	7.6	37	>500000	>55695
7100616568	TRANR	HIV+/HIV-E	Parietal cortex	32	M	16.2	77	489796	3041500
7101847783	TRANR	HIV+	Parietal cortex	59	M	11.3	8	54439	735
7101997784	TRANR	HIV+	Parietal cortex	41	M	15.3	76	711	644
7100928374	TRANR	HIV+	Parietal cortex	38	F	10.8	3	104358	93
7100598287	TRANR	HIV+	Parietal cortex	50	M	13	121	<50	<10
1093	NNTC	HIV+/possible HAD	Parietal cortex	56	M	6	365	25669	ND
2005	NNTC	HIV+	Parietal cortex	44	F	3	66	>75000	249
2012	NNTC	HIV+/HIV-E	Parietal cortex	49	M	16	273	ND	<50
5007	NNTC	HIV+/possible HAD/HIV-E	Parietal cortex	37	F	3	91	>75000	ND
5008	NNTC	HIV+/possible HAD/HIV-E	Parietal cortex	53	M	7	128	8641	54061
6081	NNTC	HIV+/probable HAD	Parietal cortex	35	M	2	ND	ND	ND
3565	HBSFRC	Cardiomyopathy	Cortex	76	M	11			
27	RMMSC	Coronary artery disease	Cortex	69	M	6.5			
712	JHSMBB	Unknown	Prefrontal cortex	44	F	20			
23895	JHSMBB	Unknown	Occipital cortex	ND	ND	ND			
000	JHSMBB	Unknown	Motor cortex	ND	ND	ND			
33	RMMSC	Pulmonary disease	Cortex	69	M	4.5			
795	JHSMBB	Huntington's disease	Sensory cortex	48	F	9			

Tissue specimens were obtained from the California NeuroAIDS Tissue Consortium (CNTC), the Texas Repository for AIDS Neuropathogenesis Research (TRANR), the National NeuroAIDS Tissue Consortium (NNTC), the Human Brain and Spinal Fluid Resource Center (HBSFRC), the Rocky Mountain MS Center (RMMSC), and the Johns Hopkins School of Medicine Brain Bank (JHSMBB). Among confirmed cases with HIV infection (as indicated by CD4 count, plasma and cerebral spinal fluid viral loads), brain tissue samples were further classified as having HIV-encephalitis (HIV-E) based of neuropathological examination or HIV-associated dementia (HAD) based on clinical history. Post-mortem interval (PMI) is indicated in hours. No data (ND).

was seen in several HIV$^+$ patients not clinically diagnosed with HIV-E/HAND. This points to pathological but modest HIV replication and/or HIV-associated neuroinflammation driving HERV-K activity within the brain, which precedes overt clinical signs and symptoms of neurocognitive impairment.

A notable finding is that the enhanced HERV-K expression was limited to neuronal cells in HIV$^+$ specimens, yet HIV is not trophic for neurons. Local neuroinflammation is likely a key driver of HERV-K expression in the brain, and is supported in a study of ALS neuropathology (Manghera et al., 2016b). Alternatively, the enhanced neuronal expression of HERV-K may be directly mediated by viral proteins released from HIV-infected cells, such as HIV Tat (Gonzalez-Hernandez et al., 2012, 2014). HIV Tat protein can be released extracellularly from infected macrophages within the brain and then taken up by neurons [reviewed in Li et al. (2009)]. In depth analysis of the HERV-K promoter suggests that several transcription factors related to inflammation, hormone regulation, and tissue-specific signaling may also modulate the transcription of this ERV (Manghera and Douville, 2013).

However, a consequence of neuronal HERV-K upregulation may be a blockade on the progression of HIV infection in the brain. Experimental evidence suggests that HERV-K expression may be a limiting factor for HIV replication in neurons. *In vitro* modeling shows that HERV-K Gag and Env proteins can play an essential role as retroviral restriction factors, thus limiting HIV replication (Monde et al., 2017; Terry et al., 2017). Furin processing of HERV-K Env impacts HIV-1 production, as well as several key amino acid residues in the surface domain altering the degree of HIV production in HERV-K108 versus HERV-Kcon Env overexpressing 293T cells (Terry et al., 2017). Furthermore, it has been demonstrated that HERV-K Env (type 2) expression in neural cells is a protective mechanism against HIV replication in these cells, and that this may confer a degree of protection against a variety of insults (Bhat et al., 2014). Despite HERV-K activity impeding HIV replication in neurons, the brain remains negatively impacted by elevated HERV-K expression in neurons. Recent data show that the expression of HERV-K in mature neurons is toxic, with data also showing a neuropathological impact of HERV-K Env on mature neurons, as transgenic mice expressing HERV-K *env* are afflicted with severe neuronal damage and progressive motor dysfunction (Li et al., 2015). Another key point is that few studies have considered the potential roles of other HERV-K-encoded proteins on the viability and function of neurons. Clearly, we need a broader view of the impact of HERV-K in neurological disorders.

THE SEARCH FOR AN HERV-K-ASSOCIATED BIOMARKER

Identification of HERV-K-associated biomarkers is a key step for both future research and clinical trials in a variety of HERV-K-associated diseases. Our previous study of patients with ALS

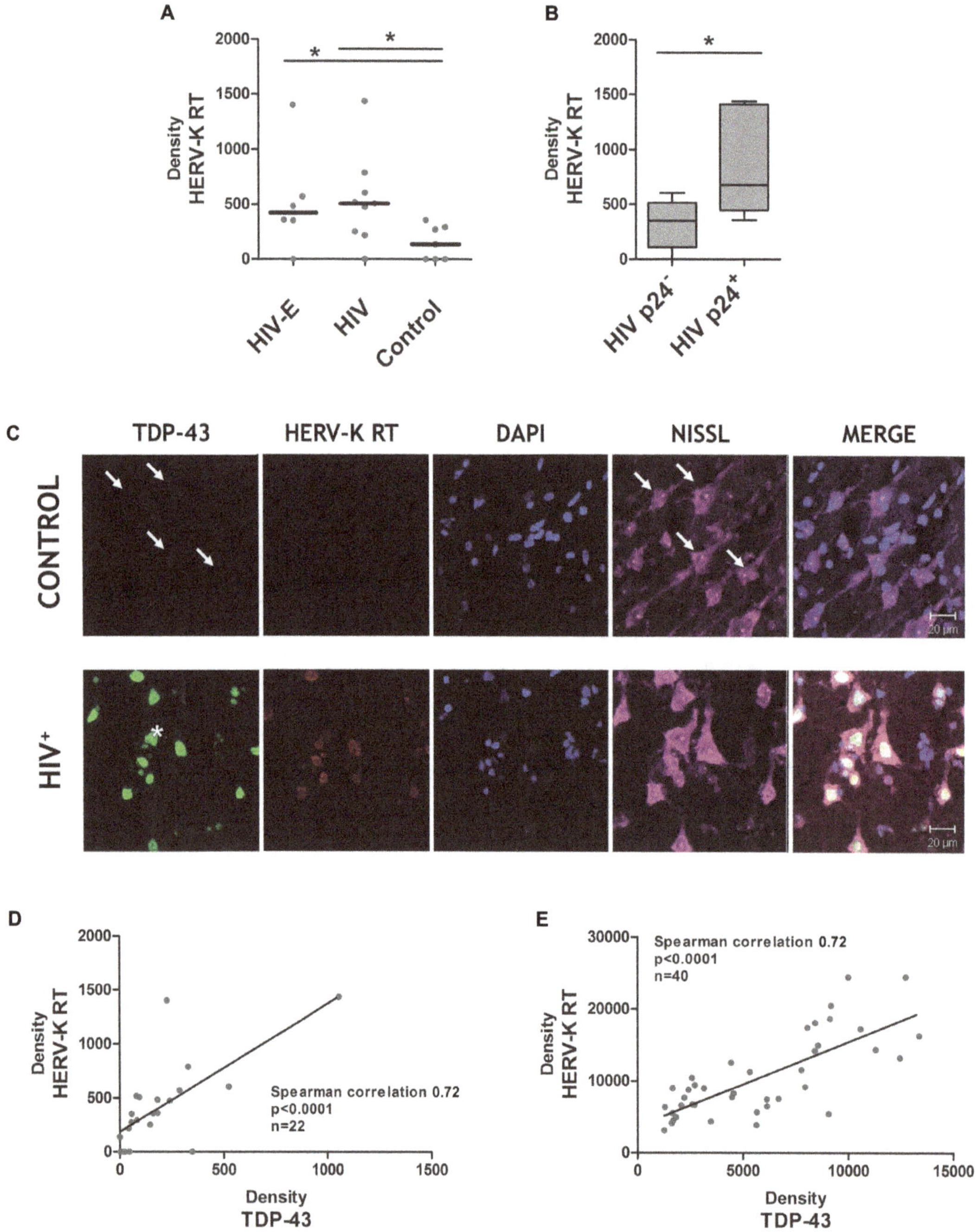

FIGURE 1 | Endogenous retrovirus-K reverse transcriptase is induced in cortical tissue during human immunodeficiency virus (HIV) infection. **(A)** HIV-infected individuals, with HAND/HIV-encephalitis (HIV-E) or without HIV-E (HIV) expressed greater levels of endogenous retrovirus-K (HERV-K) reverse transcriptase protein in their cortical tissue, as compared to patients deceased with chronic systemic disease (control). Antibodies against the HERV-K reverse transcriptase protein (AbNova #H00002087-A01) and human TDP-43 (Protein Tech #10782-2-AP) were used for immunohistochemistry as previously described (Douville et al., 2011). **(B)** HIV replication in cortical tissue, as measured by HIV p24 protein immunostaining (mouse anti-HIV p24 Gag monoclonal, #24-4 NARRRP), is associated with significantly higher HERV-K reverse transcriptase expression. Mann–Whitney derived *t*-test, $*p < 0.05$. **(C)** Significant correlation of neuronal HERV-K reverse transcriptase and TDP-43 protein levels in HIV^+ patients. Representative immunohistochemistry images of TDP-43 protein, endogenous retrovirus-K reverse transcriptase (HERV-K RT), nucleic as measured by DAPI staining, and neurons as measured by Nissl staining in the cortical brain tissue of HIV-infected patients (HIV^+) versus patients with systemic disease (control). Arrows indicate weak TDP-43 positivity in control tissue neurons. ALS-derived neuron with a TDP-43 deposit outside the nuclear boundary is indicated with an asterisk. **(D,E)** A strong correlation between HERV-K RT and TDP-43 expression in brain tissues. ImageJ analysis was used to quantify the density of HERV-K RT and TDP-43 staining within individual tissue samples **(D)** and within individual neurons **(E)** of HIV-infected and controls cortical brain specimens. Spearman correlation used to assess association between HERV-K RT and TDP-43 expression patterns.

found that the extent of HERV-K RT expression was strongly correlated with TAR DNA binding protein-43 (TDP-43) *in vivo* (Douville et al., 2011). Further, the HERV-K LTR has four binding sites for TDP-43 which have been shown to regulate its activation (Li et al., 2015). A common event in ALS is the aberrant deposit of ubiquitinated and hyper-phosphorylated TDP-43 in the cytoplasm and nucleus of neurons (Mackenzie et al., 2007; Buratti and Baralle, 2008). Further, formation of TDP-43 aggregates has been shown to alter HERV-K RT and polyprotein levels and cellular localization of these viral proteins (Manghera et al., 2016a). Measurement of TDP-43 protein expression (Protein Tech #10782-2-AP antibody) by immunohistochemistry (**Figure 1C**) or western blot analysis (data not shown) consistently show an increase in TDP-43 levels in HIV$^+$ specimens, as compared to controls. Nuclear TDP-43 expression was enhanced on average six-fold in the cortical neurons of HIV patients, and was accompanied by enhanced TDP-43 phosphorylation (data not shown). Furthermore, co-expression of HERV-K RT and TDP-43 proteins occurred in the majority of neurons (**Figure 1C**). To examine this expression pattern quantitatively, the staining density measurements for HERV-K RT and TDP-43 were performed in tissues and co-labeled neurons. **Figures 1D,E** demonstrate that there is a significant positive correlation between TDP-43 expression and HERV-K RT expression in tissue (Spearman's correlation 0.72, $p < 0.0001$, $n = 22$) and within individual neurons (Spearman's correlation 0.72, $p < 0.0001$, $n = 40$). This data supports the idea that specific post-translational modifications of TDP-43 may alter its protein turnover rate resulting in modified nuclear expression, and the inception of cytoplasmic TDP-43 aggregates (**Figure 1C**, asterisk) (Mackenzie et al., 2007; Buratti and Baralle, 2008; Brady et al., 2011). This disruption in turn can impact HERV-K expression patterns (Manghera et al., 2016a).

As to why enhanced TDP-43 expression occurs in association with HERV-K, this phenomenon may reflect a similar transcriptional responsiveness to inflammatory signals. *In silico* analysis of the TDP-43 promoter reveals that like other interferon-stimulated genes, it harbors both IRF and κB binding sites and therefore may be transcriptionally up-regulated by pro-inflammatory responses. (Douville et al., 2011). HERV-K transcription and viral protein production are also strongly associated with the activity of the transcription factor complex of IRF1, and NF-κB p50 and p65 (Manghera et al., 2016b). Moreover, TDP-43 expression has been shown to be inducible during viral infection (Brasier et al., 2004). As TDP-43 was originally described as an inhibitor of HIV transcription (Ou et al., 1995), we postulated that it may act as a retroviral restriction factor, with a potential role in repressing both HIV and HERV-K provirus expression. Subsequent studies are not in agreement as to the potential of TDP-43 as a retroviral restriction factor, with some in support (Li et al., 2015; Krug et al., 2017), and others against (Nehls et al., 2014; Manghera et al., 2016a; Prudencio et al., 2017), perhaps reflecting cell-type or model-specific effects.

Figure 1C also highlights an important neuropathological overlap between ALS and HIV-E: the formation of nuclear and cytoplasmic TDP-43 deposits in neurons. The cleavage and subsequent aggregation of TDP-43 results in neurotoxicity (Yang et al., 2010; Che et al., 2011; Ratti and Buratti, 2016). There is a preponderance of TDP-43 pathology in over 90% of ALS cases (Irwin et al., 2015; Scotter et al., 2015), despite <1% of sporadic ALS cases having a clear genetic cause (Ling et al., 2013). Similarly, we observed that all HIV$^+$ brain tissues exhibited heightened TDP-43 expression, with select neurons containing cytoplasmic TDP-43 accumulation (**Figure 1C**, asterisk). Truncated forms of TDP-43 called TDP-25 and TDP-35 are known to seed native TDP-43 aggregation (Huang et al., 2014; Xiao et al., 2015), thus altering its capacity to perform cellular functions (Che et al., 2011; Monahan et al., 2016). With sequestration of TDP-43, the cell's ability to regulate RNA splicing is compromised (Scotter et al., 2015). Thus, HIV neuroinfection and ALS may share aberrant and altered protein deposition patterns, with pathogenic consequences.

The role of retroviruses (if any) in the cell-to-cell transmission of pathogenic TDP-43 moieties has yet to be elucidated (reviewed in Hanspal et al. (2017)]. This represents an attractive hypothesis considering that cortical neurons are known to secrete exosomes (Faure et al., 2006), and that exosomes have been shown to harbor retroviral cargo (Wurdinger et al., 2012; Vargas et al., 2014). Monitoring exosome composition could be an attractive source of clinical biomarkers for future studies on ERV-associated diseases.

FUTURE DIRECTIONS

Despite repetitive association of ERVs in neurological diseases, such as ALS, multiple sclerosis, and schizophrenia, the mechanisms behind their pathological contributions remain to be resolved. Accumulating evidence suggests that HERV-K expression is a distinct pathological aspect of HIV-associated neurological disorders. Enhanced HERV-K RT expression in adult HIV$^+$ individuals was restricted to neurons, and most elevated within brain tissue exhibiting HIV replication. This is a similar pattern of neuropathology to that seen in ALS, where cortical neurons - including motor neurons - express HERV-K viral proteins (RT and envelope proteins) (Douville et al., 2011; Bhat et al., 2014; Li et al., 2015; Manghera et al., 2016b). Considering this notable association with motor neuron disease, it is important to point out the prevalence of motor disturbances in HIV infection. Perinatally-acquired HIV infection is associated with neurodevelopmental disturbances, including neurocognitive, gross motor, and psychomotor deficits (Blanchette et al., 2001; McGrath et al., 2006). Elevated rates of motor dysfunction and developmental delay is widely reported in HIV+ infants and children across socio-economic strata, with reported rates reaching 66.7% (Ferguson and Jelsma, 2009; Govender et al., 2011; Le Doare et al., 2012). Even seemingly asymptomatic HIV$^+$ children exhibit measurable motor deficits in standardized testing (Boivin et al., 1995). In adult HIV populations, motor symptoms were often found in conjunction with HAND, but in the post-HAART era it is less common to clinically observe deficits in motor skills and psychomotor speed (Heaton et al., 2011; Saylor et al., 2016). In both children and adults, early initiation of combination antiretroviral therapy (cART) has been shown to improve motor function (despite remaining subnormal), but later initiation of cART failed to yield as notable clinical improvement (Le Doare et al., 2012; Kore et al., 2015; Saylor et al., 2016). The potential role of HERV-K in mediating neurodevelopmental abnormalities in the HIV-infected children needs to be explored. Importantly, HERV-K plays a critical role in early embryogenesis (Grow et al., 2015), and hence its dysregulation by HIV could potentially alter neurodevelopment.

In rare cases, an ALS-like syndrome can occasionally be caused by retroviruses such as HIV and human T cell leukemia virus type-1 (HTLV-1) (Matsuzaki et al., 2000; Verma and Berger, 2006). Antiretroviral therapy can reverse the symptoms of this ALS-like syndrome in HIV-infected individuals (Moulignier et al., 2001; von Giesen et al., 2002), suggesting that HIV replication in the CNS can drive a pathology which symptomatically resembles ALS. Indeed, recent attempts treat HIV-associated motor neuron disease with antiretroviral therapy showed promise, with reversal of recent onset symptoms or a protracted course of the illness following treatment (Bowen et al., 2016). In these patients, the clinical improvement paralleled a decrease in HERV-K viral load in plasma (Bowen et al., 2016). Future research into HIV-associated motor deficits in pediatric and adult populations should consider the potential of HERV-K in driving motor impairment.

Our results support the concept that a failure to control HIV infection, either from a lack of response to HAART therapy, receiving a sub-optimal regimen or the inability of antiretroviral drugs to adequately penetrate the CNS, may be associated with enhanced HERV-K in the brain. The use of antiretroviral drugs to suppress HIV replication in the CNS may have an indirect (or potentially direct) neuroprotective effect by limiting HERV-K-mediated pathology. There is currently a dearth of knowledge pertaining to the identification and use of antiretrovirals customized for use against HERV-K (Tyagi et al., 2017). It remains to be seen how optimization of drug regimens more tailored to inhibition of HERV-K proteins may improve upon these clinical results.

Cognitive and psychomotor symptoms in HIV have been associated with structural changes in the brain following HIV infection, enhanced inflammation and immune activation, as well as metabolic disturbances (Saylor et al., 2016). By merging transdisciplinary expertise, our findings point to an overlapping pathological contribution of TDP-43 deregulation and HERV-K re-activation in both HAND and ALS. Exploration into the pathogenic effects of TDP-43 proteinopathy in ALS has vastly expanded potential therapeutic options for this neurological disease, including small molecule activators of autophagy, the ubiquitin-proteasome system, and chaperone proteins (Scotter et al., 2015). Indeed, therapeutics overcoming TDP-43-mediated pathology may also be clinically useful in retrovirus-associated neurological disease. An improved understanding of the role of TDP-43 in the pathogenesis of HERV-K and HIV infection may hold benefit for either ALS or HAND, in addition to other TDP-43-associated disorders such as Alzheimer's disease (Davis et al., 2017) and prefrontal dementia (Lomen-Hoerth et al., 2003; Merrilees et al., 2010). Considering the seemingly disparate human conditions associated with ERV expression, more efforts into bridging disciplines is warranted, with the goal of elucidating shared molecular pathways and pathologies. Elevating the field of ERVs into the realm of mainstream biomedical research is worthwhile given its considerable clinical relevance. New outlooks on how ERV biology fits into our understanding of human disease may bring us closer to treating some of the most clinically difficult conditions, such as HIV-associated neurological disorders and ALS.

ETHICS STATEMENT

De-identified autopsy brain samples were obtained from the National Neuro-AIDS Tissue Consortium (www.nntc.org). The use these tissues was determined to be IRB exempt.

AUTHOR CONTRIBUTIONS

RD and AN designed the study and wrote the manuscript. RD performed the experiments and analyzed the data. All authors read and approved the final manuscript.

FUNDING

This work has been supported by grants from the National Institutes of Health (NIH).

ACKNOWLEDGMENTS

We thank Dr. Wenxue Li for his advice on brain sample preparation for western blotting. We thank Marie-Josée Nadeau for careful review of the manuscript.

REFERENCES

Alfahad, T., and Nath, A. (2013). Retroviruses and amyotrophic lateral sclerosis. *Antiviral Res.* 99, 180–187. doi: 10.1016/j.antiviral.2013.05.006

Balada, E., Ordi-Ros, J., and Vilardell-Tarres, M. (2009). Molecular mechanisms mediated by human endogenous retroviruses (HERVs) in autoimmunity. *Rev. Med. Virol.* 19, 273–286. doi: 10.1002/rmv.622

Belshaw, R., Dawson, A. L., Woolven-Allen, J., Redding, J., Burt, A., and Tristem, M. (2005). Genomewide screening reveals high levels of insertional polymorphism in the human endogenous retrovirus family HERV-K(HML2): implications for present-day activity. *J. Virol.* 79, 12507–12514. doi: 10.1128/JVI.79.19.12507-12514.2005

Bhat, R. K., Rudnick, W., Antony, J. M., Maingat, F., Ellestad, K. K., Wheatley, B. M., et al. (2014). Human endogenous retrovirus-K(II) envelope induction protects neurons during HIV/AIDS. *PLOS ONE* 9:e97984. doi: 10.1371/journal.pone.0097984

Blanchette, N., Smith, M. L., Fernandes-Penney, A., King, S., and Read, S. (2001). Cognitive and motor development in children with vertically transmitted HIV infection. *Brain Cogn.* 46, 50–53. doi: 10.1016/S0278-2626(01)80032-4

Blikstad, V., Benachenhou, F., Sperber, G. O., and Blomberg, J. (2008). Evolution of human endogenous retroviral sequences: a conceptual account. *Cell Mol. Life Sci.* 65, 3348–3365. doi: 10.1007/s00018-008-8495-2

Boivin, M. J., Green, S. D., Davies, A. G., Giordani, B., Mokili, J. K., and Cutting, W. A. (1995). A preliminary evaluation of the cognitive and motor effects of pediatric HIV infection in Zairian children. *Health Psychol.* 14, 13–21. doi: 10.1037/0278-6133.14.1.13

Bowen, L. N., Tyagi, R., Li, W., Alfahad, T., Smith, B., Wright, M., et al. (2016). HIV-associated motor neuron disease: HERV-K activation and response to antiretroviral therapy. *Neurology* 87, 1756–1762. doi: 10.1212/WNL.0000000000003258

Brady, O. A., Meng, P., Zheng, Y., Mao, Y., and Hu, F. (2011). Regulation of TDP-43 aggregation by phosphorylation and p62/SQSTM1. *J. Neurochem.* 116, 248–259. doi: 10.1111/j.1471-4159.2010.07098.x

Brasier, A. R., Spratt, H., Wu, Z., Boldogh, I., Zhang, Y., Garofalo, R. P., et al. (2004). Nuclear heat shock response and novel nuclear domain 10 reorganization in respiratory syncytial virus-infected a549 cells identified by high-resolution two-dimensional gel electrophoresis. *J. Virol.* 78, 11461–11476. doi: 10.1128/JVI.78.21.11461-11476.2004

Brattas, P. L., Jonsson, M. E., Fasching, L., Nelander Wahlestedt, J., Shahsavani, M., Falk, R., et al. (2017). TRIM28 controls a gene regulatory network based on endogenous retroviruses in human neural progenitor cells. *Cell Rep.* 18, 1–11. doi: 10.1016/j.celrep.2016.12.010

Brutting, C., Emmer, A., Kornhuber, M. E., and Staege, M. S. (2017). Cooccurrences of putative endogenous retrovirus-associated diseases. *Biomed. Res. Int.* 2017:7973165. doi: 10.1155/2017/7973165

Buratti, E., and Baralle, F. E. (2008). Multiple roles of TDP-43 in gene expression, splicing regulation, and human disease. *Front. Biosci.* 13, 867–878. doi: 10.2741/2727

Che, M. X., Jiang, Y. J., Xie, Y. Y., Jiang, L. L., and Hu, H. Y. (2011). Aggregation of the 35-kDa fragment of TDP-43 causes formation of cytoplasmic inclusions and alteration of RNA processing. *FASEB J.* 25, 2344–2353. doi: 10.1096/fj.10-174482

Christensen, T. (2016). Human endogenous retroviruses in neurologic disease. *APMIS* 124, 116–126. doi: 10.1111/apm.12486

Chuong, E. B., Elde, N. C., and Feschotte, C. (2016). Regulatory evolution of innate immunity through co-option of endogenous retroviruses. *Science* 351, 1083–1087. doi: 10.1126/science.aad5497

Contreras-Galindo, R., Almodovar-Camacho, S., Gonzalez-Ramirez, S., Lorenzo, E., and Yamamura, Y. (2007a). Comparative longitudinal studies of HERV-K and HIV-1 RNA titers in HIV-1-infected patients receiving successful versus unsuccessful highly active antiretroviral therapy. *AIDS Res. Hum. Retroviruses* 23, 1083–1086.

Contreras-Galindo, R., Lopez, P., Velez, R., and Yamamura, Y. (2007b). HIV-1 infection increases the expression of human endogenous retroviruses type K (HERV-K) in vitro. *AIDS Res. Hum. Retroviruses* 23, 116–122.

Contreras-Galindo, R., Gonzalez, M., Almodovar-Camacho, S., Gonzalez-Ramirez, S., Lorenzo, E., and Yamamura, Y. (2006). A new Real-Time-RT-PCR for quantitation of human endogenous retroviruses type K (HERV-K) RNA load in plasma samples: increased HERV-K RNA titers in HIV-1 patients with HAART non-suppressive regimens. *J. Virol. Methods* 136, 51–57. doi: 10.1016/j.jviromet.2006.03.029

Davis, S. A., Gan, K. A., Dowell, J. A., Cairns, N. J., and Gitcho, M. A. (2017). TDP-43 expression influences amyloidbeta plaque deposition and tau aggregation. *Neurobiol. Dis.* 103, 154–162. doi: 10.1016/j.nbd.2017.04.012

de Mulder, M., SenGupta, D., Deeks, S. G., Martin, J. N., Pilcher, C. D., Hecht, F. M., et al. (2017). Anti-HERV-K (HML-2) capsid antibody responses in HIV elite controllers. *Retrovirology* 14, 41. doi: 10.1186/s12977-017-0365-2

Douville, R., Liu, J., Rothstein, J., and Nath, A. (2011). Identification of active loci of a human endogenous retrovirus in neurons of patients with amyotrophic lateral sclerosis. *Ann. Neurol.* 69, 141–151. doi: 10.1002/ana.22149

Faure, J., Lachenal, G., Court, M., Hirrlinger, J., Chatellard-Causse, C., Blot, B., et al. (2006). Exosomes are released by cultured cortical neurones. *Mol. Cell. Neurosci.* 31, 642–648. doi: 10.1016/j.mcn.2005.12.003

Ferguson, G., and Jelsma, J. (2009). The prevalence of motor delay among HIV infected children living in Cape Town, South Africa. *Int. J. Rehabil. Res.* 32, 108–114. doi: 10.1097/MRR.0b013e3283013b34

Gonzalez-Hernandez, M. J., Cavalcoli, J. D., Sartor, M. A., Contreras-Galindo, R., Meng, F., Dai, M., et al. (2014). Regulation of the human endogenous retrovirus K (HML-2) transcriptome by the HIV-1 Tat protein. *J. Virol.* 88, 8924–8935. doi: 10.1128/JVI.00556-14

Gonzalez-Hernandez, M. J., Swanson, M. D., Contreras-Galindo, R., Cookinham, S., King, S. R., Noel, R. J. Jr., et al. (2012). Expression of human endogenous retrovirus type K (HML-2) is activated by the Tat protein of HIV-1. *J. Virol.* 86, 7790–7805. doi: 10.1128/JVI.07215-11

Govender, R., Eley, B., Walker, K., Petersen, R., and Wilmshurst, J. M. (2011). Neurologic and neurobehavioral sequelae in children with human immunodeficiency virus (HIV-1) infection. *J. Child Neurol.* 26, 1355–1364. doi: 10.1177/0883073811405203

Grow, E. J., Flynn, R. A., Chavez, S. L., Bayless, N. L., Wossidlo, M., Wesche, D. J., et al. (2015). Intrinsic retroviral reactivation in human preimplantation embryos and pluripotent cells. *Nature* 522, 221–225. doi: 10.1038/nature14308

Hanspal, M. A., Dobson, C. M., Yerbury, J. J., and Kumita, J. R. (2017). The relevance of contact-independent cell-to-cell transfer of TDP-43 and SOD1 in amyotrophic lateral sclerosis. *Biochim. Biophys. Acta.* doi: 10.1016/j.bbadis.2017.07.007 [Epub ahead of print].

Heaton, R. K., Franklin, D. R., Ellis, R. J., McCutchan, J. A., Letendre, S. L., Leblanc, S., et al. (2011). HIV-associated neurocognitive disorders before and during the era of combination antiretroviral therapy: differences in rates, nature, and predictors. *J. Neurovirol.* 17, 3–16. doi: 10.1007/s13365-010-0006-1

Huang, C. C., Bose, J. K., Majumder, P., Lee, K. H., Huang, J. T., Huang, J. K., et al. (2014). Metabolism and mis-metabolism of the neuropathological signature protein TDP-43. *J. Cell Sci.* 127(Pt 14), 3024–3038. doi: 10.1242/jcs.136150

Hurst, T. P., and Magiorkinis, G. (2015). Activation of the innate immune response by endogenous retroviruses. *J. Gen. Virol.* 96(Pt 6), 1207–1218. doi: 10.1099/jgv.0.000017

Irwin, D. J., Cairns, N. J., Grossman, M., McMillan, C. T., Lee, E. B., Van Deerlin, V. M., et al. (2015). Frontotemporal lobar degeneration: defining phenotypic diversity through personalized medicine. *Acta Neuropathol.* 129, 469–491. doi: 10.1007/s00401-014-1380-1

Jolicoeur, P., Hu, C., Mak, T. W., Martinou, J. C., and Kay, D. G. (2003). Protection against murine leukemia virus-induced spongiform myeloencephalopathy in mice overexpressing Bcl-2 but not in mice deficient for interleukin-6, inducible nitric oxide synthetase, ICE, Fas, Fas ligand, or TNF-R1 genes. *J. Virol.* 77, 13161–13170. doi: 10.1128/JVI.77.24.13161-13170.2003

Kassiotis, G. (2014). Endogenous retroviruses and the development of cancer. *J. Immunol.* 192, 1343–1349. doi: 10.4049/jimmunol.1302972

Kore, I., Ananworanich, J., Valcour, V., Fletcher, J. L., Chalermchai, T., Paul, R., et al. (2015). Neuropsychological impairment in acute HIV and the effect of immediate antiretroviral therapy. *J. Acquir. Immune Defic. Syndr.* 70, 393–399. doi: 10.1097/QAI.0000000000000746

Kraft-Terry, S. D., Stothert, A. R., Buch, S., and Gendelman, H. E. (2010). HIV-1 neuroimmunity in the era of antiretroviral therapy. *Neurobiol. Dis.* 37, 542–548. doi: 10.1016/j.nbd.2009.12.015

Krug, L., Chatterjee, N., Borges-Monroy, R., Hearn, S., Liao, W. W., Morrill, K., et al. (2017). Retrotransposon activation contributes to neurodegeneration in a Drosophila TDP-43 model of ALS. *PLOS Genet.* 13:e1006635. doi: 10.1371/journal.pgen.1006635

Laderoute, M. P., Giulivi, A., Larocque, L., Bellfoy, D., Hou, Y., Wu, H. X., et al. (2007). The replicative activity of human endogenous retrovirus K102 (HERV-K102) with HIV viremia. *AIDS* 21, 2417–2424. doi: 10.1097/QAD.0b013e3282f14d64

Le Doare, K., Bland, R., and Newell, M. L. (2012). Neurodevelopment in children born to HIV-infected mothers by infection and treatment status. *Pediatrics* 130, e1326–e1344. doi: 10.1542/peds.2012-0405

Li, W., Lee, M. H., Henderson, L., Tyagi, R., Bachani, M., Steiner, J., et al. (2015). Human endogenous retrovirus-K contributes to motor neuron disease. *Sci. Transl. Med.* 7:307ra153. doi: 10.1126/scitranslmed.aac8201

Li, W., Li, G., Steiner, J., and Nath, A. (2009). Role of Tat protein in HIV neuropathogenesis. *Neurotox. Res.* 16, 205–220. doi: 10.1007/s12640-009-9047-8

Ling, S. C., Polymenidou, M., and Cleveland, D. W. (2013). Converging mechanisms in ALS and FTD: disrupted RNA and protein homeostasis. *Neuron* 79, 416–438. doi: 10.1016/j.neuron.2013.07.033

Lomen-Hoerth, C., Murphy, J., Langmore, S., Kramer, J. H., Olney, R. K., and Miller, B. (2003). Are amyotrophic lateral sclerosis patients cognitively normal? *Neurology* 60, 1094–1097.

Lynch, W. P., and Sharpe, A. H. (2000). Differential glycosylation of the Cas-Br-E env protein is associated with retrovirus-induced spongiform neurodegeneration. *J. Virol.* 74, 1558–1565. doi: 10.1128/JVI.74.3.1558-1565.2000

Mackenzie, I. R., Bigio, E. H., Ince, P. G., Geser, F., Neumann, M., Cairns, N. J., et al. (2007). Pathological TDP-43 distinguishes sporadic amyotrophic lateral sclerosis from amyotrophic lateral sclerosis with SOD1 mutations. *Ann. Neurol.* 61, 427–434. doi: 10.1002/ana.21147

Mager, D. L., and Stoye, J. P. (2015). Mammalian endogenous retroviruses. *Microbiol. Spectr.* 3:MDNA3-0009–2014. doi: 10.1128/microbiolspec.MDNA3-0009-2014

Manghera, M., and Douville, R. N. (2013). Endogenous retrovirus-K promoter: a landing strip for inflammatory transcription factors? *Retrovirology* 10:16. doi: 10.1186/1742-4690-10-16

Manghera, M., Ferguson, J., and Douville, R. (2014). Endogenous retrovirus-K and nervous system diseases. *Curr. Neurol. Neurosci. Rep.* 14:488. doi: 10.1007/s11910-014-0488-y

Manghera, M., Ferguson-Parry, J., and Douville, R. N. (2016a). TDP-43 regulates endogenous retrovirus-K viral protein accumulation. *Neurobiol. Dis.* 94, 226–236. doi: 10.1016/j.nbd.2016.06.017

Manghera, M., Ferguson-Parry, J., Lin, R., and Douville, R. N. (2016b). NF-kappaB and IRF1 induce endogenous retrovirus K expression via interferon-stimulated response elements in its 5' long terminal repeat. *J. Virol.* 90, 9338–9349. doi: 10.1128/JVI.01503-16

Matsuzaki, T., Nakagawa, M., Nagai, M., Nobuhara, Y., Usuku, K., Higuchi, I., et al. (2000). HTLV-I-associated myelopathy (HAM)/tropical spastic paraparesis (TSP) with amyotrophic lateral sclerosis-like manifestations. *J. Neurovirol.* 6, 544–548. doi: 10.3109/13550280009091955

McArthur, J. C., Steiner, J., Sacktor, N., and Nath, A. (2010). Human immunodeficiency virus-associated neurocognitive disorders: mind the gap. *Ann. Neurol.* 67, 699–714. doi: 10.1002/ana.22053

McGrath, N., Fawzi, W. W., Bellinger, D., Robins, J., Msamanga, G. I., Manji, K., et al. (2006). The timing of mother-to-child transmission of human immunodeficiency virus infection and the neurodevelopment of children in Tanzania. *Pediatr. Infect. Dis. J.* 25, 47–52. doi: 10.1097/01.inf.0000195638.80578.e0

Merrilees, J., Klapper, J., Murphy, J., Lomen-Hoerth, C., and Miller, B. L. (2010). Cognitive and behavioral challenges in caring for patients with frontotemporal dementia and amyotrophic lateral sclerosis. *Amyotroph. Lateral Scler.* 11, 298–302. doi: 10.3109/17482961003605788

Meyer, T. J., Rosenkrantz, J. L., Carbone, L., and Chavez, S. L. (2017). Endogenous retroviruses: with us and against us. *Front. Chem.* 5:23. doi: 10.3389/fchem.2017.00023

Monahan, Z., Shewmaker, F., and Pandey, U. B. (2016). Stress granules at the intersection of autophagy and ALS. *Brain Res.* 1649, 189–200. doi: 10.1016/j.brainres.2016.05.022

Monde, K., Terasawa, H., Nakano, Y., Soheilian, F., Nagashima, K., Maeda, Y., et al. (2017). Molecular mechanisms by which HERV-K Gag interferes with HIV-1 Gag assembly and particle infectivity. *Retrovirology* 14:27. doi: 10.1186/s12977-017-0351-8

Moulignier, A., Moulonguet, A., Pialoux, G., and Rozenbaum, W. (2001). Reversible ALS-like disorder in HIV infection. *Neurology* 57, 995–1001. doi: 10.1212/WNL.57.6.995

Nehls, J., Koppensteiner, H., Brack-Werner, R., Floss, T., and Schindler, M. (2014). HIV-1 replication in human immune cells is independent of TAR DNA binding protein 43 (TDP-43) expression. *PLOS ONE* 9:e105478. doi: 10.1371/journal.pone.0105478

Ou, S. H., Wu, F., Harrich, D., Garcia-Martinez, L. F., and Gaynor, R. B. (1995). Cloning and characterization of a novel cellular protein, TDP-43, that binds to human immunodeficiency virus type 1 TAR DNA sequence motifs. *J. Virol.* 69, 3584–3596.

Prudencio, M., Gonzales, P. K., Cook, C. N., Gendron, T. F., Daughrity, L. M., Song, Y., et al. (2017). Repetitive element transcripts are elevated in the brain of C9orf72 ALS/FTLD patients. *Hum. Mol. Genet.* 26, 3421–3431. doi: 10.1093/hmg/ddx233

Ratti, A., and Buratti, E. (2016). Physiological functions and pathobiology of TDP-43 and FUS/TLS proteins. *J. Neurochem.* 138(Suppl. 1), 95–111. doi: 10.1111/jnc.13625

Robertson, K. R., Smurzynski, M., Parsons, T. D., Wu, K., Bosch, R. J., Wu, J., et al. (2007). The prevalence and incidence of neurocognitive impairment in the HAART era. *AIDS* 21, 1915–1921. doi: 10.1097/QAD.0b013e32828e4e27

Ruprecht, K., Mayer, J., Sauter, M., Roemer, K., and Mueller-Lantzsch, N. (2008). Endogenous retroviruses and cancer. *Cell Mol. Life Sci.* 65, 3366–3382. doi: 10.1007/s00018-008-8496-1

Saylor, D., Dickens, A. M., Sacktor, N., Haughey, N., Slusher, B., Pletnikov, M., et al. (2016). HIV-associated neurocognitive disorder–pathogenesis and prospects for treatment. *Nat. Rev. Neurol.* 12, 234–248. doi: 10.1038/nrneurol.2016.27

Scotter, E. L., Chen, H. J., and Shaw, C. E. (2015). TDP-43 proteinopathy and ALS: insights into disease mechanisms and therapeutic targets. *Neurotherapeutics* 12, 352–363. doi: 10.1007/s13311-015-0338-x

Serra, C., Mameli, G., Arru, G., Sotgiu, S., Rosati, G., and Dolei, A. (2003). In vitro modulation of the multiple sclerosis (MS)-associated retrovirus by cytokines: implications for MS pathogenesis. *J. Neurovirol.* 9, 637–643. doi: 10.1080/714044485

Stetson, D. B., Ko, J. S., Heidmann, T., and Medzhitov, R. (2008). Trex1 prevents cell-intrinsic initiation of autoimmunity. *Cell* 134, 587–598. doi: 10.1016/j.cell.2008.06.032

Subramanian, R. P., Wildschutte, J. H., Russo, C., and Coffin, J. M. (2011). Identification, characterization, and comparative genomic distribution of the HERV-K (HML-2) group of human endogenous retroviruses. *Retrovirology* 8:90. doi: 10.1186/1742-4690-8-90

Terry, S. N., Manganaro, L., Cuesta-Dominguez, A., Brinzevich, D., Simon, V., and Mulder, L. C. F. (2017). Expression of HERV-K108 envelope interferes with HIV-1 production. *Virology* 509, 52–59. doi: 10.1016/j.virol.2017.06.004

Tyagi, R., Li, W., Parades, D., Bianchet, M. A., and Nath, A. (2017). Inhibition of human endogenous retrovirus-K by antiretroviral drugs. *Retrovirology* 14, 21. doi: 10.1186/s12977-017-0347-4

Vargas, A., Zhou, S., Ethier-Chiasson, M., Flipo, D., Lafond, J., Gilbert, C., et al. (2014). Syncytin proteins incorporated in placenta exosomes are important for cell uptake and show variation in abundance in serum exosomes from patients with preeclampsia. *FASEB J.* 28, 3703–3719. doi: 10.1096/fj.13-239053

Verma, A., and Berger, J. R. (2006). ALS syndrome in patients with HIV-1 infection. *J. Neurol. Sci.* 240, 59–64. doi: 10.1016/j.jns.2005.09.005

von Giesen, H. J., Kaiser, R., Koller, H., Wetzel, K., and Arendt, G. (2002). Reversible ALS-like disorder in HIV infection. An ALS-like syndrome with new HIV infection and complete response to antiretroviral therapy. *Neurology* 59, 474, author reply 474–475. doi: 10.1212/WNL.59.3.474

Wurdinger, T., Gatson, N. N., Balaj, L., Kaur, B., Breakefield, X. O., and Pegtel, D. M. (2012). Extracellular vesicles and their convergence with viral pathways. *Adv. Virol.* 2012:767694. doi: 10.1155/2012/767694

Xiao, S., Sanelli, T., Chiang, H., Sun, Y., Chakrabartty, A., Keith, J., et al. (2015). Low molecular weight species of TDP-43 generated by abnormal splicing form inclusions in amyotrophic lateral sclerosis and result in motor neuron death. *Acta Neuropathol.* 130, 49–61. doi: 10.1007/s00401-015-1412-5

Yang, C., Tan, W., Whittle, C., Qiu, L., Cao, L., Akbarian, S., et al. (2010). The C-terminal TDP-43 fragments have a high aggregation propensity and harm neurons by a dominant-negative mechanism. *PLOS ONE* 5:e15878. doi: 10.1371/journal.pone.0015878

Yu, P., Lubben, W., Slomka, H., Gebler, J., Konert, M., Cai, C., et al. (2012). Nucleic acid-sensing Toll-like receptors are essential for the control of endogenous retrovirus viremia and ERV-induced tumors. *Immunity* 37, 867–879. doi: 10.1016/j.immuni.2012.07.018

8

Intestinal Microbiome Shifts, Dysbiosis, Inflammation and Non-Alcoholic Fatty Liver Disease

Emma T. Saltzman [1,2], Talia Palacios [1,2], Michael Thomsen [1,2] and Luis Vitetta [1,2*]*

[1] *Sydney Medical School, University of Sydney, Sydney, NSW, Australia,* [2] *Medlab Clinical, Sydney, NSW, Australia*

Correspondence:
Emma T. Saltzman
esal4025@uni.sydney.edu.au
Luis Vitetta
luis.vitetta@sydney.edu.au;
luis_vitetta@medlab.co

Adverse fluctuations in the distribution of the intestinal microbiome cohort has been associated with the onset of intra- and extra-intestinal inflammatory conditions, like the metabolic syndrome (MetS) and it's hepatic manifestation, non-alcoholic fatty liver disease (NAFLD). The intestinal microbial community of obese compared to lean subjects has been shown to undergo configurational shifts in various genera, including but not limited to increased abundances of *Prevotella, Escherichia, Peptoniphilus,* and *Parabacteroides* and decreased levels of *Bifidobacteria, Roseburia,* and *Eubacteria* genera. At the phylum level, decreased *Bacteroidetes* and increased *Firmicutes* have been reported. The intestinal microbiota therefore presents an important target for designing novel therapeutic modalities that target extra-intestinal inflammatory disorders, such as NAFLD. This review hypothesizes that disruption of the intestinal–mucosal macrophage interface is a key factor in intestinal-liver axis disturbances. Intestinal immune responses implicated in the manifestation, maintenance and progression of NAFLD provide insights into the dialogue between the intestinal microbiome, the epithelia and mucosal immunity. The pro-inflammatory activity and immune imbalances implicated in NAFLD pathophysiology are reported to stem from dysbiosis of the intestinal epithelia which can serve as a source of hepatoxic effects. We posit that the hepatotoxic consequences of intestinal dysbiosis are compounded through intestinal microbiota-mediated inflammation of the local mucosa that encourages mucosal immune dysfunction, thus contributing important plausible insight in NAFLD pathogenesis. The administration of probiotics and prebiotics as a cure-all remedy for all chronic diseases is not advocated, instead, the incorporation of evidence based probiotic/prebiotic formulations as adjunctive modalities may enhance lifestyle modification management strategies for the amelioration of NAFLD.

Keywords: intestinal microbiome, intestinal epithelial cell dysbiosis, dysbiosis, macrophage, inflammation, mucosal immunity, NAFLD

INTRODUCTION

NAFLD is a growing public health concern, laying claim to both a steadily rising prevalence as well as an increasingly young age at diagnosis (Welsh et al., 2013; Nobili et al., 2014). These trends reflect the increased rates of risk factors associated with an obesogenic lifestyle and the development of type 2 diabetes mellitus (T2DM) (Targher et al., 2007; Welsh et al., 2013). The prevalence of NAFLD in obese adults or those with T2DM has been reported to be 67.5 and 74%, respectively,

(Williams et al., 2011; Paquissi, 2016) compared to only 25% in the general adult population (Younossi et al., 2016). As a spectrum of diseases, NAFLD has been associated with significant morbidity and mortality, with advanced forms of the disease expressed as fibrosis, cirrhosis, and hepatocellular carcinoma (HCC).Additionally, insulin resistance (IR) and obesity have been identified as NAFLD risk factors (Gaggini et al., 2013), with NAFLD also reported to increase the risk of T2DM and cardiovascular disease, justly classifying NAFLD as the hepatic manifestation of the metabolic syndrome (MetS) (Adams et al., 2005; Targher et al., 2007, 2010; Dunn et al., 2008; Starley et al., 2010; Gregor and Hotamisligil, 2011; Lumeng and Saltiel, 2011; Dietrich and Hellerbrand, 2014; Paolella et al., 2014; Paquissi, 2016). NAFLD hence presents as a multi-systemic disease (Starley et al., 2010; Paolella et al., 2014). In light of the potential of NAFLD to progress to an ever-increasing prevalence, an appreciation of the molecular mechanisms that facilitate the manifestation of NAFLD disease chronicity and the pathways that trigger the transition across the spectrum of diseases is a pertinent aspect in designing novel effective therapeutic modalities. With the purported pathogenic mechanisms of NAFLD being intertwined with peripheral IR, increased liver lipolysis is reported to contribute to increased levels of hepatic free fatty acids (FFAs) (Paolella et al., 2014). IR simultaneously triggers increased gluconeogenesis and reduced glyconeogenesis, which further increases the production of circulating FFAs (Paolella et al., 2014).

The definition of NAFLD covers a spectrum of liver histologies, ranging from the benign and usually non-progressive simple steatosis (SS) (Tilg and Moschen, 2010; characterized by the accumulation of lipid droplets that exceed 5% of the total weight of the liver) to non-alcoholic steatohepatitis (NASH) which is found in 30% of NAFLD patients and is described as the beginning stages of inflammation and lobular ballooning which results from persistent hepatic injury (Jiang et al., 2015). Chronic inflammation can cause the liver to respond with compensatory tissue repair, a mechanism that initiates fibrosis and even cirrhosis through collagen deposition and scarring—which eventually forms the foundation of hepatocellular cancer (HCC) in extremely rare cases (Tilg and Moschen, 2010; Bieghs and Trautwein, 2014). Systems biology continues to probe the pathophysiology of this disease and the factors that establish it's manifestation and drives disease progression across the spectrum toward severe phenotypes.

The manifestation and progression of NAFLD is tentatively attributed to a range of factors as part of the multiple *parallel hits* hypothesis, which postulates that NAFLD is the result of inflammation in the liver induced by numerous intestinal-derived or adipose tissue-derived triggers (Tilg and Moschen, 2010). With the *first hit* said to be the onset and maintenance of SS, and the additional hits of gut-derived endotoxins and pro-inflammatory cytokines from adipose tissue reported to provide the impetus for NASH development and subsequent progression (Day and James, 1998). This hypothesis is flagging the importance of aberrant innate immunity as a central pathway for NAFLD progression (Miele et al., 2009; Tilg and Moschen, 2010) along with stress signaling networks and circulating adipocytokines and pro-inflammatory cytokines (Miele et al., 2009; Tilg and Moschen, 2010).

Although the molecular pathways that lead to the pathogenesis and progression of NAFLD remain poorly understood, it is accepted that inflammation is a major factor in hepatic injury (Bieghs and Trautwein, 2014). Currently, experimental data suggests that interactions of the innate immune system with the different resident liver cell types help perpetuate and maintain adverse inflammatory responses in the liver (Starley et al., 2010; Farrell et al., 2012; Bieghs and Trautwein, 2014). Serum markers of inflammation, including C-reactive protein (CRP), interleukins (ILs), and other general immunity markers are associated with the diagnosis and prognosis of NAFLD (Chiang et al., 2010; Harley et al., 2014), whilst at the cellular level, data has implicated an imbalance in T helper 17 (Th17) cells over regulatory T (Treg) cells, that occurs from an over-differentiation of T helper cells (Hammerich et al., 2011). A disturbance to the equilibrium between Th17 and Treg cells is a key event in the initiation of pro-inflammatory activity.

The innate immune system responds to cell damage or pathogenic invasion through pattern recognition receptors (PRRs), that are expressed intracellularly or on the surface of resident liver cells (Bieghs and Trautwein, 2014). These PRRs are programmed to detect damage-associated molecular patterns (DAMPs) that are released by injured cells or pathogen-associated molecular patterns (PAMPs), which are derived from intestinal bacterial metabolites (Pedra et al., 2009; Takeuchi and Akira, 2010). From a consideration of the consequences of intestinal epithelial dysbiosis, this review hypothesizes that the cascade of signals that activate adverse innate immune system and inflammatory activity implicated in NAFLD pathophysiology are triggered by the continuous release of endotoxins and other intestinal bacterial-derived products which can reach the liver through the gut-liver axis interface.

Resident liver cells have their own PRRs in toll-like receptors (TLRs). Activating these TLRs is an important step in the development of NAFLD as they are responsible for inducing gene transcription that facilitates responses of the innate immune system (Takeuchi and Akira, 2010). Kupffer cells, stellate cells, and hepatocytes amongst others, express TLRs and recognize a large array of PAMPs, which enable pro-inflammatory activity by activating different liver cells. PAMPs and DAMPs as well as irritants from the host's environment are themselves recognized by inflammasomes, receptors of the innate immune system. In response to sensing infectious microbes, inflammasomes are responsible for the pro-inflammatory activity observed in the initiation or manifestation of inflammatory diseases, like NAFLD. NLRP3 is an inflammasome that has been reported to be specifically and critically involved in NAFLD progression, with experimental and clinical data identifying higher levels of expression in NASH-affected subjects.

The intestinal microbiome is central to the narrative that NAFLD manifestation is largely a consequence of dysregulated innate immunity in response to persistent pro-inflammatory activity. The role of the intestinal microbiome is multi-factorial, functioning as an immunological, metabolic, and protective tool for optimal host health. When the intestinal microbiome is in dysbiosis, the health of the host is compromised as the microbiome is unable to maintain control of local homeostasis, increasing intestinal permeability. Disruption to intestinal epithelial homeostasis leads to hepatic exposure to exogenous and endogenous antigens that drives hepatoxic influences via the gut-liver axis interface (Glavan et al., 2016).

THE INTESTINAL MICROBIOME AND THE EPITHELIAL BARRIER

The microbial ecosystem of the gastrointestinal tract (GIT) comprises a metabolically and immunologically complex and active organ (Vitetta et al., 2013). Recognized as the most biodiverse and dense microbial site, the intestinal microbiome is estimated to harbor over 10^{14} bacterial cells (Jiang et al., 2015). Serving as a key influence of host health, the GIT is the site that facilitates the exposure of environmental, dietary, and microbial antigens to the immune system (Vitetta et al., 2013). Existing in a state of symbiotic homeostasis, the intestinal microbiome and the immune system largely co-develop from birth (Nicholson et al., 2012). Subject to an array of complex interactions, dependent on host genetics, lifestyle, dietary and environmental cues, the microbiome and host share a bi-directional relationship, with both parties helping to shape each other's development and composition (Nicholson et al., 2012).

The intestinal epithelial barrier is a dynamic network made up of luminal and mucosal components (Paolella et al., 2014); with an epithelial cell layer interlaced with innate mucosal immunity and neuroendocrine elements, encasing the paracellular space that houses the intestinal microbiome diverse niches (Paolella et al., 2014; Ringel et al., 2015). The single layer of epithelial cells that line the intestines is bound by a tight junction protein (TJP) network, serving to form the physical barrier, which provides protection against potential pathogenic assaults and toxins that increases the risk of systemic sepsis. Intestinal epithelial cells have a rapid time of turnover of between 2 and 6 days (Ramachandran et al., 2000). The TJP network also regulates intestinal permeability, providing the pores and channels for passage of molecules (i.e., water, electrolytes, nutrients) by selective permeability (Paolella et al., 2014). The intestinal barrier is also involved in the co-ordination of responses of the innate immune system, with macrophage/dendritic cell activation contributing to host defenses against microbial-induced systemic infections (Paolella et al., 2014). The protrusions that characterize macrophages/dendritic cells allow for the sensation of potential pathogens that have breached the intestinal mucus layers, the mucosa, as well as those sensed in other parts of the intestinal lumen, resulting in the induction of responses such as phagocytosis and of the acquired immune system through B-cell activation (Kumar et al., 2011; Kinnebrew and Pamer, 2012). **Figure 1** details the maintenance of the homeostatic state of the intestinal barrier.

Intestinal microbial metabolites provide the substrate for the fermentation of complex dietary carbohydrates to produce short-chain fatty acids (SCFAs), as well as assist the host in harnessing maximal energy from dietary consumption (Jiang et al., 2015). The various metabolites exert varying effects on the host, from the beneficial production of signaling molecules (e.g., butyrate), to inducing mucus and other secretions, to provide the triggers that facilitate the innate mucosal system to maintain local homeostasis. In states of dysbiosis, the intestinal barrier increases in permeability as a result of a disruption to the regulation of the epithelial cell-to-cell tight junction protein network. A compromised intestinal barrier can be associated with bacterial translocation from the gut into the systemic circulation increasing the risk of sepsis. Lipopolysaccharides (LPS), a constituent of gram negative bacteria (Jiang et al., 2015), is found to be increased in the systemic circulation, indicative of dysbiosis (Boulangé et al., 2016). LPS has been associated with inducing apoptosis of lymphocytes under *in vivo* conditions (Norimatsu et al., 1995; Nielsen et al., 2012; Jiang et al., 2015) demonstrating an immune-modulatory effect. Studies have posited that a loss of lymphocytes in the intestinal mucosa is a consequence of intestinal epithelial dysbiosis and subsequent release of metabolic endotoxins (Jiang et al., 2015). LPS has also been implicated as an inductor of a pro-inflammatory environment which is conducive to MetS, IR and T2DM (Cani et al., 2008). Gram-negative bacteria containing LPS are therefore hypothesized to contribute to NAFLD development. Furthermore, dysbiosis and elevated systemic LPS can be envisaged as markers of intestinal toxicity (Nolan, 2010). Intestinal toxicity driven dysbiosis supports local mucosal inflammatory responses that is concomitant with an increase in intestinal permeability. This combined disruption of the intestinal barrier/mucosal immunity activity can promote and mediate NAFLD pathogenesis via the gut-liver axis (Littman and Pamer, 2011; Wieland et al., 2015).

THE GUT-LIVER AXIS

The venous system of the portal circulation defines the gut-liver axis and highlights the close anatomical proximity and functional interactions of the gastrointestinal tract and the liver (Paolella et al., 2014; Brandl et al., 2017). The axis is described as a means of enhancing interactions between metabolites of the intestinal microbiome and receptors on the liver, which can trigger a cascade of events that culminates in IR, inflammation of the liver, and eventually the development of liver fibrosis (Paolella et al., 2014). The anatomical and functional link between the gut and liver delivers 70% of hepatic blood supply via the portal vein. The portal vein is the direct venous outflow from the intestines and thus when the intestinal mucosal barrier is compromised it exposes hepatic tissue to toxic factors derived from the intestines. Therefore, various metabolites produced by intestinal bacteria that reach the liver, have been linked to the manifestation of simple steatosis and NASH (Raman et al., 2013). Dynamic shifts in the gut-liver axis, contributed by either the physical barrier, the microbiome or the liver itself, are a result of alterations to the permeability of the intestinal epithelium and or microbial composition that have been implicated in NAFLD manifestation (Mehal, 2012). Experimental and clinical evidence increasingly implicate dysfunctions of the gut-liver axis in the development

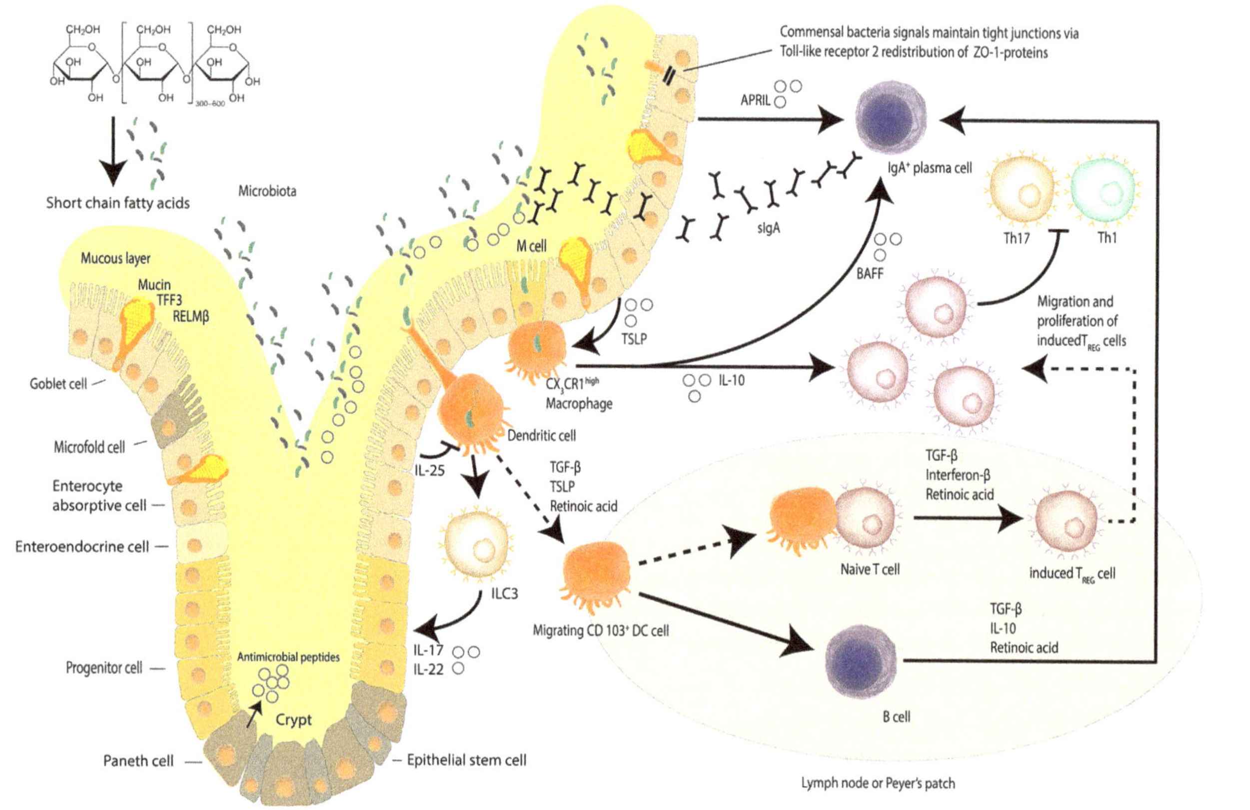

FIGURE 1 | Intestinal epithelial barrier and homeostasis. Several mechanisms, including a mucus layer, antimicrobial peptides and a tight junction protein network collaborate to ensure that the intestinal barrier is not compromised. Goblet cells secrete mucin to provide a protective coating, provide structural integrity and regulate macrophage and adaptive T cell responses during inflammation. Goblet cells also facilitate microbial translocation. The intestinal epithelia network of cells produce a range of soluble protein factors and also express the integrin ligand semaphorin 7A that modulates intestinal CX_3CR1 macrophage function. Localized CX3CR1 macrophages further release IL-10 to support the proliferation of induced Treg cells and B cell activating factor (BAFF) to further stimulate the production of migrating secretory IgA (sIgA) across the epithelium. Dendritic cells sample bacteria and present antigens to other cells including innate lymphoid cells (ILCs). Dietary starch is converted by intestinal bacteria into short chain fatty acids that serve as a source of energy for the epithelial cells but also act as signaling molecules. Signals from commensal bacteria help maintain tight junction via Toll-like receptor 2 (TLR-2) redistribution of ZO-1 proteins. (Kidd, 2003; Wahl, 2007; Hume, 2008; Ogino et al., 2011; Kayama et al., 2012; Abbas et al., 2013; Smith et al., 2013; Zheng, 2013; Ai et al., 2014; Guilliams et al., 2014; Peterson and Artis, 2014; Gottschalk and Kurts, 2015; Robinson et al., 2015; Nakahashi-Oda et al., 2016) Adapted from Peterson and Artis (2014).

and progression of NAFLD through small intestinal bacterial overgrowth (SIBO) in conjunction with intestinal dysbiosis and increased permeability (Compare et al., 2012; Li et al., 2013; Miele et al., 2013; Vajro et al., 2013; Paolella et al., 2014). Recent experimental and clinical studies suggest that the gastrointestinal microbiome affects NAFLD pathogenesis through pathways that (i) facilitate metabolism and energy harvesting (Turnbaugh et al., 2006; Jiang et al., 2015), as described from high-fat fed mice models treated with high levels of pro-inflammatory cytokines that promote NAFLD development (Le Roy et al., 2013); (ii) dynamic interactions with the host's innate immune system where NAFLD is reported consequent to disrupted local immune cell functionality (Su et al., 2012).

INTESTINAL MICROBIAL COMPOSITION AND NAFLD

Widespread biodiversity exists in the microbial ecosystems of humans, particularly in the intestinal tract. However, despite the extensive variety of bacteria, four main phylum dominate in the intestines: *Firmicutes, Bacteroidetes, Actinobacteria, and Proteobacteria* (Mokhtari et al., 2017), with up to 90% of microbes estimated to belong to the Firmicutes and Bacteroidetes phyla (Eckburg et al., 2005). In both human and experimental model based studies, NAFLD has been associated with altered microbiome abundance, composition and dysbiosis (Wigg et al., 2001; Mouzaki et al., 2013; Zhu et al., 2013). Analyses have also correlated changes in microbiota composition with change in disease severity (Shavakhi et al., 2013; Eslamparast et al., 2014, 2015; Rahimlou et al., 2015; Yari et al., 2016).

In reviewing the literature, studies that have analyzed the intestinal microbial composition of NAFLD patients in comparison to healthy controls have reported identifying patterns or trends that can be associated with NAFLD development (Harris et al., 2012).

Studies that have profiled the intestinal microbiome of NAFLD patients report that specific configurational and compositional shifts are associated with intestinal epithelial

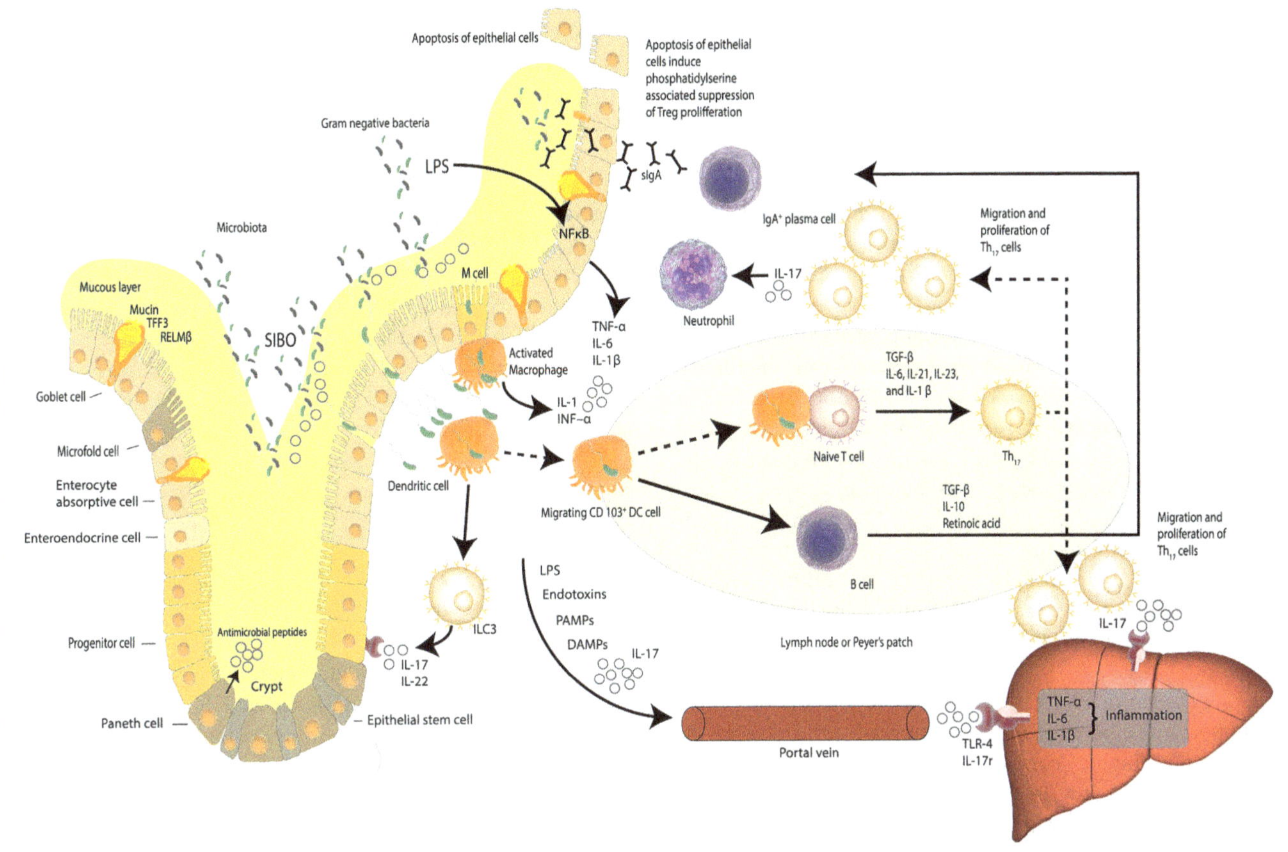

FIGURE 2 | Dysbiosis and the gut-liver axis. Increased intestinal permeability, small intestine bacterial overgrowth (SIBO) and elevated serum endotoxin like lipopolysaccharide (LPS) is found in patients with NAFLD. LPS, a hepatoxic component of gram-negative bacteria, is elevated in cases of SIBO. Increased intestinal permeability leads to increased bacterial translocation. Activated macrophages release inflammatory cytokines and dendritic cells stimulate the differentiation of naïve T cells to pro-inflammatory Th17 cells induced by TGF-β, IL-6, IL-23, and IL-1β. Th17 cells secrete neutrophil-activating IL-17. Lymphoid Th17 also migrate to the liver where IL-17 stimulates monocytes, Kupffer cells, biliary epithelial cells, and stellate cells, to secrete pro-inflammatory cytokines and chemokines—inducing liver inflammation. LPS, bacterial endotoxins, IL-17, pathogen-associated molecular patterns (PAMPs) and damage-associated molecular patterns (DAMPs) may reach the liver via the portal vein and induce inflammation via Toll-like receptor 4 (TLR-4) and interleukin-17 (IL-17) receptors. The gut-liver axis is underlined by the fact that at least 70% of the liver's blood supply is delivered directly from the intestinal tract via the portal vein outflow of the intestine. (Zheng, 2013; Carding et al., 2015; Robinson et al., 2015; Fukui, 2016; Kumar et al., 2016) Adapted from Peterson and Artis (2014).

cell dysbiosis and the elicitation of pro-inflammatory immune responses, central to NAFLD manifestation and progression (Kirpich et al., 2015). Specific bacteria have been associated with NAFLD phenotypes, serving as both antagonists and protagonists in NAFLD pathogenesis. Studies which profiled the intestinal microbiome of healthy controls and NAFLD patients across the spectrum, were able to identify families, genera and phyla that differed significantly in their abundance between the healthy controls and those with a NAFLD diagnosis. Whilst data is inconsistent regarding the association between the intestinal microbiome profile and NAFLD, patterns are emerging which highlight potential relationships between bacterial types and host health (Lau et al., 2015). A study comparing subjects diagnosed with NAFLD compared to lean adults, reported that gram negative bacteria were significantly enriched (P =0 .009) and gram positive bacteria were markedly decreased (P = 0.001) in the NAFLD cohort (Wang et al., 2016). Findings from similar studies confirm the strong relationship between the composition and configuration of the intestinal microbiome and fatty liver histologies, suggesting that adverse shifts in intestinal microbiome profiles are related to the development of NAFLD (Wang et al., 2016). In a prospective cross sectional study, a 20% increase in the *Bacteroidetes* phylum ($p = 0.005$) and a 24% decrease in *Firmicutes* ($p = 0.002$) was found in healthy controls in comparison to NAFLD patients (Wang et al., 2016). Interestingly, among the species belonging to the *Firmicutes* phylum, SCFA-producing bacteria were significantly decreased. Specific microbiome signatures of intestinal bacteria that are reported to be associated with significant reductions in butyric acid (Consolandi et al., 2015) may comprise a significant marker for the depletion of intestinal bacterial species that are important for the maintenance of intestinal barrier integrity and innate mucosal immunity equilibrium. However, currently it is difficult to identify which microbiome differences are causal and which are coincidental in the development of intestinal barrier dysbiosis and moreover NAFLD. Variations between studies, which profile microbiome composition of NAFLD patients, may in part be accounted for by different analytical techniques that have been employed. Furthermore, differences in study design, including anthropometric measures, markers used for NAFLD diagnosis as well as ultra-sonographic vs. biopsy NAFLD diagnosis adds additional discrepancies. As such Mouzaki et al. (2013), reported an inverse relationship between NASH diagnosis and the proportion of the phyla *Bacteroidetes* detected. These results were contrasted by Zhu et al (Zhu et al., 2013) who reported that NASH diagnosis was accompanied by higher levels of alcohol-producing bacteria and endogenous levels of ethanol, a result that was supported by Wong et al. (2013).

The intestinal microbial variations were also observed at the genus level, with data purporting to *Ruminococcus* and *Roseburia* genera being shown to be inconclusive. Whilst Zhu et al. (2013) and Raman et al. (2013) reported a non-significant decrease in the abundance of *Ruminococcus* in NAFLD patients compared to a group of healthy controls, whereas Del Chierico et al. (2017) and Jiang et al. (2015) found an increase in the genus' abundance in NAFLD patients.

Despite the various limitations, preliminary studies highlight and support the hypothesis that configurational shifts in the intestinal microbiome composition may contribute to the development and progression of NAFLD. Whilst further studies on a larger scale with accurate measures and controlled variables are warranted, the potential contribution of intestinal microorganisms and their metabolites are implicated in the pathophysiology of NAFLD. Studies that administer probiotics/prebiotics, which posit to encourage the intestinal microbiome to re-establish intestinal-mucosal macrophage crosstalk homeostasis that then translates to reducing the progression of NALFD are very much warranted.

MECHANISMS LINKING THE INTESTINAL MICROBIOTA AND NAFLD

Research identifies several mechanisms by which the intestinal microbiome cohort-arrangement can affect NAFLD pathogenesis and maintenance. Increased intestinal permeability (Jandhyala et al., 2015), small intestine bacterial overgrowth (SIBO) (Zhu et al., 2013) and elevated serum endotoxin like lipopolysaccharide (LPS) (Brun et al., 2007; Soares et al., 2010), have been reported by studies with NAFLD patients, with varying disease severity and staging (Elshaghabee et al., 2016). LPS, a component of gram-negative bacteria, is elevated in cases of bacterial overgrowth and increased intestinal permeability, yielding hepatoxic effects through the activation of TLR4 and initiation of a cascade of pro-inflammatory innate immune responses (Wigg et al., 2001; Soares et al., 2010).

Experimental and clinical data suggests that SIBO and a disturbed intestinal epithelial barrier are involved in NAFLD pathogenesis (Bode et al., 1987; Purohit et al., 2008; Wan et al., 2016). Furthermore, investigations have shown that the serum from NAFLD patients have elevated levels of LPS-binding protein, TLR-4, and TNF-α in hepatic tissue (Ruiz et al., 2007; Wan et al., 2016).

The gut microbiota also contributes to NAFLD pathogenesis through enriched numbers of ethanol-producing bacteria, primarily *Escherichia coli* (Small et al., 2013; Zhu et al., 2013; Jiang et al., 2015). The alcohol produced by these bacteria are reported to be involved in compromising intestinal barrier integrity which instigates inflammatory activity and ultimately hepatoxic events. Ethanol is a common and dominant metabolite of numerous resident intestinal microbes. As a product of hetero-lactic organisms, endogenously produced ethanol is implicated as a pro-inflammatory hepatoxic factor in NAFLD pathogenesis (Cope et al., 2000; Baker et al., 2010). Linked with increased concentrations of serum ethanol, enrichment in the presence of alcohol-producing intestinal bacteria, like *E. coli*, has been demonstrated to increase intestinal epithelial permeability (Aron-Wisnewsky et al., 2013; Jiang et al., 2015).

A prelude to the liver's averseness to excessive accumulation of FFAs, is intestinal dysbiosis. Dysbiosis is the concept that describes compositional alterations away from the conventional symbiotic intestinal microbiota that may be associated with pathology within the host and is visually described in **Figure 2**. Herein we further posit that compositional alterations in the intestinal microbiota adversely affect the intestinal epithelial barrier exacerbating *epithelial cell dysbiosis*. It has been shown that intestinal epithelial cell disruption can directly adversely affect intestinal resident macrophages and act as critical effector cells in the initiation of inflammation in the pathogenesis of metabolic diseases (Chawla et al., 2011). Disturbances of the TJP network which link the epithelial cells to form the intestinal barrier is a central regulatory mechanism, facilitating selective permeability across the intestinal mucosa and limiting bacterial translocation. Examining the duodenum of NAFLD patients and healthy adults has revealed that in comparison to NAFLD patients, (Jiang et al., 2015) the TJP network was significantly more intact in the duodenum of a healthy adult, with regular alignment and extensive abundance of the microvilli(Jiang et al., 2015). These observations are in stark contrast to the significantly wider gaps and disrupted TJPs reported in NAFLD patients, suggesting a loss of barrier integrity with a consequent increase in bacterial translocation through increased intestinal permeability (Briskey et al., 2016). Additional assessment of the serum biomarkers of the TJPs, including occludin proteins, which are structural components of the tight junctions, have been reported with significantly higher levels in the intestinal mucosa of healthy adults compared to NAFLD patients (Jiang et al., 2015). Measuring the serum levels of the proteins that comprise the structural backbone of the intestinal TJP network lends further supportive data to the hypothesis that intestinal mucosal permeability is greater in NAFLD patients than lean subjects or controls, suggesting intestinal epithelial dysbiosis is a causal factor in NAFLD pathogenesis.

With the establishment of the intestinal microbiota as a participant in the onset and maintenance of low-grade systemic inflammation, the probing of the intestinal microbiome as a potential therapeutic target for extra-intestinal inflammatory conditions, such as NAFLD begun.

The supposition that the intestinal microbiome could indirectly and adversely influence the physiological function of an end–organ such as the liver, by contributing pro–inflammatory activity in the intestinal mucosa, is a novel concept with biological plausibility. As an example, the uptake of Shiga-toxin from the pathogen enterohemorrhagic *E. coli* by M cells and the underlying macrophages in the Peyer's patches is a critical step that teaches about bacterial translocation. This step has been correlated to the efficiency of the infection by the pathogen (Etienne-Mesmin et al., 2011). Numerous bacterial pathogens and their products cross the epithelial barrier though M cell junctions that are then subsequently captured by intestinal resident macrophages (Alisi et al., 2017). Moreover, the LPS components of bacteria are ligands of TLR4 that are expressed on various immune cells, including intestinal macrophages (Vijayan et al., 2017). TLR4 in the M1 configuration is a mediator of inflammation that may imply that increased LPS/TLR4 signaling could be a driving factor in the accelerated inflammation process in patients with NAFLD (Alisi et al., 2017). LPS also induces activation of genes on macrophages such as the early growth response gene 1 (EGR1) as well as the LPS-induced expression of TNF-α, an action that is directly mediated through EGR1 and NF-kB (Xu et al., 2001). Therefore bacterial products that activate macrophages and other immune cells to produce pro-inflammatory mediators can trigger inflammation in an end organ such as the liver (Tateya et al., 2013). Signals released in response to microbial dangers are absorbed on a backgorund of increased and dysregulated intestinal barrier permeability. These signals are recognized by PRRs, including TLR-4 (Szabo et al., 2010; Wan et al., 2016), and when sensed by NLRP3, support the hypothesis that inflammasome-driven microflora are potential drivers of NAFLD onset (Wan et al., 2016).

Intestinal homeostasis is pivotal in optimal functionality of the innate immune system and hinges on macrophages eliminating pathogenic bacteria and their particles (Vitetta, 2016). Activated macrophages play a dual role within the innate immune system (Sansonetti, 2002; Vitetta, 2016). Firstly, they help to elicit appropriate immune responses to detected microbial proteins by facilitating the presentation of antigens to T lymphocytes (Sansonetti, 2002; Vitetta, 2016). Secondly, activated macrophages serve as a secretory source for an array of cytokines that regulate the activation of T cell lymphocytes, including IL-1, INF–α, and cytotoxic proteins (Sansonetti, 2002; Vitetta, 2016). The overall action of the macrophage within the immune responses rely on their ability to neutralize exogenous antigens, cellular debris, insoluble particles, and activated clotting factors via phagocytic activity (Tacke, 2017).

REPRISE

NAFLD's pathway to pathogenicity is characterized by the presence of ectopic fat within hepatocytes that results from an imbalance in the levels of lipogenesis and lipolysis (Machado and Cortez-Pinto, 2014). Triglycerides are synthesized from FFAs that are reported to accumulate in the liver. Therefore, it is envisaged that the concentration of FFAs function as a regulator of lipogenesis in the liver.

Previous studies have associated bacterial phyla, families, or even single genera with obese or lean phenotypes, with an increased lactobacilli count and decreased *Bacteroidetes* presence associated with leanness (Armougom et al., 2009). In support of this, an increased abundance of genus' of the *Bifidobacterium animalis* or *Lactobacillus* species were associated with weight management and a healthy body weight (Million et al., 2012). *Lactobacillus reuteri* has specifically been identified as being associated with an obese phenotype (Million et al., 2012). Assessing intestinal microorganisms for possible correlations with NAFLD is a biologically plausible next step in progressing an understanding of how much influence the intestinal microbiome as a metabolic and immunological organ may have on the development and progression of NAFLD.

Methodological and technological difficulties have largely prevented robust and definitive data from studies that specifically assess the intestinal microbiota of adults with NAFLD and the health of the intestinal mucosal barrier as well as a need for further knowledge into what constitutes a healthy microbiota. When the mucosal barrier of the intestine, which also serves as the largest immune area of the intestinal immune system, is impaired and disrupted, the liver is exposed to intestinal-derived bacterial factors, which are potentially hepatoxic through the gut-liver axis.

A majority of the current literature details the involvement of the innate branch of the immune system in pro-inflammatory pathways leading to NAFLD pathogenesis and progression. However, the adaptive immune system is also implicated in NAFLD development (Ganz and Szabo, 2013; Sutti et al., 2016). Linking the innate and adaptive branches, natural killer (NK) cells are abundant in hepatic tissue and have been reported to influence the development of liver injury and fibrotic deposition that spark NASH materialization (Ganz and Szabo, 2013). Studies in both animal and human models have found a decrease in circulating NK cells in obese subjects compared to lean counterparts (Ganz and Szabo, 2013), with further exploratory investigations suggesting a reduction in their levels and thus activity may in turn increase the sensitivity of obese patients to develop progressive forms of NAFLD, including cirrhosis (Radaeva et al., 2006). A subset of NK cells, the natural killer T (NKT) cells, also known for their exhibition of both innate and adaptive immunity features, serve to regulate hepatic immune responses by secreting both Th1 and Th2 cytokines (Godfrey et al., 2000). Experimental and clinical data indicates that a depletion in NKT cells can lead to the chronic pro-inflammatory environment that can accompanies hepatic steatosis (Li et al., 2005; Ronchi and Falcone, 2008).

With no effective medication having yet been tested for managing or treating NAFLD and the only universally accepted treatment strategy being lifestyle modifications that focus of weight loss, novel therapeutic agents are being pursued in an endeavor to address the rise of NAFLD as one of the most common non-communicable liver disease world-wide (Volynets et al., 2012).

Whilst lifestyle modification recommendations encourage weight loss, this approach requires significant commitment and efficiency decreases over the long term due to waning dedication. Intestinal microbial manipulation through the administration of probiotics presents as an attractive therapeutic adjunct. In an attempt to reduce intestinal epithelial inflammation, probiotics shift the intestinal microbial community toward beneficial bacterial communities such as the *Parabacteroides, Prevotella,* and *Oscillibacter* (Ohland and MacNaughton, 2010). These microbial communities are well known to produce anti-inflammatory metabolites such as SCFAs (Schwiertz et al., 2010). SCFAs, such as butyrate, serve as important facilitators in the harvesting of energy and harnessing it for peripheral tissues and the intestinal epithelia (Elshaghabee et al., 2016). *Oscillibacter* and *Parabacteroides* are associated with T-cell differentiation by enhancing and maintaining the IL-10 producing Treg cells (Arpaia et al., 2013). Moreover, a probiotic formulation that attenuated hepatocellular carcinoma in a murine model offered further insight on how the intestinal microbiota influences the regulation of T-cell differentiation of mucosal immunity in the intestines and in turn, there is down-regulation of the level of pro-inflammatory cytokines (Li et al., 2016). A recently completed murine study by our group reported attenuation of steatosis by 60% in a high fat diet model of NAFLD (Briskey et al., 2016). As such the administration of probiotics to attenuate the progression of NAFLD is both clinically plausible and very much warranted.

Despite increasing focus and attention directed at identifying the mechanisms by which NAFLD develops and progresses, ambiguity remains surrounding the driving factors and molecular pathways that result in NAFLD onset. Immunological mechanisms, including the collaboration of the consequences of innate immunity, adaptive immunity, and TLR receptor signaling dysfunction with the gut-liver axis are each posited to contribute to disease pathogenesis and maintenance.

This narrative review has highlighted the requisite for the completion of a systematic literature review detailing the association between innate immune responses triggered by intestinal epithelial inflammation and dysbiosis and the onset of extra-intestinal pathologies, such as NAFLD. The intestinal microbiome is a significant environmental factor in NAFLD pathogenesis, specifically through effects on intestinal barrier integrity. A review of the literature which explores the correlation between changes in intestinal integrity, intestinal permeability, and therefore endotoxin translocation will help elucidate the specific patterns or profiles of intestinal microorganisms that are of interest in NAFLD manifestation and therefore relevant for therapeutic target purposes. Furthermore, such a review may also define bacterial species that elicit a hepatoprotective effect on the microbiome and extra-intestinal inflammation.

AUTHOR CONTRIBUTIONS

ES and LV: Conception and design of commentary, review; ES, LV, MT, and TP: Read, amended and approved final version of manuscript.

FUNDING

LV has received National Institute of Complementary Medicine and National Health and Medical Research Council of Australia competitive funding and Industry support for research into biocompounds and probiotics. ES, LV, and MT participate in research on probiotics in Medlab Clinical's research laboratory facility in Sydney, Australia.

REFERENCES

Abbas, A. K., Benoist, C., Bluestone, J. A., Campbell, D. J., Ghosh, S., Hori, S., et al. (2013). Regulatory T cells: recommendations to simplify the nomenclature. *Nat. Immunol.* 14, 307–308. doi: 10.1038/ni.2554

Adams, L. A., Lymp, J. F., St Sauver, J., Sanderson, S. O., Lindor, K. D., Feldstein, A., et al. (2005). The natural history of nonalcoholic fatty liver disease: a population-based cohort study. *Gastroenterology* 129, 113–121. doi: 10.1053/j.gastro.2005.04.014

Ai, T. L., Solomon, B. D., and Hsieh, C. S. (2014). T-cell selection and intestinal homeostasis. *Immunol. Rev.* 259, 60–74. doi: 10.1111/imr.12171

Alisi, A., Carpino, G., Oliveira, F. L., Panera, N., Nobili, V., and Gaudio, E. (2017). The role of tissue macrophage-mediated inflammation on nafld pathogenesis and its clinical implications. *Mediators Inflamm.* 2017:8162421. doi: 10.1155/2017/8162421

Armougom, F., Henry, M., Vialettes, B., Raccah, D., and Raoult, D. (2009). Monitoring bacterial community of human gut microbiota reveals an increase in Lactobacillus in obese patients and methanogens in anorexic patients. *PLoS ONE* 4:e7125. doi: 10.1371/journal.pone.0007125

Aron-Wisnewsky, J., Gaborit, B., Dutour, A., and Clement, K. (2013). Gut microbiota and non-alcoholic fatty liver disease: new insights. *Clin. Microbiol. Infect.* 19, 338–348. doi: 10.1111/1469-0691.12140

Arpaia, N., Campbell, C., Fan, X., Dikiy, S., van der Veeken, J., deRoos, P., et al. (2013). Metabolites produced by commensal bacteria promote peripheral regulatory T-cell generation. *Nature* 504, 451–455. doi: 10.1038/nature12726

Baker, S. S., Baker, R. D., Liu, W., Nowak, N. J., and Zhu, L. (2010). Role of alcohol metabolism in non-alcoholic steatohepatitis. *PLoS ONE* 5:e9570. doi: 10.1371/journal.pone.0009570

Bieghs, V., and Trautwein, C. (2014). Innate immune signaling and gut-liver interactions in non-alcoholic fatty liver disease. *Hepatobiliary Surg. Nutr.* 3, 377–385. doi: 10.3978/j.issn.2304-3881.2014.12.04

Bode, C., Kugler, V., and Bode, J. C. (1987). Endotoxemia in patients with alcoholic and non-alcoholic cirrhosis and in subjects with no evidence of chronic liver disease following acute alcohol excess. *J. Hepatol.* 4, 8–14. doi: 10.1016/S0168-8278(87)80003-X

Boulangé, C. L., Neves, A. L., Chilloux, J., Nicholson, J. K., and Dumas, M.-E. (2016). Impact of the gut microbiota on inflammation, obesity, and metabolic disease. *Genome Med.* 8:42. doi: 10.1186/s13073-016-0303-2

Brandl, K., Kumar, V., and Eckmann, L. (2017). Gut-liver axis at the frontier of host-microbial interactions. *Am. J. Physiol. Gastrointest. Liver physiol.* 312, G413–g9. doi: 10.1152/ajpgi.00361.2016

Briskey, D., Heritage, M., Jaskowski, L. A., Peake, J., Gobe, G., Subramaniam, V. N., et al. (2016). Probiotics modify tight-junction proteins in an animal model of nonalcoholic fatty liver disease. *Therap. Adv. Gastroenterol.* 9, 463–472. doi: 10.1177/1756283X16645055

Brun, P., Castagliuolo, I., Di Leo, V., Buda, A., Pinzani, M., Palù, G., et al. (2007). Increased intestinal permeability in obese mice: new evidence in the pathogenesis of nonalcoholic steatohepatitis. *Am. J. Physiol. Gastrointestinal Liver Physiol.* 292, G518–G525. doi: 10.1152/ajpgi.00024.2006

Cani, P. D., Bibiloni, R., Knauf, C., Waget, A., Neyrinck, A. M., Delzenne, N. M., et al. (2008). Changes in gut microbiota control metabolic endotoxemia-induced inflammation in high-fat diet-induced obesity and diabetes in mice. *Diabetes* 57, 1470–1481. doi: 10.2337/db07-1403

Carding, S., Verbeke, K., Vipond, D. T., Corfe, B. M., and Owen, L. J. (2015). Dysbiosis of the gut microbiota in disease. *Microb. Ecol. Health Dis.* 26:26191. doi: 10.3402/mehd.v26.26191

Chawla, A., Nguyen, K. D., and Goh, Y. P. (2011). Macrophage-mediated inflammation in metabolic disease. *Nat. Rev. Immunol.* 11, 738–749. doi: 10.1038/nri3071

Chiang, C. H., Huang, C. C., Chan, W. L., Chen, J. W., and Leu, H. B. (2010). The severity of non-alcoholic fatty liver disease correlates with high sensitivity C-reactive protein value and is independently associated with increased cardiovascular risk in healthy population. *Clin. Biochem.* 43, 1399–1404. doi: 10.1016/j.clinbiochem.2010.09.003

Compare, D., Coccoli, P., Rocco, A., Nardone, O. M., De Maria, S., Cartenì, M., et al. (2012). Gut–liver axis: the impact of gut microbiota on non alcoholic fatty liver disease. *Nutr. Metab. Cardiovasc. Dis.* 22, 471–476. doi: 10.1016/j.numecd.2012.02.007

Consolandi, C., Turroni, S., Emmi, G., Severgnini, M., Fiori, J., Peano, C., et al. (2015). Behcet's syndrome patients exhibit specific microbiome signature. *Autoimmun. Rev.* 14, 269–276. doi: 10.1016/j.autrev.2014.11.009

Cope, K., Risby, T., and Diehl, A. M. (2000). Increased gastrointestinal ethanol production in obese mice: implications for fatty liver disease pathogenesis. *Gastroenterology* 119, 1340–1347. doi: 10.1053/gast.2000.19267

Day, C. P., and James, O. F. (1998). Steatohepatitis: a tale of two "hits"? *Gastroenterology* 114, 842–845. doi: 10.1016/S0016-5085(98)70599-2

Del Chierico, F., Nobili, V., Vernocchi, P., Russo, A., Stefanis, C., Gnani, D., et al. (2017). Gut microbiota profiling of pediatric nonalcoholic fatty liver disease and obese patients unveiled by an integrated meta-omics-based approach. *Hepatology* 65, 451–464. doi: 10.1002/hep.28572

Dietrich, P., and Hellerbrand, C. (2014). Non-alcoholic fatty liver disease, obesity and the metabolic syndrome. *Best Pract. Res. Clin. Gastroenterol.* 28, 637–653. doi: 10.1016/j.bpg.2014.07.008

Dunn, W., Xu, R., Wingard, D. L., Rogers, C., Angulo, P., Younossi, Z. M., et al. (2008). Suspected nonalcoholic fatty liver disease and mortality risk in a population-based cohort study. *Am. J. Gastroenterol.* 103, 2263–2271. doi: 10.1111/j.1572-0241.2008.02034.x

Eckburg, P. B., Bik, E. M., Bernstein, C. N., Purdom, E., Dethlefsen, L., Sargent, M., et al. (2005). Diversity of the human intestinal microbial flora. *Science* 308, 1635–1638. doi: 10.1126/science.1110591

Elshaghabee, F. M., Bockelmann, W., Meske, D., de Vrese, M., Walte, H.-G., Schrezenmeir, J., et al. (2016). Ethanol production by selected intestinal microorganisms and lactic acid bacteria growing under different nutritional conditions. *Front. Microbiol.* 7:47. doi: 10.3389/fmicb.2016.00047

Eslamparast, T., Eghtesad, S., Poustchi, H., and Hekmatdoost, A. (2015). Recent advances in dietary supplementation, in treating non-alcoholic fatty liver disease. *World J. Hepatol.* 7, 204–212. doi: 10.4254/wjh.v7.i2.204

Eslamparast, T., Poustchi, H., Zamani, F., Sharafkhah, M., Malekzadeh, R., and Hekmatdoost, A. (2014). Synbiotic supplementation in nonalcoholic fatty liver disease: a randomized, double-blind, placebo-controlled pilot study. *Am. J. Clin. Nutr.* 99, 535–542. doi: 10.3945/ajcn.113.068890

Etienne-Mesmin, L., Chassaing, B., Sauvanet, P., Denizot, J., Blanquet-Diot, S., Darfeuille-Michaud, A., et al. (2011). Interactions with M cells and macrophages as key steps in the pathogenesis of enterohemorrhagic *Escherichia coli* infections. *PLoS ONE* 6:e23594. doi: 10.1371/journal.pone.0023594

Farrell, G. C., van Rooyen, D., Gan, L., and Chitturi, S. (2012). NASH is an inflammatory disorder: pathogenic, prognostic and therapeutic implications. *Gut Liver* 6, 149–171. doi: 10.5009/gnl.2012.6.2.149

Fukui, H. (2016). Increased intestinal permeability and decreased barrier function: does it really influence the risk of inflammation? *Inflamm. Intest. Dis.* 1, 135–145. doi: 10.1159/000447252

Gaggini, M., Morelli, M., Buzzigoli, E., DeFronzo, R. A., Bugianesi, E., and Gastaldelli, A. (2013). Non-Alcoholic Fatty Liver Disease (NAFLD) and its connection with insulin resistance, dyslipidemia, atherosclerosis and coronary heart disease. *Nutrients* 5, 1544–1560. doi: 10.3390/nu5051544

Ganz, M., and Szabo, G. (2013). Immune and inflammatory pathways in NASH. *Hepatol. Int.* 7, 771–781. doi: 10.1007/s12072-013-9468-6

Glavan, T. W., Gaulke, C. A., Santos Rocha, C., Sankaran-Walters, S., Hirao, L. A., Raffatellu, M., et al. (2016). Gut immune dysfunction through impaired innate pattern recognition receptor expression and gut microbiota dysbiosis in chronic SIV infection. *Mucosal Immunol.* 9, 677–688. doi: 10.1038/mi.2015.92

Godfrey, D. I., Hammond, K. J., Poulton, L. D., Smyth, M. J., and Baxter, A. G. (2000). NKT cells: facts, functions and fallacies. *Immunol. Today* 21, 573–583. doi: 10.1016/S0167-5699(00)01735-7

Gottschalk, C., and Kurts, C. (2015). The debate about dendritic cells and macrophages in the kidney. *Front. Immunol.* 6:435. doi: 10.3389/fimmu.2015.00435

Gregor, M. F., and Hotamisligil, G. S. (2011). Inflammatory mechanisms in obesity. *Annu. Rev. Immunol.* 29, 415–445. doi: 10.1146/annurev-immunol-031210-101322

Guilliams, M., Ginhoux, F., Jakubzick, C., Naik, S. H., Onai, N., Schraml, B. U., et al. (2014). Dendritic cells, monocytes and macrophages: a unified nomenclature based on ontogeny. *Nat. Rev. Immunol.* 14, 571–578. doi: 10.1038/nri3712

Hammerich, L., Heymann, F., and Tacke, F. (2011). Role of IL-17 and Th17 cells in liver diseases. *Clin. Dev. Immunol.* 2011:345803. doi: 10.1155/2011/345803

Harley, I. T., Stankiewicz, T. E., Giles, D. A., Softic, S., Flick, L. M., Cappelletti, M., et al. (2014). IL-17 signaling accelerates the progression of nonalcoholic fatty liver disease in mice. *Hepatology* 59, 1830–1839. doi: 10.1002/hep.26746

Harris, K., Kassis, A., Major, G., and Chou, C. J. (2012). Is the gut microbiota a new factor contributing to obesity and its metabolic disorders? *J. Obes.* 2012:879151. doi: 10.1155/2012/879151

Hume, D. A. (2008). Macrophages as APC and the dendritic cell myth. *J. Immunol.* 181, 5829–5835. doi: 10.4049/jimmunol.181.9.5829

Jandhyala, S. M., Talukdar, R., Subramanyam, C., Vuyyuru, H., Sasikala, M., and Nageshwar Reddy, D. (2015). Role of the normal gut microbiota. *World J. Gastroenterol.* 21, 8787–8803. doi: 10.3748/wjg.v21.i29.8787

Jiang, W., Wu, N., Wang, X., Chi, Y., Zhang, Y., Qiu, X., et al. (2015). Dysbiosis gut microbiota associated with inflammation and impaired mucosal immune function in intestine of humans with non-alcoholic fatty liver disease. *Sci. Rep.* 5:8096. doi: 10.1038/srep08096

Kayama, H., Ueda, Y., Sawa, Y., Jeon, S. G., Ma, J. S., Okumura, R., et al. (2012). Intestinal CX3C chemokine receptor 1(high) (CX3CR1(high)) myeloid cells prevent T-cell-dependent colitis. *Proc. Natl. Acad. Sci. U.S.A.* 109, 5010–5015. doi: 10.1073/pnas.1114931109

Kidd, P. (2003). Th1/Th2 balance: the hypothesis, its limitations, and implications for health and disease. *Altern. Med. Rev.* 8, 223–246.

Kinnebrew, M. A., and Pamer, E. G. (2012). Innate immune signaling in defense against intestinal microbes. *Immunol. Rev.* 245, 113–131. doi: 10.1111/j.1600-065X.2011.01081.x

Kirpich, I. A., Parajuli, D., and McClain, C. J. (2015). Microbiome in NAFLD and ALD. *Clin. Liver Dis.* 6, 55–58. doi: 10.1002/cld.494

Kumar, H., Kawai, T., and Akira, S. (2011). Pathogen recognition by the innate immune system. *Int. Rev. Immunol.* 30, 16–34. doi: 10.3109/08830185.2010.529976

Kumar, P., Monin, L., Castillo, P., Elsegeiny, W., Horne, W., Eddens, T., et al. (2016). Intestinal interleukin-17 receptor signaling mediates reciprocal control of the gut microbiota and autoimmune inflammation. *Immunity* 44, 659–671. doi: 10.1016/j.immuni.2016.02.007

Lau, E., Carvalho, D., and Freitas, P. (2015). Gut microbiota: association with NAFLD and metabolic disturbances. *Biomed Res. Int.* 2015:979515. doi: 10.1155/2015/979515

Le Roy, T., Llopis, M., Lepage, P., Bruneau, A., Rabot, S., Bevilacqua, C., et al. (2013). Intestinal microbiota determines development of non-alcoholic fatty liver disease in mice. *Gut* 62, 1787–1794. doi: 10.1136/gutjnl-2012-303816

Li, D. Y., Yang, M., Edwards, S., and Ye, S. Q. (2013). Nonalcoholic fatty liver disease: for better or worse, blame the gut microbiota? *J. Parenteral Enteral Nutr.* 37, 787–793. doi: 10.1177/0148607113481623

Li, J., Sung, C. Y., Lee, N., Ni, Y., Pihlajamäki, J., Panagiotou, G., et al. (2016). Probiotics modulated gut microbiota suppresses hepatocellular carcinoma growth in mice. *Proc. Natl. Acad. Sci. U.S.A.* 113, E1306–E1315. doi: 10.1073/pnas.1518189113

Li, Z., Soloski, M. J., and Diehl, A. M. (2005). Dietary factors alter hepatic innate immune system in mice with nonalcoholic fatty liver disease. *Hepatology* 42, 880–885. doi: 10.1002/hep.20826

Littman, D. R., and Pamer, E. G. (2011). Role of the commensal microbiota in normal and pathogenic host immune responses. *Cell Host Microbe* 10, 311–323. doi: 10.1016/j.chom.2011.10.004

Lumeng, C. N., and Saltiel, A. R. (2011). Inflammatory links between obesity and metabolic disease. *J. Clin. Invest.* 121, 2111–2117. doi: 10.1172/JCI57132

Machado, M. V., and Cortez-Pinto, H. (2014). Non-alcoholic fatty liver disease: what the clinician needs to know. *World J. Gastroenterol.* 20, 12956–12980. doi: 10.3748/wjg.v20.i36.12956

Mehal, W. Z. (2012). The gut-liver axis: a busy two-way street. *Hepatology* 55, 1647–1649. doi: 10.1002/hep.25704

Miele, L., Marrone, G., Lauritano, C., Cefalo, C., Gasbarrini, A., Day, C., et al. (2013). Gut-liver axis and microbiota in NAFLD: insight pathophysiology for novel therapeutic target. *Curr. Pharm. Des.* 19, 5314–5324. doi: 10.2174/1381612811319290011

Miele, L., Valenza, V., La Torre, G., Montalto, M., Cammarota, G., Ricci, R., et al. (2009). Increased intestinal permeability and tight junction alterations in nonalcoholic fatty liver disease. *Hepatology* 49, 1877–1887. doi: 10.1002/hep.22848

Million, M., Maraninchi, M., Henry, M., Armougom, F., Richet, H., Carrieri, P., et al. (2012). Obesity-associated gut microbiota is enriched in *Lactobacillus reuteri* and depleted in *Bifidobacterium animalis* and *Methanobrevibacter smithii*. *Int. J. Obes.* 36, 817–825. doi: 10.1038/ijo.2011.153

Mokhtari, Z., Gibson, D. L., and Hekmatdoost, A. (2017). Nonalcoholic fatty liver disease, the gut microbiome, and diet. *Adv. Nutr.* 8, 240–252. doi: 10.3945/an.116.013151

Mouzaki, M., Comelli, E. M., Arendt, B. M., Bonengel, J., Fung, S. K., Fischer, S. E., et al. (2013). Intestinal microbiota in patients with nonalcoholic fatty liver disease. *Hepatology* 58, 120–127. doi: 10.1002/hep.26319

Nakahashi-Oda, C., Udayanga, K. G., Nakamura, Y., Nakazawa, Y., Totsuka, N., Miki, H., et al. (2016). Apoptotic epithelial cells control the abundance of Treg cells at barrier surfaces. *Nat. Immunol.* 17, 441–450. doi: 10.1038/ni.3345

Nicholson, J. K., Holmes, E., Kinross, J., Burcelin, R., Gibson, G., Jia, W., et al. (2012). Host-gut microbiota metabolic interactions. *Science* 336, 1262–1267. doi: 10.1126/science.1223813

Nielsen, J. S., Larsson, A., Ledet, T., Turina, M., Tønnesen, E., and Krog, J. (2012). Rough-form lipopolysaccharide increases apoptosis in human CD4(+) and CD8(+) T lymphocytes. *Scand. J. Immunol.* 75, 193–202. doi: 10.1111/j.1365-3083.2011.02613.x

Nobili, V., Giorgio, V., Liccardo, D., Bedogni, G., Morino, G., Alisi, A., et al. (2014). Vitamin D levels and liver histological alterations in children with nonalcoholic fatty liver disease. *Eur. J. Endocrinol.* 170, 547–553. doi: 10.1530/EJE-13-0609

Nolan, J. P. (2010). The role of intestinal endotoxin in liver injury: a long and evolving history. *Hepatology* 52, 1829–1835. doi: 10.1002/hep.23917

Norimatsu, M., Ono, T., Aoki, A., Ohishi, K., Takahashi, T., Watanabe, G., et al. (1995). Lipopolysaccharide-induced apoptosis in swine lymphocytes *in vivo*. *Infect. Immun.* 63, 1122–1126.

Ogino, H., Nakamura, K., Ihara, E., Akiho, H., and Takayanagi, R. (2011). CD4+CD25+ regulatory T cells suppress Th17-responses in an experimental colitis model. *Dig. Dis. Sci.* 56, 376–386. doi: 10.1007/s10620-010-1286-2

Ohland, C. L., and Macnaughton, W. K. (2010). Probiotic bacteria and intestinal epithelial barrier function. *Am. J. Physiol. Gastrointest. Liver Physiol.* 298, G807–G819. doi: 10.1152/ajpgi.00243.2009

Paolella, G., Mandato, C., Pierri, L., Poeta, M., Di Stasi, M., and Vajro, P. (2014). Gut-liver axis and probiotics: Their role in non-alcoholic fatty liver disease. *World J. Gastroenterol.* 20, 15518–15531. doi: 10.3748/wjg.v20.i42.15518

Paquissi, F. C. (2016). Immune imbalances in non-alcoholic fatty liver disease: from general biomarkers and neutrophils to interleukin-17 axis activation and new therapeutic targets. *Front. Immunol.* 7:490. doi: 10.3389/fimmu.2016.00490

Pedra, J. H., Cassel, S. L., and Sutterwala, F. S. (2009). Sensing pathogens and danger signals by the inflammasome. *Curr. Opin. Immunol.* 21, 10–16. doi: 10.1016/j.coi.2009.01.006

Peterson, L. W., and Artis, D. (2014). Intestinal epithelial cells: regulators of barrier function and immune homeostasis. *Nat. Rev. Immunol.* 14, 141–153. doi: 10.1038/nri3608

Purohit, V., Bode, J. C., Bode, C., Brenner, D. A., Choudhry, M. A., Hamilton, F., et al. (2008). Alcohol, intestinal bacterial growth, intestinal permeability to endotoxin, and medical consequences: summary of a symposium. *Alcohol* 42, 349–361. doi: 10.1016/j.alcohol.2008.03.131

Radaeva, S., Sun, R., Jaruga, B., Nguyen, V. T., Tian, Z., and Gao, B. (2006). Natural killer cells ameliorate liver fibrosis by killing activated stellate cells in NKG2D-dependent and tumor necrosis factor-related apoptosis-inducing ligand-dependent manners. *Gastroenterology* 130, 435–452. doi: 10.1053/j.gastro.2005.10.055

Rahimlou, M., Ahmadnia, H., and Hekmatdoost, A. (2015). Dietary supplements and pediatric non-alcoholic fatty liver disease: present and the future. *World J. Hepatol.* 7, 2597–2602. doi: 10.4254/wjh.v7.i25.2597

Ramachandran, A., Madesh, M., and Balasubramanian, K. A. (2000). Apoptosis in the intestinal epithelium: its relevance in normal and pathophysiological conditions. *J. Gastroenterol. Hepatol.* 15, 109–120. doi: 10.1046/j.1440-1746.2000.02059.x

Raman, M., Ahmed, I., Gillevet, P. M., Probert, C. S., Ratcliffe, N. M., Smith, S., et al. (2013). Fecal microbiome and volatile organic compound metabolome in obese humans with nonalcoholic fatty liver disease. *Clin. Gastroenterol. Hepatol.* 11, 868.e1-3–875.e1-3. doi: 10.1016/j.cgh.2013.02.015

Ringel, Y., Maharshak, N., Ringel-Kulka, T., Wolber, E. A., Sartor, R. B., and Carroll, I. M. (2015). High throughput sequencing reveals distinct microbial populations within the mucosal and luminal niches in healthy individuals. *Gut Microbes* 6, 173–181. doi: 10.1080/19490976.2015.1044711

Robinson, K., Deng, Z., Hou, Y., and Zhang, G. (2015). Regulation of the intestinal barrier function by host defense peptides. *Front. Vet. Sci.* 2:57. doi: 10.3389/fvets.2015.00057

Ronchi, F., and Falcone, M. (2008). Immune regulation by invariant NKT cells in autoimmunity. *Front. Biosci.* 13, 4827–4837. doi: 10.2741/3042

Ruiz, A. G., Casafont, F., Crespo, J., Cayón, A., Mayorga, M., Estebanez, A., et al. (2007). Lipopolysaccharide-binding protein plasma levels and liver TNF-alpha gene expression in obese patients: evidence for the potential role of endotoxin in the pathogenesis of non-alcoholic steatohepatitis. *Obes. Surg.* 17, 1374–1380. doi: 10.1007/s11695-007-9243-7

Sansonetti, P. (2002). Host-pathogen interactions: the seduction of molecular cross talk. *Gut* 50 (Suppl. 3):Iii2–Iii8. doi: 10.1136/gut.50.suppl_3.iii2

Schwiertz, A., Taras, D., Schäfer, K., Beijer, S., Bos, N. A., Donus, C., et al. (2010). Microbiota and SCFA in lean and overweight healthy subjects. *Obesity* 18, 190–195. doi: 10.1038/oby.2009.167

Shavakhi, A., Minakari, M., Firouzian, H., Assali, R., Hekmatdoost, A., and Ferns, G. (2013). Effect of a probiotic and metformin on liver aminotransferases in non-alcoholic steatohepatitis: a double blind randomized clinical trial. *Int. J. Prev. Med.* 4, 531–537.

Small, C. L., Reid-Yu, S. A., McPhee, J. B., and Coombes, B. K. (2013). Persistent infection with Crohn's disease-associated adherent-invasive *Escherichia coli* leads to chronic inflammation and intestinal fibrosis. *Nat. Commun.* 4:1957. doi: 10.1038/ncomms2957

Smith, P. M., Howitt, M. R., Panikov, N., Michaud, M., Gallini, C. A., Bohlooly, Y. M., et al. (2013). The microbial metabolites, short-chain fatty acids, regulate colonic Treg cell homeostasis. *Science* 341, 569–573. doi: 10.1126/science.1241165

Soares, J. B., Pimentel-Nunes, P., Roncon-Albuquerque, R., and Leite-Moreira, A. (2010). The role of lipopolysaccharide/toll-like receptor 4 signaling in chronic liver diseases. *Hepatol. Int.* 4, 659–672. doi: 10.1007/s12072-010-9219-x

Starley, B. Q., Calcagno, C. J., and Harrison, S. A. (2010). Nonalcoholic fatty liver disease and hepatocellular carcinoma: a weighty connection. *Hepatology* 51, 1820–1832. doi: 10.1002/hep.23594

Su, L., Wang, J. H., Cong, X., Wang, L. H., Liu, F., Xie, X. W., et al. (2012). Intestinal immune barrier integrity in rats with nonalcoholic hepatic steatosis and steatohepatitis. *Chin. Med. J.* 125, 306–311.

Sutti, S., Bruzzì, S., and Albano, E. (2016). The role of immune mechanisms in alcoholic and nonalcoholic steatohepatitis: a 2015 update. *Expert Rev. Gastroenterol. Hepatol.* 10, 243–253. doi: 10.1586/17474124.2016.1111758

Szabo, G., Bala, S., Petrasek, J., and Gattu, A. (2010). Gut-liver axis and sensing microbes. *Dig. Dis.* 28, 737–744. doi: 10.1159/000324281

Tacke, F. (2017). Targeting hepatic macrophages to treat liver diseases. *J. Hepatol.* 66, 1300–1312. doi: 10.1016/j.jhep.2017.02.026

Takeuchi, O., and Akira, S. (2010). Pattern recognition receptors and inflammation. *Cell* 140, 805–820. doi: 10.1016/j.cell.2010.01.022

Targher, G., Bertolini, L., Padovani, R., Rodella, S., Tessari, R., Zenari, L., et al. (2007). Prevalence of nonalcoholic fatty liver disease and its association with cardiovascular disease among type 2 diabetic patients. *Diabetes Care* 30, 1212–1218. doi: 10.2337/dc06-2247

Targher, G., Bertolini, L., Padovani, R., Rodella, S., Zoppini, G., Pichiri, I., et al. (2010). Prevalence of non-alcoholic fatty liver disease and its association with cardiovascular disease in patients with type 1 diabetes. *J. Hepatol.* 53, 713–718. doi: 10.1016/j.jhep.2010.04.030

Tateya, S., Kim, F., and Tamori, Y. (2013). Recent advances in obesity-induced inflammation and insulin resistance. *Front. Endocrinol.* 4:93. doi: 10.3389/fendo.2013.00093

Tilg, H., and Moschen, A. R. (2010). Evolution of inflammation in nonalcoholic fatty liver disease: the multiple parallel hits hypothesis. *Hepatology* 52, 1836–1846. doi: 10.1002/hep.24001

Turnbaugh, P. J., Ley, R. E., Mahowald, M. A., Magrini, V., Mardis, E. R., and Gordon, J. I. (2006). An obesity-associated gut microbiome with increased capacity for energy harvest. *Nature* 444, 1027–1031. doi: 10.1038/nature05414

Vajro, P., Paolella, G., and Fasano, A. (2013). Microbiota and gut-liver axis: their influences on obesity and obesity-related liver disease. *J. Pediatr. Gastroenterol. Nutr.* 56, 461–468. doi: 10.1097/MPG.0b013e318284abb5

Vijayan, V., Srinu, T., Karnati, S., Garikapati, V., Linke, M., Kamalyan, L., et al. (2017). A new immunomodulatory role for peroxisomes in macrophages activated by the TLR4 ligand lipopolysaccharide. *J. Immunol.* 198, 2414–2425. doi: 10.4049/jimmunol.1601596

Vitetta, L. (2016). *Lactobacillus acidophilus* restores functionality in uremic macrophages: plausible or lacking evidence? *Dig. Dis. Sci.* 61, 1417–1419. doi: 10.1007/s10620-016-4084-7

Vitetta, L., Coulson, S., Linnane, A. W., and Butt, H. (2013). The gastrointestinal microbiome and musculoskeletal diseases: a beneficial role for probiotics and prebiotics. *Pathogens* 2, 606–626. doi: 10.3390/pathogens2040606

Volynets, V., Küper, M. A., Strahl, S., Maier, I. B., Spruss, A., Wagnerberger, S., et al. (2012). Nutrition, intestinal permeability, and blood ethanol levels are altered in patients with Nonalcoholic Fatty Liver Disease (NAFLD). *Dig. Dis. Sci.* 57, 1932–1941. doi: 10.1007/s10620-012-2112-9

Wahl, S. M. (2007). Transforming growth factor-beta: innately bipolar. *Curr. Opin. Immunol.* 19, 55–62. doi: 10.1016/j.coi.2006.11.008

Wan, X., Xu, C., Yu, C., and Li, Y. (2016). Role of NLRP3 inflammasome in the progression of NAFLD to NASH. *Can. J. Gastroenterol. Hepatol.* 2016:6489012. doi: 10.1155/2016/6489012

Wang, B., Jiang, X., Cao, M., Ge, J., Bao, Q., Tang, L., et al. (2016). Altered fecal microbiota correlates with liver biochemistry in nonobese patients with non-alcoholic fatty liver disease. *Sci. Rep.* 6:32002. doi: 10.1038/srep32002

Welsh, J. A., Karpen, S., and Vos, M. B. (2013). Increasing prevalence of nonalcoholic fatty liver disease among United States adolescents, 1988-1994 to 2007-2010. *J. Pediatr.* 162, 496.e1–500.e1. doi: 10.1016/j.jpeds.2012.08.043

Wieland, A., Frank, D. N., Harnke, B., and Bambha, K. (2015). Systematic review: microbial dysbiosis and nonalcoholic fatty liver disease. *Aliment. Pharmacol. Ther.* 42, 1051–1063. doi: 10.1111/apt.13376

Wigg, A. J., Roberts-Thomson, I. C., Dymock, R. B., McCarthy, P. J., Grose, R. H., and Cummins, A. G. (2001). The role of small intestinal bacterial overgrowth, intestinal permeability, endotoxaemia, and tumour necrosis factor alpha in the pathogenesis of non-alcoholic steatohepatitis. *Gut* 48, 206–211. doi: 10.1136/gut.48.2.206

Williams, C. D., Stengel, J., Asike, M. I., Torres, D. M., Shaw, J., Contreras, M., et al. (2011). Prevalence of nonalcoholic fatty liver disease and nonalcoholic steatohepatitis among a largely middle-aged population utilizing ultrasound and liver biopsy: a prospective study. *Gastroenterology* 140, 124–131. doi: 10.1053/j.gastro.2010.09.038

Wong, V. W., Tse, C., Lam, T. T., Wong, G. L., Chim, A. M., Chu, W. C., et al. (2013). Molecular characterization of the fecal microbiota in patients with nonalcoholic steatohepatitis – a longitudinal study. *PLoS ONE* 8:e62885. doi: 10.1371/journal.pone.0062885

Xu, Z., Dziarski, R., Wang, Q., Swartz, K., Sakamoto, K. M., and Gupta, D. (2001). Bacterial peptidoglycan-induced tnf-alpha transcription is mediated through the transcription factors Egr-1, Elk-1, and NF-kappaB. *J. Immunol.* 167, 6975–6982. doi: 10.4049/jimmunol.167.12.6975

Yari, Z., Rahimlou, M., Eslamparast, T., Ebrahimi-Daryani, N., Poustchi, H., and Hekmatdoost, A. (2016). Flaxseed supplementation in non-alcoholic fatty liver disease: a pilot randomized, open labeled, controlled study. *Int. J. Food Sci. Nutr.* 67, 461–469. doi: 10.3109/09637486.2016.1161011

Younossi, Z. M., Koenig, A. B., Abdelatif, D., Fazel, Y., Henry, L., and Wymer, M. (2016). Global epidemiology of nonalcoholic fatty liver disease-Meta-analytic assessment of prevalence, incidence, and outcomes. *Hepatology* 64, 73–84. doi: 10.1002/hep.28431

Zheng, S. G. (2013). Regulatory T cells vs Th17: differentiation of Th17 versus Treg, are the mutually exclusive? *Am. J. Clin. Exp. Immunol.* 2, 94–106.

Zhu, L., Baker, S. S., Gill, C., Liu, W., Alkhouri, R., Baker, R. D., et al. (2013). Characterization of gut microbiomes in nonalcoholic steatohepatitis (NASH) patients: a connection between endogenous alcohol and NASH. *Hepatology* 57, 601–609. doi: 10.1002/hep.26093

9

Modulation of Lipid Droplet Metabolism—A Potential Target for Therapeutic Intervention in *Flaviviridae* Infections

Jingshu Zhang[1†], *Yun Lan*[1†] *and Sumana Sanyal*[1, 2*]

[1] HKU-Pasteur Research Pole, School of Public Health, Li Ka Shing Faculty of Medicine, University of Hong Kong, Hong Kong, China, [2] School of Biomedical Sciences, Li Ka Shing Faculty of Medicine, University of Hong Kong, Hong Kong, China

***Correspondence:**
Sumana Sanyal
sanyal@hku.hk

† These authors have contributed equally to this work.

Lipid droplets (LDs) are endoplasmic reticulum (ER)-related dynamic organelles that store and regulate fatty acids and neutral lipids. They play a central role in cellular energy storage, lipid metabolism and cellular homeostasis. It has become evident that viruses have co-evolved in order to exploit host lipid metabolic pathways. This is especially characteristic of the *Flaviviridae* family, including hepatitis C virus (HCV) and several flaviviruses. Devoid of an appropriate lipid biosynthetic machinery of their own, these single-strand positive-sense RNA viruses can induce dramatic changes in host metabolic pathways to establish a favorable environment for viral multiplication and acquire essential components to facilitate their assembly and traffic. Here we have reviewed the current knowledge on the intracellular life cycle of those from the *Flaviviridae* family, with particular emphasis on HCV and dengue virus (DENV), and their association with the biosynthesis and metabolism of LDs, with the aim to identify potential antiviral targets for development of novel therapeutic interventions.

Keywords: lipid droplet, lipid metabolism, HCV, flavivirus, dengue

INTRODUCTION

Cellular homeostasis is maintained by a constant metabolic energy flux. As one of the major energy sources, lipids are synthesized, modified and utilized through various pathways. Lipid droplets (LDs) are ubiquitous and conserved cytoplasmic compartments delineated by a phospholipid monolayer, and serve as energy reservoirs in almost all living organisms. Excess lipids are packaged, stored and distributed in LDs, an organelle which is not only important in lipid storage and metabolism, but protein quality control, pathogenesis, and immune responses (Walther and Farese, 2012).

Since viruses lack the appropriate machinery to conduct their own lipid synthesis, most have evolved mechanisms to hijack host lipid metabolic pathways (including LDs) for completing their intracellular replication cycles. Hepatitis C virus (HCV) has long been demonstrated to do so (Paul et al., 2014). Apart from the cell biology underlying infection, the interplay between viral infection and host lipid metabolic pathways is important not only to elucidate the pathogenicity of this category of viruses but also to assess how they can be targeted as a general means of combating infections.

As a consequence of development of gene editing and mass spectrometry based lipidomics and proteomics technologies, an increasing body of evidence indicates the involvement of host LDs at different steps of the intracellular life cycle of HCV and flaviviruses (Martín-Acebes et al., 2016b). Here, we have cataloged these interactions and anticipate that this knowledge will be beneficial for identification of host factors as suitable targets for antiviral interventions.

LIPID DROPLET—A MULTIFUNCTIONAL ORGANELLE

Morphology and Composition of LDs

LDs are essentially the emulsion phase of insoluble oil droplets dispersed in aqueous cytoplasm. Compared to other cellular organelles with double-layered membranes, the structure of LDs is rather unique, containing a hydrophobic core and a single layer of amphipathic phospholipids. The neutral lipid core contains predominantly triacylglycerols (TAGs) and cholesterol esters (CEs) (Thiam et al., 2013). Although the composition of the phospholipid monolayer varies in different cell types, phosphatidylcholine (PC) and phosphatidylethanolamine (PE) are the two major phospholipids. The morphology and consumption of LDs are drastically altered by the composition of their phospholipid monolayer (Guo et al., 2008). The surface of the monolayer is decorated with LD-associated proteins, including lipolytic enzymes such as hormone-sensitive lipase (HSL), adipose triglyceride lipase (ATGL), and PAT-domain family (perilipin, adipophilin and TIP47) (Tauchi-Sato et al., 2002; Ohsaki et al., 2006; Wilfling et al., 2014a). Despite being present in nearly all cell types across different organisms, LDs are highly heterogeneous and dynamic with varied numbers and sizes (ranging from 100 nm to 100 mm in diameter) in otherwise identical cells. Even within the same cell, LDs expand or shrink in response to cellular signals.

Biogenesis of LDs

In eukaryotes, LDs respond to increased cellular fatty acid levels and emerge from the accumulation of neutral lipids in the ER, which harbors enzymes necessary for neutral lipid synthesis in most cell types (Buhman et al., 2001; Pol et al., 2004). First established as an oil-in-water emulsion, the small nascent LDs undergo a series of well-organized processes and grow into larger, mature LDs. The final steps of TAG and CE synthesis are catalyzed by ER-localized diacylglycerol acyltransferases (DGATs) and acyl-CoA:cholesterol acyltranserases (ACATs), respectively. The continuous accumulation of the newly synthesized TAGs and CEs at specific sites at the ER results in separation of two phases, where globules of TAGs arise between the two leaflets of the bilayer and eventually dissociate. DGAT2, which is inserted into one leaflet of the ER membrane, is transported to LDs where it continues to catalyze synthesis of TAGs, hence promoting further growth of LDs (Kassan et al., 2013; Wilfling et al., 2013). This process is thermodynamically enabled by the unique phospholipid monolayer structure of LDs.

Abbreviations: 769662, 6,7-Dihydro-4-hydroxy-3-(2′-hydroxy[1,1′-biphenyl]-4-yl)-6-oxo-thieno[2,3-b]pyridine-5-carbonitrile; AADAC, arylacetamide deacetylase; ACAT, acyl-CoA, cholesterol acyltranserases; ACC, acetyl coenzyme a carboxylase; ADRP, adipose differentiation-related protein; AICAR, aminoimidazole carboxamide ribonucleotide; AMPK, 5′ AMP-activated protein kinase; ApoB100, apolipoprotein B100; ARF, ADP-ribosylation factor; ARF1-COP I, ADP-ribosylation factor-coat protein I; ATGL, adipose triglyceride lipase; AUP1, ancient ubiquitous protein 1; AY9944, trans-1,4-bis(2-Chlorobenzylaminoethyl) cyclohexane dihydrochloride; BA, 2-chloro-5-nitro-N-(pyridyl)benzamide; BAPTA-AM, 1,2-Bis(2-aminophenoxy)ethane-*N,N,N′,N′*-tetraacetic acid tetrakis(acetoxymethyl ester); BMS-200150, 2-[1-(3,3-diphenylpropyl)-4-piperidinyl]-2,3-dihydro-1H-isoindol-1-one; C75, 4-Methylene-2-octyl-5-oxotetrahydrofuran-3-carboxylic acid; CD2AP, CD2 associated protein; CE, cholesterol ester; CerS, ceramide synthase; CGI58, comparative gene identification-58; CHO, cholesterol; CMA, chaperone-mediated autophagy; COP, coat protein; CPT-1, carnitine palmitoyltransferase 1; D609, tricyclodecan-9-yl-xanthogenate; DAG, diacylyglycerol; DCI, 3,2-trans-enoyl-CoA iosmerase; DDX3X, DEAD box polypeptide 3 X-linked; DENV, dengue virus; DGAT, diacylglycerol acyltransferases; DHCR, dehydrocholesterol reductase; DHF, dengue hemorrhagic fever; DMV, double-membrane vesicle; DNJ, 1-deoxynojirimycin; dsRNA, double-stranded RNA; DSS, dengue shock syndrome; E protein, envelope protein; ER, endoplasmic reticulum; ERAD, ER-associated degradation; ERGIC, ER-Golgi intermediate compartment; FAPP2, Golgi-associated four-phosphate adaptor protein 2; FASN, fatty acid synthase; GBF1, golgi-specific brefeldin A-resistance guanine nucleotide exchange factor 1; GGTase I, geranylgeranyltransferase; GGTI-286, *N*-4-[2(*R*)-Amino-3-mercaptopropyl]amino-2-phenylbenzoyl-(L)-leucine methyl ester; GGTI-298, *N*-4-[2(*R*)-Amino-3-mercaptopropyl]amino-2-naphthylbenzoyl-(L)-leucine methyl ester trifluoroacetate salt; GW4869, N,N′-Bis[4-(4,5-dihydro-1H-imidazol-2-yl)phenyl]-3,3′-*p*-phenylene-bis-acrylamide dihydrochloride; HCV, hepatitis C virus; HMGCoA, 3-hydroxy-3-methylglutaryl CoA; HMGCR, 3-hydroxy-methyglutaryl-Coenzyme A reductase; HMGCS, hydroxymethylglutaryl-CoA synthase; HSL, hormone-sensitive lipase; IKK, IkB kinase; JEV, Japanese encephalitis virus; LD, lipid droplet; LY294002, 2-(4-Morpholinyl)-8-phenyl-4*H*-1-benzopyran-4-one; MAPK, mitogen-activated protein kinases; MEDICA 16:3,3,14,14-Tetramethylhexadecanedioic acid; MGL, monoglyceride lipase; MS-209, dofequidar fumarate; MTase, methyltransferase; MTOC, microtubule-organizing center; MTP, microsomal triglyceride transfer protein large subunit; MVD, mevalonate (diphospho) decarboxylase; MβCD, methyl-β-cyclodextrin; NIM811, *N*-methyl-4-isoleucine cyclosporine; NB-DNJ, N-Butyldeoxynojirimycin; NIs, nucleoside/nucleotide analog inhibitors; NNIs, non-nucleoside inhibitors; NS, non-structural; nSMase2, neutral sphingomyelinase 2; OSBP, oxysterol-binding protein; OSC, oxidosqualene cyclase; OSW-1, 3β,16β,17α-trihydroxycholest-5-en-22-one 16-*O*-(2-*O*-4-methoxybenzoyl-β-*D*-xylopyranosyl)-(1→ 3)-(2-*O*-acetyl-α-l-arabinopyranoside); PC, phosphatidylcholine; PDMP, D,L-*threo*-1-phenyl-2-decanoylamino-3-morpholino-1-propanol; PE, phosphatidylethanolamine; PERL, polyunsaturated ER liposomes; PF-429242, 4-[(Diethylamino)methyl]-*N*-[2-(2-methoxyphenyl)ethyl]-*N*-(3*R*)-3-pyrrolidinyl-benzamide; PI3K, phosphatidylinositide 3-kinases; PI4KA, phosphatidylinositol 4-kinases; PI4P, phosphatidylinositol 4-phosphate; PLA2G4A, cytosolic phospholipase A2; PNPLA5, patatin-like phospholipase domain-containing protein 5; PPARα, peroxisome proliferator-activated receptor α; RdRp, RNA-dependent RNA polymerase; S1P, site 1 protease; SAM, S-adenosylmethionine; SCAP, Sterol regulatory element-binding protein cleavage-activating protein; SCPI-1, [*N*-(4-{[4-(3,4-dichlorophenyl)-1,3-thiazol-2-yl]amino}-phenyl)acetamidehydrobromide]; SCP-2, sterol carrier protein 2; SKI-1, subtilisin/kexin-isozyme-1; Smase, sphingomyelinase; SphK, sphingosine kinase; SPP, signal peptide peptidase; SPT, serine palmitoyltransferase; SQS, squalene synthetase; SRB1, scavenger receptor class B member 1; SREBP, sterol regulatory element-binding protein; TAG, triacylglycerol; TBEV, tick-borne encephalitis virus; TOFA,5-tetradecyl-oxy-2-furoic acid; U0126, 1,4-Diamino-2,3-dicyano-1,4-*bis*(2-aminophenylthio)butadiene; U18666A, 3β-(2-Diethylaminoethoxy)androst-5-en-17-one; VAP, vesicle-associated membrane protein-associated protein; VLDL, very low-density lipoprotein; WNV, West Nile virus; YFV, yellow fever virus; ZIKV, Zika virus.

The Multifunctionality of LDs

Long been regarded as simple and passive lipid storage compartments, LDs are currently considered highly dynamic and complex. They play a central role in lipid metabolism and are connected to diverse cellular processes like fatty acid trafficking, cellular signaling, protein storage, autophagy, immunity, and virus replication (Singh et al., 2009; Saka and Valdivia, 2012; Rambold et al., 2015; Welte, 2015; Velázquez et al., 2016).

LDs as the Central Regulator for Cellular Homeostasis

As metabolically active organelles, LDs regulate the balance between host lipid synthesis and mobilization to maintain cellular homeostasis. Catalyzed by DGAT1 and DGAT2, cellular fatty acids together with diacylglycerols (DAGs) are converted into TAGs and stored in LDs. TAGs can be further hydrolyzed to generate DAGs or phosphatidic acid (PA) for membrane phospholipid synthesis and free fatty acids (FFAs) for energy production (Pol et al., 2014).

LDs as Transient Protein Storage Compartments for Degradation

Due to unique structural features and proximity to the ER, the surface of LDs can also serve as transient storage depots for proteins that are destined for degradation via the ER-associated degradation (ERAD) pathway (Gao and Goodman, 2015). Misfolded proteins in the ER are removed and degraded by the ubiquitin–proteasome system. Current evidence suggests that ubiquitinated apolipoprotein B100 (ApoB100) (Ohsaki et al., 2008) and 3-hydroxy-3-methylglutaryl CoA reductase (HMGCR) (Hartman et al., 2010) are likely degraded on the surface of LDs through proteasomal and autophagic pathways (Ohsaki et al., 2006). HMGCR is one of the rate-limiting enzymes for cholesterol synthesis in mammalian cells. Ubiquitination of HMGCR is mediated by ancient ubiquitous protein 1 (AUP1), a highly conserved monotopic membrane protein localized to both LDs and the ER membrane (Spandl et al., 2011). AUP1 recruits the ubiquitin-conjugating enzyme UBE2G2 to LDs and facilitates its binding with the ER ubiquitin ligases gp78 and Trc8, which subsequently initiates the ubiquitination/degradation of HMGCR resulting in inhibition of cholesterol synthesis (Jo et al., 2013). Apart from providing a molecular link between LDs and the ubiquitination machinery, monoubiquitinated AUP1 was reported to induce LD clustering, a widespread phenomenon observed in multiple cell types across all species (Lohmann et al., 2013). LDs may also provide sequestration platforms for protein storage (Cermelli et al., 2006), such as during the synthesis of eicosanoids, a class of signaling molecules that use LDs as distinct sites for eicosanoid generation (Bozza et al., 2011).

Mobilization of Lipids from LDs

Depending on the cell type, starvation and/or physiological conditions, eukaryotic cells mobilize lipids stored in LDs via two major pathways termed lipolysis and lipophagy. In mammalian adipocytes, lipolysis is activated in response to changes in cellular energy and hormone levels. This allows transient docking and activation of three major lipolytic enzymes, ATGL, HSL, and monoglyceride lipase (MGL) which co-ordinate the hydrolysis of TAGs for energy production (Karlsson et al., 1997; Zimmermann et al., 2004; Dugail and Hajduch, 2007; Lass et al., 2011). Perilipins localize to LD surfaces and under basal conditions shield TAGs from cytosolic lipases. During starvation, perilipins are degraded via the chaperone-mediated autophagy (CMA) pathway to facilitate lipolysis by HSL and ATGL (Brasaemle, 2007; Sztalryd and Kimmel, 2014; Kaushik and Cuervo, 2015). Apart from LD-associated proteins, the ADP-ribosylation factor-coat protein I (ARF1-COPI) vesicular trafficking machinery is likely to play an important role in mediating lipolysis by regulating LD composition and targeting ATGL to LDs (Soni et al., 2009; Wilfling et al., 2014b).

The role of autophagy in regulating lipid metabolism has been intensively studied in recent years (Singh et al., 2009; Singh and Cuervo, 2012). Various cell types have been used to demonstrate the process of LD mobilization via the autophagy pathway, such as hypothalamic neurons (Kaushik et al., 2011), glial cells (Martinez-Vicente et al., 2010), and enterocytes (Narabayashi et al., 2015). Autophagy is a conserved cellular process that delivers cytoplasmic contents, including dysfunctional proteins, and excess or damaged organelles to lytic compartments for degradation and recycling. The process can be induced by a number of factors such as ER stress, cellular starvation, and pathogenic infection. Available data support that three distinct types of autophagy can be triggered: macro-, micro- and chaperone-mediated autophagy , amongst which, macroautophagy is the best characterized (Yoshimori, 2004; Mizushima, 2007). Upon activation, cytoplasmic components are first enclosed by a double-layered vesicular structure termed autophagosome, which fuse with lysosomes where internal cargos are degraded (Mizushima, 2007). Multiple factors such as nutrient deprivation, virus infection, and sterol (cholesterol) depletion, can trigger degradation of LDs through the autophagic machinery (Ouimet and Marcel, 2012). LC3II, a structural component of the autophagosomes, and autophagy-related proteins Atg2, Atg5, and Atg7 are recruited to the surface of LDs to form autophagosomes. LDs are engulfed for lysosomal degradation to release stored lipids, which undergo mitochondrial β-oxidation for energy production. This process is frequently manipulated by flaviviruses to promote their replication (see Usage of LD as an energy reservoir during viral life cycle) (Singh et al., 2009; Heaton and Randall, 2010; Fujimoto and Parton, 2011; Velikkakath et al., 2012). The level and distribution of cellular cholesterol is tightly regulated; excess free cholesterol stored as cholesteryl esters in LDs are hydrolyzed during sterol starvation through autophagy (Cheng et al., 2006; Ouimet and Marcel, 2012). Sterol regulatory element-binding proteins (SREBPs) are the central transcriptional regulators of cholesterol metabolism and lipogenesis. In the presence of high cholesterol content in the cytoplasm, SREBP binds to sterol regulatory element-binding protein cleavage-activating protein (SCAP) and the ER-associated protein Insig. Upon reduction of cellular cholesterol below a threshold, Insig is degraded through the ERAD pathway, the SCAP-SREBP complex is transported to the Golgi, where SREBP undergoes intramembrane proteolysis and translocates to the nucleus. This mature form of SREBP initiates transcription of a series of down-stream genes involved in the biosynthesis of cholesterol (Brown and Goldstein, 1997; Yang et al., 2002).

THE *FLAVIVIRIDAE* FAMILY

Viruses of the *Flaviviridae* family are enveloped single-strand positive-sense RNA viruses, with the nucleocapsids surrounded by two or more types of envelope glycoproteins and lipid bilayers (Lindenbach et al., 2007; Paul and Bartenschlager, 2015). It comprises several different genera including *Hepacivirus* (e.g., HCV), *Flavivirus* [e.g., Zika virus (ZIKV), dengue virus (DENV)], *Pegivirus*, and *Pestivirus*.

Persistent infection with HCV in humans can develop into serious liver diseases, including fibrosis and liver cirrhosis, which could further progress into hepatocellular carcinoma (Bartenschlager et al., 2013). Medically-relevant flaviviruses, including yellow fever virus (YFV), ZIKV, DENV, West Nile virus (WNV), and Japanese encephalitis virus (JEV), are usually arboviruses (viz., transmitted by arthropods, mainly mosquitoes and ticks) that are responsible for severe mortality in humans and animals worldwide. DENV and YFV infections are known to cause vascular leakage and hemorrhage in some infected patients (Siqueira et al., 2005; Garske et al., 2014; Thanachartwet et al., 2015). JEV and WSN infections on the other hand, tend to cause neurological diseases (Sarkari et al., 2012; Samaan et al., 2016). ZIKV infection is associated with serious birth defects—microcephaly in particular—and other neurological disorders (Petersen et al., 2016). Although there has been significant progress in therapeutic interventions for HCV and some other flaviviruses (for example YFV), there is still an urgent need for vaccines and medications against others such as DENV and ZIKV. Additionally, the ever-increasing geographical spread and number of outbreaks caused by these pathogens pose a considerable threat to public health (Gould and Solomon, 2008).

Despite significant differences in transmission, tissue tropism and pathogenesis, viruses of the *Flaviviridae* family employ similar intracellular replication strategies. After receptor-mediated endocytosis, the acidic environment in the endosomes triggers fusion between the virion lipid envelope and cellular membranes, followed by viral uncoating. The viral RNA is subsequently released into the cytoplasm and used directly as mRNA for translation of the viral polyprotein. Host and viral proteases cleave the newly synthesized viral polyprotein to generate the structural and non-structural (NS) proteins (Lindenbach et al., 2007). Viral replicase proteins together with other host factors induce massive rearrangements of intracellular membranes to form organelle-like membrane-delineated compartments for efficient RNA replication. At the replication sites, the positive-sense RNA is used as template to generate the negative-sense RNA intermediate, while multiple positive-sense progeny RNAs are produced to be incorporated into nascent virus particles (Paul and Bartenschlager, 2015). Progeny virions are assembled in close proximity to the ER and LDs, and appear to bud into the ER-lumen, followed by transport through the host secretory pathway where they undergo further maturation, and are eventually released from the cell surface (Lindenbach et al., 2007; Paul and Bartenschlager, 2015; **Figure 1**).

INFLUENCE OF LD METABOLISM ON THE VIRUS LIFE CYCLE

HCV has historically been used for studying interactions between LD metabolism and the viral life cycle. Others from the same family, such as DENV, have recently started receiving more attention in this regard. The magnitude and complexity of these interactions underscore the significance of targeting LD metabolism to control viral infection. As a dynamic cellular lipid storage organelle, LDs participate in the viral life cycle by providing intracellular membrane surface area, lipids, energy, and proteins.

Contribution of LDs in Virus Replication and Assembly

Upon infection massive intracellular membrane rearrangements are induced by perturbing lipid biosynthetic pathways to spatially segregate the replication and assembly sites (Welsch et al., 2009; Romero-Brey et al., 2012). On the one hand, the two sites need to be separated to avoid competition between the capsid protein and the viral replicase complex at the level of RNA binding. On the other hand, newly synthesized positive-sense progeny RNAs need to be transported from the replication to the assembly sites, where the capsid protein is concentrated. For maximum efficiency in virus assembly the two sites require close proximity to each other (Welsch et al., 2009; Romero-Brey et al., 2012; **Figure 2**).

Association of LDs to Viral Replication Compartments

LDs have been reported to associate with virus-induced membrane bound compartments believed to be replication sites. Despite belonging to the same family, HCV and DENV induce morphologically distinctive replication compartments. In the case of HCV infection, the double-membrane vesicles (DMVs) are derived from the ER (Romero-Brey et al., 2012; **Figure 2A**). DMVs are composed of active viral replicase proteins and double-stranded RNA (dsRNA), along with several host components including vesicle-associated membrane protein-associated protein A (VAP-A) and VAP-B that are crucial for viral RNA replication (Evans et al., 2004; Gao et al., 2004). The highly hydrophobic NS4B of HCV, together with NS5A, are the major viral factors that contribute to DMV formation (Lundin et al., 2006). These virus-induced compartments use cholesterol as a structural component and can be visualized in close proximity to LDs (Romero-Brey et al., 2012; Paul et al., 2013). While DMVs are considered as replication factories of HCV, their association to LDs is still unclear. The interferon-induced antiviral protein viperin, which inhibits HCV RNA replication, localizes to LDs using a similar mechanism as HCV NS5A, indicating the importance of LD-NS5A association during HCV replication (Jiang et al., 2008; Hinson and Cresswell, 2009). LDs release free cholesterol from the esterified form for membrane biogenesis as per the host cellular requirements (Maxfield and Tabas, 2005) and, therefore, may serve as reservoirs for lipids required for

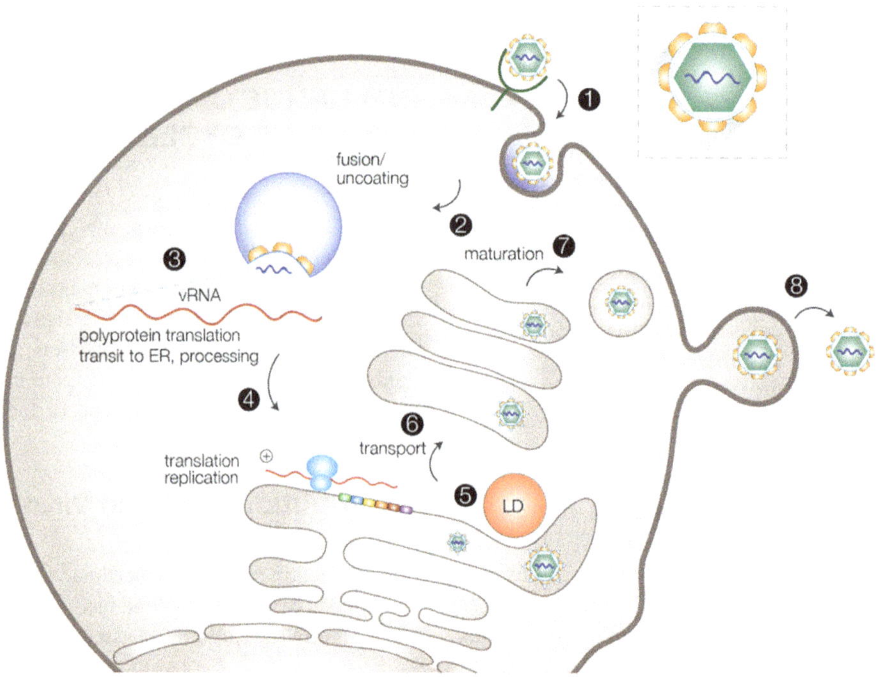

FIGURE 1 | Intracellular life cycle of flaviviruses. Viral particles are internalized via receptor-mediated endocytosis (1). After the uncoating of viral particles (2), viral RNA is released into cytosol for translation and replication (3,4). Progeny virions are assembled in close proximity to the ER and LDs (5). Virions are transported through the host secretory pathway and undergo maturation (6,7). Mature virions are released from the cell surface (8).

expanding the intracellular membrane surface to form DMVs (see Association of LDs to Viral Replication Compartments). Besides, HCV replication triggers the activation of the cellular SREBP pathway for *de novo* synthesis of membrane lipids, which, in turn, regulate biogenesis of LDs (see Manipulation of LD Reserves during Viral life Cycle) (Li et al., 2013). Another possibility is that LDs themselves provide a platform for virus assembly and, therefore, require close proximity to the replication sites for efficient recruitment of newly synthesized viral proteins and subsequent virion packaging (see LDs as a Platform for Virion Assembly) (Miyanari et al., 2007).

Unlike HCV, DENV infection induces formation of single-membrane in-folding into the ER lumen and unstructured convoluted membranes (Welsch et al., 2009; **Figure 2B**). These DENV-induced vesicle-like structures contain viral replicase and dsRNA. Pore-like openings on these structures enable release of newly synthesized viral RNA, facilitating replication and efficient encapsidation (Welsch et al., 2009). Other flaviviruses, such as WNV and tick-borne encephalitis virus (TBEV) share similar features of intracellular membrane rearrangements (Gillespie et al., 2010; Miorin et al., 2013). DENV replication activates the autophagy pathway to mobilize FFAs from LDs and co-opts FA synthase (FASN). FFAs released from LDs are consumed by oxidation in mitochondria to generate ATP, which is required for viral RNA replication (see Usage of LD as an Energy Reservoir during Viral life Cycle) (Heaton and Randall, 2010). Moreover, DENV NS3 recruits FASN to virus replication sites during membrane remodeling in a Rab18-dependent fashion, engaging both LDs and the viral replication complexes in the process (Heaton et al., 2010; Tang et al., 2014). Regardless of the distinct membrane compartmentalization strategies of HCV and DENV both require close juxtaposition of LDs for energy supply and subsequent virion assembly, as reviewed below.

LDs as a Platform for Virion Assembly

In the case of HCV infection, after being generated at the ER, the capsid protein localizes to LDs via its domain 2 in a time-dependent manner. They accumulate on discrete regions of LDs before fully covering the surface of LDs (Boulant et al., 2007; Shavinskaya et al., 2007). Host DGAT1 that synthesizes triglycerides stored within LDs, binds to the HCV capsid protein, which in turn acquires access to DGAT1-generated LDs. Viral RNA replication complexes are subsequently recruited to appropriate sites of virus assembly. LD-localized capsid protein provides stability to these structures via interfering with TAG turnover and inducing aggregation of LDs (Boulant et al., 2008; Herker et al., 2010; Harris et al., 2011). Additionally, by replacing LD-localized ADRP, the capsid protein induces imbalance between the minus-end-directed and the plus-end-directed motors, causing movement of LDs on microtubules toward the nucleus so as to enhance interactions between sites of HCV RNA replication and virion assembly (Boulant et al., 2008). The capsid protein recruits viral NS5A, while the N-terminal of NS5A engages viral replication complexes to LD-associated membranes (Boulant et al., 2007; Appel et al., 2008). HCV NS5A also associates with Rab18, a member of the Rab

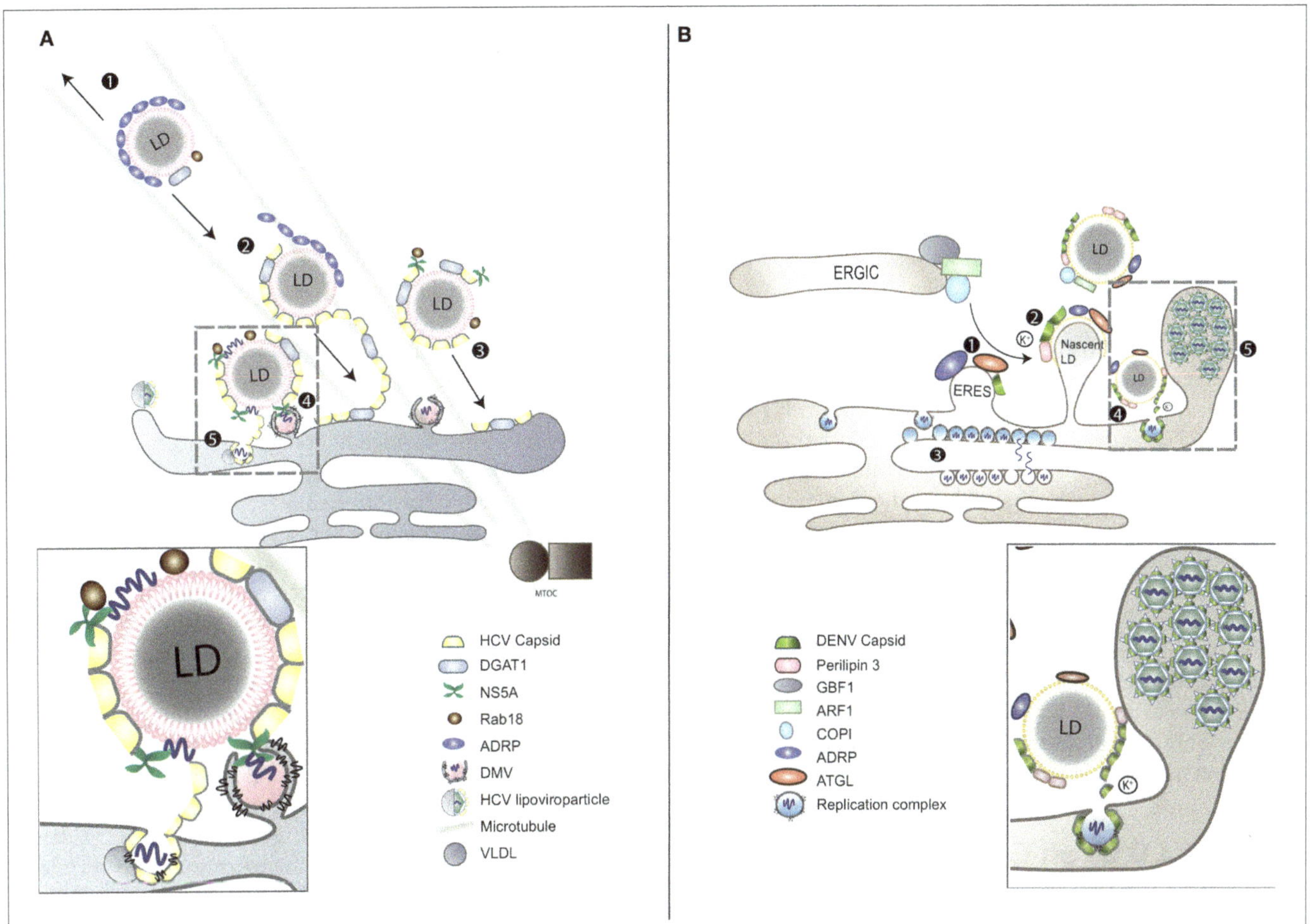

FIGURE 2 | LDs as platforms for virion assembly in **(A)** HCV and **(B)** DENV infection. **(A)** (1) ADRP-coated LDs are able to interact with microtubules and move toward both plus and minus ends. (2) During HCV infection, viral capsid protein replaces ADRP from LD surface with the assistance of DGAT1. (3) As the consequence of losing ADRP, LD losses the balance of mobility, moving toward MTOC and nucleus. (4) Clustering of LDs at the peripheral of nucleus enables the contact between LDs and the replication complex of HCV. HCV RNA is delivered from ER-bound replication complexes to NS5A, obtaining access to LD surface, followed by nucleocapsid formation (gray-dashed frame and enlarged panel). (5) The nucleocapsid fuses with VLDL to form viral lipoviroparticle in ER. **(B)** (1) At the ER–Golgi intermediate compartment (ERGIC), ARF1 and its guanine nucleotide exchange factor (GEF) GBF1 together with COPI deliver ATGL and ADRP from ER export sites (ERES) to the surface of LD. DENV subverts this process for the transportation of capsid protein to LD surface. (2) The accumulation of DENV capsid protein on LDs associates with cellular perilipin 3 and intracellular K^+ concentration. (3) Replicated DENV genomes are released through the vesicle pore and then engaged into nucleocapsids that bud through the ER membrane in close proximity. (4) Capsid protein can be released from LDs to the cytosol or other cellular compartments for subsequent viral assembly (gray-dashed frame and enlarged panel). (5) Packed virions accumulate within the lumen of the vesicle packets-containing ER network before transported to Golgi (Boulant et al., 2008; Chatel-Chaix and Bartenschlager, 2014).

GTPase family that plays an essential role in membrane traffic (Salloum et al., 2013). Rab18 localizes directly to the monolayer surface of LDs in response to lipolytic stimulation (Martin et al., 2005), and facilitates association of NS5A and other replicase components with LDs (Salloum et al., 2013; **Figure 2A**). HCV infection increases the expression of apolipoprotein J, which further stabilizes LD-associated capsid protein and NS5A, thereby facilitating virion assembly (Lin et al., 2014). Cellular CD2 associated protein (CD2AP) also regulates HCV assembly by interacting with HCV NS5A while modulating LD biogenesis at the same time (Li, 2017). Dissociation of HCV capsid protein from LDs has no effect on viral RNA replication but decreases production of infectious virions, indicating that LDs either directly provide a platform for HCV assembly or facilitate transport of the capsid protein from RNA translation/replication to the assembly sites (Boulant et al., 2007, 2008; Miyanari et al., 2007). Additionally, during chronic HCV infection, LDs in liver tissues increase in number and size, causing pathological accumulation of liver lipids, also known as hepatic steatosis. The interaction between the HCV capsid protein and LDs is critical for this development. An LD membrane protein, perilipin 3, regulates the capsid-induced steatosis, indicating host LD-associated proteins as an effective preventive measure of HCV-induced pathology (Ferguson et al., 2017).

The DENV capsid protein also interacts with LDs but in a mechanistically distinct manner as compared to HCV. DENV capsid protein accumulates on the surface of LDs via its center domain and the N-terminal disordered region (Samsa et al., 2009;

Martins et al., 2012). Additionally, the binding between DENV capsid protein and LDs may also be attributed to the association between capsid protein and LD membrane protein perilipin 3 in a potassium ion-dependent fashion. Changing the concentration of potassium ion concentration regulates the binding and release of capsid protein from LDs. This phenomenon indicates that DENV may manipulate specific intracellular ion concentrations to favor viral replication (Carvalho et al., 2012). HCV may use the same potassium ion-dependent strategy to interact with LDs via its p7 and NS5A proteins (Carvalho et al., 2012). Contrary to DGAT1-dependent trafficking to LDs, the DENV capsid protein utilizes host Golgi-specific brefeldin A-resistance guanine nucleotide exchange factor 1 (GBF1)-ARF-COPI pathway to localize to the surface of LDs (Iglesias et al., 2015; **Figure 2B**). Similar to HCV infection, inhibiting the association between DENV capsid protein and LDs results in attenuated infectious virion production but not viral RNA replication, underscoring the function of LDs as a scaffold for DENV assembly through exposure of the protein cationic surface toward the aqueous environment (Carvalho et al., 2012).

DENV and HCV capsid proteins use distinct mechanisms for LD association. The process by which LDs gain or release viral capsid proteins remain unknown. However, current evidence on the involvement of LDs provides several possible targets for developing antiviral approaches (**Table 1**) (section Targeting LD Metabolism as Antiviral Strategies).

Usage of LD as an Energy Reservoir during Viral Life Cycle

Replication of the viral genome is an energy-consuming process. In HCV infected cells, cytoplasmic ATP levels decrease dramatically, as a result of active energy consumption. Meanwhile, elevated ATP levels at replication compartments within infected cells have also been reported (Ando et al., 2012). This would involve either incorporation of ATP-generating machinery into the membrane-associated replication site, or transport of ATP though membrane-to-membrane communication between mitochondria and replication compartments (Ando et al., 2012). The C terminus of *Flaviviridae* NS3 encodes a DExH/D-box RNA helicase that functions to unwind dsRNA molecules through ATP-hydrolysis (Tai et al., 1996; Dumont et al., 2006). Many of the cellular signaling events activated during viral infection are also regulated by ATP levels (Hardie, 2011). Given the highly reduced and hydrophobic lipids at the core, LDs serve as an efficient storage for energy (Walther and Farese, 2012). FA hydrolysis releases 2.5 times more ATPs per gram compared to glucose, which provides a tremendous reservoir for supplying energy during viral replication. Not surprisingly, many other pathogens also manipulate LD metabolism to acquire fuel for replication.

Energy stored in LDs is released through lipolysis. Mobilization of TAG stores from LDs by lipases produces significant amounts of FFAs that can be used in β-oxidation, generating ATP and other intermediates for the cell. In addition to lipolysis, an alternative route through autophagy, commonly referred to as lipophagy, can also take up and deliver LDs to lytic compartments for lipid hydrolysis (see Mobilization of Lipids from LDs) (Wang, 2016).

A model proposed by Randall and Heaton suggested that DENV infection triggers lipophagy to deplete LDs, releasing FFAs. DENV also induces cellular β-oxidation to consume the FFAs released from lipophagy for energy production. Exogenously supplemented FAs can replace the need for lipophagy during DENV replication, suggesting that flaviviruses manipulate cellular lipid metabolism to create an environment that favors virus replication (Heaton and Randall, 2010). Our own data support this model. AUP1, a monotopic membrane protein localized to both LDs and ER membranes, was identified as a key component in DENV biogenesis. Expression of AUP1 was up-regulated during DENV infection and was found to be necessary for virus-triggered lipophagy to proceed (Zhang et al., 2016). The requirement of lipophagy during other flavivirus infections is still to be investigated.

Virus-induced lipophagy for energy production remains unclear in the context of HCV infection. HCV uses membranes of autophagic vacuoles for viral RNA replication. The induction of autophagosomes is nutrient starvation-independent. An impaired autophagy pathway results in attenuated virion production (Dreux et al., 2009; Sir et al., 2012). Proteomic and lipidomic studies showed an up-regulation of lipogenic enzymes and proteins related to β-oxidation, such as 3,2-trans-enoyl-CoA isomerase (DCI) (Diamond et al., 2010). In line with this study, DCI was reported to be essential for productive HCV infection through regulation of mitochondrial FA oxidation (Rasmussen et al., 2011). Another microarray analysis revealed a down-regulation of genes involved in degradation and oxidation of FAs, and an elevation of genes that control metabolism and transport of FAs (Blackham et al., 2010). Although a direct experimental evidence of lipophagy induced by HCV is still missing, data from several indirect sources strongly suggest the utilization of cellular pathways for β-oxidation of FFAs.

Manipulation of LD Reserves during Viral Life Cycle

Apart from providing FFAs for β-oxidation during *Flaviviridae* infection, LDs also function as a reservoir for lipids that are essential for viral replication.

Flaviviridae replication organelles consist of FAs, specific phospholipids, sphingolipids, and cholesterol (Heaton et al., 2010; Perera et al., 2012; Paul et al., 2013; Martín-Acebes et al., 2016a). While DENV obtains FAs by breakdown of LDs via lipophagy (Heaton and Randall, 2010), HCV controls the transcriptional induction of lipid biosynthetic and related genes through SREBP signaling (Olmstead et al., 2012). HCV infection activates the SREBP precursor that localizes to the ER, and triggers its trafficking to the Golgi. Thereafter, the SREBP precursor is proteolytically processed by site 1 protease (S1P) and S2P at Golgi, releasing its N-terminal fragment that is transported into the nucleus and initiates transcription of lipogenic factors such as FASN and 3-hydroxy-3-methylglutaryl CoA (HMGCoA). The 3′ untranslated region of the HCV RNA genome with DEAD

TABLE 1 | Examples antiviral strategies against HCV and flaviviruses interfering with lipid metabolism-related processes.

Step	HCV				Flaviviruses			
	Lipid biogenesis process	Inhibitory target	Drug/inhibitor	References	Lipid biogenesis process	Inhibitory target	Drug/inhibitor	References
Replication	FA synthesis	FASN	C75	Yang et al., 2008	FA synthesis	FASN	Cerulenin, C75	Heaton et al., 2010; Martín-Acebes et al., 2011; Perera et al., 2012; Poh et al., 2012
		ACC	TOFA	Kapadia and Chisari, 2005		ACC	TOFA, MEDICA 16	Merino-Ramos et al., 2016
	FA β-oxidation	DCI	Etomoxir	Rasmussen et al., 2011	FA β-oxidation	CPT-1	Etomoxir	Heaton and Randall, 2010
	Sphingolipids synthesis	SPT	NA808, myriocin, NA255, ISP-1, HPA-12	Sakamoto et al., 2005; Umehara et al., 2006; Aizaki et al., 2008; Amemiya et al., 2008; Weng et al., 2010; Hirata et al., 2012; Katsume et al., 2013	Sphingolipids synthesis	SMase	D609, MS-209	Martín-Acebes et al., 2016a
						SPT	Myriocin	Aktepe et al., 2015
						CerS	Fumonisin B1	Aktepe et al., 2015
						SphK	SKI/SK1-II	Carr et al., 2013; Clarke et al., 2016
	CHO synthesis	OSBP	OSW-1	Wang et al., 2014	CHO synthesis	SCP-2	SCPI-1	Fu et al., 2015
		PI4KA	AL-9	Wang et al., 2014		SQS	Zaragozic acid A	Rothwell et al., 2009
		SREBPs	BAPTA-AM, pyrrolidine dithiocarbamate	Waris et al., 2007		HMGCS	Hymeglusin	Rothwell et al., 2009
		PI3K	LY294002	Waris et al., 2007; Park et al., 2009		OSC	U18666A	Poh et al., 2012
		CHO	MβCD	Sagan et al., 2006		HMGCR	Lovastatin, paravastatin, hymeglusin, fluvastatin	Mackenzie et al., 2007; Rothwell et al., 2009; Soto-Acosta et al., 2013
		HMGCR	25-hydroxycholesterol, cerulenin, lovastatin, simvastatin, mevastatin, fluvastatin	Ye et al., 2003; Sagan et al., 2006; Amemiya et al., 2008; Delang et al., 2009				
						S1P	PF-429242	Uchida et al., 2016
						DHCR7	AY-9944	Mackenzie et al., 2007
		GGTase I	GGTI-286	Sagan et al., 2006		GGTase I	GGTI-298	Mackenzie et al., 2007
	Glycosphingolipids synthesis	FAPP2	NB-DNJ, PDMP	Khan et al., 2014	Lipophagy	PI3K	3-methyladenine	Heaton and Randall, 2010
	TAG and CHO synthesis	PPARα	BA	Lyn et al., 2009				
	Lipid biosynthesis	AMPK	Metformin, AICAR, A769662	Mankouri et al., 2010				

(Continued)

TABLE 1 | Continued

Step	HCV				Flaviviruses			
	Lipid biogenesis process	**Inhibitory target**	**Drug/inhibitor**	**References**	**Lipid biogenesis process**	**Inhibitory target**	**Drug/inhibitor**	**References**
Assembly	LD-viral capsid protein binding	DGAT1	DGAT1 inhibitor	Herker et al., 2010; Harris et al., 2011	LD-viral capsid protein binding	Perilipin 3	Ouabain	Carvalho et al., 2012
		MAPK, PLA2G4A	U0126	Menzel et al., 2012		MAPK, PLA2G4A	U0126	Menzel et al., 2012
	CHO synthesis	SRB1	PERL	Pollock et al., 2010		GBF1	Brefeldin A	Iglesias et al., 2015
	LDs formation	IKK	Wedelolactone, Inhibitor XII	Li et al., 2013				
		SKI-1/S1P	Spn4A-RRLL	Olmstead et al., 2012				
	LDs redistribution	Microtubule	Nocodazole	Boulant et al., 2008				
Budding	VLDL pathway, LDs lipids transfer	Cyclophilins	NIM811	Anderson et al., 2011	Sphingolipids synthesis	Smase	Amitriptyline	Tani et al., 2010
	Apolipoproteins	MTP	BMS-200150	Perlemuter et al., 2002; Gastaminza et al., 2008		nSmase2	GW4869	Menzel et al., 2012; Martín-Acebes et al., 2014
		MTP/ ACAT2/ HMGCR	Naringenin	Nahmias et al., 2008				

Underlined, antiviral strategies targeting host lipids and lipid biogenesis processes that directly relate to LDs.

box polypeptide 3 X-linked (DDX3X) further activates IκB kinase (IKK)-α, which translocates to the nucleus and stimulates SREBP transcriptional activity, thus modulating LD biogenesis (Olmstead et al., 2012; Li et al., 2013).

HCV replication organelles use cholesterol as a structural component (Romero-Brey et al., 2012; Paul et al., 2013). Cellular oxysterol-binding protein (OSBP) and phosphatidylinositol 4-kinases (PI4KA) facilitate trafficking of cholesterol to the HCV-rearranged membrane-like structures during replication, highlighting the need for both factors in supporting HCV replication (Wang et al., 2014). OSBPs are speculated to be sterol carriers and might function to transport sterols out of the ER and incorporate them into LDs in a phosphatidylinositol 4-phosphate (PI(4)P)-dependent manner. Sterols and cholesterol are exchanged by OSBP at the ER-Golgi interface (Mesmin et al., 2013). OSBP-related protein 2 that resides on the surface of LDs may also participate in the process of lipid exchange (Hynynen et al., 2009). Notwithstanding its cellular function, the activity of OSBP appears to be dispensable for DENV replication (Hynynen et al., 2009). DENV replication is regulated by endogenous cholesterol production that is controlled by mevalonate (diphospho) decarboxylase (MVD) and exogenous cholesterol uptake (Rothwell et al., 2009). Similarly, WNV also hijacks cellular cholesterol and redistributes it to viral RNA replication compartments (Mackenzie et al., 2007).

Besides cholesterol, sphingomyelin is another essential membrane component of HCV replication organelles. An active role for sphingolipids in HCV RNA replication has been reported. Sphingomyelin enhances binding of the RNA dependent RNA polymerase NS5B to the template RNA and is therefore important for HCV replication (Weng et al., 2010; Hirata et al., 2012). Expression of genes that encode sphingomyelin synthases 1 and 2 is up-regulated upon HCV infection, resulting in enhanced synthesis of sphingomyelin (Hirata et al., 2012). Dynamic pools of sphingomyelin were observed in LDs, with the high affinity sphingomyelin-binding protein ADRP on the surface of LDs (McIntosh et al., 2010). It is likely that LDs participate in the biogenesis of sphingolipids necessary for HCV replication.

In addition to consumption of lipids that are stored in LDs, HCV can also obstruct the turnover of LDs to establish a microenvironment that is more favorable to viral infection. Release of infectious HCV particles relies on secretion of hepatic very low-density lipoprotein (VLDL)—a TAG-rich lipoprotein. For hijacking VLDL secretion, HCV inhibits the function of the putative TAG lipase, arylacetamide deacetylase (AADAC), thus, further impairing TAG lipolysis (Nourbakhsh et al., 2013). Moreover, HCV capsid protein that localizes to LDs through the activity of DGAT1 (Harris et al., 2011), restrains lipolysis of TAG by interacting with ATGL and its activator comparative gene identification-58 (CGI-58) (Camus et al., 2014).

As with LD association, distinct strategies are employed by HCV and DENV for mobilizing lipids within LDs, hence providing insights into LD catabolism and cellular factors as possible targets (**Table 1**).

TARGETING LD METABOLISM AS ANTIVIRAL STRATEGIES

Although viruses of the *Flaviviridae* family cause severe human diseases, there are currently no clinically approved drugs available for treatment against them, other than for HCV. Historically, the development of antiviral therapy has largely focused on directly targeting viral components involved in multiple stages of the virus life cycle.

Entry of flaviviruses is mediated by fusion of the viral envelope (E) protein with the host membrane. Blocking virus entry via targeting the viral E protein offers a means to suppress the onset of infection. A few heterocyclic compounds, such as compound 6, NITD-448 and P02, have been identified to directly bind to the hydrophobic pocket of viral E protein and block its conformational change, which is essential for virus-host fusion (Modis et al., 2003, 2004; Zhou et al., 2008; Poh et al., 2009; Wang et al., 2009). Due to the multifunctional nature of the E protein, its inhibitors may potentially block multiple steps in the viral life cycle, including entry and virion assembly/maturation. More importantly, these inhibitors can exert their effect through direct binding to virions without the need to cross the hydrophobic membrane bilayer and be delivered into infected cells. However, due to the complexity and high variability of flaviviral E protein, it is challenging to develop pan-serotype inhibitors (Wang and Shi, 2015).

During replication, the viral genome is translated into a single polyprotein which is cleaved into individual proteins by a viral protease complex. Since polyprotein processing is a prerequisite for viral replication and assembly, these virally encoded proteases are one of the most attractive antiviral targets (Chambers et al., 1990, 1993; Luo et al., 2015). Two HCV NS3/4A serine protease inhibitors, boceprevir and telaprevir, have been approved in combination with PEG-interferon plus ribavirin for treatment of chronic HCV genotype 1 (Ghany et al., 2011). Recent study by Shiryaev and colleagues have identified a group of small molecule antiviral inhibitors that interfering with the productive fold of the NS2B cofactor in the two-component protease, inhibit its cleavage activity and therefore suppress ZIKV infection. The most potent inhibitor NSC157058 was shown to inhibit ZIKV infection in both cultured hfNPCs and mice without significant toxicity (Shiryaev et al., 2017). Despite these advances, resistance to protease inhibitors can occur rapidly, especially for chronic infections such as HCV due to the genetic variability of the virus and high mutation rate (Rong et al., 2010; Wu et al., 2013). Another concern in developing protease-based antiviral therapy is toxicity. Similarities in viral and host cellular serine proteases would presumably create problems in specificity while targeting the virus.

The flaviviral NS3 RNA helicase is located adjacent to the C terminal of the NS3 protease (Luo et al., 2008). The RNA helicase is believed to be required for several different functions such as initiation of RNA synthesis, separating dsRNA structures formed during viral RNA synthesis and as a translocase that eliminates proteins bound to the viral RNA (Sampath and Padmanabhan, 2009). Viruses with a mutated NS3 helicase are unable to replicate properly (Matusan et al., 2001). Several RNA helicase inhibitors have been identified. The antiparasitic drug ivermectin was shown to inhibit WNV, YFV, and DENV at submicromolar levels, and a small molecule inhibitor ST-610 was found to potently and selectively inhibit all four serotypes of DENV *in vivo* (Mastrangelo et al., 2012; Lim et al., 2013). However, due to a lack of specific binding pockets for RNA and NTPs, molecules that target the RNA helicase via these binding sites might also non-selectively bind to other cellular proteins with helicase/NTPase activities, resulting in significant toxicity (Luo et al., 2015).

The NS5 RNA-dependent RNA polymerase (RdRp) is the most conserved amongst the flavivirus proteins, and is essential for viral RNA synthesis. Since host cells lack these enzymes, the specificity makes them one of the most promising and intensively studied classes of antiviral targets. RdRp can be targeted by non-nucleoside inhibitors (NNIs) and nucleoside/nucleotide analog inhibitors (NIs) (Malet et al., 2008). NNIs directly target the binding pocket of the polymerase and block its conformational change from its inactive to active form (Biswal et al., 2005). Although a number of NNI candidates for HCV are under clinical development, there hasn't been any FDA approved NNIs for flaviviruses yet. The major challenge in the use of NNIs in antiviral therapy is the structural variability of the binding pockets across different serotypes or genotypes as well as the resistant mutation in or near the binding pocket which results in resistance to the NNIs (Sofia et al., 2012). NIs have been widely used in clinics for treatment of hepatitis, HIV and herpesvirus infections (Jordheim et al., 2013; Menéndez-Arias et al., 2014). Compared to other classes of inhibitors, NIs have a higher threshold for developing resistance, and a relatively broad-antiviral spectrum due to the relatively conserved polymerase structure (Delang et al., 2011; Lim et al., 2013). Unlike NNIs which directly bind to RNA polymerase, NIs have to convert into its triphosphate form inside cells by host kinases before exerting their antiviral effects (Stein and Moore, 2001). However, the kinase activity varies significantly in different cell types/hosts, causing variable efficacy of the same NI. Another major issue associated with NIs is the unpredictable toxicity *in vitro*. Although the toxicity of NIs is often associated with the inhibition of mitochondrial polymerases (Arnold et al., 2012), other mitochondrial perturbations may also attribute to toxicity (Selvaraj et al., 2014).

The N-terminal domain of NS5 contains one methyltransferase (MTase) that catalyzes guanine N-7 and ribose 2′-*O*-methylations using S-adenosylmethionine (SAM) as a methyl donor during viral cap formation (Zhou et al., 2007). Non-selective competitive inhibitors, such as S-adenosylhomocysteine and sinefungin bind to SAM binding sites and inhibit its function (Boldescu et al., 2017). Using virtual screening, a group of small compound molecules have been identified with broad-spectrum activity against the MTase proteins of multiple flaviviruses, including DENV2, DENV3, and YFV (Brecher et al., 2015). Apart from the most important antiviral targets such as E protein, NS3 protease and NS5 polymerase, other viral targets such as capsid protein, NS1 and NS4 proteins are also under evaluation. The details of different

TABLE 2 | Comparison of advantages and disadvantages of different antiviral strategies against HCV and flaviviruses.

	Host Target		Viral Target			
	Host factors in lipid metabolism	**Other cellular factors (host protease, glucosidase, kinases)**	**Viral entry**	**Viral proteasome**	**RNA helicase**	**RdRp**
Advantages	• Higher barrier to resistance • Broad-spectrum antiviral effects, e.g., Statin • Effective control of emerging and novel pathogens • Fast development process with known inhibitors • Can impair both genome replication and particle morphogenesis	• Higher barrier to resistance • Broad-spectrum antiviral effects, e.g., DNJ • Effective control of emerging and novel pathogens • Fast development process with known inhibitors • Target different steps of viral life cycle • Target specific manifestations, e.g., DHF/DSS	• Effective in early steps of viral life cycle • Fast inhibition for acute infection • No need for penetration into the host cells • Blocking multiple steps of viral cycle (entry and virion assembly/maturation)	• Broad-spectrum of antiviral activity • Potential of combination therapy	• Broad-spectrum of antiviral activity	**Non-nucleoside inhibitors (NNIs)** • Lower off-target effects • Lower cytotoxicity **Nucleoside/nucleotide analog inhibitors (NIs)** • Higher barrier to resistance • Broad spectrum of antiviral activity • Lower off-target effects
Disadvantages	• Not effective in early steps of viral life cycle (entry and fusion) • Enhanced cellular toxicities, e.g., PI4KIIIα inhibitors	• Enhanced cellular toxicities, e.g., NITD008 and Balapiravir • Drug resistance induced by viral substrate mutation, e.g., kinase inhibitor AZD0530	• Low barrier to resistance • Difficult to develop pan-serotype inhibitors	• Low barrier to resistance • Cross inhibition against human enzymes	• Enhanced toxicity due to lack of specific binding pockets for RNA and NTP binding sites	**Non-nucleoside inhibitors (NNIs)** • Low barrier to resistance • Difficult to develop pan-serotype inhibitors **Nucleoside/nucleotide analog inhibitors (NIs)** • Unpredictable structure-activity relationship • Varied efficacy across different cell types and hosts • Unpredictable toxicity *in vivo*

viral targets have been reviewed elsewhere (Boldescu et al., 2017; García et al., 2017).

Due to extensive dependence of viruses (replication, assembly, and budding) on host LDs, the interface of virus-host interactions with LDs and/or LD metabolism provides a rich source for potential antiviral interventions (**Table 1**). First, targeting host factors may produce potential broad-spectrum activity against multiple viral infections due to similar intracellular pathways employed by viruses within the same genus or family. Second, given the high replication and mutation rates of viruses, long-term antiviral therapy against chronic infections inevitably selects for the resistant variants which alter the drug target and therefore are less susceptible to the inhibitory effects of the treatment. The resistant mutants eventually become the dominant species and lead to treatment failure and persistent infection. Development of drug-resistance has become a major challenge with direct-acting antivirals when treating chronic infections (Rong et al., 2010). Unlike viral elements, host cellular factors are much less prone to mutation; thus targeting host lipid metabolism provides an attractive approach for long-term treatment of diseases caused by viral infection. However, since LDs play a role in lipid metabolism *in-vivo*, manipulating a major metabolic pathway may have a more pleiotropic impact on cellular homeostasis (Georgel et al., 2010). Such consequences need to be carefully assessed to hit the right balance between causing host toxicity while preventing viral pathogenesis. Third, several inhibitors targeting host lipid metabolic pathways are well characterized, which can greatly accelerate the process of drug development. Moreover, targeting specific steps of LD biosynthesis, distribution, trafficking, and metabolism which viruses routinely exploit, allows us to design antiviral strategies with an enhanced therapeutic window. For example, triglyceride-synthesizing enzyme DGAT1 has been identified as an important host factor which is required for trafficking of viral capsid protein to LDs, facilitating early steps of viral assembly. Of note, RNAi-mediated silencing of DGAT1 resulted in impaired viral particle production without affecting LD composition (Herker et al., 2010). Currently, novel classes of pharmacological inhibitors targeting DGAT1 have been developed for clinical applications (DeVita and Pinto, 2013). In addition, regulating enzymes in the FA synthesis pathway has been shown to inhibit production of different viruses. C75, a FA synthase inhibitor, displayed a strong inhibitory effect on HCV replication (Yang et al., 2008), DENV production (Samsa et al., 2009), as well as WNV and YFV replication (Martín-Acebes et al., 2011) without causing significant toxicity to host cells. A series of chemical probes (ML-206, ML-219 and ML-220) has been shown to reduce the biogenesis and consumption of LDs without toxicity to mammalian cells (Boxer et al., 2013). These probes may prove to be beneficial in inhibiting virus production. A noteworthy and indirect strategy to interrupt the association between virus and LDs during viral replication and assembly is to target involved viral proteins. During the biosynthesis of the HCV polyproteins, an internal signal sequence between the capsid protein and envelope protein E1 can be preceded by cellular signal peptide peptidase (SPP). This process releases the capsid protein from the ER, followed by its transport to LDs. SPP inhibitor $(Z\text{-}LL)_2$-ketone abolishes the cleavage of capsid protein by SPP and thereby inhibits production of infectious HCV (McLauchlan et al., 2002).

Ideally, antiviral treatments should exert their effects as early as possible after infection. This is particularly true for acute flaviviral infections such as DENV. Targeting intracellular host factors, however, is perhaps less effective in preventing the onset of an infection compared to other inhibitors, which block viral entry. The advantages and disadvantages of antiviral strategies against HCV and flaviviruses by targeting viral components and host factors including those involved in LD metabolism are summarized in **Table 2**.

CONCLUSION

Despite being an immense global health problem, there are no affordable and efficient prophylactic or therapeutic treatments for some pathogenic flaviviruses. It is imperative to have alternative therapeutic strategies of inhibiting specific steps in the intracellular virus life cycle to combat infection. Viruses from the *Flaviviridae* family often cause perturbations in cellular energy and lipid homeostasis during infection. This has been reported for DENV, WNV, and HCV infection. Therefore, targeting cellular LDs offers possibilities for such interventions, including inhibition of lipid metabolism and disruption of interactions with viral components. Although knowledge on the participation of LDs during infection of HCV and flaviviruses has significantly progressed, comparative studies that aim to determine the shared or specific requirements of LD components for these pathogens are still lacking. In addition, much of the information available is from *in-vitro* studies, while the *in-vivo* relevance remains unexplored. Therefore, a more comprehensive understanding of the molecular biology of viruses and their dependence on host LD metabolism is of utmost priority for development of broad-spectrum and specific anti-flaviviral strategies.

AUTHOR CONTRIBUTIONS

JZ and YL drafted the manuscript and contributed equally to this work. SS supervised, evaluated, and edited the manuscript.

ACKNOWLEDGMENTS

This work was funded by Research Grants Council (GRF grants 17117914 and 17113915), and partially supported by Health and Medical Research Funds (16150592), theme based research grant from the Research Grants Council (Project No. T11-705/14N) and research funds from Institut Pasteur (PTR 546). SS is supported by the Croucher Foundation.

REFERENCES

Aizaki, H., Morikawa, K., Fukasawa, M., Hara, H., Inoue, Y., Tani, H., et al. (2008). Critical role of virion-associated cholesterol and sphingolipid in hepatitis C virus infection. *J. Virol.* 82, 5715–5724. doi: 10.1128/JVI.02530-07

Aktepe, T. E., Pham, H., and Mackenzie, J. M. (2015). Differential utilisation of ceramide during replication of the flaviviruses West Nile and dengue virus. *Virology* 484, 241–250. doi: 10.1016/j.virol.2015.06.015

Amemiya, F., Maekawa, S., Itakura, Y., Kanayama, A., Matsui, A., Takano, S., et al. (2008). Targeting lipid metabolism in the treatment of hepatitis C virus infection. *J. Infect. Dis.* 197, 361–370. doi: 10.1086/525287

Anderson, L. J., Lin, K., Compton, T., and Wiedmann, B. (2011). Inhibition of cyclophilins alters lipid trafficking and blocks hepatitis C virus secretion. *Virol. J.* 8:329. doi: 10.1186/1743-422X-8-329

Ando, T., Imamura, H., Suzuki, R., Aizaki, H., Watanabe, T., Wakita, T., et al. (2012). Visualization and measurement of ATP levels in living cells replicating hepatitis C virus genome RNA. *PLoS Pathog.* 8:e1002561. doi: 10.1371/journal.ppat.1002561

Appel, N., Zayas, M., Miller, S., Krijnse-Locker, J., Schaller, T., Friebe, P., et al. (2008). Essential role of domain III of nonstructural protein 5A for hepatitis C virus infectious particle assembly. *PLoS Pathog.* 4:e1000035. doi: 10.1371/journal.ppat.1000035

Arnold, J. J., Sharma, S. D., Feng, J. Y., Ray, A. S., Smidansky, E. D., Kireeva, M. L., et al. (2012). Sensitivity of mitochondrial transcription and resistance of RNA polymerase II dependent nuclear transcription to antiviral ribonucleosides. *PLoS Pathog.* 8:e1003030. doi: 10.1371/journal.ppat.1003030

Bartenschlager, R., Lohmann, V., and Penin, F. (2013). The molecular and structural basis of advanced antiviral therapy for hepatitis C virus infection. *Nat. Rev. Microbiol.* 11, 482–496. doi: 10.1038/nrmicro3046

Biswal, B. K., Cherney, M. M., Wang, M., Chan, L., Yannopoulos, C. G., Bilimoria, D., et al. (2005). Crystal structures of the RNA-dependent RNA polymerase genotype 2a of hepatitis C virus reveal two conformations and suggest mechanisms of inhibition by non-nucleoside inhibitors. *J. Biol. Chem.* 280, 18202–18210. doi: 10.1074/jbc.M413410200

Blackham, S., Baillie, A., Al-Hababi, F., Remlinger, K., You, S., Hamatake, R., et al. (2010). Gene expression profiling indicates the roles of host oxidative stress, apoptosis, lipid metabolism, and intracellular transport genes in the replication of hepatitis C virus. *J. Virol.* 84, 5404–5414. doi: 10.1128/JVI.02529-09

Boldescu, V., Behnam, M. A. M., Vasilakis, N., and Klein, C. D. (2017). Broad-spectrum agents for flaviviral infections: dengue, Zika and beyond. *Nat. Rev. Drug Discov.* 16, 565–586. doi: 10.1038/nrd.2017.33

Boulant, S., Douglas, M. W., Moody, L., Budkowska, A., Targett-Adams, P., and McLauchlan, J. (2008). Hepatitis C virus core protein induces lipid droplet redistribution in a microtubule- and dynein-dependent manner. *Traffic* 9, 1268–1282. doi: 10.1111/j.1600-0854.2008.00767.x

Boulant, S., Targett-Adams, P., and McLauchlan, J. (2007). Disrupting the association of hepatitis C virus core protein with lipid droplets correlates with a loss in production of infectious virus. *J. Gen. Virol.* 88(Pt 8), 2204–2213. doi: 10.1099/vir.0.82898-0

Boxer, M. B., Shen, M., Zhang, Y. Q., Liu, L., Auld, D. S., and Beller, M. (2013). *Modulators of Lipid Storage.* Probe Reports from the NIH Molecular Libraries Program. Bethesda, MD: National Center for Biotechnology Information (US).

Bozza, P. T., Bakker-Abreu, I., Navarro-Xavier, R. A., and Bandeira-Melo, C. (2011). Lipid body function in eicosanoid synthesis: an update. *Prostaglandins Leukot. Essent. Fatty Acids* 85, 205–213. doi: 10.1016/j.plefa.2011.04.020

Brasaemle, D. L. (2007). Thematic review series: adipocyte biology. The perilipin family of structural lipid droplet proteins: stabilization of lipid droplets and control of lipolysis. *J. Lipid Res.* 48, 2547–2559. doi: 10.1194/jlr.R700014-JLR200

Brecher, M., Chen, H., Liu, B., Banavali, N. K., Jones, S. A., Zhang, J., et al. (2015). Novel broad spectrum inhibitors targeting the flavivirus methyltransferase. *PLoS ONE* 10:e0130062. doi: 10.1371/journal.pone.0130062

Brown, M. S., and Goldstein, J. L. (1997). The SREBP pathway: regulation of cholesterol metabolism by proteolysis of a membrane-bound transcription factor. *Cell* 89, 331–340. doi: 10.1016/S0092-8674(00)80213-5

Buhman, K. K., Chen, H. C., and Farese, R. V. (2001). The enzymes of neutral lipid synthesis. *J. Biol. Chem.* 276, 40369–40372. doi: 10.1074/jbc.R100050200

Camus, G., Schweiger, M., Herker, E., Harris, C., Kondratowicz, A. S., Tsou, C. L., et al. (2014). The hepatitis C virus core protein inhibits adipose triglyceride lipase (ATGL)-mediated lipid mobilization and enhances the ATGL interaction with comparative gene identification 58 (CGI-58) and lipid droplets. *J. Biol. Chem.* 289, 35770–35780. doi: 10.1074/jbc.M114.587816

Carr, J. M., Kua, T., Clarke, J. N., Calvert, J. K., Zebol, J. R., Beard, M. R., et al. (2013). Reduced sphingosine kinase 1 activity in dengue virus type-2 infected cells can be mediated by the 3′ untranslated region of dengue virus type-2 RNA. *J. Gen. Virol.* 94, 2437–2448. doi: 10.1099/vir.0.055616-0

Carvalho, F. A., Carneiro, F. A., Martins, I. C., Assunção-Miranda, I., Faustino, A. F., Pereira, R. M., et al. (2012). Dengue virus capsid protein binding to hepatic lipid droplets (LD) is potassium ion dependent and is mediated by ld surface proteins. *J. Virol.* 86, 2096–2108. doi: 10.1128/JVI.06796-11

Cermelli, S., Guo, Y., Gross, S. P., and Welte, M. A. (2006). The lipid-droplet proteome reveals that droplets are a protein-storage depot. *Curr. Biol.* 16, 1783–1795. doi: 10.1016/j.cub.2006.07.062

Chambers, T. J., Nestorowicz, A., Amberg, S. M., and Rice, C. M. (1993). Mutagenesis of the yellow fever virus NS2B protein: effects on proteolytic processing, NS2B-NS3 complex formation, and viral replication. *J. Virol.* 67, 6797–6807.

Chambers, T. J., Weir, R. C., Grakoui, A., McCourt, D. W., Bazan, J. F., Fletterick, R. J., et al. (1990). Evidence that the N-terminal domain of nonstructural protein NS3 from yellow fever virus is a serine protease responsible for site-specific cleavages in the viral polyprotein. *Proc. Natl. Acad. Sci. U.S.A.* 87, 8898–8902. doi: 10.1073/pnas.87.22.8898

Chatel-Chaix, L., and Bartenschlager, R. (2014). Dengue virus- and hepatitis C virus-induced replication and assembly compartments: the enemy inside-caught in the web. *J. Virol.* 88, 5907–5911. doi: 10.1128/JVI.03404-13

Cheng, J., Ohsaki, Y., Tauchi-Sato, K., Fujita, A., and Fujimoto, T. (2006). Cholesterol depletion induces autophagy. *Biochem. Biophys. Res. Commun.* 351, 246–252. doi: 10.1016/j.bbrc.2006.10.042

Clarke, J. N., Davies, L. K., Calvert, J. K., Gliddon, B. L., Al Shujari, W. H., Aloia, A. L., et al. (2016). Reduction in sphingosine kinase 1 influences the susceptibility to dengue virus infection by altering antiviral responses. *J. Gen. Virol.* 97, 95–109. doi: 10.1099/jgv.0.000334

Delang, L., Paeshuyse, J., Vliegen, I., Leyssen, P., Obeid, S., Durantel, D., et al. (2009). Statins potentiate the *in vitro* anti-hepatitis C virus activity of selective hepatitis C virus inhibitors and delay or prevent resistance development. *Hepatology* 50, 6–16. doi: 10.1002/hep.22916

Delang, L., Vliegen, I., Froeyen, M., and Neyts, J. (2011). Comparative study of the genetic barriers and pathways towards resistance of selective inhibitors of hepatitis C virus replication. *Antimicrob. Agents Chemother.* 55, 4103–4113. doi: 10.1128/AAC.00294-11

DeVita, R. J., and Pinto, S. (2013). Current status of the research and development of diacylglycerol O-acyltransferase 1 (DGAT1) inhibitors: miniperspective. *J. Med. Chem.* 56, 9820–9825. doi: 10.1021/jm4007033

Diamond, D. L., Syder, A. J., Jacobs, J. M., Sorensen, C. M., Walters, K. A., Proll, S. C., et al. (2010). Temporal proteome and lipidome profiles reveal hepatitis C virus-associated reprogramming of hepatocellular metabolism and bioenergetics. *PLoS Pathog.* 6:e1000719. doi: 10.1371/journal.ppat.1000719

Dreux, M., Gastaminza, P., Wieland, S. F., and Chisari, F. V. (2009). The autophagy machinery is required to initiate hepatitis C virus replication. *Proc. Natl. Acad. Sci. U.S.A.* 106, 14046–14051. doi: 10.1073/pnas.0907344106

Dugail, I., and Hajduch, E. (2007). A new look at adipocyte lipid droplets: towards a role in the sensing of triacylglycerol stores. *Cell. Mol. Life Sci.* 64, 2452–2458. doi: 10.1007/s00018-007-7277-6

Dumont, S., Cheng, W., Serebrov, V., Beran, R. K., Tinoco, I. Jr., Pyle, A. M., et al. (2006). RNA translocation and unwinding mechanism of HCV NS3 helicase and its coordination by ATP. *Nature* 439, 105–108. doi: 10.1038/nature04331

Evans, M. J., Rice, C. M., and Goff, S. P. (2004). Phosphorylation of hepatitis C virus nonstructural protein 5A modulates its protein interactions and viral RNA replication. *Proc. Natl. Acad. Sci. U.S.A.* 101, 13038–13043. doi: 10.1073/pnas.0405152101

Ferguson, D., Zhang, J., Davis, M. A., Helsley, R. N., Vedin, L. L., Lee, R. G., et al. (2017). The lipid droplet-associated protein perilipin 3 facilitates hepatitis C virus-driven hepatic steatosis. *J. Lipid Res.* 58, 420–432. doi: 10.1194/jlr.M073734

Fu, Q., Inankur, B., Yin, J., Striker, R., and Lan, Q. (2015). Sterol carrier protein 2, a critical host factor for dengue virus infection, alters the cholesterol distribution in mosquito Aag2 cells. *J. Med. Entomol.* 52, 1124–1134. doi: 10.1093/jme/tjv101

Fujimoto, T., and Parton, R. G. (2011). Not just fat: the structure and function of the lipid droplet. *Cold Spring Harb. Perspect. Biol.* 3:a004838. doi: 10.1101/cshperspect.a004838

Gao, L., Aizaki, H., He, J. W., and Lai, M. M. (2004). Interactions between viral nonstructural proteins and host protein hVAP-33 mediate the formation of hepatitis C virus RNA replication complex on lipid raft. *J. Virol.* 78, 3480–3488. doi: 10.1128/JVI.78.7.3480-3488.2004

Gao, Q., and Goodman, J. M. (2015). The lipid droplet—a well-connected organelle. *Front. Cell Dev. Biol.* 3:49. doi: 10.3389/fcell.2015.00049

García, L. L., Padilla, L., and Castano, J. C. (2017). Inhibitors compounds of the flavivirus replication process. *Virol. J.* 14:95. doi:10.1186/s12985-017-0761-1

Garske, T., Van Kerkhove, M. D., Yactayo, S., Ronveaux, O., Lewis, R. F., Staples, J. E., et al. (2014). Yellow Fever in Africa: estimating the burden of disease and impact of mass vaccination from outbreak and serological data. *PLoS Med.* 11:e1001638. doi: 10.1371/journal.pmed.1001638

Gastaminza, P., Cheng, G., Wieland, S., Zhong, J., Liao, W., and Chisari, F. V. (2008). Cellular determinants of hepatitis C virus assembly, maturation, degradation, and secretion. *J. Virol.* 82, 2120–2129. doi: 10.1128/JVI.02053-07

Georgel, P., Schuster, C., Zeisel, M. B., Stoll-Keller, F., Berg, T., Bahram, S., et al. (2010). Virus–host interactions in hepatitis C virus infection: implications for molecular pathogenesis and antiviral strategies. *Trends Mol. Med.* 16, 277–286. doi: 10.1016/j.molmed.2010.04.003

Ghany, M. G., Nelson, D. R., Strader, D. B., Thomas, D. L., and Seeff, L. B. (2011). An update on treatment of genotype 1 chronic hepatitis C virus infection: 2011 practice guideline by the American Association for the Study of Liver Diseases. *Hepatology* 54, 1433–1444. doi: 10.1002/hep.24641

Gillespie, L. K., Hoenen, A., Morgan, G., and Mackenzie, J. M. (2010). The endoplasmic reticulum provides the membrane platform for biogenesis of the flavivirus replication complex. *J. Virol.* 84, 10438–10447. doi: 10.1128/JVI.00986-10

Gould, E. A., and Solomon, T. (2008). Pathogenic flaviviruses. *Lancet* 371, 500–509. doi: 10.1016/S0140-6736(08)60238-X

Guo, Y., Walther, T. C., Rao, M., Stuurman, N., Goshima, G., Terayama, K., et al. (2008). Functional genomic screen reveals genes involved in lipid-droplet formation and utilization. *Nature* 453, 657–661. doi: 10.1038/nature06928

Hardie, D. G. (2011). AMP-activated protein kinase-an energy sensor that regulates all aspects of cell function. *Genes Dev.* 25, 1895–1908. doi: 10.1101/gad.17420111

Harris, C., Herker, E., Farese, R. V. Jr., and Ott, M. (2011). Hepatitis C virus core protein decreases lipid droplet turnover: a mechanism for core-induced steatosis. *J. Biol. Chem.* 286, 42615–42625. doi: 10.1074/jbc.M111.285148

Hartman, I. Z., Liu, P., Zehmer, J. K., Luby-Phelps, K., Jo, Y., Anderson, R. G., et al. (2010). Sterol-induced dislocation of HMG CoA reductase from ER membranes into the cytosol through a subcellular compartment resembling lipid droplets. *J Biol Chem.* 110:134213. doi: 10.1074/jbc.M110.134213

Heaton, N. S., Perera, R., Berger, K. L., Khadka, S., Lacount, D. J., Kuhn, R. J., et al. (2010). Dengue virus nonstructural protein 3 redistributes fatty acid synthase to sites of viral replication and increases cellular fatty acid synthesis. *Proc. Natl. Acad. Sci. U.S.A.* 107, 17345–17350. doi: 10.1073/pnas.1010811107

Heaton, N. S., and Randall, G. (2010). Dengue virus-induced autophagy regulates lipid metabolism. *Cell Host Microbe* 8, 422–432. doi: 10.1016/j.chom.2010.10.006

Herker, E., Harris, C., Hernandez, C., Carpentier, A., Kaehlcke, K., Rosenberg, A. R., et al. (2010). Efficient hepatitis C virus particle formation requires diacylglycerol acyltransferase-1. *Nat. Med.* 16, 1295–1298. doi: 10.1038/nm.2238

Hinson, E. R., and Cresswell, P. (2009). The antiviral protein, viperin, localizes to lipid droplets via its N-terminal amphipathic alpha-helix. *Proc. Natl. Acad. Sci. U.S.A.* 106, 20452–20457. doi: 10.1073/pnas.0911679106

Hirata, Y., Ikeda, K., Sudoh, M., Tokunaga, Y., Suzuki, A., Weng, L., et al. (2012). Self-enhancement of hepatitis C virus replication by promotion of specific sphingolipid biosynthesis. *PLoS Pathog.* 8:e1002860. doi: 10.1371/journal.ppat.1002860

Hynynen, R., Suchanek, M., Spandl, J., Bäck, N., Thiele, C., and Olkkonen, V. M. (2009). OSBP-related protein 2 is a sterol receptor on lipid droplets that regulates the metabolism of neutral lipids. *J. Lipid Res.* 50, 1305–1315. doi: 10.1194/jlr.M800661-JLR200

Iglesias, N. G., Mondotte, J. A., Byk, L. A., De Maio, F. A., Samsa, M. M., Alvarez, C., et al. (2015). dengue virus uses a non-canonical function of the host GBF1-Arf-COPI system for capsid protein accumulation on lipid droplets. *Traffic* 16, 962–977. doi: 10.1111/tra.12305

Jiang, D., Guo, H., Xu, C., Chang, J., Gu, B., Wang, L., et al. (2008). Identification of three interferon-inducible cellular enzymes that inhibit the replication of hepatitis C virus. *J. Virol.* 82, 1665–1678. doi: 10.1128/JVI.02113-07

Jo, Y., Hartman, I. Z., and DeBose-Boyd, R. A. (2013). Ancient ubiquitous protein-1 mediates sterol-induced ubiquitination of 3-hydroxy-3-methylglutaryl CoA reductase in lipid droplet–associated endoplasmic reticulum membranes. *Mol. Biol. Cell* 24, 169–183. doi: 10.1091/mbc.E12-07-0564

Jordheim, L. P., Durantel, D., Zoulim, F., and Dumontet, C. (2013). Advances in the development of nucleoside and nucleotide analogues for cancer and viral diseases. *Nat. Rev. Drug Discov.* 12, 447–464. doi: 10.1038/nrd4010

Kapadia, S. B., and Chisari, F. V. (2005). Hepatitis C virus RNA replication is regulated by host geranylgeranylation and fatty acids. *Proc. Natl. Acad. Sci. U.S.A.* 102, 2561–2566. doi: 10.1073/pnas.0409834102

Karlsson, M., Contreras, J. A., Hellman, U., Tornqvist, H., and Holm, C. (1997). cDNA cloning, tissue distribution, and identification of the catalytic triad of monoglyceride lipase evolutionary relationship to esterases, lysophospholipases, and haloperoxidases. *J. Biol. Chem.* 272, 27218–27223. doi: 10.1074/jbc.272.43.27218

Kassan, A., Herms, A., Fernández-Vidal, A., Bosch, M., Schieber, N. L., Reddy, B. J., et al. (2013). Acyl-CoA synthetase 3 promotes lipid droplet biogenesis in ER microdomains. *J. Cell Biol.* 203, 985–1001. doi: 10.1083/jcb.201305142

Katsume, A., Tokunaga, Y., Hirata, Y., Munakata, T., Saito, M., Hayashi, H., et al. (2013). A serine palmitoyltransferase inhibitor blocks hepatitis C virus replication in human hepatocytes. *Gastroenterology* 145, 865–873. doi: 10.1053/j.gastro.2013.06.012

Kaushik, S., and Cuervo, A. M. (2015). Degradation of lipid droplet-associated proteins by chaperone-mediated autophagy facilitates lipolysis. *Nat. Cell Biol.* 17, 759–770. doi: 10.1038/ncb3166

Kaushik, S., Rodriguez-Navarro, J. A., Arias, E., Kiffin, R., Sahu, S., Schwartz, G. J., et al. (2011). Autophagy in hypothalamic AgRP neurons regulates food intake and energy balance. *Cell Metab.* 14, 173–183. doi: 10.1016/j.cmet.2011.06.008

Khan, I., Katikaneni, D. S., Han, Q., Sanchez-Felipe, L., Hanada, K., Ambrose, R. L., et al. (2014). Modulation of hepatitis C virus genome replication by glycosphingolipids and four-phosphate adaptor protein 2. *J. Virol.* 88, 12276–12295. doi: 10.1128/JVI.00970-14

Lass, A., Zimmermann, R., Oberer, M., and Zechner, R. (2011). Lipolysis–a highly regulated multi-enzyme complex mediates the catabolism of cellular fat stores. *Prog. Lipid Res.* 50, 14–27. doi: 10.1016/j.plipres.2010.10.004

Li, C. Y. (2017). CD2AP facilitates HCV production by targeting NS5A to lipid droplets and regulating lipid droplet biogenesis. *FASEB J.* 31(1 Suppl. 184.181). doi: 10.1096/fj.1530-6860

Li, Q., Pène, V., Krishnamurthy, S., Cha, H., and Liang, T. J. (2013). Hepatitis C virus infection activates an innate pathway involving IKK-alpha in lipogenesis and viral assembly. *Nat. Med.* 19, 722–729. doi: 10.1038/nm.3190

Lim, S. P., Wang, Q. Y., Noble, C. G., Chen, Y. L., Dong, H., Zou, B., et al. (2013). Ten years of dengue drug discovery: progress and prospects. *Antiviral Res.* 100, 500–519. doi: 10.1016/j.antiviral.2013.09.013

Lin, C. C., Tsai, P., Sun, H. Y., Hsu, M. C., Lee, J. C., Wu, I. C., et al. (2014). Apolipoprotein J, a glucose-upregulated molecular chaperone, stabilizes core and NS5A to promote infectious hepatitis C virus virion production. *J. Hepatol.* 61, 984–993. doi: 10.1016/j.jhep.2014.06.026

Lindenbach, B. D., Thiel, H.-J., and Rice, C. M. (2007). "Flaviviridae: the viruses and their replication," in *Fields Virology, 5th Edn.*, eds D. M. Knipe and P. M. Howley (Philadelphia, PA: Lippincott-Raven Publishers), 1101–1152.

Lohmann, D., Spandl, J., Stevanovic, A., Schoene, M., Philippou-Massier, J., and Thiele, C. (2013). Monoubiquitination of ancient ubiquitous protein 1 promotes lipid droplet clustering. *PLoS ONE* 8:e72453. doi: 10.1371/journal.pone.0072453

Lundin, M., Lindström, H., Grönwall, C., and Persson, M. A. (2006). Dual topology of the processed hepatitis C virus protein NS4B is influenced by the NS5A protein. *J. Gen. Virol.* 87(Pt 11), 3263–3272. doi: 10.1099/vir.0.82211-0

Luo, D., Vasudevan, S. G., and Lescar, J. (2015). The flavivirus NS2B-NS3 protease-helicase as a target for antiviral drug development. *Antiviral Res.* 118, 148–158. doi: 10.1016/j.antiviral.2015.03.014

Luo, D., Xu, T., Hunke, C., Grüber, G., Vasudevan, S. G., and Lescar, J. (2008). Crystal structure of the NS3 protease-helicase from dengue virus. *J. Virol.* 82, 173–183. doi: 10.1128/JVI.01788-07

Lyn, R. K., Kennedy, D. C., Sagan, S. M., Blais, D. R., Rouleau, Y., Pegoraro, A. F., et al. (2009). Direct imaging of the disruption of hepatitis C virus replication complexes by inhibitors of lipid metabolism. *Virology* 394, 130–142. doi: 10.1016/j.virol.2009.08.022

Mackenzie, J. M., Khromykh, A. A., and Parton, R. G. (2007). Cholesterol manipulation by west nile virus perturbs the cellular immune response. *Cell Host Microbe* 2, 229–239. doi: 10.1016/j.chom.2007.09.003

Malet, H., Massé, N., Selisko, B., Romette, J. L., Alvarez, K., Guillemot, J. C., et al. (2008). The flavivirus polymerase as a target for drug discovery. *Antiviral Res.* 80, 23–35. doi: 10.1016/j.antiviral.2008.06.007

Mankouri, J., Tedbury, P. R., Gretton, S., Hughes, M. E., Griffin, S. D., Dallas, M. L., et al. (2010). Enhanced hepatitis C virus genome replication and lipid accumulation mediated by inhibition of AMP-activated protein kinase. *Proc. Natl. Acad. Sci. U.S.A.* 107, 11549–11554. doi: 10.1073/pnas.0912426107

Martin, S., Driessen, K., Nixon, S. J., Zerial, M., and Parton, R. G. (2005). Regulated localization of Rab18 to lipid droplets: effects of lipolytic stimulation and inhibition of lipid droplet catabolism. *J. Biol. Chem.* 280, 42325–42335. doi: 10.1074/jbc.M506651200

Martín-Acebes, M. A., Blázquez, A. B., Jiménez de Oya, N., Escribano-Romero, E., and Saiz, J. C. (2011). West Nile virus replication requires fatty acid synthesis but is independent on phosphatidylinositol-4-phosphate lipids. *PLoS ONE* 6:e24970. doi: 10.1371/journal.pone.0024970

Martín-Acebes, M. A., Gabandé-Rodríguez, E., García-Cabrero, A. M., Sánchez, M. P., Ledesma, M. D., Sobrino, F., et al. (2016a). Host sphingomyelin increases West Nile virus infection *in vivo*. *J. Lipid Res.* 57, 422–432. doi: 10.1194/jlr.M064212

Martín-Acebes, M. A., Merino-Ramos, T., Blázquez, A. B., Casas, J., Escribano-Romero, E., Sobrino, F., et al. (2014). The composition of West Nile virus lipid envelope unveils a role of sphingolipid metabolism in flavivirus biogenesis. *J. Virol.* 88, 12041–12054. doi: 10.1128/JVI.02061-14

Martín-Acebes, M. A., Vázquez-Calvo, Á., and Saiz, J. C. (2016b). Lipids and flaviviruses, present and future perspectives for the control of dengue, Zika, and West Nile viruses. *Prog. Lipid Res.* 64, 123–137. doi: 10.1016/j.plipres.2016.09.005

Martinez-Vicente, M., Talloczy, Z., Wong, E., Tang, G., Koga, H., Kaushik, S., et al. (2010). Cargo recognition failure is responsible for inefficient autophagy in Huntington's disease. *Nat. Neurosci.* 13, 567–576. doi: 10.1038/nn.2528

Martins, I. C., Gomes-Neto, F., Faustino, A. F., Carvalho, F. A., Carneiro, F. A., Bozza, P. T., et al. (2012). The disordered N-terminal region of dengue virus capsid protein contains a lipid-droplet-binding motif. *Biochem. J.* 444, 405–415. doi: 10.1042/BJ20112219

Mastrangelo, E., Pezzullo, M., De Burghgraeve, T., Kaptein, S., Pastorino, B., Dallmeier, K., et al. (2012). Ivermectin is a potent inhibitor of flavivirus replication specifically targeting NS3 helicase activity: new prospects for an old drug. *J. Antimicrob. Chemother.* 67, 1884–1894. doi: 10.1093/jac/dks147

Matusan, A. E., Pryor, M. J., Davidson, A. D., and Wright, P. J. (2001). Mutagenesis of the Dengue virus type 2 NS3 protein within and outside helicase motifs: effects on enzyme activity and virus replication. *J. Virol.* 75, 9633–9643. doi: 10.1128/JVI.75.20.9633-9643.2001

Maxfield, F. R., and Tabas, I. (2005). Role of cholesterol and lipid organization in disease. *Nature* 438, 612–621. doi: 10.1038/nature04399

McIntosh, A. L., Storey, S. M., and Atshaves, B. P. (2010). Intracellular lipid droplets contain dynamic pools of sphingomyelin: ADRP binds phospholipids with high affinity. *Lipids* 45, 465–477. doi: 10.1007/s11745-010-3424-1

McLauchlan, J., Lemberg, M. K., Hope, G., and Martoglio, B. (2002). Intramembrane proteolysis promotes trafficking of hepatitis C virus core protein to lipid droplets. *Embo J.* 21, 3980–3988. doi: 10.1093/emboj/cdf414

Menéndez-Arias, L., Álvarez, M., and Pacheco, B. (2014). Nucleoside/nucleotide analog inhibitors of hepatitis B virus polymerase: mechanism of action and resistance. *Curr. Opin. Virol.* 8, 1–9. doi: 10.1016/j.coviro.2014.04.005

Menzel, N., Fischl, W., Hueging, K., Bankwitz, D., Frentzen, A., Haid, S., et al. (2012). MAP-kinase regulated cytosolic phospholipase A2 activity is essential for production of infectious hepatitis C virus particles. *PLoS Pathog.* 8:e1002829. doi: 10.1371/journal.ppat.1002829

Merino-Ramos, T., Vázquez-Calvo Á., Casas, J., Sobrino, F., Saiz, J. C., and Martín-Acebes, M. A. (2016). Modification of the Host cell lipid metabolism induced by hypolipidemic drugs targeting the acetyl coenzyme A carboxylase impairs west nile virus replication. *Antimicrob. Agents Chemother.* 60, 307–315. doi: 10.1128/AAC.01578-15

Mesmin, B., Bigay, J., Moser von Filseck, J., Lacas-Gervais, S., Drin, G., and Antonny, B. (2013). A four-step cycle driven by PI(4)P hydrolysis directs sterol/PI(4)P exchange by the ER-Golgi tether OSBP. *Cell* 155, 830–843. doi: 10.1016/j.cell.2013.09.056

Miorin, L., Romero-Brey, I., Maiuri, P., Hoppe, S., Krijnse-Locker, J., Bartenschlager, R., et al. (2013). Three-dimensional architecture of tick-borne encephalitis virus replication sites and trafficking of the replicated RNA. *J. Virol.* 87, 6469–6481. doi: 10.1128/JVI.03456-12

Miyanari, Y., Atsuzawa, K., Usuda, N., Watashi, K., Hishiki, T., Zayas, M., et al. (2007). The lipid droplet is an important organelle for hepatitis C virus production. *Nat. Cell Biol.* 9, 1089–1097. doi: 10.1038/ncb1631

Mizushima, N. (2007). Autophagy: process and function. *Genes Dev.* 21, 2861–2873. doi: 10.1101/gad.1599207

Modis, Y., Ogata, S., Clements, D., and Harrison, S. C. (2003). A ligand-binding pocket in the dengue virus envelope glycoprotein. *Proc. Natl. Acad. Sci. U.S.A.* 100, 6986–6991. doi: 10.1073/pnas.0832193100

Modis, Y., Ogata, S., Clements, D., and Harrison, S. C. (2004). Structure of the dengue virus envelope protein after membrane fusion. *Nature* 427, 313–319. doi: 10.1038/nature02165

Nahmias, Y., Goldwasser, J., Casali, M., van Poll, D., Wakita, T., Chung, R. T., et al. (2008). Apolipoprotein B-dependent hepatitis C virus secretion is inhibited by the grapefruit flavonoid naringenin. *Hepatology* 47, 1437–1445. doi: 10.1002/hep.22197

Narabayashi, K., Ito, Y., Eid, N., Maemura, K., Inoue, T., Takeuchi, T., et al. (2015). Indomethacin suppresses LAMP-2 expression and induces lipophagy and lipoapoptosis in rat enterocytes via the ER stress pathway. *J. Gastroenterol.* 50, 541–554. doi: 10.1007/s00535-014-0995-2

Nourbakhsh, M., Douglas, D. N., Pu, C. H., Lewis, J. T., Kawahara, T., Lisboa, L. F., et al. (2013). Arylacetamide deacetylase: a novel host factor with important roles in the lipolysis of cellular triacylglycerol stores, VLDL assembly and HCV production. *J. Hepatol.* 59, 336–343. doi: 10.1016/j.jhep.2013.03.022

Ohsaki, Y., Cheng, J., Fujita, A., Tokumoto, T., and Fujimoto, T. (2006). Cytoplasmic lipid droplets are sites of convergence of proteasomal and autophagic degradation of apolipoprotein B. *Mol. Biol. Cell* 17, 2674–2683. doi: 10.1091/mbc.E05-07-0659

Ohsaki, Y., Cheng, J., Suzuki, M., Fujita, A., and Fujimoto, T. (2008). Lipid droplets are arrested in the ER membrane by tight binding of lipidated apolipoprotein B-100. *J. Cell Sci.* 121, 2415–2422. doi: 10.1242/jcs.025452

Olmstead, A. D., Knecht, W., Lazarov, I., Dixit, S. B., and Jean, F. (2012). Human subtilase SKI-1/S1P is a master regulator of the hcv lifecycle and a potential host cell target for developing indirect-acting antiviral agents. *PLoS Pathog.* 8:e1002468. doi: 10.1371/journal.ppat.1002468

Ouimet, M., and Marcel, Y. L. (2012). Regulation of lipid droplet cholesterol efflux from macrophage foam cells. *Arterioscler. Thromb. Vasc. Biol.* 32, 575–581. doi: 10.1161/ATVBAHA.111.240705

Park, C. Y., Jun, H. J., Wakita, T., Cheong, J. H., and Hwang, S. B. (2009). Hepatitis C virus nonstructural 4B protein modulates sterol regulatory element-binding protein signaling via the AKT pathway. *J. Biol. Chem.* 284, 9237–9246. doi: 10.1074/jbc.M808773200

Paul, D., and Bartenschlager, R. (2015). Flaviviridae replication organelles: oh, what a tangled web we weave. *Annu. Rev. Virol.* 2, 289–310. doi: 10.1146/annurev-virology-100114-055007

Paul, D., Hoppe, S., Saher, G., Krijnse-Locker, J., and Bartenschlager, R. (2013). Morphological and biochemical characterization of the membranous hepatitis C virus replication compartment. *J. Virol.* 87, 10612–10627. doi: 10.1128/JVI.01370-13

Paul, D., Madan, V., and Bartenschlager, R. (2014). Hepatitis C virus RNA replication and assembly: living on the fat of the land. *Cell Host Microbe* 16, 569–579. doi: 10.1016/j.chom.2014.10.008

Perera, R., Riley, C., Isaac, G., Hopf-Jannasch, A. S., Moore, R. J., Weitz, K. W., et al. (2012). Dengue virus infection perturbs lipid homeostasis in infected mosquito cells. *PLoS Pathog.* 8:e1002584. doi: 10.1371/journal.ppat.1002584

Perlemuter, G., Sabile, A., Letteron, P., Vona, G., Topilco, A., Chrétien, Y., et al. (2002). Hepatitis C virus core protein inhibits microsomal triglyceride transfer protein activity and very low density lipoprotein secretion: a model of viral-related steatosis. *FASEB J.* 16, 185–194. doi: 10.1096/fj.01-0396com

Petersen, L. R., Jamieson, D. J., and Honein, M. A. (2016). Zika virus. *N. Engl. J. Med.* 375, 294–295. doi: 10.1056/NEJMra1602113

Poh, M. K., Shui, G., Xie, X., Shi, P. Y., Wenk, M. R., and Gu, F. (2012). U18666A, an intra-cellular cholesterol transport inhibitor, inhibits dengue virus entry and replication. *Antiviral Res.* 93, 191–198. doi: 10.1016/j.antiviral.2011.11.014

Poh, M. K., Yip, A., Zhang, S., Priestle, J. P., Ma, N. L., Smit, J. M., et al. (2009). A small molecule fusion inhibitor of dengue virus. *Antiviral Res.* 84, 260–266. doi: 10.1016/j.antiviral.2009.09.011

Pol, A., Gross, S. P., and Parton, R. G. (2014). Biogenesis of the multifunctional lipid droplet: lipids, proteins, and sites. *J. Cell Biol.* 204, 635–646. doi: 10.1083/jcb.201311051

Pol, A., Martin, S., Fernandez, M. A., Ferguson, C., Carozzi, A., Luetterforst, R., et al. (2004). Dynamic and regulated association of caveolin with lipid bodies: modulation of lipid body motility and function by a dominant negative mutant. *Mol. Biol. Cell* 15, 99–110. doi: 10.1091/mbc.E03-06-0368

Pollock, S., Nichita, N. B., Böhmer, A., Radulescu, C., Dwek, R. A., and Zitzmann, N. (2010). Polyunsaturated liposomes are antiviral against hepatitis B and C viruses and HIV by decreasing cholesterol levels in infected cells. *Proc. Natl. Acad. Sci. U.S.A.* 107, 17176–17181. doi: 10.1073/pnas.1009445107

Rambold, A. S., Cohen, S., and Lippincott-Schwartz, J. (2015). Fatty acid trafficking in starved cells: regulation by lipid droplet lipolysis, autophagy, and mitochondrial fusion dynamics. *Dev. Cell* 32, 678–692. doi: 10.1016/j.devcel.2015.01.029

Rasmussen, A. L., Diamond, D. L., McDermott, J. E., Gao, X., Metz, T. O., Matzke, M. M., et al. (2011). Systems virology identifies a mitochondrial fatty acid oxidation enzyme, dodecenoyl coenzyme A delta isomerase, required for hepatitis C virus replication and likely pathogenesis. *J. Virol.* 85, 11646–11654. doi: 10.1128/JVI.05605-11

Romero-Brey, I., Merz, A., Chiramel, A., Lee, J. Y., Chlanda, P., Haselman, U., et al. (2012). Three-dimensional architecture and biogenesis of membrane structures associated with hepatitis C virus replication. *PLoS Pathog.* 8:e1003056. doi: 10.1371/journal.ppat.1003056

Rong, L., Dahari, H., Ribeiro, R. M., and Perelson, A. S. (2010). Rapid emergence of protease inhibitor resistance in hepatitis C virus. *Sci. Transl. Med.* 2:30ra32. doi: 10.1126/scitranslmed.3000544

Rothwell, C., Lebreton, A., Young Ng, C., Lim, J. Y., Liu, W., Vasudevan, S., et al. (2009). Cholesterol biosynthesis modulation regulates dengue viral replication. *Virology* 389, 8–19. doi: 10.1016/j.virol.2009.03.025

Sagan, S. M., Rouleau, Y., Leggiadro, C., Supekova, L., Schultz, P. G., Su, A. I., et al. (2006). The influence of cholesterol and lipid metabolism on host cell structure and hepatitis C virus replication. *Biochem. Cell Biol.* 84, 67–79. doi: 10.1139/o05-149

Saka, H. A., and Valdivia, R. (2012). Emerging roles for lipid droplets in immunity and host-pathogen interactions. *Annu. Rev. Cell Dev. Biol.* 28, 411–437. doi: 10.1146/annurev-cellbio-092910-153958

Sakamoto, H., Okamoto, K., Aoki, M., Kato, H., Katsume, A., Ohta, A., et al. (2005). Host sphingolipid biosynthesis as a target for hepatitis C virus therapy. *Nat. Chem. Biol.* 1, 333–337. doi: 10.1038/nchembio742

Salloum, S., Wang, H., Ferguson, C., Parton, R. G., and Tai, A. W. (2013). Rab18 binds to hepatitis C virus NS5A and promotes interaction between sites of viral replication and lipid droplets. *PLoS Pathog.* 9:e1003513. doi: 10.1371/journal.ppat.1003513

Samaan, Z., McDermid Vaz, S., Bawor, M., Potter, T. H., Eskandarian, S., and Loeb, M. (2016). Neuropsychological impact of West Nile virus infection: an extensive neuropsychiatric assessment of 49 cases in Canada. *PLoS ONE* 11:e0158364. doi: 10.1371/journal.pone.0158364

Sampath, A., and Padmanabhan, R. (2009). Molecular targets for flavivirus drug discovery. *Antiviral Res.* 81, 6–15. doi: 10.1016/j.antiviral.2008.08.004

Samsa, M. M., Mondotte, J. A., Iglesias, N. G., Assunçã, I., Barbosa-Lima, G., Da Poian, A. T., et al. (2009). Dengue virus capsid protein usurps lipid droplets for viral particle formation. *PLoS Pathog.* 5:e1000632. doi: 10.1371/journal.ppat.1000632

Sarkari, N. B., Thacker, A. K., Barthwal, S. P., Mishra, V. K., Prapann, S., Srivastava, D., et al. (2012). Japanese encephalitis (JE). Part I: clinical profile of 1,282 adult acute cases of four epidemics. *J. Neurol.* 259, 47–57. doi: 10.1007/s00415-011-6118-6

Selvaraj, S., Ghebremichael, M., Li, M., Foli, Y., Langs-Barlow, A., Ogbuagu, A., et al. (2014). Antiretroviral therapy-induced mitochondrial toxicity: potential mechanisms beyond polymerase-gamma inhibition. *Clin. Pharmacol. Ther.* 96, 110–120. doi: 10.1038/clpt.2014.64

Shavinskaya, A., Boulant, S., Penin, F., McLauchlan, J., and Bartenschlager, R. (2007). The lipid droplet binding domain of hepatitis C virus core protein is a major determinant for efficient virus assembly. *J. Biol. Chem.* 282, 37158–37169. doi: 10.1074/jbc.M707329200

Shiryaev, S. A., Farhy, C., Pinto, A., Huang, C. T., Simonetti, N., Ngono, A. E., et al. (2017). Characterization of the Zika virus two-component NS2B-NS3 protease and structure-assisted identification of allosteric small-molecule antagonists. *Antiviral Res.* 143, 218–229. doi: 10.1016/j.antiviral.2017.04.015

Singh, R., and Cuervo, A. M. (2012). Lipophagy: connecting autophagy and lipid metabolism. *Int. J. Cell Biol.* 2012:282041. doi: 10.1155/2012/282041

Singh, R., Kaushik, S., Wang, Y., Xiang, Y., Novak, I., Komatsu, M., et al. (2009). Autophagy regulates lipid metabolism. *Nature* 458, 1131–1135. doi: 10.1038/nature07976

Siqueira, J. B. Jr., Martelli, C. M., Coelho, G. E., Simplicio, A. C., and Hatch, D. L. (2005). Dengue and dengue hemorrhagic fever, Brazil, 1981-2002. *Emerg. Infect. Dis.* 11, 48–53. doi: 10.3201/eid1101.031091

Sir, D., Kuo, C. F., Tian, Y., Liu, H. M., Huang, E. J., Jung, J. U., et al. (2012). Replication of hepatitis C virus RNA on autophagosomal membranes. *J. Biol. Chem.* 287, 18036–18043. doi: 10.1074/jbc.M111.320085

Sofia, M. J., Chang, W., Furman, P. A., Mosley, R. T., and Ross, B. S. (2012). Nucleoside, nucleotide, and non-nucleoside inhibitors of hepatitis C virus NS5B RNA-dependent RNA-polymerase. *J. Med. Chem.* 55, 2481–2531. doi: 10.1021/jm201384j

Soni, K. G., Mardones, G. A., Sougrat, R., Smirnova, E., Jackson, C. L., and Bonifacino, J. S. (2009). Coatomer-dependent protein delivery to lipid droplets. *J. Cell Sci.* 122, 1834–1841. doi: 10.1242/jcs.045849

Soto-Acosta, R., Mosso, C., Cervantes-Salazar, M., Puerta-Guardo, H., Medina, F., Favari, L., et al. (2013). The increase in cholesterol levels at early stages after dengue virus infection. correlates with an augment in LDL particle uptake and HMG-CoA reductase activity. *Virology* 442, 132–147. doi: 10.1016/j.virol.2013.04.003

Spandl, J., Lohmann, D., Kuerschner, L., Moessinger, C., and Thiele, C. (2011). Ancient ubiquitous protein 1 (AUP1) localizes to lipid droplets and binds the E2 ubiquitin conjugase G2 (Ube2g2) via its G2 binding region. *J. Biol. Chem.* 286, 5599–5606. doi: 10.1074/jbc.M110.190785

Stein, D. S., and Moore, K. H. (2001). Phosphorylation of nucleoside analog antiretrovirals: a review for clinicians. *Pharmacotherapy* 21, 11–34. doi: 10.1592/phco.21.1.11.34439

Sztalryd, C., and Kimmel, A. R. (2014). Perilipins: lipid droplet coat proteins adapted for tissue-specific energy storage and utilization, and lipid cytoprotection. *Biochimie* 96, 96–101. doi: 10.1016/j.biochi.2013.08.026

Tai, C. L., Chi, W. K., Chen, D. S., and Hwang, L. H. (1996). The helicase activity associated with hepatitis C virus nonstructural protein 3 (NS3). *J. Virol.* 70, 8477–8484.

Tang, W. C., Lin, R. J., Liao, C. L., and Lin, Y. L. (2014). Rab18 facilitates dengue virus infection by targeting fatty acid synthase to sites of viral replication. *J. Virol.* 88, 6793–6804. doi: 10.1128/JVI.00045-14

Tani, H., Shiokawa, M., Kaname, Y., Kambara, H., Mori, Y., Abe, T., et al. (2010). Involvement of ceramide in the propagation of japanese encephalitis virus. *J. Virol.* 84, 2798–2807. doi: 10.1128/JVI.02499-09

Tauchi-Sato, K., Ozeki, S., Houjou, T., Taguchi, R., and Fujimoto, T. (2002). The surface of lipid droplets is a phospholipid monolayer with a unique fatty acid composition. *J. Biol. Chem.* 277, 44507–44512. doi: 10.1074/jbc.M207712200

Thanachartwet, V., Oer-Areemitr, N., Chamnanchanunt, S., Sahassananda, D., Jittmittraphap, A., Suwannakudt, P., et al. (2015). Identification of clinical factors associated with severe dengue among Thai adults: a prospective study. *BMC Infect. Dis.* 15:420. doi:10.1186/s12879-015-1150-2

Thiam, A. R., Farese, R. V. Jr., and Walther, T. C. (2013). The biophysics and cell biology of lipid droplets. *Nat. Rev. Mol. Cell Biol.* 14, 775–786. doi: 10.1038/nrm3699

Uchida, L., Urata, S., Ulanday, G. E., Takamatsu, Y., Yasuda, J., Morita, K., et al. (2016). Suppressive effects of the Site 1 Protease (S1P) inhibitor, PF-429242, on dengue virus propagation. *Viruses* 8:e46. doi: 10.3390/v8020046

Umehara, T., Sudoh, M., Yasui, F., Matsuda, C., Hayashi, Y., Chayama, K., et al. (2006). Serine palmitoyltransferase inhibitor suppresses HCV replication in a mouse model. *Biochem. Biophys. Res. Commun.* 346, 67–73. doi: 10.1016/j.bbrc.2006.05.085

Velázquez, A. P., Tatsuta, T., Ghillebert, R., Drescher, I., and Graef, M. (2016). Lipid droplet-mediated ER homeostasis regulates autophagy and cell survival during starvation. *J. Cell Biol.* 212, 621–631. doi: 10.1083/jcb.201508102

Velikkakath, A. K., Nishimura, T., Oita, E., Ishihara, N., and Mizushima, N. (2012). Mammalian Atg2 proteins are essential for autophagosome formation and important for regulation of size and distribution of lipid droplets. *Mol. Biol. Cell* 23, 896–909. doi: 10.1091/mbc.E11-09-0785

Walther, T. C., and Farese, R. V. Jr. (2012). Lipid droplets and cellular lipid metabolism. *Annu. Rev. Biochem.* 81, 687–714. doi: 10.1146/annurev-biochem-061009-102430

Wang, C. W. (2016). Lipid droplets, lipophagy, and beyond. *Biochim. Biophys. Acta* 1861(8 Pt B), 793–805. doi: 10.1016/j.bbalip.2015.12.010

Wang, H., Perry, J. W., Lauring, A. S., Neddermann, P., De Francesco, R., and Tai, A. W. (2014). Oxysterol-binding protein is a phosphatidylinositol 4-kinase effector required for HCV replication membrane integrity and cholesterol trafficking. *Gastroenterology* 146, 1373–1385. doi: 10.1053/j.gastro.2014.02.002

Wang, Q. Y., Patel, S. J., Vangrevelinghe, E., Xu, H. Y., Rao, R., Jaber, D., et al. (2009). A small-molecule dengue virus entry inhibitor. *Antimicrob. Agents Chemother.* 53, 1823–1831. doi: 10.1128/AAC.01148-08

Wang, Q. Y., and Shi, P. Y. (2015). Flavivirus entry inhibitors. *ACS Infect. Dis.* 1, 428–434. doi: 10.1021/acsinfecdis.5b00066

Waris, G., Felmlee, D. J., Negro, F., and Siddiqui, A. (2007). Hepatitis C virus induces proteolytic cleavage of sterol regulatory element binding proteins and stimulates their phosphorylation via oxidative stress. *J. Virol.* 81, 8122–8130. doi: 10.1128/JVI.00125-07

Welsch, S., Miller, S., Romero-Brey, I., Merz, A., Bleck, C. K., Walther, P., et al. (2009). Composition and three-dimensional architecture of the dengue virus replication and assembly sites. *Cell Host Microbe* 5, 365–375. doi: 10.1016/j.chom.2009.03.007

Welte, M. A. (2015). Expanding roles for lipid droplets. *Curr. Biol.* 25, R470–R481. doi: 10.1016/j.cub.2015.04.004

Weng, L. Y., Hirata, Y., Arai, M., Kohara, M., Wakita, T., Watashi, K., et al. (2010). Sphingomyelin activates hepatitis C virus RNA polymerase in a genotype-specific manner. *J. Virol.* 84, 11761–11770. doi: 10.1128/JVI.00638-10

Wilfling, F., Haas, J. T., Walther, T. C., and Farese, R. V. Jr. (2014a). Lipid droplet biogenesis. *Curr. Opin. Cell Biol.* 29, 39–45. doi: 10.1016/j.ceb.2014.03.008

Wilfling, F., Thiam, A. R., Olarte, M. J., Wang, J., Beck, R., Gould, T. J., et al. (2014b). Arf1/COPI machinery acts directly on lipid droplets and enables their connection to the ER for protein targeting. *Elife* 3:e01607. doi: 10.7554/eLife.01607

Wilfling, F., Wang, H., Haas, J. T., Krahmer, N., Gould, T. J., Uchida, A., et al. (2013). Triacylglycerol synthesis enzymes mediate lipid droplet growth by relocalizing from the ER to lipid droplets. *Dev. Cell* 24, 384–399. doi: 10.1016/j.devcel.2013.01.013

Wu, S., Kanda, T., Nakamoto, S., Imazeki, F., and Yokosuka, O. (2013). Hepatitis C virus protease inhibitor-resistance mutations: our experience and review. *World J. Gastroenterol.* 19, 8940–8948. doi: 10.3748/wjg.v19.i47.8940

Yang, T., Espenshade, P. J., Wright, M. E., Yabe, D., Gong, Y., Aebersold, R., et al. (2002). Crucial step in cholesterol homeostasis: sterols promote binding of SCAP to INSIG-1, a membrane protein that facilitates retention of SREBPs in ER. *Cell* 110, 489–500. doi: 10.1016/S0092-8674(02)00872-3

Yang, W., Hood, B. L., Chadwick, S. L., Liu, S., Watkins, S. C., Luo, G., et al. (2008). Fatty acid synthase is up-regulated during hepatitis C virus infection and regulates hepatitis C virus entry and production. *Hepatology* 48, 1396–1403. doi: 10.1002/hep.22508

Ye, J., Wang, C., Sumpter, R., Brown, M. S., Goldstein, J. L., and Gale, M. (2003). Disruption of hepatitis C virus RNA replication through inhibition of host protein geranylgeranylation. *Proc. Natl. Acad. Sci. U.S.A.* 100, 15865–15870. doi: 10.1073/pnas.2237238100

Yoshimori, T. (2004). Autophagy: a regulated bulk degradation process inside cells. *Biochem. Biophys. Res. Commun.* 313, 453–458. doi: 10.1016/j.bbrc.2003.07.023

Zhang, J. S., Lamers, M. M., Li, M. Y., Angyal, D., Ashour, J., and Sanyal, S. (2016). "Lipid droplet associated membrane protein Aup1 facilitates dengue virus release through induction of lipophagy," in *12th GERLI Lipidomics meeting "Microbe and host lipids"* (Toulouse).

Zhou, Y., Ray, D., Zhao, Y., Dong, H., Ren, S., Li, Z., et al. (2007). Structure and function of flavivirus NS5 methyltransferase. *J. Virol.* 81, 3891–3903. doi: 10.1128/JVI.02704-06

Zhou, Z., Khaliq, M., Suk, J. E., Patkar, C., Li, L., Kuhn, R. J., et al. (2008). Antiviral compounds discovered by virtual screening of small-molecule libraries against dengue virus E protein. *ACS Chem. Biol.* 3, 765–775. doi: 10.1021/cb800176t

Zimmermann, R., Strauss, J. G., Haemmerle, G., Schoiswohl, G., Birner-Gruenberger, R., Riederer, M., et al. (2004). Fat mobilization in adipose tissue is promoted by adipose triglyceride lipase. *Science* 306, 1383–1386. doi: 10.1126/science.1100747

10

Real-Time qPCR as a Method for Detection of Antibody-Neutralized Phage Particles

*Anna Kłopot[1], Adriana Zakrzewska[1], Dorota Lecion[1], Joanna M. Majewska[1], Marek A. Harhala[1], Karolina Lahutta[1], Zuzanna Kaźmierczak[1], Łukasz Łaczmański[1,2], Marlena Kłak[2] and Krystyna Dąbrowska[1,2]**

[1] Bacteriophage Laboratory, Institute of Immunology and Experimental Therapy, Polish Academy of Sciences, Wrocław, Poland, [2] Research and Development Center, Regional Specialist Hospital, Wrocław, Poland

***Correspondence:**
Krystyna Dąbrowska
dabrok@iitd.pan.wroc.pl

The most common method for phage quantitation is the plaque assay, which relies on phage ability to infect bacteria. However, non-infective phage particles may preserve other biological properties; specifically, they may enter interactions with the immune system of animals and humans. Here, we demonstrate real-time quantitative polymerase chain reaction (qPCR) detection of bacteriophages as an alternative to the plaque assay. The closely related staphylococcal bacteriophages A3R and 676Z and the coliphage T4 were used as model phages. They were tested *in vivo* in mice, *ex vivo* in human sera, and on plastic surfaces designed for ELISAs. T4 phage was injected intravenously into pre-immunized mice. The phage was completely neutralized by specific antibodies within 5 h (0 pfu/ml of serum, as determined by the plaque assay), but it was still detected by qPCR in the amount of approximately 10^7 pfu/ml of serum. This demonstrates a substantial timelapse between "microbiological disappearance" and true clearance of phage particles from the circulation. In human sera *ex vivo*, qPCR was also able to detect neutralized phage particles that were not detected by the standard plaque assay. The investigated bacteriophages differed considerably in their ability to immobilize on plastic surfaces: this difference was greater than one order of magnitude, as shown by qPCR of phage recovered from plastic plates. The ELISA did not detect differences in phage binding to plates. Major limitations of qPCR are possible inhibitors of the PCR reaction or free phage DNA, which need to be considered in procedures of phage sample preparation for qPCR testing. We propose that phage pharmacokinetic and pharmacodynamic studies should not rely merely on detection of antibacterial activity of a phage. Real-time qPCR can be an alternative for phage detection, especially in immunological studies of bacteriophages. It can also be useful for studies of phage-based drug nanocarriers or biosensors.

Keywords: qPCR, plaque assay, phage, quantitation, antibody, neutralizing, humoral response, immune response

INTRODUCTION

Bacteriophages can be used in multiple medical applications (Międzybrodzki et al., 2012; Kutter et al., 2015; Vandenheuvel et al., 2015; Karimi et al., 2016; Saeed et al., 2017), veterinary (Grant et al., 2016), biotechnology (Oślizło et al., 2011; Lee et al., 2012; O'Sullivan et al., 2016), agriculture (Żaczek et al., 2015), or food processing (Endersen et al., 2014). Development of all these phage applications relies on experimental testing with the accurate detection of phage particles in various conditions. Specifically, phage quantitation is the key step in comparisons between different phage strains, different health status of animals or humans, and different experimental design. The most common and prevalent method for phage quantitation is the plaque assay. It simply employs a microbiological culture, where a sensitive bacterial host is cultured with a phage in a double layer plate, eventually allowing for direct counting of plaques as soon as bacteria become visible in the plate (Adams, 1959). There are important limitations of this method. The most important one is the fact that microbiological detection of phage activity does not meet the real count of bacteriophage particles in samples; it in fact allows for testing how many phages were able to infect their host effectively. Phage capability of infection, in turn, may be dependent on a myriad of factors: from simple ion content in the environment and presence of organic compounds or detergents, to the presence of specific antibodies, complement system elements or competitive phages of other types (Ishiguro et al., 1983; Matsushita et al., 2011; Refardt, 2011; Cheng et al., 2013, 2016; Hodyra-Stefaniak et al., 2015; Szermer-Olearnik et al., 2017). Once inactivated, phage cannot be detected by the plaque assay, which makes quantitation of real phage particle content very difficult or even impossible.

Non-infective phage particles may preserve other biological or technological properties that are not related to their ability to infect bacteria. Phage immunoreactivity, i.e., the potency of phage to interact with antibodies and other elements of the immune system, is a phenomenon independent on phage infectivity (Kirsch et al., 2008; Samoylova et al., 2012; Dąbrowska et al., 2014). Most bacteriophages are complex, multi-protein structures where the infection apparatus is only a fraction of the whole particle. Other structural proteins can interact with mammalian system (Dąbrowska et al., 2006, 2007; Barr et al., 2013) regardless phage infectivity. Therefore, phage pharmacokinetics/pharmacodynamics studies should not rely merely on detection of antibacterial activity of a phage.

Techniques that rely on nucleic acid amplification and detection are among the most valuable tools in biological research. Real-time quantitative polymerase chain reaction (qPCR) detection of eukaryotic viruses in environmental and human or animal samples is a standard and commercialized method (Watzinger et al., 2004; Hmaied et al., 2015). Bacteriophages have been quantitatively analyzed and discriminated by real-time qPCR directly in microbiological cultures, and the authors found this method to be a good alternative to the plaque assay (Edelman and Barletta, 2003; Clokie, 2009; Anderson et al., 2011; Refardt, 2012; Dieterle et al., 2016). Real-time PCR has been further demonstrated as applicable for a rapid screening allowing phage detection in food (milk, fruits, vegetables, seafood, meat) (Imamovic and Muniesa, 2011; Flannery et al., 2014; Perrin et al., 2015; Parente et al., 2016; Hartard et al., 2017) and water samples (Farkas et al., 2015; Kunze et al., 2015; Unnithan et al., 2015; Mankiewicz-Boczek et al., 2016) or in feces (Imamovic et al., 2010; Chehoud et al., 2016). However, potential applicability of real-time qPCR for detection of inactivated (non-infective) but still biologically active (e.g., immunoreactive) phage has never been investigated.

Here we propose real-time qPCR as a quantitative method for phage detection in immunological studies of bacteriophages. Specifically, it was tested in comparisons between different phage strains, different immunological statuses of animals or humans, and different experimental designs. Two closely related staphylococcal bacteriophages, A3R and 676Z, together with the coliphage T4, were used as the model phage strains. We assessed and validated a real-time qPCR-based method for immunological studies of samples derived from animals and humans (*in vivo* and *ex vivo* experiments), as well as for optimization of comparative ELISAs of different phages.

MATERIALS AND METHODS

Preparation of Phages T4, A3R, and 676Z and Determination of Phage Titers Using Plaque Assay

T4 phage was purchased from American Type Culture Collection (ATCC, Manassas, VA, United States) and phages A3R and 676Z are part of the IIET Microorganisms Collection (Institute of Immunology and Experimental Therapy, Polish Academy of Sciences, Wroclaw, Poland). Enriched broth cultures of phages were purified by filtration through polysulfone membranes and by fast protein liquid chromatography: gel filtration on Sepharose 4B (Sigma–Aldrich, Poland). The final preparation was dialyzed using 1000 kDa-pore membranes against PBS to remove the bacterial residuals and lipopolysaccharide (LPS), and filtered through 0.22 μm PVDF filters (Millipore, Europe). Prior to dialysis of T4 phage we used LPS-affinity chromatography EndoTrap HD according to the manufacturer's instructions (Hyglos GmbH, Bernried, Germany) in order to further remove LPS. LPS removal was done by three successive incubations of the preparation with the slurry followed by centrifugations. Each purified phage T4 preparation was tested for phage concentration by determining phage titer after serial dilution with PBS (dilutions from 10^{-1} to 10^{-9}), 25 μl of each dilution was spotted on a culture plate pre-covered with susceptible bacteria, two spots for each dilution. The plate was incubated overnight at 37°C to obtain visible plaques. The plaques were counted, mean values of two spots were calculated, and the phage concentration was calculated per milliliter with regard to the dilution and spot volume. For phages A3R and 676Z we used double layer agar plates according to Adams in order to determine phage titer (Adams, 1959).

Isolation of Genomic DNA from T4, A3R, and 676Z Phages and Preparation of DNA Standards

Phage genomic DNA was isolated using GenElute Mammalian Genomic DNA Miniprep (Sigma–Aldrich, Poznan, Poland). For this procedure we used phage lysates each containing 10^8 pfu. After incubating samples with DNase and RNase (Sigma–Aldrich, Poland) (50 μg of each, 10 min, 37°C), 40 μg of proteinase K (Sigma–Aldrich, Poland) as well as 100 μl of Resuspension Buffer was added to each sample. Samples were then incubated for 5 min at 70°C. Next, 200 μl of Lysis Solution C was added to the samples and samples were incubated for 10 min at 70°C. Afterward 200 μl of 96% ethanol (Sigma–Aldrich, Poland) was added to each sample. Samples were applied to the columns provided with the kit and prepared in advance using Column Preparation Solution. Following column centrifugation (6500 × *g*, 1 min, room temperature) 500 μl of wash buffer was applied to the columns and the columns were centrifuged (12,000 × *g*, 1 min, room temperature). The washing step was repeated twice. Finally phage genomic DNA was eluted using 60 μl of DNase-free water. DNA was quantified using NanoDrop (Wilmington, DE, United States). Based on this we prepared 10 ng/μl stocks of phage genomic DNA. In order to prepare a standard curve for each phage genomic DNA we used 10 ng/μl stock solutions to prepare the following dilutions of phage genomic DNA: 1, 0.1, and 0.01 ng/μl. For the phages A3R, 676Z, and T4 the highest standard equals approximately 6.5×10^7, 8.6×10^7, and 5×10^7 phage particles per microliter, respectively. Numbers of virus particles were calculated as genomic equivalents. In order to calculate genomic equivalents based on the amount of nanograms of DNA in qPCR samples we used an online calculator (Stothard, 2000) to calculate the molecular weight of a single phage genome from the exact genomic sequences of the bacteriophages (accession numbers for A3R, 676Z, and T4, are JX080301, JX080302, and NC_000866, respectively). The following molecular weights were calculated for single phage DNA molecules: 87108105.24 Da for A3R, 91769200.84 Da for 676Z, and 104340909.87 Da for T4 phage. These molecular weights of phage genomes were used to calculate numbers of single genomic DNA molecules in investigated samples (1 Da weighs approximately 1.67×10^{-24} g), resulting in the values called *genomic equivalents*. The standard solutions were used in duplicate to prepare the standard curve for qPCR. For the purpose of absolute quantifications, standard curves were created by plotting quantification cycle (*Cq*) values against the number of genomic equivalents.

Primer Design and qPCR Reaction

The genome sequences of T4, A3R, and 676Z phages were obtained from the GenBank (accession numbers for T4, A3R, and 676Z are NC_000866, JX080301, and JX080302, respectively). Based on the genome sequence, qPCR primers were designed using the Primer-BLAST software at the National Center for Biotechnology Information (National Center for Biotechnology Information, 2017).

To detect T4 phage we used forward primer 5′-ACT GGC CAG GTA TTC GCA-3′ and reverse primer 5′-ATG CTT CTT TAG CAC CGG CA-3′. To detect A3R and 676Z phages the following primers were used: forward primer 5′-TGA AGA AGA CCG TGC AGG ATT-3′ and reverse primer 5′-TCA GAA GGA GCT GAT TGA GCG-3′.

The amount of genomic DNA in each test sample was determined using 5× HOT FIREPolEvaGreen qPCR Mix Plus (Solis BioDyne, Tartu, Estonia) following the manufacturer's recommendations. Briefly, each PCR reaction contained 1 μl of DNA template and 15 pM of each primer as well as 2 μl of 5× HOT FIREPolEvaGreen qPCR Mix Plus in a final volume of 10 μl. Cycling conditions were as described by 5× HOT FIREPolEvaGreen qPCR Mix Plus's manufacturer. The amount of phage genomic DNA in test samples was calculated based on the standard curve generated using standard solutions prepared as outlined above. qPCR normalization was performed according to MIQE Guidelines (Bustin et al., 2009).

ELISA

A MaxiSorp flat-bottom 96-well plate (Nunc, Thermo Scientific, Poznań, Poland) was covered with purified phage preparations obtained by chromatography as described above (100 μl per well, as indicated in the figures) sterilely, at 4°C, overnight. Plates were washed five times with PBS and blocked with five times diluted Superblock (Thermo Fisher Scientific Inc., Rockford, IL, United States) for 1 h (100 μl per well) at room temperature. Blocking solution was removed and the plate was washed five times with PBS with 0.05% Tween 20 (Serva, Heidelberg, Germany). Serum diluted 1:100 was applied to the wells in 100 μl per well. Each sample was processed in duplicate. The plate was incubated at 37°C for 2 h. Plates were washed five times with PBS with 0.05% Tween 20 (Sigma–Aldrich, Poland). Diluted detection antibody was added in the amount of 100 μl per well: peroxidase-conjugated AffiniPure goat anti-mouse IgM (Jackson ImmunoResearch Laboratories, West Grove, PA, United States) or peroxidase-conjugated AffiniPure goat anti-mouse IgG (Jackson ImmunoResearch Laboratories, West Grove, PA, United States) at a final dilution of 200,000. The detection antibody was incubated in the wells for 1 h at room temperature in the dark, removed, and the plate was washed five times with PBS with 0.05% Tween 20. TMB X-Treme (Nordic BioSite AB, Sweden) substrate reagent for peroxidase was used (50 μl) according to the manufacturer's instructions (ImmunO4, Westminster, MD, United States). Twenty-five microliters of 2 N H_2SO_4 (Sigma–Aldrich, Poland) was added to each well without substrate removal, then absorbance was measured at 450 (main reading) and 550 nm (background). The background values were subtracted from the main readings and the average value of each duplicate was calculated. In the case of relative increases of antibody levels OD values are presented.

Experimental Design

Experiment 1: Comparison of qPCR and Plaque Assay Method for T4 Phage Detection in Human Sera *ex Vivo*

In this experiment equal volumes of T4 phage (50 μl, titer 10^7 pfu/ml) were mixed with equal volumes of human serum samples. We specifically used serum samples from three healthy donors that contained high amounts of antibodies against T4 phage as well as samples from three healthy donors that contained low amounts of such antibodies. The serum samples mixed with T4 phage were incubated for 1 h at 37°C in order to allow for antibody-mediated destruction of T4 phage followed by detection of the amount of live phage in serum samples using the plaque method. In addition we used the qPCR method described above to detect genomic DNA.

Experiment 2: Comparison of qPCR and Plaque Assay Method for T4 Phage Detection in Serum of Mice Immunized to T4 Phage

Three BALB/c female mice were injected intraperitoneally on day 0 with 1×10^{11} pfu T4 phage/mouse and three BALB/c female mice were injected with an equal volume of sterile PBS. Eleven days after the challenge animals were bled from the tail and serum was separated from the blood by double centrifugation at $2250 \times g$. The serum samples were subjected to the ELISA test in order to determine the amount of antibodies specific for T4 phage belonging to classes IgM and IgG. Thirteen days after the challenge mice were injected i.v. with T4 phage 1×10^{11} pfu/mouse determined by the plaque method and bled from the tail 0.5 and 5 h later. Serum was separated as outlined above. A portion of each serum was used to detect the amount of T4 phage via the plaque method, whereas a 50 μl portion of serum was subjected to isolation of viral nucleic acid using a viral RNA and DNA kit (Macherey Nagel, Duren, Germany) according to the protocol outlined by the manufacturer. Obtained DNA was used to detect the amount of T4 phage via the qPCR method.

Experiment 3: Quantitation of Phage Particles on Plastic Surfaces

We used dilutions of each phage (T4, A3R, and 676Z) that contained 1×10^9, 5×10^9, and 1×10^{10} pfu/ml as determined by the plaque assay, six replicates each. Hundred microliters of each dilution for each phage was used to coat a 96-well Maxisorp plate (Nunc). As a negative control we used PBS solution that was also used as a diluent for phage solutions. The plate was incubated overnight at 4°C. The next day the plate was washed five times with 150 μl of PBS per well and non-specific binding was blocked with fivefold diluted Superblock (Thermo Fisher Scientific Inc., Rockford, IL, United States) for 45 min at room temperature. Then, 10 μg of proteinase K (A&A Biotechnology, Gdynia, Poland) diluted in Tris-EDTA buffer pH 8.0 (final volume 100 μl) was added to each well and the plate was incubated for 4 h at 50°C. After incubation the content of each well was transferred to a single tube. Tubes were incubated for 20 min at 85°C in order to inactivate proteinase K. Following brief centrifugation samples were frozen at −80°C before further use for qPCR reactions as described above.

Experiment 4: Comparison of the Amount of Phage Detectable by qPCR and the Relative Signal from the ELISA

In this experiment A3R and 676Z phages at 1×10^9, 5×10^9, and 1×10^{10} pfu/ml dilutions as determined by the plaque assay as well as PBS were used in triplicate to coat Maxisorp plates. One plate was processed for qPCR analysis of adhered phage particles as described above (see Experiment 1), and the other identical plate was processed for ELISA. In the ELISA experiment we used mouse serum specific to major capsid protein (AFN38316) as the first antibody source and goat anti-mouse IgG as the detection antibody. The ELISA test was conducted as outlined above.

Ethics Statement

The female 6- to 8-week-old BALB/c mice were purchased from Mossakowski Medical Research Centre, Polish Academy of Sciences, Warsaw, Poland and kept in specific pathogen-free (SPF) conditions in the Animal Breeding Centre of the IIET. The experiments were approved by the First Local Committee for Experiments with the Use of Laboratory Animals, Wroclaw, Poland (no. 92/2016). The Bioethics Committee of Wrocław Medical University approved obtaining blood samples from healthy donors. All study subjects gave written informed consent for participation in the study.

Data Analysis and Statistics

Each experiment was repeated at least twice and the results of one experiment are shown. The data are presented as mean ± SE. Statistical analysis was done by one-way ANOVA followed by Tukey's multiple comparison test with a significance level of $p = 0.05$ or two-tailed unpaired t-test with a significance level of $p = 0.05$. The graphs and statistical analysis were performed using GraphPad Prism software.

RESULTS

Characterization of qPCR Reaction

We determined efficiency and specificity of qPCR reactions performed with primers specifically recognizing genomic DNA of staphylococcal phages A3R and 676Z and coliphage T4. In all investigated phages, primers were specific to genes coding for major head proteins. It should be noted that these genes are 100% homologous in A3R and 676Z phages [overall homology of the genomes is 94.6% (Łobocka et al., 2012)]; thus, the same set of primers was used in both phages. Sample standard curves obtained for phages A3R, 676Z, and T4 are presented in **Figure 1**. These curves together with corresponding correlation coefficients (**Table 1**) show a strong correlation between the Cq value and the genomic equivalents representing numbers of phage particles. The efficiency of amplification reaction for any phage genomic DNA was higher than 75%.

The sensitivity of phage detection by qPCR reaction was determined by Cq values of the PCR reaction performed with the phage concentration range from 0 to 10^{11} pfu/ml, for all three investigated phages. We propose the range from 10^3 to 10^{11} pfu/ml as a reliable correlation between phage concentration and Cq value; in this range we observed a linear relationship between Cq values and the number of each phage particles (**Figure 2**). For the lower phage titers Cq values were characterized by high deviations: in a range between 35.36 ± 0.3 and 35.57 ± 1.32 for A3R phage, between 33.4 ± 0.85 and 34 ± 0.923 for 676Z phage, and 31.32 ± 0.69 and 32.57 ± 0.064 for T4 phage.

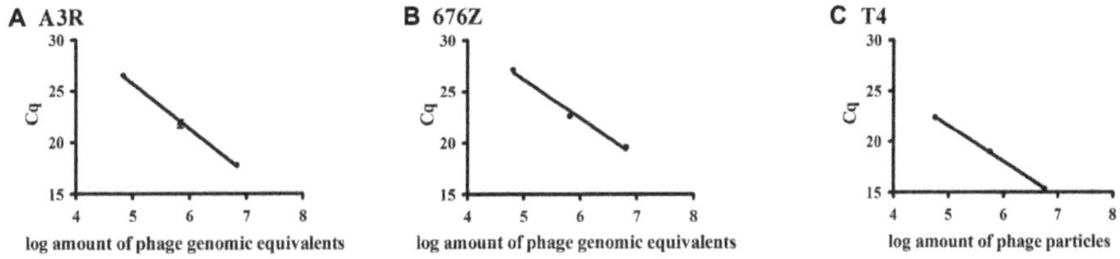

FIGURE 1 | Standard curves representing the correlation between number of phage particles and *Cq* values of real-time PCR detection of **(A)** A3R phage, **(B)** 676Z phage, and **(C)** T4 phage (representative examples are presented).

Comparison of qPCR and Plaque Assay Method for T4 Phage Detection in Serum of Mice Immunized to T4 Phage

Optimized qPCR detection of phage (see above) was used to detect the phage in *in vivo* model with animals eliciting phage-neutralizing antibodies. Mice were challenged with T4 to develop a specific antibody response as previously described (Dąbrowska et al., 2014); a high antibody level was confirmed by ELISA (**Supplementary Figure S1**). The mice specifically immunized to T4 phage and control mice were injected intravenously with the phage; phage concentration in blood serum was assessed 0.5 and 5 h after injection by the plaque assay or by qPCR. The amounts of phage detected in murine sera are compared in **Figure 3**. Both methods showed that the presence of specific antibodies results in a decrease of phage concentration in animals' sera, but there was a striking difference in the demonstrated levels of the decrease. Half an hour after phage administration to mice, the difference between phage concentration in phage-immunized mice and control mice as detected by the plaque assay was more than five orders of magnitude, but only two orders of magnitude by qPCR. Five hours after phage administration to mice, this difference as detected by the plaque assay was more than 10 orders of magnitude (no active phage was detected in immunized mice) but less than three orders of magnitude by qPCR (still approximately 10^7 genomic equivalents/ml of phage particles detected). This demonstrates that the phage, even when neutralized in terms of antibacterial activity, can still be present in the circulation in high amounts and it can be detected and quantitatively assessed by qPCR.

Comparison of qPCR and Plaque Assay Method for T4 Phage Detection in Human Sera *ex Vivo*

The potency of qPCR to detect immunologically inactivated phage was further verified in human sera *ex vivo*. T4

TABLE 1 | Correlation coefficients calculated for qPCR reaction (corresponding to **Figure 1**).

PCR reaction specific for	R^2	Slope	Reaction efficiency (%)	T_m
A3R	0.993	−4.083	75.76	77.6
676Z	0.986	−3.77	84.18	78.02
T4	0.999	−3.533	91.89	84.3

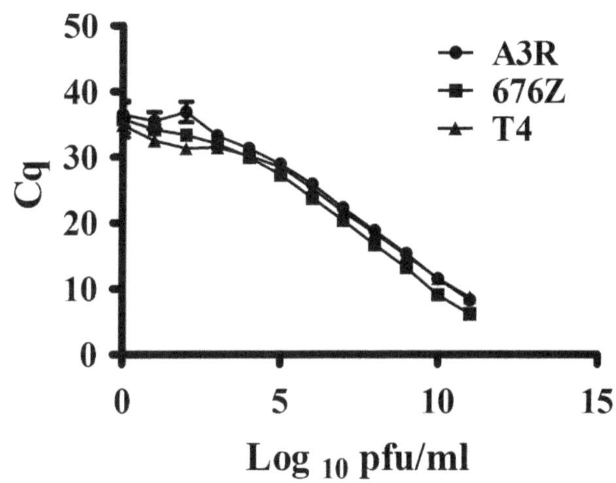

FIGURE 2 | Correlation between *Cq* values of qPCR reaction and the amount of phage particles used as a template in qPCR reaction. Three independent serial dilutions (*N* = 3) containing from 0 to 10^{11} pfu/ml of 676Z phage, A3R phage, or T4 phage were used as templates in qPCR reactions. The *X*-axis presents the logarithm of phage titers used as template DNA in the qPCR reaction and the *Y*-axis presents *Cq* values of the qPCR reactions.

bacteriophage was incubated with human sera, both with those containing a high concentration of phage-specific antibodies (positive sera) and with those with a low content of phage-specific IgG (negative sera); a previously described collection of positive and negative sera was used (Dąbrowska et al., 2014). After incubation, the phage was detected either by plaque assay or by qPCR and the results were compared. The plaque assay revealed statistically significantly lower (70% decrease) activity of phage after incubation with positive sera than that after incubation with negative sera ($p = 0.037$). In the qPCR method the amount of phage detected in both groups was not statistically different ($p = 0.39$) (**Figure 4**). This is in line with the proposition of qPCR as a method for detection of phage whose antibacterial activity has been neutralized.

Quantitation of Phage Particles on Plastic Surfaces

Due to the devastating effect that antibodies may exert on phage activity, probably the major area of immunological studies of bacteriophages is identification of phage-specific

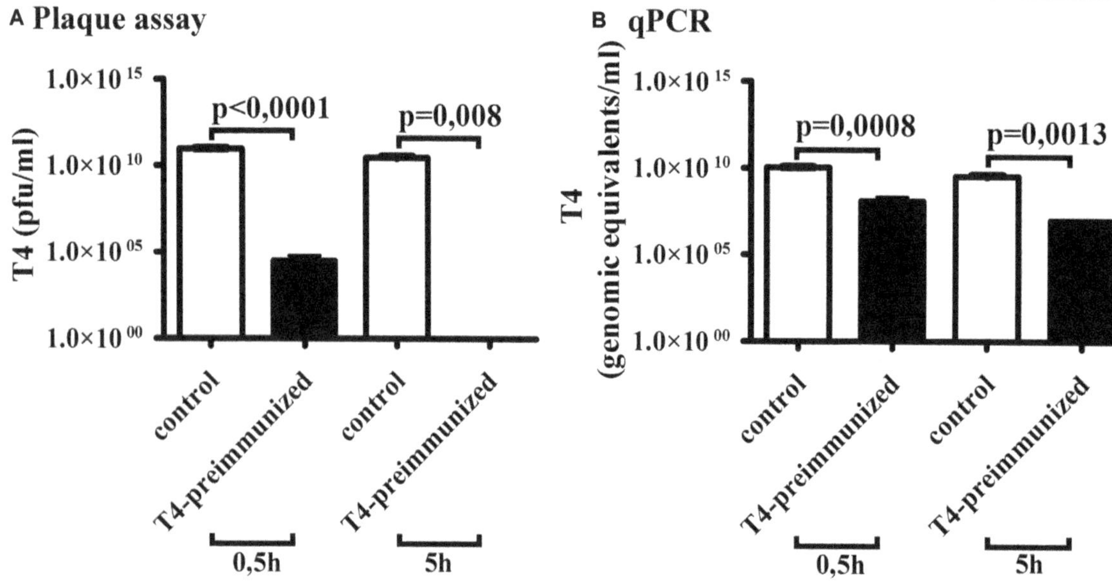

FIGURE 3 | Comparison of qPCR and plaque assay method for T4 phage detection in serum of mice immunized to T4 phage. Control and pre-immunized BALB/c mice were injected i.v. with T4 phage 10^{11} pfu/mouse, murine sera were collected 0.5 and 5 h after and phage concentration in the sera was tested by **(A)** plaque assay method or **(B)** qPCR method.

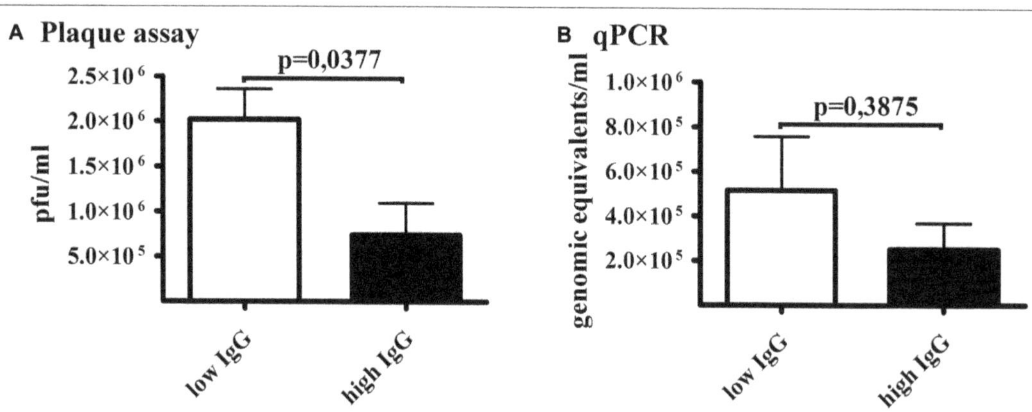

FIGURE 4 | Comparison of qPCR and plaque assay method for T4 phage detection in human sera *ex vivo*. T4 phage 10^7 pfu/ml was incubated for 1 h with human sera (1:1); the sera had either a high or low concentration of T4 phage-neutralizing antibodies. After the incubation samples were directly used for testing phage concentration by **(A)** plaque assay method or **(B)** qPCR method.

antibodies. Comparative studies of bacteriophages as different antigens by ELISA need to include quantitation of phage particles immobilized on ELISA plates. Here, quantitation of T4, A3R, and 676Z phage particles adhering to 96-well plates was conducted by qPCR, using the developed standard curves (see section Characterization of qPCR Reaction).

In general, all investigated bacteriophages were detectable by qPCR when immobilized on ELISA plates. We further observed that the amount of immobilized phage correlated positively with concentration of the phage that was used for incubation with the plate (**Figure 5**). Comparison of the three investigated phages revealed that their individual affinity to plastic surfaces was markedly different. Incubation with the highest phage concentration (1×10^{10} pfu/ml) allowed for the following approximated amounts of recovered bacteriophages (as genome equivalents): 1×10^8 for T4, 3×10^9 for A3R, and 6×10^9 for 676Z (**Figure 5**).

We further compared the amount of phage detectable by qPCR and the relative signal from the ELISA, to assess the reliability of ELISA for comparisons between phages. ELISA plates covered with two very similar bacteriophages, A3R and 676Z, were processed either for adhering phage quantitation by qPCR or for immunodetection of phage by major capsid protein-specific antibody (ELISA). Although the qPCR method revealed approximately two times more 676Z phage adhering to the ELISA plate (in comparison to A3R phage), no differences were detected by ELISA (**Figure 6**).

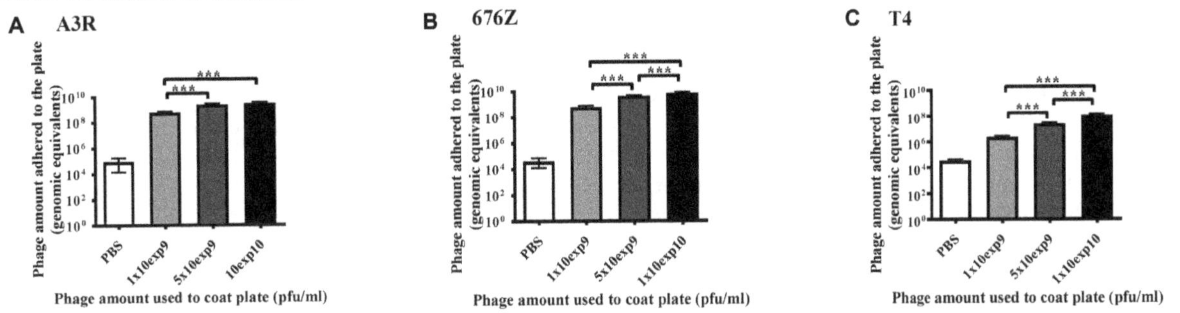

FIGURE 5 | Quantitation of phage particles on plastic surfaces by RT-qPCR. A standard ELISA plate was covered with three dilutions of A3R **(A)**, 676Z **(B)**, or T4 **(C)** phage. The amount of phage used to coat the plate was determined by plaque assay and it is indicated on the *X*-axis of each graph. The amount of genomic equivalents recovered from the plate was determined by qPCR reaction and it is presented on the *Y*-axis. $^{***}p < 0.001$.

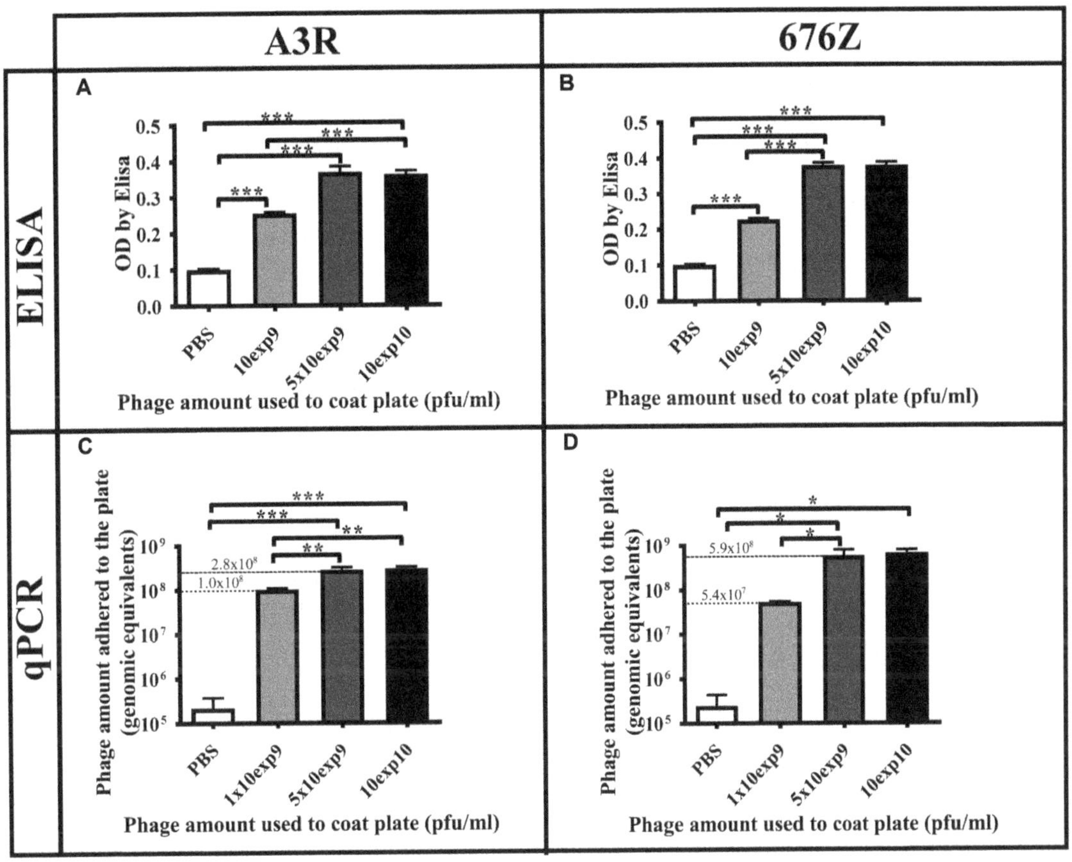

FIGURE 6 | Comparison of the amount of phage detectable by qPCR and the relative signal from ELISA. ELISA plates were coated with three dilutions of A3R or 676Z phage. The plates were processed either for **(A,B)** immunodetection of phage by ELISA with major capsid protein-specific antibodies, or **(C,D)** for qPCR detection of phage immobilized on the plate, with PCR primers specific to the genes coding for major capsid proteins. $^{*}p < 0.05$, $^{**}p < 0.01$, $^{***}p < 0.001$.

Estimation of the efficiency of phage immobilization in the well was calculated from the total amount of phage DNA in the solution that was applied to the wells and from the amount of phage DNA recovered from the wells. It revealed that when 1×10^{10} pfu/ml solutions of phages A3R and 676Z were applied to the wells we recovered 4.5 and 9.67%, respectively.

DISCUSSION

In this work we investigated qPCR as a useful alternative for phage detection, in comparison to standard methods based on phage cultures with bacteria. We focused on immunological studies of bacteriophages, since antibodies are probably the most efficient biological factors able to neutralize phages.

We demonstrated that the phage, even when neutralized in terms of antibacterial activity, can still be present in the circulation in high amounts and it can be detected and quantitatively assessed by qPCR (**Figure 3**). This implies that the phage may exert biological effects much longer than it can be detected by standard microbiological methods. Phage effects that are independent of its antibacterial activity may apply to phage use as drug nanocarriers (Karimi et al., 2016; Bashari et al., 2017), vaccine platforms (Aghebati-Maleki et al., 2016; Pires et al., 2016; Tao et al., 2016), as well as to possible immunomodulation exerted by the phage (Barr, 2017; Górski et al., 2017). Our observations demonstrate that the time lapse between "microbiological disappearance" and true clearance of phage particles from the circulation can be substantial. This particularly applies to common phages that may run up against a frequent and strong anti-phage immune response in the population, such as T4 (Dąbrowska et al., 2014).

A further consequence of the strong influence of antibodies on the results of microbiological detection of phages is the fact that standard attempts to detect phages in human and animal sera can be unsuccessful even when the phages are highly represented there. Phage translocation and "phagoviremia" has been postulated as an important physiological phenomenon (Górski et al., 2006), although not demonstrated yet. There are still not enough data to assess levels of immunization of humans and animals to phages naturally belonging to their gut- (or other) microbiota. However, a model phage was demonstrated as able to induce a specific systemic response and a high serum level of specific IgG (Majewska et al., 2015). Assuming that phages of the microbiome eventually induce antibody production, it may be impossible to detect true phage translocation to the circulation only by microbiological methods. We propose the qPCR method as an appropriate and reliable method for studies of phage translocation to blood. This method can also be applied in other experiments that require detection of a "neutralized" phage, which is merely a phage that is not active against bacteria. Notably, qPCR has already been applied for phage detection in other (than phage neutralizing) conditions: in phage cultures (Edelman and Barletta, 2003; Clokie, 2009; Anderson et al., 2011; Refardt, 2012; Dieterle et al., 2016), food (Imamovic and Muniesa, 2011; Flannery et al., 2014; Perrin et al., 2015; Parente et al., 2016; Hartard et al., 2017; Muhammed et al., 2017), environmental samples (Farkas et al., 2015; Kunze et al., 2015; Unnithan et al., 2015; Mankiewicz-Boczek et al., 2016), and in feces (Imamovic et al., 2010; Chehoud et al., 2016), where some interference from antibodies cannot be excluded (Majewska et al., 2015).

We have also shown that different bacteriophages may differ strongly in their ability to immobilize on plastic surfaces. Here, we report more than one order of magnitude difference between phage recovery from plastic that was covered by different phages in the same conditions (**Figure 5**). This should be considered in any comparative studies of bacteriophages that include phage immobilization on various surfaces, e.g., in biosensor constructing or in the ELISA assay for phage immune-reactivity. As demonstrated by comparison of the ELISA signal to qPCR phage detection, differences in phage ability to adhere to a plastic surface can be missed by immunodetection (**Figure 5**). Notably, the two staphylococcal bacteriophages investigated in this work are highly similar. They have identical genes coding for major capsid proteins (the ones detected by qPCR here) (Łobocka et al., 2012), but minor structural elements of their virions differ. Eventually, their adherence to plastic also differs as much as twofold (**Figures 5, 6**).

Quantitative analysis of phage by real-time PCR as a method has a few limitations that should be considered when planning its use. First, although qPCR can detect even those phage particles that are not able to infect bacteria, it is sensitive to inhibitors of the PCR reaction. Thus, in conditions where these inhibitors cannot be removed, phage detection may be more efficient in the plaque assay that in qPCR. For example, our *post hoc* analysis indicated that the animals in this study were challenged with 5.8×10^{11} pfu/ml of T4 as measured by plaque assay and 1.56×10^{11} of T4 as measured by qPCR. We also observed an inhibitory effect of raw human sera when applied into the composition of the qPCR reaction (data not shown). Thus, we isolated phage DNA from murine sera by a standard isolation kit to compare phage circulation between immunized and non-immunized mice. This approach turned out to be appropriate to overcome the problem of PCR reaction inhibitors in serum samples. The second considerable requirement for experiments employing qPCR is to use phage preparations without free phage DNA. In the qPCR method, free phage DNA present in phage solution can easily produce a false positive signal mimicking phage particles. It means that production of phage preparations, including often complex procedures of phage purification, need to be gentle enough not to destroy phage particles releasing phage nucleic acids.

Concluding Remarks

This study demonstrates a substantial time lapse between inactivation of antibacterial activity and true clearance of phage particles from the circulation of pre-immunized individuals. qPCR allows for detection of inactivated bacteriophages that cannot be detected by plaque assay. Further, qPCR demonstrated marked differences in the ability of investigated bacteriophages to immobilize on plastic surfaces, while the ELISA did not detect differences in phage binding to plates. We propose that phage pharmacokinetic and pharmacodynamic studies should not rely merely on detection of antibacterial activity of a phage; real-time qPCR can be an extension for phage detection methods.

AUTHOR CONTRIBUTIONS

AK performed most of the experiments, analyzed the results, and participated in writing the manuscript. AZ, DL, JM, MH, KL, MK, and ZK participated in experimental work. ŁŁ participated in experimental design, data analysis, and reviewed the manuscript. KD conceived and designed the experiments, participated in experimental work and in data analysis, and wrote the paper.

FUNDING

This work was supported by the National Science Centre in Poland grant UMO-2012/05/E/NZ6/03314, and by Wroclaw Centre of Biotechnology, program The Leading National Research Centre (KNOW) for years 2014–2018.

ACKNOWLEDGMENTS

We are grateful to Professor Andrzej Gorski, Bacteriophage Laboratory, IIET, for valuable scientific discussions and for his continuous, valuable support for immunological studies of phages.

SUPPLEMENTARY MATERIAL

FIGURE S1 | T4-specific antibody detection in mice pre-immunized with T4. Significant induction of serum IgM and IgG specific for T4 phage was detected by ELISA (IgM level: T4-challenged mice vs. PBS control, $p = 0.005$; IgG level: T4-challenged mice vs. PBS control, $p < 0.0001$).

REFERENCES

Adams, M. H. (1959). "Enumeration of bacteriophage particles," in *The Bacteriophages*, ed. M. H. Adams (New York, NY: Interscience publishers, Inc.), 27–34.

Aghebati-Maleki, L., Bakhshinejad, B., Baradaran, B., Motallebnezhad, M., Aghebati-Maleki, A., Nickho, H., et al. (2016). Phage display as a promising approach for vaccine development. *J. Biomed. Sci.* 23, 66. doi: 10.1186/s12929-016-0285-9

Anderson, B., Rashid, M. H., Carter, C., Pasternack, G., Rajanna, C., Revazishvili, T., et al. (2011). Enumeration of bacteriophage particles: comparative analysis of the traditional plaque assay and real-time QPCR- and nanosight-based assays. *Bacteriophage* 1, 86–93. doi: 10.4161/bact.1.2.15456

Barr, J. J. (2017). A bacteriophages journey through the human body. *Immunol. Rev.* 279, 106–122. doi: 10.1111/imr.12565

Barr, J. J., Auro, R., Furlan, M., Whiteson, K. L., Erb, M. L., Pogliano, J., et al. (2013). Bacteriophage adhering to mucus provide a non-host-derived immunity. *Proc. Natl. Acad. Sci. U.S.A.* 110, 10771–10776. doi: 10.1073/pnas.1305923110

Bashari, O., Redko, B., Cohen, A., Luboshits, G., Gellerman, G., and Firer, M. A. (2017). Discovery of peptide drug carrier candidates for targeted multi-drug delivery into prostate cancer cells. *Cancer Lett.* 408, 164–173. doi: 10.1016/j.canlet.2017.08.040

Bustin, S. A., Benes, V., Garson, J. A., Hellemans, J., Huggett, J., Kubista, M., et al. (2009). The MIQE guidelines: minimum information for publication of quantitative real-time PCR experiments. *Clin. Chem.* 55, 611–622. doi: 10.1373/clinchem.2008.112797

Chehoud, C., Dryga, A., Hwang, Y., Nagy-Szakal, D., Hollister, E. B., Luna, R. A., et al. (2016). Transfer of viral communities between human individuals during fecal microbiota transplantation. *mBio* 7:e00322-16. doi: 10.1128/mBio.00322-16

Cheng, R., Li, G., Shi, L., Xue, X., Kang, M., and Zheng, X. (2016). The mechanism for bacteriophage f2 removal by nanoscale zero-valent iron. *Water Res.* 105, 429–435. doi: 10.1016/j.watres.2016.09.025

Cheng, X., Imai, T., Teeka, J., Hirose, M., Higuchi, T., and Sekine, M. (2013). Inactivation of bacteriophages by high levels of dissolved CO2. *Environ. Technol.* 34, 539–544. doi: 10.1080/09593330.2012.704403

Clokie, M. R. (2009). Quantification of host and phage mRNA expression during infection using real-time PCR. *Methods Mol. Biol.* 502, 177–191. doi: 10.1007/978-1-60327-565-1_11

Dąbrowska, K., Miernikiewicz, P., Piotrowicz, A., Hodyra, K., Owczarek, B., Lecion, D., et al. (2014). Immunogenicity studies of proteins forming the T4 phage head surface. *J. Virol.* 88, 12551–12557. doi: 10.1128/JVI.02043-14

Dąbrowska, K., Switała-Jeleń, K., Opolski, A., and Górski, A. (2006). Possible association between phages, Hoc protein, and the immune system. *Arch. Virol.* 151, 209–215. doi: 10.1007/s00705-005-0641-7

Dąbrowska, K., Zembala, M., Boratynski, J., Switala-Jelen, K., Wietrzyk, J., Opolski, A., et al. (2007). Hoc protein regulates the biological effects of T4 phage in mammals. *Arch. Microbiol.* 187, 489–498. doi: 10.1007/s00203-007-0216-y

Dieterle, M. E., Fina Martin, J., Durán, R., Nemirovsky, S. I., Sanchez Rivas, C., Bowman, C., et al. (2016). Characterization of prophages containing "evolved" Dit/Tal modules in the genome of *Lactobacillus casei* BL23. *Appl. Microbiol. Biotechnol.* 100, 9201–9215. doi: 10.1007/s00253-016-7727-x

Edelman, D. C., and Barletta, J. (2003). Real-time PCR provides improved detection and titer determination of bacteriophage. *BioTechniques* 35, 368–375.

Endersen, L., O'Mahony, J., Hill, C., Ross, R. P., McAuliffe, O., and Coffey, A. (2014). Phage therapy in the food industry. *Annu. Rev. Food Sci. Technol.* 5, 327–349. doi: 10.1146/annurev-food-030713-092415

Farkas, K., Varsani, A., Marjoshi, D., Easingwood, R., McGill, E., and Pang, L. (2015). Size exclusion-based purification and PCR-based quantitation of MS2 bacteriophage particles for environmental applications. *J. Virol. Methods* 213, 135–138. doi: 10.1016/j.jviromet.2014.11.024

Flannery, J., Rajko-Nenow, P., Winterbourn, J. B., Malham, S. K., and Jones, D. L. (2014). Effectiveness of cooking to reduce norovirus and infectious F-specific RNA bacteriophage concentrations in *Mytilus edulis*. *J. Appl. Microbiol.* 117, 564–571. doi: 10.1111/jam.12534

Górski, A., Dąbrowska, K., Międzybrodzki, R., Weber-Dąbrowska, B., Łusiak-Szelachowska, M., Jończyk-Matysiak, E., et al. (2017). Phages and immunomodulation. *Future Microbiol.* 12, 905–914. doi: 10.2217/fmb-2017-0049

Górski, A., Wazna, E., Dabrowska, B. W., Dabrowska, K., Switała-Jeleń, K., and Miedzybrodzki, R. (2006). Bacteriophage translocation. *FEMS Immunol. Med. Microbiol.* 46, 313–319. doi: 10.1111/j.1574-695X.2006.00044.x

Grant, A., Hashem, F., and Parveen, S. (2016). *Salmonella* and Campylobacter: antimicrobial resistance and bacteriophage control in poultry. *Food Microbiol.* 53(Pt B), 104–109. doi: 10.1016/j.fm.2015.09.008

Hartard, C., Banas, S., Rivet, R., Boudaud, N., and Gantzer, C. (2017). Rapid and sensitive method to assess human viral pollution in shellfish using infectious F-specific RNA bacteriophages: application to marketed products. *Food Microbiol.* 63, 248–254. doi: 10.1016/j.fm.2016.12.002

Hmaied, F., Keskes, S., Jebri, S., Amri, I., Yahya, M., Loisy-Hamon, F., et al. (2015). Removal of rotavirus and bacteriophages by Membrane Bioreactor Technology from Sewage. *Curr. Microbiol.* 71, 540–545. doi: 10.1007/s00284-015-0882-y

Hodyra-Stefaniak, K., Miernikiewicz, P., Drapała, J., Drab, M., Jończyk-Matysiak, E., Lecion, D., et al. (2015). Mammalian Host-Versus-Phage immune response determines phage fate in vivo. *Sci. Rep.* 5:14802. doi: 10.1038/srep14802

Imamovic, L., Ballesté, E., Jofre, J., and Muniesa, M. (2010). Quantification of Shiga toxin-converting bacteriophages in wastewater and in fecal samples by real-time quantitative PCR. *Appl. Environ. Microbiol.* 76, 5693–5701. doi: 10.1128/AEM.00107-10

Imamovic, L., and Muniesa, M. (2011). Quantification and evaluation of infectivity of shiga toxin-encoding bacteriophages in beef and salad. *Appl. Environ. Microbiol.* 77, 3536–3540. doi: 10.1128/AEM.02703-10

Ishiguro, E. E., Ainsworth, T., Shaw, D. H., Kay, W. W., and Trust, T. J. (1983). A lipopolysaccharide-specific bacteriophage for *Aeromonas salmonicida*. *Can. J. Microbiol.* 10, 1458–1461. doi: 10.1139/m83-223

Karimi, M., Mirshekari, H., Moosavi Basri, S. M., Bahrami, S., Moghoofei, M., and Hamblin, M. R. (2016). Bacteriophages and phage-inspired nanocarriers for targeted delivery of therapeutic cargos. *Adv. Drug Deliv. Rev.* 106(Pt A), 45–62. doi: 10.1016/j.addr.2016.03.003

Kirsch, M. I., Hülseweh, B., Nacke, C., Rülker, T., Schirrmann, T., Marschall, H. J., et al. (2008). Development of human antibody fragments using antibody phage display for the detection and diagnosis of Venezuelan equine encephalitis virus (VEEV). *BMC Biotechnol.* 8:66. doi: 10.1186/1472-6750-8-66

Kunze, A., Pei, L., Elsässer, D., Niessner, R., and Seidel, M. (2015). High performance concentration method for viruses in drinking water. *J. Virol. Methods* 222, 132–137. doi: 10.1016/j.jviromet.2015.06.007

Kutter, E. M., Kuhl, S. J., and Abedon, S. T. (2015). Re-establishing a place for phage therapy in western medicine. *Future Microbiol.* 10, 685–688. doi: 10.2217/fmb.15.28

Lee, B. Y., Zhang, J., Zueger, C., Chung, W. J., Yoo, S. Y., Wang, E., et al. (2012). Virus-based piezoelectric energy generation. *Nat. Nanotechnol.* 7, 351–356. doi: 10.1038/nnano.2012.69

Łobocka, M., Hejnowicz, M. S., Dąbrowski, K., Gozdek, A., Kosakowski, J., Witkowska, M., et al. (2012). Genomics of staphylococcal Twort-like phages–potential therapeutics of the post-antibiotic era. *Adv. Virus Res.* 83, 143–216. doi: 10.1016/B978-0-12-394438-2.00005-0

Majewska, J., Beta, W., Lecion, D., Hodyra-Stefaniak, K., Kłopot, A., Kaźmierczak, Z., et al. (2015). Oral application of T4 phage induces weak antibody production in the gut and in the blood. *Viruses* 7, 4783–4799. doi: 10.3390/v7082845

Mankiewicz-Boczek, J., Jaskulska, A., Pawełczyk, J., Gągała, I., Serwecińska, L., and Dziadek, J. (2016). Cyanophages infection of microcystis bloom in lowland dam reservoir of Sulejów, Poland. *Microb. Ecol.* 71, 315–325. doi: 10.1007/s00248-015-0677-5

Matsushita, T., Shirasaki, N., Matsui, Y., and Ohno, K. (2011). Virus inactivation during coagulation with aluminum coagulants. *Chemosphere* 85, 571–576. doi: 10.1016/j.chemosphere.2011.06.083

Międzybrodzki, R. J., Borysowski, B., Weber-Dąbrowska, W., Fortuna, S., Letkiewicz, K., Szufnarowski, Z., et al. (2012). Clinical aspects of phage therapy. *Adv. Virus Res.* 83, 73–121. doi: 10.1016/B978-0-12-394438-2.00003-7

Muhammed, M. K., Krych, L., Nielsen, D. S., and Vogensen, F. K. (2017). A high-throughput qPCR system for simultaneous quantitative detection of dairy *Lactococcus lactis* and Leuconostoc bacteriophages. *PLOS ONE* 12:e0174223. doi: 10.1371/journal.pone.0174223

National Center for Biotechnology Information (2017) Available at: https://www.ncbi.nlm.nih.gov/tools/primer-blast/

Oślizło, A., Miernikiewicz, P., Piotrowicz, A., Owczarek, B., Kopciuch, A., Figura, G., et al. (2011). Purification of phage display-modified bacteriophage T4 by affinity chromatography. *BMC Biotechnol.* 11:59. doi: 10.1186/1472-6750-11-59

O'Sullivan, L., Buttimer, C., McAuliffe, O., Bolton, D., and Coffey, A. (2016). Bacteriophage-based tools: recent advances and novel applications. *F1000Res.* 5, 2782. doi: 10.12688/f1000research.9705.1

Parente, E., Guidone, A., Matera, A., De Filippis, F., Mauriello, G., and Ricciardi, A. (2016). Microbial community dynamics in thermophilic undefined milk starter cultures. *Int. J. Food Microbiol.* 217, 59–67. doi: 10.1016/j.ijfoodmicro.2015.10.014

Perrin, A., Loutreul, J., Boudaud, N., Bertrand, I., and Gantzer, C. (2015). Rapid, simple and efficient method for detection of viral genomes on raspberries. *J. Virol. Methods* 224, 95–101. doi: 10.1016/j.jviromet.2015.08.005

Pires, D. P., Cleto, S., Sillankorva, S., Azeredo, J., and Lu, T. K. (2016). Genetically engineered phages: a review of advances over the last decade. *Microbiol. Mol. Biol. Rev.* 80, 523–543. doi: 10.1128/MMBR.00069-15

Refardt, D. (2011). Within-host competition determines reproductive success of temperate bacteriophages. *ISME J.* 5, 1451–1460. doi: 10.1038/ismej.2011.30

Refardt, D. (2012). Real-time quantitative PCR to discriminate and quantify lambdoid bacteriophages of *Escherichia coli* K-12. *Bacteriophage* 2, 98–104. doi: 10.4161/bact.20092

Saeed, A. F., Wang, R., Ling, S., and Wang, S. (2017). Antibody engineering for pursuing a healthier future. *Front. Microbiol.* 8:495. doi: 10.3389/fmicb.2017.00495

Samoylova, T. I., Norris, M. D., Samoylov, A. M., Cochran, A. M., Wolfe, K. G., Petrenko, V. A., et al. (2012). Infective and inactivated filamentous phage as carriers for immunogenic peptides. *J. Virol. Methods* 183, 63–68. doi: 10.1016/j.jviromet.2012.03.032

Stothard, P. (2000). The sequence manipulation suite: JavaScript programs for analyzing and formatting protein and DNA sequences. *Biotechniques* 28, 1102–1104.

Szermer-Olearnik, B., Drab, M., Mąkosa, M., Zembala, M., Barbasz, J., Dąbrowska, K., et al. (2017). Aggregation/dispersion transitions of T4 phage triggered by environmental ion availability. *J. Nanobiotechnology* 15, 32. doi: 10.1186/s12951-017-0266-5

Tao, P., Mahalingam, M., and Rao, V. B. (2016). Highly effective soluble and bacteriophage T4 nanoparticle plague vaccines against *Yersinia pestis*. *Methods Mol. Biol.* 1403, 499–518. doi: 10.1007/978-1-4939-3387-7_28

Unnithan, V. V., Unc, A., and Smith, G. B. (2015). enzymatic pre-treatment of wastewater to minimize recovery by reverse transcriptase PCR of RNA from inactive bacteriophages. *Curr. Microbiol.* 71, 49–53. doi: 10.1007/s00284-015-0830-x

Vandenheuvel, D., Lavigne, R., and Brüssow, H. (2015). Bacteriophage therapy: advances in formulation strategies and human clinical trials. *Annu. Rev. Virol.* 2, 599–618. doi: 10.1146/annurev-virology-100114-054915

Watzinger, F., Suda, M., Preuner, S., Baumgartinger, R., Ebner, K., Baskova, L., et al. (2004). Real-time quantitative PCR assays for detection and monitoring of pathogenic human viruses in immunosuppressed pediatric patients. *J. Clin. Microbiol.* 42, 5189–5198. doi: 10.1128/JCM.42.11.5189-5198.2004

Żaczek, M., Weber-Dąbrowska, B., and Górski, A. (2015). Phages in the global fruit and vegetable industry. *J. Appl. Microbiol.* 118, 537–556. doi: 10.1111/jam.12700

11

Infectious Agents and Inflammation: The Role of Microbiota in Autoimmune Arthritis

*Andrea Picchianti-Diamanti[1], Maria M. Rosado[2] and Raffaele D'Amelio[1]**

[1] *Department of Clinical and Molecular Medicine, Sant'Andrea University Hospital, Sapienza University of Rome, Rome, Italy,*
[2] *Independent Researcher, Rome, Italy*

***Correspondence:**
Raffaele D'Amelio
raffaele.damelio@uniroma1.it

In higher vertebrates, mucosal sites at the border between the internal and external environments, directly interact with bacteria, viruses, and fungi. Through co-evolution, hosts developed mechanisms of tolerance or ignorance toward some infectious agents, because hosts established "gain of function" interactions with symbiotic bacteria. Indeed, some bacteria assist hosts in different functions, among which are digestion of complex carbohydrates, and absorption and supply of vitamins. There is no doubt that microbiota modulate innate and acquired immune responses starting at birth. However, variations in quality and quantity of bacterial species interfere with the equilibrium between inflammation and tolerance. In fact, correlations between gut bacteria composition and the severity of inflammation were first described for inflammatory bowel diseases and later extended to other pathologies. The genetic background, environmental factors (e.g., stress or smoking), and diet can induce strong changes in the resident bacteria which can expose the intestinal epithelium to a variety of different metabolites, many of which have unknown functions and consequences. In addition, alterations in gut permeability may allow pathogens entry, thereby triggering infection and/or chronic inflammation. In this context, a local event occurring at a mucosal site may be the triggering cause of an autoimmune reaction that eventually involves distant sites or organs. Recently, several studies attributed a pathogenic role to altered oral microbiota in rheumatoid arthritis (RA) and to gut dysbiosis in spondyloarthritis (SpA). There is also growing evidence that different drugs, such as antibiotics and immunosuppressants, can influence and be influenced by the diversity and composition of microbiota in RA and SpA patients. Hence, in complex disorders such RA and SpA, not only the genetic background, gender, and immunologic context of the individual are relevant, but also the history of infections and the structure of the microbial community at mucosal sites should be considered. Here the role of the microbiota and infections in the initiation and progression of chronic arthritis is discussed, as well as how these factors can influence a patient's response to synthetic and biologic immunosuppressive therapy.

Keywords: microbiota, autoimmune arthritis, infections, immunosuppressive therapy, biologics

MICROBIOTA AND THE IMMUNE SYSTEM

Host–microbe interactions are the result of a co-evolution process, in which both partners have set borders and have developed mechanisms of tolerance or ignorance. In this context, hosts were able to establish a continuous connection with symbiotic bacteria, representing for the host a "gain of function." Bacteria provide help for different functions, including the digestion of complex carbohydrates as well as the absorption and supply of vitamins (LeBlanc et al., 2013). Worth mentioning is that, in the complex network of interactions of the microbiome, the environment should be taken into account since the outbreak of an infection and/or an inflammatory disease relies on the complex relationships between the microorganisms, the host, and the environment (such as dietary components, pollutants and even drugs) (Kim et al., 2016).

Microbiota are composed of archaea, bacteria, fungi, and viruses forming a complex ecosystem of which bacteria are the most well-characterized member. Any microbial imbalance resulting in a shift (i.e., loss or overgrowth of a species) and/or reduction in microbial diversity is defined as dysbiosis.

The mucosa has a dual function in our body. It works as a physical barrier, promoting pathogen exclusion, and is an absorption site that allows entry of food-derived metabolites and gas exchange. The mucosal immune system is not fully developed when we are born because many of the lymphoid structures, especially in the gut, are formed only upon stimulation through exposure to microorganisms. In fact, mice bred and maintained in germ-free conditions have small Payer's patches and lack isolated lymphoid follicles (ILF) in their bowel. Furthermore, serum levels of IgM natural antibodies and IgA secreting cells in the spleen and intestine are reduced in germ free mice (Rhee et al., 2004). This phenotype is rescued by gut colonization once the animals are transferred from isolators to conventional housing and food. At birth, colonization plays a crucial role in inducing and shaping the development of the secondary lymphoid organs as well as setting-up thresholds of reactivity for both innate and acquired immune responses. Thus, the neonate microbiota intervenes with the fine balance amongst infection, inflammation, and tolerance that may "imprint" the immune system for life.

Recently, Vatanen et al. (2016) followed-up the gut colonization of children from birth to 3 years of age. Children from Finland, Estonia and Russia were selected who shared a human leukocyte antigen (HLA) distribution typical of individuals at risk for autoimmunity (Vatanen et al., 2016). The study showed that, depending on the lipopolysaccharide (LPS) subtype produced by different *Bacteroides* species, Toll-like receptor-4 (TLR4) could be either activated or inhibited. This had an impact on tolerance to endotoxin, and, consequently, strongly conditioned the genetic predisposition of the infants to type I diabetes (T1D). Thus, the presence of different LPS subtypes in the gut could partially explain the difference in prevalence of early onset autoimmune diseases in Finland and Estonia compared to Russia. In line with the hygiene hypothesis, this work adds another clue to the correlation between exposure or lack of exposure to specific microorganisms in early life and the increase of autoimmune diseases in western countries.

The microbiota is comprised of both pathogenic and non-pathogenic bacteria, however, this distinction is not absolute. A microorganism may behave as commensal or as pathogenic with regards to the dietary components, nutritional milieu, broad-spectrum antibiotic treatment, co-infection or genetic background of its host. Moreover, even though commensals are by definition not supposed to induce immune responses, and lamina propria-derived antigen-presenting cells traffic preferentially to mucosal-associated lymphoid tissue (MALT) in order to restrict systemic immune responses against the microbiota, it is possible to find antibodies specific to commensals in the serum of healthy people, as well as circulating T cells reactive against non-pathogenic bacteria (Macpherson et al., 1996; Ergin et al., 2011). Also, in specific genetic conditions, such as in individuals with defects in interleukin-17 (IL17) signaling pathway, commensal microorganisms become pathogenic through invasion, causing fungal disease (Puel et al., 2011). Another condition in which commensals may be harmful is in mucosal leakage. Changes of permeability at mucosal sites or altered immune functions strongly condition the persistence of antigenic stimulation, not only at the place of microbial entry but also in faraway locations, such as articular sites (Asquith et al., 2014). Moreover, in frail patients, the administration of *Saccharomyces cerevisiae* as a probiotic has been anecdotally reported to induce sepsis (Montineri et al., 2008; Eren et al., 2014).

It is worth mentioning here that the microbiota itself plays a role in regulating the growth of opportunistic enteric infections, a mechanism termed colonization resistance (Stecher and Hardt, 2011). Often antibiotic administration, by altering the equilibrium of the gut microbiota, leads to overgrowth of *Clostridium difficile*. This infection represents, nowadays, a major clinical problem because *C. difficile* is one of the bacterial species with higher antibiotic resistance. Microbiota transplantation from healthy donors, by rescuing microbial equilibrium, has been one of the most successful strategies to treat serious *C. difficile* infection (Hand, 2016).

Bacterial products, such as the previously mentioned LPS, are sensed by enterocytes through TLRs. Microbial stimulation of enterocytes induce the production of antimicrobial peptides (AMPs) and the fucosylation of small intestinal epithelial cells by Fucosyltransferase 2 (Fut2), both of which can limit specific infections (Pickard et al., 2014). TLRs regulate innate immune responses but are also crucial for epithelial cell homeostasis at mucosal sites. Altered immune function of TLRs, for example due to different polymorphisms, may change binding to bacterial products, secretion of cytokines or chemokines, which consequently interferes with acquired immune cell generation/migration and inflammation. Thus, it can contribute to the persistence of inflammatory diseases such as rheumatoid arthritis (RA) (Rogier et al., 2015).

In addition to bacteria, bacterial-derived products can also control, directly or indirectly, the function of both epithelial and inflammatory cells. For example, two important metabolites are the short-chain fatty acids (SCFAs) and the lipid mediator prostaglandin E2 (PGE2). Recognition of the SCFAs by innate immune cells is important to modulate inflammation in response not only to intestinal but even to articular damage (Maslowski et al., 2009). Commensals are also able to regulate the inflammatory activity of monocytes, by promoting the release of PGE2 that, in turn, down-modulates the activation of tissue-damaging neutrophils (Grainger et al., 2013).

The gut is the main site for the generation of the two most important T cell populations, the inducible regulatory T cells (iTregs) and CD4IL17-producing cells (Th17), both of which play critical roles in the development and persistence of autoimmune disorders. Colonization of the distal small intestine, by segmented filamentous bacteria (SFB), is fundamental to development of resident lamina propria dendritic cells (DCs) able to release IL6 and IL22 that trigger the loop of Th17-Treg cell in the newborn gut (Ivanov et al., 2009; Maslowski et al., 2009). Although many studies have addressed gut microbiota composition in humans, we still do not know which would be the "best/healthiest" microbial composition for the maintenance of the balance between regulatory (iTregs) and inflammatory (Th17) cells (Hand, 2016). Recent studies revealed that the homeostasis of the colonic Treg compartment relies more on the synergistic effects of different bacterial strains than on a single species of that strain. This observation strongly suggests the importance of the entire bacterial community in shaping the appropriate microenvironment that is able to sustain the production and maintenance of the anti-inflammatory environment (Atarashi et al., 2013).

ORAL/GUT DYSBIOSIS AND ARTHRITIS

Rheumatoid arthritis and Spondyloarthritis (SpA) are chronic inflammatory autoimmune diseases potentially leading to quality of life impairment and reduction in life expectancy. RA is characterized by the presence of autoantibodies [rheumatoid factor (RF) and anti-citrullinated protein antibodies (ACPAs)] and is characterized clinically by the emergence of erosive synovitis predominantly involving small joints, such as hands, wrists, and feet. The reported prevalence of the disease is 0.5–1% in the general population (Hayter and Cook, 2012).

Spondyloarthritis is a pleomorphic group of conditions that includes ankylosing spondylitis (AS), psoriatic arthritis (PsA), reactive arthritis (ReA), SpA associated to inflammatory bowel disease (IBD), acute anterior uveitis and axial non-radiographic SpA. The reported prevalence for AS is 2.4/1,000 (Dean et al., 2014). Arthritis is the most frequent extra-intestinal disease manifestation in patients with IBD (range 15–40%); conversely, up to 60% of patients with SpA present subclinical gut inflammation and 10% overt inflammation evolving to Crohn's disease (Mielants et al., 1995; De Vos et al., 1996; Olivieri et al., 2014).

The evidence of a direct role for the gut microbiota in the development of autoimmune arthritis arises from experimental studies on germ-free mice in which a reduced severity and/or incidence of arthritis has been demonstrated (Carding et al., 2015).

However, in man, a direct correlation between gut dysfunction and systemic inflammation has been clearly established only in AS. Some studies by Ciccia et al. (2012) have identified several alterations of the ileum architecture in AS patients that may be the cause for chronic inflammation, both local and systemic. AS patients showed disruption of the basal membrane with compromised epithelial cell permeability, hyperplasia of goblet cells (with increased mucins production) (Ciccia et al., 2012) and activation of Paneth cells, producing high levels of adenosine monophosphate, such as α-defensin 5 (Ciccia et al., 2010) and proinflammatory cytokines, such as IL23 (Ciccia et al., 2009). These characteristics may be the cause or the consequence of dysbiosis, with changes in the diversity of the commensal bacteria (Costello et al., 2015). Increased intestinal permeability, probably determined by genetic factors such as HLA-B27 expression (Rosenbaum and Davey, 2011; Lin et al., 2014; Bowness, 2015), results in continuous antigenic stimulation with activation of effector T cells. These effector cells do not show a clearly defined Th17, Th1, and/or Th9 polarization, due to the over-expression of an IL23 response by Paneth cells (Ciccia et al., 2009). Worth noting is that IL23 can regulate the maturation of autoreactive Th17 cells but can also induce chronic inflammation by stimulating IL17, IL6, IL8, and tumour necrosis factor (TNF)-α production in neutrophils and macrophages. Furthermore, a link between IL23R polymorphisms and susceptibility to psoriasis, PsA and AS have been shown (Liu et al., 2008).

In patients with PsA, subclinical gut inflammation is characterized by the overexpression of IL9 and the generation of Th9, Th17, and Th22 responses. Th9 cells produced in the gut are found to be increased in the peripheral blood and they are able to migrate, enter synovial tissues and become established. In the meantime, gut-activated Paneth cells express both IL9 and IL9 receptors, creating a positive autocrine loop that perpetuates local inflammation (Ciccia et al., 2016).

Solid data suggest that alterations in the oral microbiota can influence both progression and disease outcome in RA patients (Diamanti et al., 2016; **Table 1**). It has been speculated that certain species of bacteria, mainly *Porphyromonas gingivalis* (PG) which may be present in the oral cavity, and are increased in patients affected by periodontitis, can induce loss of tolerance and lead to citrullination of several peptides and proteins (Wegner et al., 2010; Quirke et al., 2014; Ciccia et al., 2016).

Citrullination is a post-translational modification that converts arginine residues into citrulline leading to relevant changes in the protein structure, charge and function. *Porphyromonas gingivalis* peptidyl-arginine-deiminases enzyme (PPAD) can catalyze citrullination on different self-proteins (mainly α-enolase and fibrinogen) thus resulting in immune evasion by these neo-epitopes and the production of ACPAs (McInnes and Schett, 2011).

Indeed, it has been reported a direct correlation exists between the serum level of antibodies to PG and ACPAs in RA patients (Mercado et al., 2001; Dissick et al., 2010; Scher et al., 2012; Lange et al., 2016). This observation has been confirmed by the increased prevalence of PG-induced periodontitis in RA patients as compared to healthy individuals. Likewise, other studies

TABLE 1 | Most frequently reported dysbiosis in RA and SpA patients and the proposed pathogenic mechanisms.

Autoimmune arthritis	Dysbiosis		Pathogenic mechanisms
	Increased amount	**Decreased amount**	
Rheumatoid arthritis	*Porphyromonas gingivalis* (PG) (periodontitis induced by PG is a poor prognostic factor of response to anti-TNFα therapy) *Lactobacillus salivarius* (active RA) *Prevotella copri* spp. (RA) *Mycoplasma fermentans*, *Escherichia coli*, *Proteus mirabilis* (early RA) *Collinsella, Eggerthella, Faecalibacterium* (long-standing RA)	*Haemophilus* spp. (active RA) Bacteroidetes *phylum* members (RA) Common commensals such as: *Bifidobacteria and Bacteroides* (early RA)	PG peptidyl-arginine-deaminase enzyme can catalyze citrullination on different self-proteins (mainly α-enolase and fibrinogen) thus resulting in the immune evasion to these neo-epitopes and production of ACPAs.
Spondyloarthritis	*Lachnospiraceae*, *Ruminococcaceae*, *Rikenellaceae, Porphyromonadaceae*, *Bacteroidaceae* (SpA) *Bifidobacterium* genus (children with enthesitis) The *genus Dialister* positively correlated with SpA activity Sulphate-reducing bacteria (AS) Firmicutes (skin of PsA patients)	*Veillonellaceae* and *Prevotellaceae* (SpA) *Faecalibacterium prausnitzii* spp. and *Lachnospiraceae* (children with enthesitis) *Akkermansia*, *Ruminococcus* and *Pseudobutyrivibrio* (stool of PsA patients) Actinobacteria, *Propionibacteria* spp (skin of PsA patients)	Disruption of the gut basal membrane with compromised epithelial cell permeability, hyperplasia of goblet cells and activation of Paneth cells. Continuous antigenic stimulation with activation of effector T cells.

RA, rheumatoid arthritis; SpA, spondyloarthritis; PsA, psoriatic arthritis; ACPAs, anti-citrullinated protein antibodies.

have demonstrated that the presence of periodontitis is a poor prognostic factor in RA patients treated with anti-TNFα agents. The clearing of a periodontal infection can reduce the severity of active RA and lead to a better disease outcome during synthetic and biologic immunosuppressant treatment (Ortiz et al., 2009; Savioli et al., 2012; Kaur et al., 2014).

In line with the above described observations, a case of complete and long-lasting recovery in a patient with early RA after PD treatment has been recently reported, suggesting that, at the onset of disease, periodontitis treatment may avoid the development of a chronic and progressive arthritis (Salemi et al., 2014).

The influence of the intestinal microbiota on RA is still a matter of debate. A lower representation of common commensals such as *Bifidobacteria and Bacteroides* species (Vaahtovuo et al., 2008) and an increase in *Mycoplasma fermentans* (Johnson et al., 2000), *Escherichia coli* (Newkirk et al., 2010) and *Proteus mirabilis* (Senior et al., 1999) has been reported in early RA patients, whereas another study showed that stool samples from early RA patients had significantly more *Lactobacillus* communities than healthy subjects (Liu et al., 2013). In patients with long-standing RA a decreased gut microbial diversity seems to correlate with disease duration and autoantibody levels as well as expansion of rare genera, *Collinsella, Eggerthella,* and *Faecalibacterium* (Chen et al., 2016). Other authors have reported, in the fecal microbiota of RA patients, an increase of *Prevotella copri* spp. with concomitant reduction of Bacteroidetes phylum members (Scher et al., 2013). Recently Zhang et al. (2015) described a dysbiosis of both fecal and oral samples from RA patients using metagenomic shotgun sequencing and a metagenome-wide association study; these concordant abnormalities in mouth and gut microflora were restored after immunosuppressive treatment. In particular, *Haemophilus spp.* was strongly reduced, whereas *Lactobacillus salivarius* was increased especially in oral microbiota of patients with active RA disease (Zhang et al., 2015; **Table 1**).

The role of the gastrointestinal tract in the pathogenesis of SpA was proposed by Costello et al. (2015) who have evaluated biopsy specimens from 9 early SpA patients finding a higher abundance of five families of bacteria (*Lachnospiraceae, Ruminococcaceae, Rikenellaceae, Porphyromonadaceae,* and *Bacteroidaceae*), accompanied by a reduction of *Veillonellaceae* and *Prevotellaceae* with respect to healthy controls. Tito et al analyzed the gut microbiota (colon biopsy specimens) of 27 patients with SpA and 15 healthy controls and showed that the intestinal inflammation was associated with the mucosal microbiota composition. Of particular interest, they found that the genus *Dialister* positively correlated with the SpA activity (Tito et al., 2016). Stebbings et al. (2002) were the first group that reported differences in the fecal samples of AS patients compared to healthy controls by using molecular analysis. They did not find significant differences in the microbiota composition but did find a higher proportion of sulfate-reducing bacteria in AS patients (Stebbings et al., 2002). Fecal samples and blood specimens obtained from children with enthesitis showed less *Faecalibacterium prausnitzii* spp. and *Lachnospiraceae* family members and a significant increase in the *Bifidobacterium* genus (Stoll et al., 2014). Finally, other authors have reported a significant increase in Firmicutes associated with a reduction in members of Actinobacteria *phylum* and *Propionibacteria* spp in the skin samples of patients with psoriasis, compared to healthy controls (Fahlén et al., 2012). The gut microbiota observed in patients with PsA also showed limited diversity compared to healthy controls. In particular, it has been demonstrated that there is a decrease in the bacterial genus *Akkermansia, Ruminococcus,* and *Pseudobutyrivibrio* in fecal samples from PsA patients (Scher et al., 2015; **Table 1**).

There is a growing awareness that the microbiota diversity and composition can influence a patient's response to synthetic and biologic immunosuppressive therapy. Immunosuppressive drugs, such as cyclophosphamide and methotrexate (MTX), can induce a diffuse depletion of the gut microbiota associated with a decrease in the commensal anaerobic species in favor of potential pathogens that can damage the gut barrier, altering epithelial cell permeability with consequent bacterial translocation (Viaud et al., 2013; Karin et al., 2014). Different authors have underlined the importance of an intact intestinal microbiota in the response to sulphasalazine (SSA), a synthetic drug frequently used in autoimmune arthritis. They found a decreased efficacy of SSA therapy in patients with ulcerative colitis previously treated with severe antibiotic regimens (Das et al., 1973; Peppercorn and Goldman, 1972). Conversely, the use of a multi-strain probiotic regimen does not seem to interfere with the metabolism of SSA in RA patients (Lee et al., 2010).

By now, data on the impact of microbiota in patients receiving immunosuppressive biologics are limited and only refer to IBD patients. One research group has found a reduction in the bacterial species Firmicutes *phylum* in patients affected by relapsing Crohn's disease as compared to clinically stable patients with administration of anti-TNFα agents. This modification in gut microbiota was associated with a reduction in *F. prausnitzii* spp. predicting clinical relapse of the Crohn's disease (Rajca et al., 2014). More recently, Busquets et al. (2015) have demonstrated that adalimumab (fully human anti-TNFα monoclonal antibody) could partially restore a healthy microbiota in a small group of patients affected by Crohn's disease. Treatment resulted in the recovery of Firmicutes, Bacteroides and Actinobacteria diversity species whereas *E. coli* spp. was decreased (Busquets et al., 2015).

INFECTIONS AND ARTHRITIS

In autoimmune arthritis, such as RA and SpA, the hypothesis of an infectious event as the cause for disease induction and relapse has been under consideration for a long time. Arleevskaya et al. (2014) have shown during a 10-year follow-up study that minor infections are more frequent and prolonged in RA patients and their relatives than in families without a history of autoimmunity. This study suggests a role for some predisposing defects of anti-bacterial defense mechanisms, more than for a specific microorganism. However, although by now no causative pathogen has been clearly identified nor a direct correlation with a specific infection has been established, it does not imply its absence. In fact, many pathogens have been indicated as possible triggers for RA disease but heterogeneity of the studies impairs forming any conclusions (Arleevskaya et al., 2016).

The most intriguing and supported idea for a role of infection in triggering RA, is that the microorganism can enter to and be located in the intestine, lungs or mouth; where it can interact with environmental factors such as smoke and drugs and, with a genetic predisposition, lead to mucosal inflammation. This, in turn, results in increased immune activation and spreading of inflammatory mediators, which locally perpetuate the disease. Exacerbated immune activation may also lead to aberrant migration of intestinal macrophages and lymphocytes from inflamed mucosa to the joints (Salmi et al., 1995).

The complex and interwoven link between microbes and joint inflammation is a frequent challenge for clinicians.

A severe increase in the serologic inflammatory parameters (i.e., erythrocyte sedimentation rate and C reactive protein), induced by a concomitant infection in a patient with autoimmune arthritis under immunosuppressive therapy is commonly encountered in the rheumatologic clinical practice. Indeed, the stimulation of systemic inflammation induced by the infectious pathogen can resemble a reactivation of the autoimmune arthritis, leading clinicians to increase the immunosuppressive therapy with a consequent worsening and dissemination of the infection.

The link between microbes and arthritis also has a broad spectrum of clinical expression. In fact, it can range from septic arthritis, in which the pathogen is directly responsible for joint inflammation and damage, to ReA. In the latter, infections by microorganisms, mainly Gram negative, such as *Chlamydia trachomatis, Yersinia, Salmonella, Shigella, and Campylobacter* (Espinoza and García-Valladares, 2013), find a genetically predisposed background (i.e., HLAB27) eventually resulting in chronic inflammation. However, the mechanism underlying the immune stimulation and consequent migration to distant synovial tissue is poorly understood (Keat et al., 1978; Granfors et al., 1990; Merilahti-Palo et al., 1991). It is worth mentioning that T cell clones specific for enteric bacteria have been found in synovial tissue of patients with ReA (Hermann et al., 1990; Probst et al., 1993).

It can be argued that the early recognition and eradication of the infective focus can lead to a resolution of the inflammatory stimulus and consequent interruption of the chronic immune loop. This can be the case of periodontal treatment in early RA, antibiotic therapy for beta-hemolytic *Streptococcus* in rheumatic fever and anti-hepatitis C virus (HCV) treatment for mixed cryoglobulinemia.

Recently, Campisi et al. (2016) using a complex and elegant set of experiments in mice, demonstrated that microbial infection at mucosal sites can elicit a break in tolerance by promoting the presentation of self-antigens derived from epithelial cell apoptotic bodies. Apoptosis of infected colonic cells leads to the generation of both anti-pathogen and autoreactive T cells, mainly Th17 cells, with production of auto-antibodies and inflammation (Campisi et al., 2016). These results have important implications for understanding how infections can stimulate the development of autoimmunity in an immunological context different from bystander activation of autoreactive T cells or epitope mimicry. Further studies are needed to establish similar correlations in humans.

The risk of infections in autoimmune patients is higher than in healthy individuals, due to endogenous (dysfunctional immune system) and external factors (i.e., comorbidities and immunosuppressive therapy). The risk has been reported to be approximately double for infections of bone and joints, skin, soft tissues and respiratory tract (Myllykangas-Luosujarvi et al., 1995). Moreover, it is known that infections can induce disease relapses, present a more severe clinical outcome and can be a frequent cause of death in immune-suppressed subjects (Gonzalez et al., 2007).

Immunosuppressive treatment is the main exogenous factor contributing to the increased risk of infections in autoimmune patients. TNFα blocking agents are the first biological immunosuppressive therapy approved for both RA and SpA. Currently five different drugs targeting TNFα are available: infliximab (the first antibody to be approved) is a chimeric monoclonal antibody (mAb) with approximately one third murine and two thirds human sequences; adalimumab, a fully human mAb produced by chinese hamster ovary (CHO) cells; golimumab a fully human mAb; certolizumab pegol, a poly-etyhlene-glycol (PEG)ylated humanized Fab' fragment; and etanercept a fusion protein that consists of the p75 part of TNFR2 and a human IgG1 Fc domain (Salemi et al., 2015; Dieterich et al., 2016). Although these agents have shown a good safety and efficacy profile, up to 40% of the patients may present a primary or secondary drug failure or treatment-related adverse events (Day, 2002).

In the last decade, several research groups have studied in depth the molecular pathways involved in the development of autoimmune arthritis, allowing identification of new therapeutic targets. Among those, the anti-CD20 chimeric mAb (rituximab) (de la Torre et al., 2012); the humanized anti-human IL6 receptor mAb (tocilizumab) (Nishimoto et al., 2007), and the CTLA-4-Ig (abatacept), a fusion protein that works as an inhibitor of T cell activation (Moreland et al., 2006), are currently available for RA patients. More recently, mAb against the p40 subunit of interleukin 12/23 ustekinumab (Gottlieb et al., 2009) and the mAb against the IL17A, secukinumab have been introduced for the treatment of patients with SpA (Patel et al., 2013).

Different authors have evaluated the infection risk induced by corticosteroids (CS) as well as synthetic and biologic immunosuppressant drugs in SpA and RA patients. Studies generally showed that synthetic immunosuppressive therapy (mainly MTX), is relatively safe, whereas data on the possible increase in the number and/or severity of infections in patients taking TNFα blocking agents are contrasting. Doran et al. (2002) showed that the use of CS, older age, extra-articular manifestations of RA, leukopenia, and comorbidities, are strong predictors of infections, whereas the use of synthetic immunosuppressive agents was not associated with increased risk. These results were partially confirmed by Lacaille et al. (2008), who reported an increased risk of infections in RA patients taking CS, but not synthetic immunosuppressive therapy. Data on the infection risk for biologic drugs derives mainly from national registries among which are the British Biologics Register and the RABBIT German Registry. Data from these registries estimated a two-fold increased risk of serious infections which was directly related to the dose of CS, mainly when CS were associated with TNFα inhibitors (Dixon et al., 2006; Zink et al., 2014). Results obtained from meta-analysis studies have also indicated a significant increase in the occurrence of serious infections (40%), in patients receiving anti-TNFα agents, while the data for opportunistic infections were not conclusive (Bongartz et al., 2006; Minozzi et al., 2016).

We have recently described, in a retrospective observational cohort study, that the combination of anti-TNFα with CS appears to be the most "pro-infective" treatment, whereas synthetic immunosuppressant drugs, either alone or associated with CS, were relatively safe in both patients with RA or with SpA (Germano et al., 2014). In contrast with these real-life data, the placebo-controlled trials evaluating TNFα blockers in RA patients, did not find a higher rate of infections in treated patients with respect to the placebo group (Lipsky et al., 2000; Klareskog et al., 2004; Weinblatt et al., 2005).

CONCLUSION

Patients with autoimmune arthritis are at high risk of infections, due to endogenous (dysfunctional immune system) and external factors (i.e., comorbidities, drugs).

Infections can induce disease relapses and be characterized by a severe clinical outcome in these patients, representing a frequent cause of death. Furthermore, the stimulation of systemic inflammation induced by the infectious pathogen, mimicking a reactivation of the autoimmune arthritis, frequently represents a confounding and dangerous factor for clinicians.

In the last few years the efforts of several researchers have focused on the gut and mouth microflora leading to the identification of specific abnormalities in both its composition and diversity. In susceptible individuals, the presence of PG could be a trigger factor for RA development by inducing the generation of citrullinated proteins via a PPAD enzyme on different self-proteins that results in the production of ACPAs. In SpA patients the increased intestinal permeability, probably induced by genetic factors (e.g., HLA-B27) could lead to a disruption of the basal membrane, hyperplasia of goblet cells and activation of Paneth cells producing high levels of AMPs and IL23. It would result in a continuous antigenic stimulation with activation of effector T cells.

Careful monitoring for infectious foci, especially in the mouth and intestine, should be recommended in order to allow their early recognition and eradication, thus resulting in removal of the inflammatory stimulus, inhibition of the chronic immune loop and improvement of the arthritis.

AUTHOR CONTRIBUTIONS

AP-D and MR drafted the manuscript and performed the revision of the literature. RD critically revised the manuscript giving important intellectual contribution.

REFERENCES

Arleevskaya, M. I., Gabdoulkhakova, A. G., Filina, Y. V., Miftakhova, R. R., Bredberg, A., and Tsybulkin, A. P. (2014). A transient peak of infections during onset of rheumatoid arthritis: a 10-year prospective cohort study. *BMJ Open* 4:e005254. doi: 10.1136/bmjopen-2014-005254

Arleevskaya, M. I., Kravtsova, O. A., Lemerle, J., Renaudineau, Y., and Tsibulkin, A. P. (2016). How rheumatoid arthritis can result from provocation of the immune system by microorganisms and viruses. *Front. Microbiol.* 7:1296 doi: 10.3389/fmicb.2016.01296

Asquith, M., Elewaut, D., Lin, P., and Rosenbaum, J. T. (2014). The role of the gut and microbes in the pathogenesis of spondyloarthritis. *Best Pract. Res. Clin. Rheumatol.* 28, 687–702. doi: 10.1016/j.berh.2014.10.018

Atarashi, K., Tanoue, T., Oshima, K., Suda, W., Nagano, Y., Nishikawa, H., et al. (2013). Treg induction by a rationally selected mixture of Clostridia strains from the human microbiota. *Nature* 500, 232–236. doi: 10.1038/nature12331

Bongartz, T., Sutton, A. J., Sweeting, M. J., Buchan, I., Matteson, E. L., and Montori, V. (2006). Anti-TNF antibody therapy in rheumatoid arthritis and the risk of serious infections and malignancies: systematic review and meta-analysis of rare harmful effects in randomized controlled trials. *JAMA* 295, 2275–2285. doi: 10.1001/jama.295.19.2275

Bowness, P. (2015). HLA-B27. *Ann. Rev. Immunol.* 33, 29–48. doi: 10.1146/annurev-immunol-032414-112110

Busquets, D., Mas-de-Xaxars, T., López-Siles, M., Martínez-Medina, M., Bahí, A., et al. (2015). Anti-tumour necrosis factor. treatment with adalimumab induces changes in the microbiota of Crohn's disease. *J. Crohns Colitis* 9, 899–906 doi: 10.1093/ecco-jcc/jjv119

Campisi, L., Barbet, G., Ding, Y., Esplugues, E., Flavell, R. A., and Blander, J. M. (2016). Apoptosis in response to microbial infection induces autoreactive TH17 cells. *Nat. Immunol.* 17, 1084–1092. doi: 10.1038/ni.3512

Carding, A., Verbeke, K., Vipond, D. T., Corfe, B. M., and Owen, L. J. (2015). Dysbiosis of the gut microbiota in disease. *Microb. Ecol. Health Dis.* 26:26191 doi: 10.3402/mehd.v26.26191

Chen, J., Wright, K., Davis, J. M., Jeraldo, P., Marietta, E. V., Murray, J., et al. (2016). An expansion of rare lineage intestinal microbes characterizes rheumatoid arthritis. *Genome Med.* 8:43. doi: 10.1186/s13073-016-0299-7

Ciccia, F., Accardo-Palumbo, A., Alessandro, R., Rizzo, A., Principe, S., Peralta, S., et al. (2012). Interleukin-22 and interleukin-22-producing NKp44Þ NK cells in the subclinical gut inflammation of patients with ankylosing spondylitis. *Arthritis Rheum.* 64, 1869–1878. doi: 10.1002/art.34355

Ciccia, F., Bombardieri, M., Principato, A., Giardina, A., Tripodo, C., Porcasi, R., et al. (2009). Overexpression of interleukin-23, but not interleukin-17, as an immunologic signature of subclinical intestinal inflammation in ankylosing spondylitis. *Arthritis Rheum.* 60, 955–965. doi: 10.1002/art.24389

Ciccia, F., Bombardieri, M., Rizzo, A., Principato, A., Giardina, A. R., Raiata, F., et al. (2010). Over expression of paneth cell derived antimicrobial peptides in the gut of patients with ankylosing spondylitis and subclinical intestinal inflammation. *Rheumatology* 49, 2076–2083. doi: 10.1093/rheumatology/keq239

Ciccia, F., Guggino, G., Ferrante, A., Raimondo, S., Bignone, R., Rodolico, V., et al. (2016). Interleukin-9 overexpression and Th9 polarization characterize the inflamed gut,the synovial tissue, and the peripheral blood of patients with psoriatic arthritis. *Arthritis Rheumatol.* 68, 1922–1931. doi: 10.1002/art.39649

Costello, M. E., Ciccia, F., Willner, D., Warrington, N., Robinson, P. C., Gardiner, B., et al. (2015). Intestinal dysbiosis in ankylosing & spondylitis. *Arthritis Rheumatol.* 67, 686–691. doi: 10.1002/art.38967

Das, K. M., Eastwood, M. A., McManus, J. P., and Sircus, W. (1973). The metabolism of salicylazosulphapyridine in ulcerative colitis. I. The relationship between metabolites and the response to treatment in inpatients. *Gut* 14, 631–641

Day, R. (2002). Adverse reactions to TNF-alpha inhibitors in rheumatoid arthritis. *Lancet* 359, 540–541. doi: 10.1016/S0140-6736(02)07718-8

de la Torre, I., Leandro, M. J., Edwards, J. C., and Cambridge, G. (2012). Baseline serum immunoglobulin levels in patients with rheumatoid arthritis: relationships with clinical parameters and with B-cell dynamics following rituximab. *Clin. Exp. Rheumatol.* 30, 554–560.

De Vos, M., Mielants, H., Cuvelier, C., Elewaut, A., and Veys, E. (1996). Long term evolution of gut inflammation in patients with spondyloarthropathy. *Gastroenterology* 110, 1696–1703. doi: 10.1053/gast.1996.v110.pm8964393

Dean, L. E., Jones, G. T., MacDonald, A. G., Downham, C., Sturrock, R. D., and Macfarlane, G. J. (2014). Global prevalence of ankylosing spondylitis. *Rheumatology* 53, 650–657. doi: 10.1093/rheumatology/ket387

Diamanti, A. P., Manuela Rosado, M., Laganà, B., and D'Amelio, R. (2016). Microbiota and chronic inflammatory arthritis: an interwoven link. *J. Transl. Med.* 14:233 doi: 10.1186/s12967-016-0989-3

Dieterich, W., Neurath, M. F., and Atreya, R. (2016). Molecular mechanism of action of anti-tumor necrosis factor antibodies in inflammatory bowel diseases. *World J. Gastroenterol.* 22, 9300–9313

Dissick, A., Redman, R. S., Jones, M., Rangan, B. V., Reimold, A., Griffiths, G. R., et al. (2010). Association of periodontitis with rheumatoid arthritis: a pilot study. *J. Periodontol.* 81, 223–230. doi: 10.1902/jop.2009.090309

Dixon, W. G., Watson, K., and Lunt, M. (2006). Rates of serious infection, including site-specific and bacterial intracellular infection, in rheumatoid arthritis patients receiving anti-tumor necrosis factor therapy. Results from the British society for rheumatology biologics register. *Arthritis Rheum.* 54, 2368–2376

Doran, M. F., Crowson, C. S., Pond, G. R., O'Fallon, W. M., and Gabriel, S. E. (2002). Predictors of infection in Rheumatoid arthritis. *Arthritis Rheum.* 49, 2294–2300. doi: 10.1002/art.10529

Eren, Z., Gurol, Y., Sonmezoglu, M., Eren, H. S., Celik, G., and Kantarci, G., (2014). Saccharomyces cerevisiae fungemia in an elderly patient following probiotic treatment. *Mikrobiyol. Bul.* 48, 351–355 doi: 10.5578/mb.6970

Ergin, A., Syrbe, U., and Scheer, R. et al. (2011). Impaired peripheral Th1 $CD4^+$ T cell response to *Escherichia coli* proteins in patients with Crohn's disease and ankylosing spondylitis. *J. Clin. Immunol.* 31, 998–1009. doi: 10.1007/s10875-011-9575-x

Espinoza, L. R., and García-Valladares, I. (2013). Of bugs and joints: the relationship between infection and joints. *Reumatol Clin.* 9, 229–238 doi: 10.1016/j.reuma.2012.06.008

Fahlén, A., Engstrand, L., Baker, B. S., Powles, A., and Fry, L. (2012). Comparison of bacterial microbiota in skin biopsies from normal and psoriatic skin. *Arch. Dermatol. Res.* 304, 15–22. doi: 10.1007/s00403-011-1189-x

Germano, V., Cattaruzza, M. S., Osborn, J., Tarantino, A., Di Rosa, R., Salemi, S., et al. (2014). Infection risk in rheumatoid arthritis and spondyloarthropathy patients under treatment with DMARDs, corticosteroids and TNF-α antagonists. *J. Transl. Med.* 12:77 doi: 10.1186/1479-5876-12-77

Gonzalez, A., Kremers, M. H., Crowson, C. S., Nicola, P. J., Davis, J. M., III., Therneau, T. M. et al. (2007). The widening mortality gap, between rheumatoid arthritis patients and the general population. *Arthritis Rheum.* 56, 3583–3587. doi: 10.1002/art.22979

Gottlieb, A., Menter, A., Mendelsohn, A., Shen, Y. K., Li, S., Guzzo, C., et al. (2009). Ustekinumab, a human interleukin 12/23 monoclonal antibody, for psoriatic arthritis: randomised, double-blind, placebo-controlled, crossover trial. *Lancet* 373, 633–640. doi: 10.1016/S0140-6736(09)60140-9

Grainger, J. R., Wohlfert, E. A., Fuss, I. J., Bouladoux, N., Askenase, M. H., Legrand, F., et al. (2013). Inflammatory monocytes regulate pathologic responses to commensals during acute gastrointestinal infection. *Nat. Med.* 19, 713–721. doi: 10.1038/nm.3189

Granfors, K., Jalkanen, S., Lindberg, A. A., Mäki-Ikola, O., von Essen, R., Lahesmaa-Rantala, R., et al. (1990). *Salmonella* lipopolysaccharide in synovial cells from patients with reactive arthritis. *Lancet* 335, 685–688; doi: 10.1016/0140-6736(90)90804-E

Hand, T. W. (2016). The role of the microbiota in shaping infectious immunity. Trends Immunol. 37, 647–658. doi: 10.1016/j.it.2016.08.007

Hayter, S. M., and Cook, M. C. (2012). Updated assessment of the prevalence, spectrum and case definition of autoimmune disease. *Autoimmun. Rev.* 11, 754–765. doi: 10.1016/j.autrev.2012.02.001

Hermann, E., Mayet, W. J., Poralla, T., Meyer zum Büschenfelde, K. H., and Fleischer, B. (1990). *Salmonella*-reactive synovial fluid T-cell clones in a patient with post-infectious *Salmonella* arthritis. *Scand. J. Rheumatol.* 19, 350–355 doi: 10.3109/03009749009096790

Ivanov, I. I., Atarashi, K., and Manel, N., Brodie, E. L., Shima, T., Karaoz, U., et al. (2009). Induction of intestinal Th17 cells by segmented filamentous bacteria. *Cell* 139, 485–498. doi: 10.1016/j.cell.2009.09.033

Johnson, S., Sidebottom, D., Bruckner, F., and Collins, D. (2000). Identification of *Mycoplasma fermentans* in synovial fluid samples from arthritis patients with inflammatory disease. *J. Clin. Microbiol.* 38, 90–93.

Karin, M., Jobin, C., and Balkwill, F. (2014). Chemotherapy, immunity and microbiota–a new triumvirate? *Nat. Med.* 20, 126–127. doi: 10.1038/nm.3473

Kaur, S., Bright, R., Proudman, S. M., and Bartold, P. M. (2014). Does periodontal treatment influence clinical and biochemical measures for rheumatoid arthritis? A systematic review and meta-analysis. *Semin. Arthritis Rheum.* 44, 113–122. doi: 10.1016/j.semarthrit.2014.04.009

Keat, A. C., Maini, R. N., Nkwazi, G. C., Pegrum, G. D., Ridgway, G. L., and Scott, J. T. (1978). Role of Chlamydia trachomatis and HLA-B27 in sexually acquired reactive arthritis. *Br. Med. J.* 1, 605–607 doi: 10.1136/bmj.1.6113.605

Kim, K. S., Hong, S. W., Han, D., Yi, J., Jung, J., Yang, B. G., Lee, J. Y., et al. (2016). Dietary antigens limit mucosal immunity by inducing regulatory T cells in the small intestine. *Science* 351, 858–863. doi: 10.1126/science.aac5560

Klareskog, L., van der Heijde, D., De Jager, J. P., Gough, A., Kalden, J., Malaise, M., et al. (2004). Therapeutic effect of the combination of etanercept and methotrexate compared with each treatment alone in patients with rheumatoid arthritis: double-blind randomised controlled trial. *Lancet* 363, 675–681. doi: 10.1016/S0140-6736(04)15640-7

Lacaille, D., Guh, D. P., Abrahamowicz, M., Anis, A. H., and Esdaile, J. M. (2008). Use of non biologic disease-modifying antirheumatic drugs and risk of infection in patients with rheumatoid arthritis. *Arthritis Rheum.* 59, 1074–1081. doi: 10.1002/art.23913

Lange, L., Thiele, G. M., McCracken, C., Wang, G., Ponder, L. A., Angeles-Han, S. T., et al. (2016). Symptoms of periodontitis and antibody responses to *Porphyromonas gingivalis* in juvenile idiopathic arthritis. *Pediatr. Rheumatol. Online J.* 14:8. doi: 10.1186/s12969-016-0068-6

LeBlanc, J. G., Milani, C., de Giori, G. S., Sesma, F., van Sinderen, D., and Ventura, M. (2013). Bacteria as vitamin suppliers to their host: a gut microbiota perspective. *Curr. Opin. Biotechnol.* 24, 160–168. doi: 10.1016/j.copbio.2012.08.005

Lee, H. J., Waller, R. D., Stebbings, S., Highton, J., Orlovich, D. A., Schmierer, D., et al. (2010). The effects of an orally administered probiotic on sulfasalazine metabolism in individuals with rheumatoid arthritis: a preliminary study. *Int. J. Rheum. Dis.* 13, 48–54 doi: 10.1111/j.1756-185X.2009.01449.x

Lin, P., Bach, M., Asquith, M., Lee, A. Y., Akileswaran, L., Stauffer, P., et al. (2014). HLA-B27 and human beta2-microglobulin affect the gut microbiota of transgenic rats. *PLOS ONE* 9:e105684. doi: 10.1371/journal.pone.0105684

Lipsky, P. E., van der Heijde, D. M., St Clair, E. W., Furst, D. E., Breedveld, F. C., Kalden, J. R., et al. (2000). Anti-tumor necrosis factor trial in rheumatoid arthritis with concomitant therapy study group infliximab and methotrexate in the treatment of rheumatoid arthritis. *N. Engl. J. Med.* 343:1594–1602.

Liu, X., Zou, Q., Zeng, B., Fang, Y., and Wei, H. (2013). Analysis of fecal lactobacillus community structure in patients with early rheumatoid arthritis. *Curr. Microbiol.* 67, 170–176. doi: 10.1007/s00284-013-0338-1

Liu, Y., Helms, C., Liao, W., Zaba, L. C., Duan, S., Gardner, J., et al. (2008). A genome-wide association study of psoriasis and psoriatic arthritis identifies new disease loci. *PLOS Genet.* 4:e1000041 doi: 10.1371/journal.pgen.1000041

Macpherson, A., Khoo, U. Y., Forgacs, I., Philpott-Howard, J., and Bjarnason, I. (1996). Mucosal antibodies in inflammatory bowel disease are directed against intestinal bacteria. *Gut* 38, 365–375. doi: 10.1136/gut.38.3.365

Maslowski, K. M., Vieira, A. T., Ng, A., Kranich, J., Sierro, F., Yu, D., et al. (2009). Regulation of inflammatory responses by gut microbiota and chemoattractant receptor GPR43. *Nature* 461, 1282–1286 doi: 10.1038/nature08530

McInnes, I. B., and Schett, G. (2011). The pathogenesis of rheumatoid arthritis. *N. Engl. J. Med.* 365, 2205–2219. doi: 10.1056/NEJMra1004965

Mercado, F. B., Marshall, R. I., Klestov, A. C., and Bartold, P. M. (2001). Relationship between rheumatoid arthritis and periodontitis. *J. Periodontol.* 72, 779–787. doi: 10.1902/jop.2001.72.6.779

Merilahti-Palo, R., Söderström, K. O., Lahesmaa-Rantala, R., Granfors, K., and Toivanen, A. (1991). Bacterial antigens in synovial biopsy specimens in yersinia triggered reactive arthritis. *Ann. Rheum. Dis.* 50, 87–90 doi: 10.1136/ard.50.2.87

Mielants, H., Veys, E. M., Cuvelier, C., De Vos, M., Goemaere, S., De Clercq, L., et al. (1995). The evolution of spondyloarthropathies in relation to gut histology. II. Histological aspects. *J. Rheumatol.* 22, 2273–2278.

Minozzi, S., Bonovas, S., Lytras, T., Pecoraro, V., González-Lorenzo, M., Bastiampillai A. J., et al. (2016). Risk of infections using anti-TNF agents in rheumatoid arthritis, psoriatic arthritis, and ankylosing spondylitis: a systematic review and meta-analysis. *Expert Opin. Drug Saf.* 15 (Suppl.1), 11–34. doi: 10.1080/14740338.2016.1240783

Montineri, A., Iacobello, C., Larocca, L., La Rosa, R., Nigro, L., and Fatuzzo, F. (2008). Saccharomyces cerevisiae fungemia associated with multifocal pneumonia in a patient with alcohol-related hepatic cirrhosis. *Infez. Med.* 16, 227–229.

Moreland, L., Bate, G., and Kirkpatrick, P. (2006). Abatacept. *Nat. Rev. Drug Discov.* 5, 185–186. doi: 10.1038/nrd1989

Myllykangas-Luosujarvi, R., Aho, K., Kautiainen, H., and Isomaki, H. (1995). Shortening of life span and causes of excess mortality in a population-based series of subjects with rheumatoid arthritis. *Clin. Exp. Rheumatol.* 13, 149–153.

Newkirk, M. M., Zbar, A., Baron, M., Manges, A. R. (2010). Distinct bacterial colonization patterns of Escherichia coli subtypes associate with rheumatoid factor status in early inflammatory arthritis. *Rheumatology (Oxford)* 49, 1311–1316. doi: 10.1093/rheumatology/keq088

Nishimoto, N., Hashimoto, J., Miyasaka, N., Yamamoto, K., Kawai, S., Takeuchi, T., et al. (2007). Study of active controlled monotherapy used for rheumatoid arthritis, an IL-6 inhibitor (SAMURAI): evidence of clinical and radiographic benefit from an x-ray reader-blinded radnomised controlled trial of tocilizumab. *Ann. Rheum. Dis.* 66, 1162–1167. doi: 10.1136/ard.2006.068064

Olivieri, I., Cantini, F., Castiglione, F., Felice, C., Gionchetti, P., Orlando, A., et al. (2014). Italian Expert Panel on the management of patients with coexisting spondyloarthritis and inflammatory bowel disease. *Autoimmun. Rev.* 13, 822–830. doi: 10.1016/j.autrev.2014.04.003

Ortiz, P., Bissada, N. F., Palomo, L., Han, Y. W., Al-Zahrani, M. S., Panneerselvam, A., et al. (2009). Periodontal therapy reduces the severity of active rheumatoid arthritis in patients treated with or without tumor necrosis factor inhibitors. *J. Periodontol.* 80, 535–540. doi: 10.1902/jop.2009.080447

Patel, D. D., Lee, D. M., Kolbinger, F., and Antoni, C. (2013). Effect of IL-17A blockade with secukinumab in autoimmune diseases. *Ann. Rheum. Dis.* 72(Suppl. 2), 116–123. doi: 10.1136/annrheumdis-2012-202371

Peppercorn, M. A., and Goldman, P. (1972). The role of intestinal bacteria in the metabolism of salicylazosulfapyridine. *J. Pharmacol. Exp. Ther.* 181, 555–562.

Pickard, J. M., Maurice, C. F., Kinnebrew, M. A., Abt, M. C., Schenten, D., Golovkina, T. V., et al. (2014). Rapid fucosylation of intestinal epithelium sustains host-commensal symbiosis in sickness. *Nature* 514:638–641 doi: 10.1038/nature13823

Probst, P., Hermann, E., Meyer zum Büschenfelde, K. H., and Fleischer, B. (1993). Multiclonal synovial T cell response to Yersinia enterocolitica in reactive arthritis: the Yersinia 61-kDa heat-shock protein is not the major target antigen. *J. Infect. Dis.* 167, 385–391

Puel, A., Cypowyj, S., Bustamante, J., Wright, J. F., Liu, L., Lim, H. K., et al. (2011). Chronic mucocutaneous candidiasis in humans with inborn errors of interleukin-17 immunity. *Science* 332, 65–68. doi: 10.1126/science.1200439

Quirke, A. M., Lugli, E. B., Wegner, N., Hamilton, B. C., Charles, P., Chowdhury, M., et al. (2014). Heightened immune response to autocitrullinated *Porphyromonas gingivalis* peptidylarginine deiminase: a potential mechanism for breaching immunologic tolerance in rheumatoid arthritis. *Ann. Rheum. Dis.* 73, 263–269. doi: 10.1136/annrheumdis-2012-202726

Rajca, S., Grondin, V., Louis, E., Vernier-Massouille, G., Grimaud, J. C., Bouhnik, Y., et al. (2014). Alterations in the intestinal microbiome (dysbiosis) as a predictor of relapse after infliximab withdrawal in Crohn's disease. *Inflamm. Bowel Dis.* 20, 978–986. doi: 10.1097/MIB.0000000000000036

Rhee, K. J., Sethupathi, P., Driks, A., Lanning, D. K., and Knight, K. L. (2004). Role of commensal bacteria in development of gut-associated lymphoid tissues and preimmune antibody repertoire. *J. Immunol.* 172, 1118–1124. doi: 10.4049/jimmunol.172.2.1118

Rogier, R., Koenders, M. I., and Abdollahi-Roodsaz, S. (2015). Toll-like receptor mediated modulation of T cell response by commensal intestinal microbiota as a trigger for autoimmune arthritis. *J. Immunol. Res.* 2015:527696. doi: 10.1155/2015/527696

Rosenbaum, J. T., and Davey, M. P. (2011). Time for a gut check: evidence for the hypothesis that HLA-B27 predisposes to ankylosing spondylitis by altering the microbiome. *Arthritis Rheum.* 63, 3195–3198. doi: 10.1002/art.30558

Salemi, S., Biondo, M. I., Fiorentino, C., Argento, G., Paolantonio, M., Di Murro, C., et al. (2014). Could early rheumatoid arthritis resolve after periodontitis treatment only? Case report and review of the literature. *Medicine* 93:e195. doi: 10.1097/MD.0000000000000195

Salemi, S., Markovic, M., Martini, G., and D'Amelio, R. (2015). The expanding role of therapeutic antibodies. *Int. Rev. Immunol.* 34, 202–264 doi: 10.3109/08830185.2013.863304

Salmi, M., Andrew, D. P., Butcher, E. C., and Jalkanen, S. (1995). Dual binding capacity of mucosal immunoblasts to mucosal and synovial endothelium in humans: dissection of the molecular mechanisms. *J. Exp. Med.* 181, 137–149. doi: 10.1084/jem.181.1.137

Savioli, C., Ribeiro, A. C., Fabri, G. M., Calich, A. L., Carvalho, J., Silva, C. A., et al. (2012). Persistent periodontal disease hampers anti-tumor necrosis factor treatment response in rheumatoid arthritis. *J. Clin. Rheumatol.* 18, 180–184. doi: 10.1097/RHU.0b013e31825828be

Scher, J. U., Sczesnak, A., Longman, R. S., Segata, N., Ubeda, C., Bielski, C., et al. (2013). Expansion of intestinal prevotella copri correlates with enhanced susceptibility to arthritis. *Elife* 2:e01202. doi: 10.7554/eLife.01202

Scher, J. U., Ubeda, C., Artacho, A., Attur, M., Isaac, S., Reddy, S. M., et al. (2015). Decreased bacterial diversity characterizes the altered gut microbiota in patients with psoriatic arthritis, resembling dysbiosis in inflammatory bowel disease. *Arthritis Rheumatol.* 67, 128–139. doi: 10.1002/art.38892

Scher, J. U., Ubeda, C., Equinda, M., Khanin, R., Buischi, Y., Viale, A., et al. (2012). Periodontal disease and the oral microbiota in new-onset rheumatoid arthritis. *Arthritis Rheum.* 64, 3083–3094. doi: 10.1002/art.34539

Senior, B. W., Anderson, G. A., Morley, K. D., and Kerr, M. A. (1999). Evidence that patients with rheumatoid arthritis have asymptomatic 'non-significant' *Proteus mirabilis* bacteriuria more frequently than healthy controls. *J. Infect.* 38, 99–106. doi: 10.1016/S0163-4453(99)90076-2

Stebbings, S., Munro, K., Simon, M. A., Tannock, G., Highton, J., Harmsen, H., et al. (2002). Comparison of the fecal microflora of patients with ankylosing spondylitis and controls using molecular methods of analysis. *Rheumatology* 41, 1395–1401. doi: 10.1093/rheumatology/41.12.1395

Stecher, B., and Hardt, W. D. (2011). Mechanisms controlling pathogen colonization of the gut. *Curr. Opin. Microbiol.* 14, 82–91. doi: 10.1016/j.mib.2010.10.003

Stoll, M. L., Kumar, R., Morrow, C. D., Lefkowitz, E. J., Cui, X., Genin, A., et al. (2014). Altered microbiota associated with abnormal humoral immune responses to commensal organisms in enthesitis-related arthritis. *Arthritis Res. Ther.* 16:486. doi: 10.1186/s13075-014-0486-0

Tito, R. Y., Cypers, H., Joossens, M., Varkas, G., Van Praet, L., Glorieus, E., et al. (2016). *Dialister* as a microbial marker of disease activity in spondyloarthritis. *Arthritis Rheumatol.* 69, 114–121. doi: 10.1002/art.39802

Vaahtovuo, J., Munukka, E., Korkeamäki, M., Luukkainen, R., and Toivanen, P. (2008). Fecal microbiota in early rheumatoid arthritis. *J. Rheumatol.* 35, 1500–1505.

Vatanen, T., Kostic, A. D., and d'Hennezel, E., Siljander, H., Franzosa, E. A., Yassour, M., et al. (2016). Variation in microbiome LPS immunogenicity contributes to autoimmunity in humans. *Cell* 165, 842–853 doi: 10.1016/j.cell.2016.04.007

Viaud, S., Saccheri, F., Mignot, G., Yamazaki, T., Daillère, R., Hannani, D., et al. (2013). The intestinal microbiota modulates the anticancer immune effects of cyclophosphamide. *Science* 342, 971–976. doi: 10.1126/science.1240537

Wegner, N., Wait, R., Sroka, A., Eick, S., Nguyen, K. A., Lundberg, K., et al. (2010). Peptidylarginine deiminase from *Porphyromonas gingivalis* citrullinates human fibrinogen and α-enolase: implications for autoimmunity in rheumatoid arthritis. *Arthritis Rheum.* 62, 2662–2672. doi: 10.1002/art.27552

Weinblatt, M. E., Keystone, E. C., and Furst, D. E. (2005). Long-term efficacy and safety of adalimumab plus methotrexate in patients with rheumatoid arthritis: ARMADA 4-year extended study. *Ann. Rheum. Dis.* 65, 753–759. doi: 10.1136/ard.2005.044404

Zhang, X., Zhang, D., Jia, H., Feng, Q., Wang, D., Liang, D., et al. 2015. The oral and gut microbiomes are perturbed in rheumatoid arthritis and partly normalized after treatment. *Nat. Med.* 21, 895–905. doi: 10.1038/nm.3914

Zink, A., Manger, B., Kaufmann, J., Eisterhues, C., Krause, A., Listing, J., et al. (2014). Evaluation of the RABBIT risk score for serious infections. *Ann. Rheum. Dis.* 73, 1673–1676. doi: 10.1136/annrheumdis-2013-203341

12

Gut Dysbiosis and Adaptive Immune Response in Diet-Induced Obesity vs. Systemic Inflammation

Jana Pindjakova[1], *Claudio Sartini*[2], *Oriana Lo Re*[1], *Francesca Rappa*[3], *Berengere Coupe*[4], *Benjamin Lelouvier*[4], *Valerio Pazienza*[5] *and Manlio Vinciguerra*[1,6]*

[1] *Center for Translational Medicine, International Clinical Research Center, St. Anne's University Hospital, Brno, Czechia,* [2] *Department of Primary Care and Population Health, University College London, London, United Kingdom,* [3] *Section of Human Anatomy, Department of Experimental Biomedicine and Clinical Neurosciences, University of Palermo, Palermo, Italy,* [4] *Vaiomer, Labège, France,* [5] *Gastroenterology Unit, IRCCS "Casa Sollievo della Sofferenza" Hospital, San Giovanni Rotondo, Italy,* [6] *Division of Medicine, Institute for Liver and Digestive Health, University College London, London, United Kingdom*

***Correspondence:**
Manlio Vinciguerra
manliovinciguerra@gmail.com

A mutual interplay exists between adaptive immune system and gut microbiota. Altered gut microbial ecosystems are associated with the metabolic syndrome, occurring in most obese individuals. However, it is unknown why 10–25% of obese individuals are metabolically healthy, while normal weight individuals can develop inflammation and atherosclerosis. We modeled these specific metabolic conditions in mice fed with a chow diet, an obesogenic but not inflammatory diet—mimicking healthy obesity, or Paigen diet—mimicking inflammation in the lean subjects. We analyzed a range of markers and cytokines in the aorta, heart, abdominal fat, liver and spleen, and metagenomics analyses were performed on stool samples. T lymphocytes infiltration was found in the aorta and in the liver upon both diets, however a significant increase in CD4+ and CD8+ cells was found only in the heart of Paigen-fed animals, paralleled by increased expression of IL-1, IL-4, IL-6, IL-17, and IFN-γ. Bacteroidia, Deltaproteobacteria, and Verrucomicrobia dominated in mice fed Paigen diet, while Gammaproteobacteria, Delataproteobacteria, and Erysipelotrichia were more abundant in obese mice. Mice reproducing human metabolic exceptions displayed gut microbiota phylogenetically distinct from normal diet-fed mice, and correlated with specific adaptive immune responses. Diet composition thus has a pervasive role in co-regulating adaptive immunity and the diversity of microbiota.

Keywords: obesity, inflammation, gut microbiota, adaptive immune system

INTRODUCTION

The main feature of obesity is an excess of adipose tissue, which is the result of an imbalance existing between the intake and the expenditure of energy. The causes of obesity are both genetic and environmental; the diseases often comes along with the establishment of several chronic co-morbidities, such as high fasting hyperglycaemia, hypertriglyceridemia, dyslipidaemia, and hypertension (Alberti et al., 2005). Clinical diagnosis of metabolic syndrome is defined by the co-presence of at least three of the above criteria (Alberti et al., 2005). Metabolic syndrome enhances the odds of having type 2 diabetes and of developing diseases of the cardiovascular system. The majority of people with the metabolic syndrome are in obese, suggesting that the excess mass of adipose tissue may play a causative role in this cluster of diseases (Despres et al., 2008). However, this hypothesis has been strongly debated because several epidemiological analyses have evidenced people with a normal body mass index (BMI) who nevertheless display markers of inflammation and metabolic diseases [here termed metabolic syndrome leans (MSL)], such as high levels of triglycerides and accumulation of fat in the liver (Alberti et al., 2005); in fact, independently of BMI, and with variability linked to race and geographical areas, approximately 1 adult in every 4 or 5 had metabolic syndrome (Alberti et al., 2005). Conversely, a lack of clinical consistency for several or all metabolic syndrome components is found in some individuals with long-established and morbid obesity, which is actually recognized as healthy despite a high BMI. These subjects are referred to as metabolically healthy obese (MHO), and their prevalence has been estimated to be between 10 and 40% of the obese population, notwithstanding design differences between studies, such as age, ethnicity, geography, sample size, and the lack of a standardization (Munoz-Garach et al., 2016). As the prevalence of obesity and metabolic syndrome rises continuously with enormous economic and social costs, innovative countermeasures on the biological mechanisms, beyond prevention and lifestyle interventions, are required. In particular, the biological and disease mechanisms underlying the pathology of MSL and the health of MHO are not understood. Inflammation has been persistently associated with both obesity-associated diseases and the metabolic syndrome, indicating that low-grade inflammation is a potential and modifiable risk factor (Cox et al., 2015). The gut microbiota can be considered a distinct organ with endocrine properties; gut microbiota is involved, through a tight molecular interplay with the host organism, in the homeostasis of host organism energy and in stimulating of its immune system (Clarke et al., 2014). It has been proposed that gut microbiota participates to the establishment of metabolic diseases via the onset of low-grade inflammatory processes (Zupancic et al., 2012; Marchesi et al., 2016), and its composition is rapidly and heavily modulated by the diet (David et al., 2014). However, under healthy conditions commensal bacteria colonizing the gut interplay with the host immunity to maintain a state of

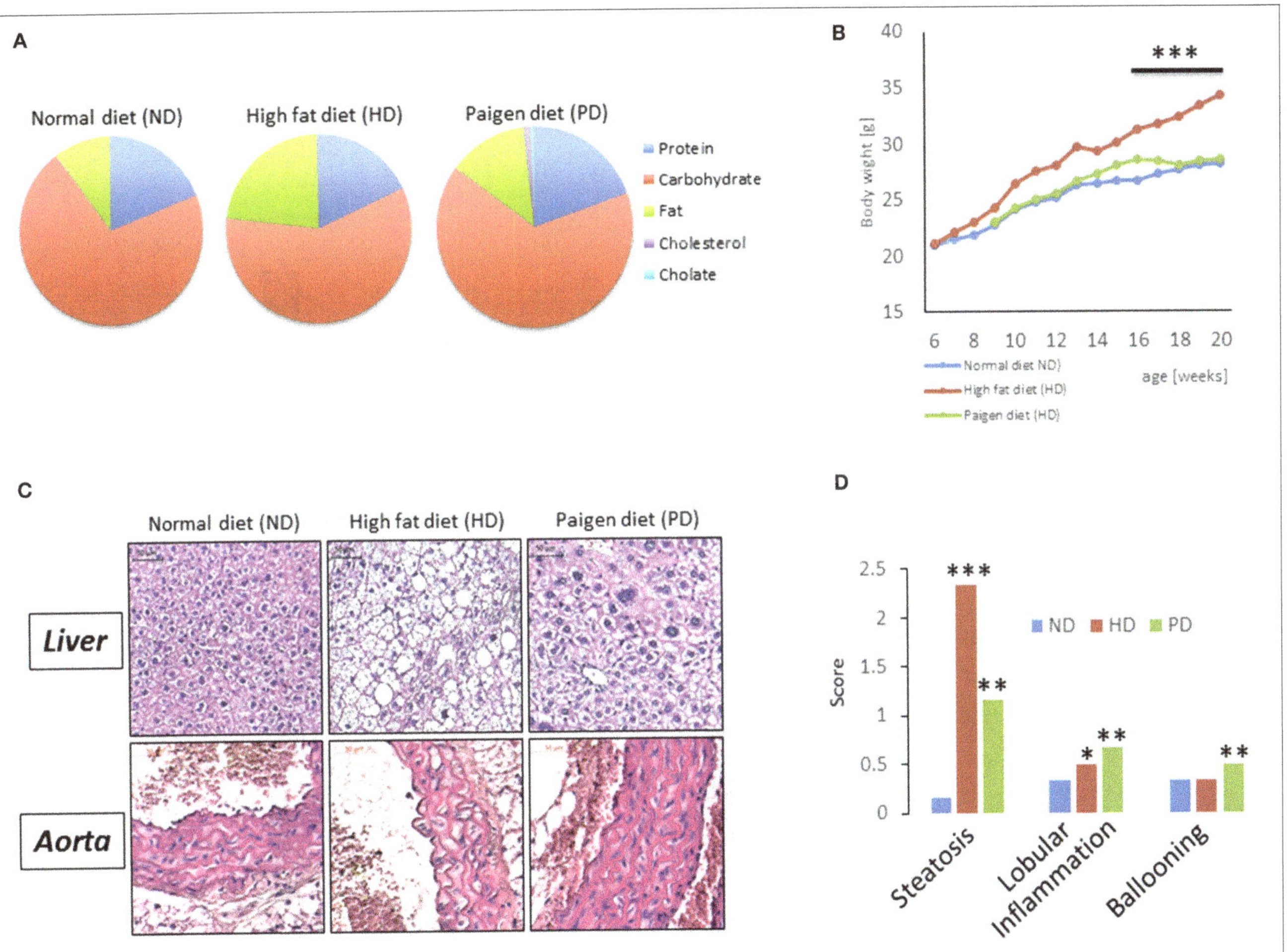

FIGURE 1 | (A) Pie chart representing diet compositions in terms of fat, carbohydrates, choline, cholesterol, proteins. **(B)** Body weight of C57/BL6 mice fed for 20 weeks with a normal chow diet (ND), high fat diet (HD), or Paigen diet (PD). **(C)** Representative pictures from hematoxylin and eosin staining of liver sections (upper panels) and aorta sections (lower panels) in C57/BL6 mice fed with ND, HD, or PD. **(D)** Steatosis, lobular inflammation, and ballooning were scored semi quantitatively (0–4). $^{*}p < 0.05$; $^{**}p < 0.01$; $^{***}p < 0.001$ vs. ND.

homeostasis. In this respect, an immune system–gut microbiota cooperation which operates at optimal levels is instrumental for setting protective mechanisms against pathogenic agents and, at the same time, for keeping in check the regulatory pathways implicated in the avoidance of triggering immune responses to harmless antigens (Belkaid and Hand, 2014). This reciprocal interaction involves both innate (Thaiss et al., 2014) and adaptive immunity (Kato et al., 2014; Zhang and Luo, 2015). In this respect, signals from gut microbiome play crucial role in maturation (or differentiation) of IL-17 expressing Th17 cells as well as IFN-γ expressing Th1 cells (Ivanov et al., 2008; Gaboriau-Routhiau et al., 2009). Although, it has been suggested that dysbiosis can cause immune dysfunctions by activating B and T cells regardless of their distance from the location of their induction (Honda and Littman, 2016), there is scarce knowledge on the relationship between distinct immune cell populations, more in particular those belonging to the adaptive immunity, and the heterogeneity of digestive system-residing and symbiotic bacteria.

Here we modeled the metabolic and clinical features of MSL and MHO humans in C57/BL6 mice fed for 20 weeks with a chow diet, a high fat obesogenic but not inflammatory diet (mimicking healthy obesity) or a hypercholesteraemic, pro-atherogenic, low fat diet (Paigen diet, mimicking systemic inflammation, and fatty liver in the lean subjects; Getz and Reardon, 2006), under the same housing environment. We then analyzed possible interactions among adaptive immune system in multiple tissues, and gut microbiota. Mice fed these distinct "unhealthy" diets reproducing human metabolic exceptions, MSL and MHO, had a gut microbiota with phylogenetic characteristics significantly divergent from normal diet-fed littermates, and displayed specific intra-tissue adaptive immune responses.

MATERIALS AND METHODS

Dietary Mice Models

Four week old male C57BL/6 (B6) mice were purchased from Velaz, Ltd. (Prague, Czech Republic). Animals ($n = 10$ per experimental group) were housed in specific pathogen-free facilities and fed *ad libitum* with basal (normal) or specific (Paigen or Western) diet for 20 weeks with fresh, clean water available at all time. Diet compositions were as following: normal diet (ND): proteins % 18.6, fat % 10 (Linoleic Acid, % 3.34, Linolenic Acid, % 0.07 Arachidonic Acid, % 0.01, Omega-3 FA, % 0.07, Saturated FA % 2.72, Monounsaturated FA, % 3.31, Polyunsaturated FA, % 3.42), carbohydrates % 60.6, cholesterol % 0, choline chloride % 0; High fat diet (HD): proteins % 17.3, fat % 21.2 (Linoleic Acid, % 1.70, Linolenic Acid, % 0.16

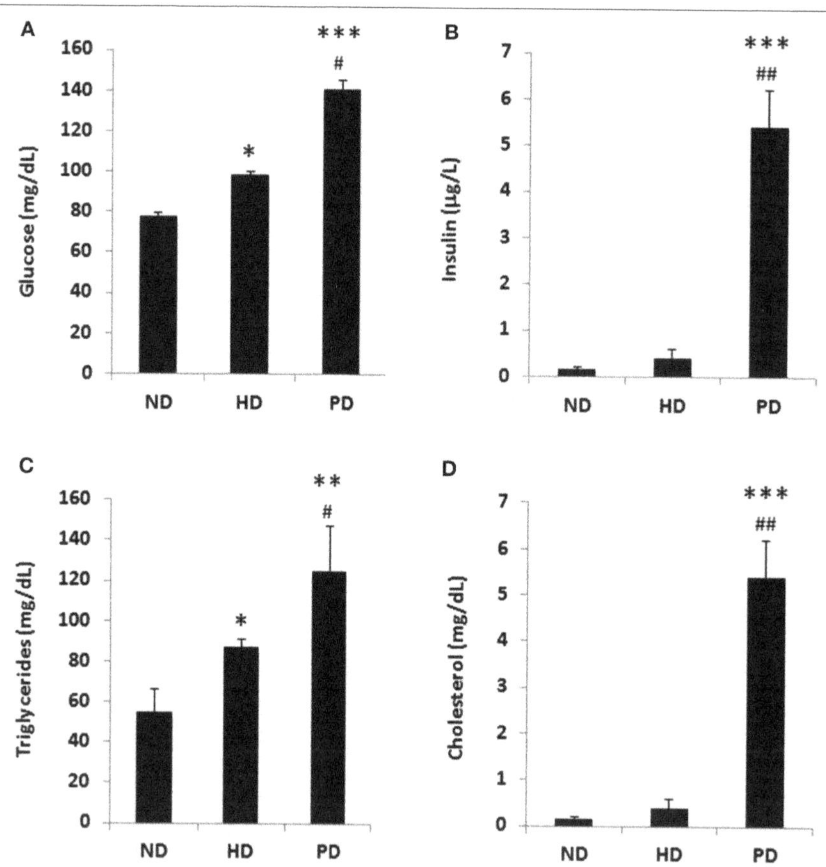

FIGURE 2 | Metabolic parameters of C57BL/6 mice fed a standard normal chow (ND) or a high fat diet (HD) or a Paigen diet (PD) for 15 weeks. **(A)** fasting glucose; **(B)** fasting insulin; **(C)** serum triglycerides; **(D)** serum cholesterol. $N = 4$. $^{*}p < 0.05$, $^{**}p < 0.01$, $^{***}p < 0.001$ vs. ND; $^{\#}p < 0.05$, $^{\#\#}p < 0.01$ vs. HD.

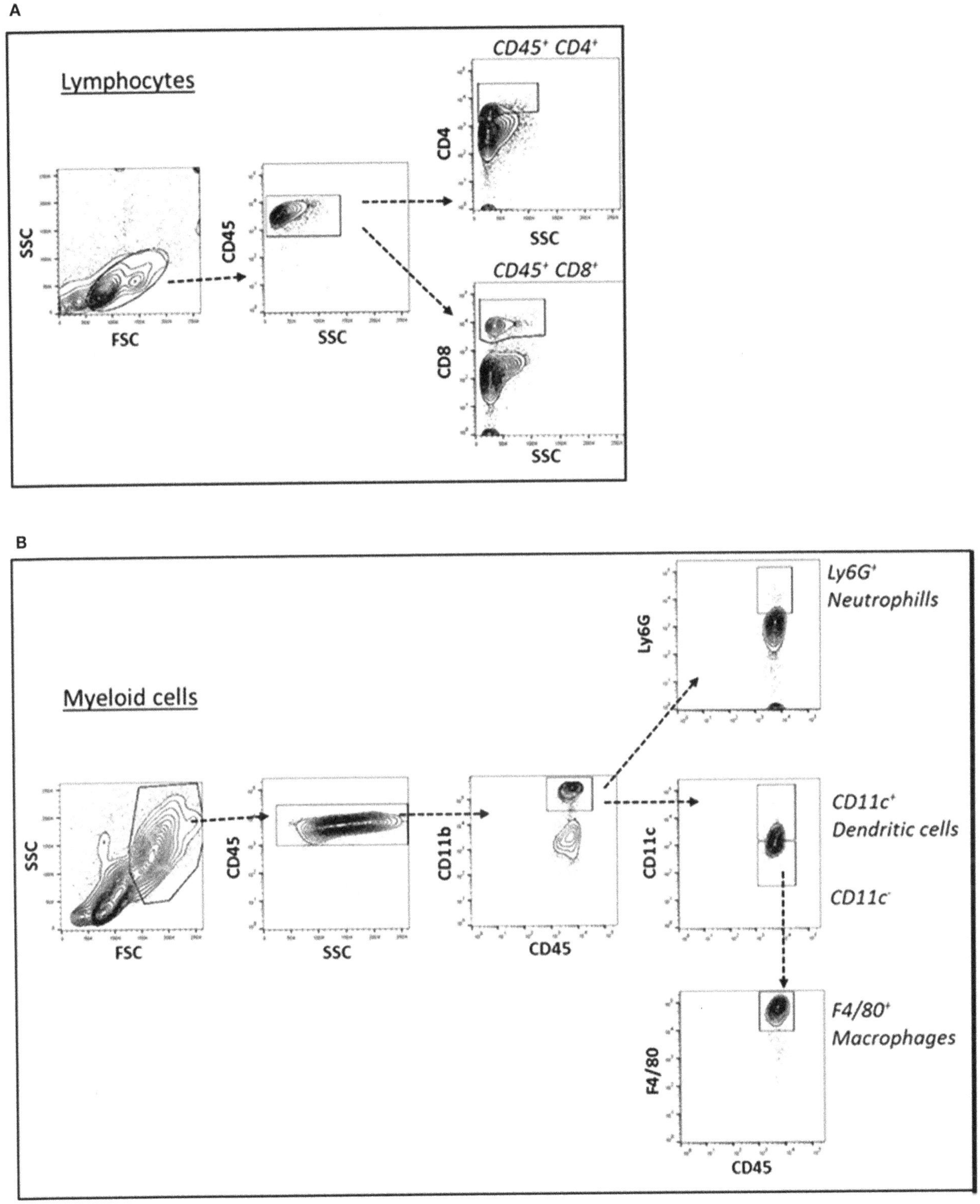

FIGURE 3 | (A) Cell suspension obtained from tissues were surface-stained for T lymphocyte markers with antibody combination CD45, CD4, and CD8 **(A)** and gated for CD45+ CD4+ T lymphocytes and CD45+ CD8+ T lymphocytes. **(B)** For myeloid cell subsets, the cell suspensions were surface-stained with antibody against CD45, CD11b, CD11c, Ly6G, and F4/80 **(B)** and gated for CD45+ CD11b+ Ly6G+ neutrophils, CD45+ CD11b+ CD11c+ dendritic cells, CD45+ CD11b+ CD11c- F4/80+ macrophages.

Arachidonic Acid, % 0.02 Omega-3 FA, % 0.23, Saturated FA, % 7.92 Monounsaturated FA, 6.28, Polyunsaturated FA, % 3.14), carbohydrate % 48.5, cholesterol % 0, choline chloride % 0.2); Paigen diet (PD): proteins % 20.8, fat % 15 (Linoleic Acid, % 1.70, Linolenic Acid, % 0.14, Arachidonic Acid, % 0.01, Omega-3 FA, % 0.16, Saturated FA % 7.18 Monounsaturated FA, % 5.34, Polyunsaturated FA, % 1.91), carbohydrate % 61, cholesterol % 1.25, choline chloride % 0.5. The experiments were performed in accordance with the law governing the protection of animals and the principles derived from the requirements of the Act No. 359/2012 Sb., on the protection of animals against cruelty and the decree 419/2012 Sb. Ministry of Agriculture of Czech Republic on the protection of experimental animals (including relevant EU regulations). The experiments were approved by the local Animal Ethics Committee on the Welfare of Experimental Animals and by the Ministry of Education of Czech Republic (MSMT-2582/2016-14)—project number 66-2015. Serum levels of fasting glucose, fasting insulin, triglycerides, and cholesterol were measured as we have previously described (Cederroth et al., 2008; Pazienza et al., 2016).

Histology

Samples of liver, aorta, and heart from each mouse and were fixed in formalin and embedded in paraffin for histological analysis. Sections with a thickness of 4 μm were obtained from paraffin blocks and stained with hematoxylin and eosin for histological examinations (Benegiamo et al., 2013). Histological classification of NAFLD was performed by applying a semiquantitative scoring system grouping histological traits into broad classes (steatosis, fibrosis, portal inflammation, hepatocellular injury, and miscellaneous features; Kleiner et al., 2005).

Tissue Digestion and Single Cell Suspension Preparation

To prepare single cell suspension from solid tissue (aorta, heart, and abdominal fat), required digestion, the tissue was minced with a sterile scissors and placed in 1 ml DMEM containing: for heart and aorta—2.5 mg/ml Collagenase type XI, 0.25 mg/ml Hyaluronidase type I-s, 0.25 mg/ml DNase I, 2.5 mg Collagenase type I; for abdominal fat – 1 mg/ml Collagenase IV of 3% DMEM. Tissues were incubated in water bath for 1 h with vortex every

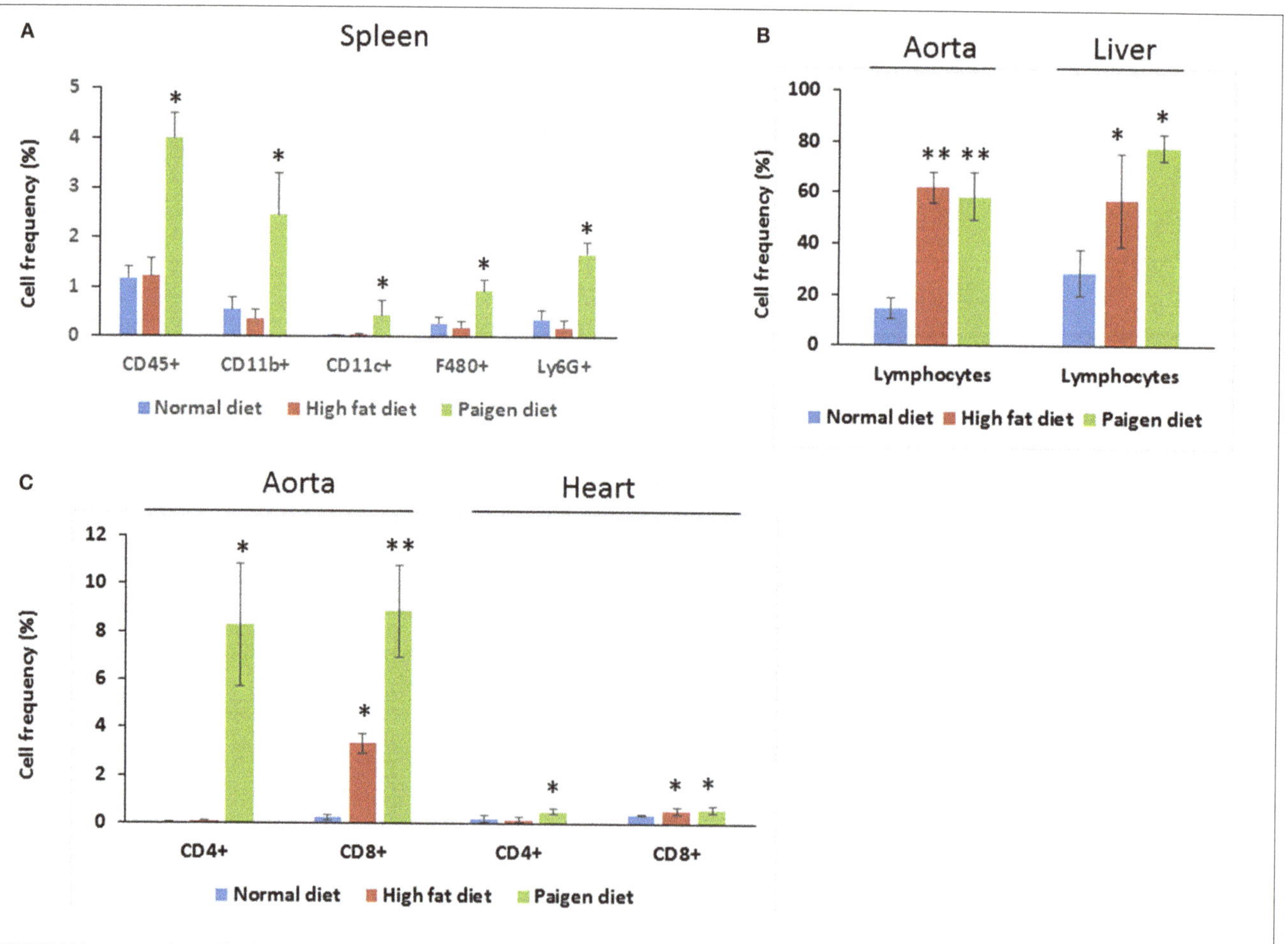

FIGURE 4 | Immune cells profiling in the tissues of Normal diet (ND)-, High fat diet (HD)-, and Paigen diet (PD)-fed mice. Single cell suspensions were prepared from solid tissues (aorta, heart, and liver) and processed for FACS analyses. Combination of surface markers for T-lymphocytes was CD45, CD4, and CD8 and myeloid cells were stained for CD45, CD11b, CD11c, F4/80, and Ly6G. **(A)** Frequency of total myeloid cells and cells positive gated for CD45, CD11b, CD11c, F4/80, and Ly6G in the spleen. **(B)** Frequency of lymphocytes in the aorta and in the liver, of gated cells. **(C)** Frequency of cells gated for CD4 and CD8 in the aorta and in the heart. $N = 3.4$. $^{*}p < 0.05$; $^{**}p < 0.01$.

15 min and washed by cold PBS. Erythrocytes were removed by RBC lysis buffer (Biolegend), cells were washed by PBS and transferred to fresh tubes through 70 mm nylon mesh. Finally, the cell suspension was resuspended in 1 ml PBS per sample. Spleen and liver were cut into small pieces and passed through tissue grinder to Petri dish, and then the cell suspension was passed through the 70 μm cell strainers and processed as mentioned above. Peripheral blood was collected into heparinized syringe, resuspend in PBS and spin down. Erythrocytes were removed by RBC lysis buffer and cells passed through the 70 μm cell strainer. Single cell suspensions were used for flow cytometry or PCR.

Flow Cytometry

Cells in single cell suspensions were stained in 100 μl aliquots of FACS buffer (2% FBS in PBS) after incubation with fluorochrome-labeled antibodies for 30 min at 4°C followed by washing in FACS buffer. Combination of surface markers for T-lymphocytes was CD45, CD4, and CD8 and myeloid cell subsets were stained for CD45, CD11b, CD11c, F4/80, and Ly6G using specific antibodies (Biolegend). Analysis was performed using a BD Biosciences FACSCanto® flow cytometer and FlowJo® software (TreeStar Inc., Olten, Switzerland).

Gene Expression

Total RNA was isolated from cell suspensions using Trizol LS Reagent (Life Technologies). RNA was converted to cDNA using gb Reverse Transcription Kit (Generi-Biotech, Czech Republic). Equal amounts of cDNA were analyzed by Real-Time quantitative PCR using gb Elite PCR Master Mix (Generi-Biotech, Czech Republic) on a LightCycler® 480 Real Time PCR System (Roche). Relative quantifications were performed using the comparative CT method with normalization to GAPDH and results expressed as fold difference relative to a relevant control sample. Primers and probes were from Qiagen: GAPDH (Mm99999915_g1), IL-17A (Mm00439618_m1), IFN-γ (Mm01168134_m1), IL-4 (Mm00445259_m1), TGF-β (Mm01178820_m1), IL-6 (Mm00446190_m1), IL-12 p35 (Mm00434165_m1).

Metagenomics Profiling

The microbial population present in the fecal samples from mice was determined using next generation high throughput sequencing of variable regions of the 16S rRNA bacterial gene. The workflow performed at VAIOMER (France) includes the steps of (i) Library construction and sequencing; (ii)

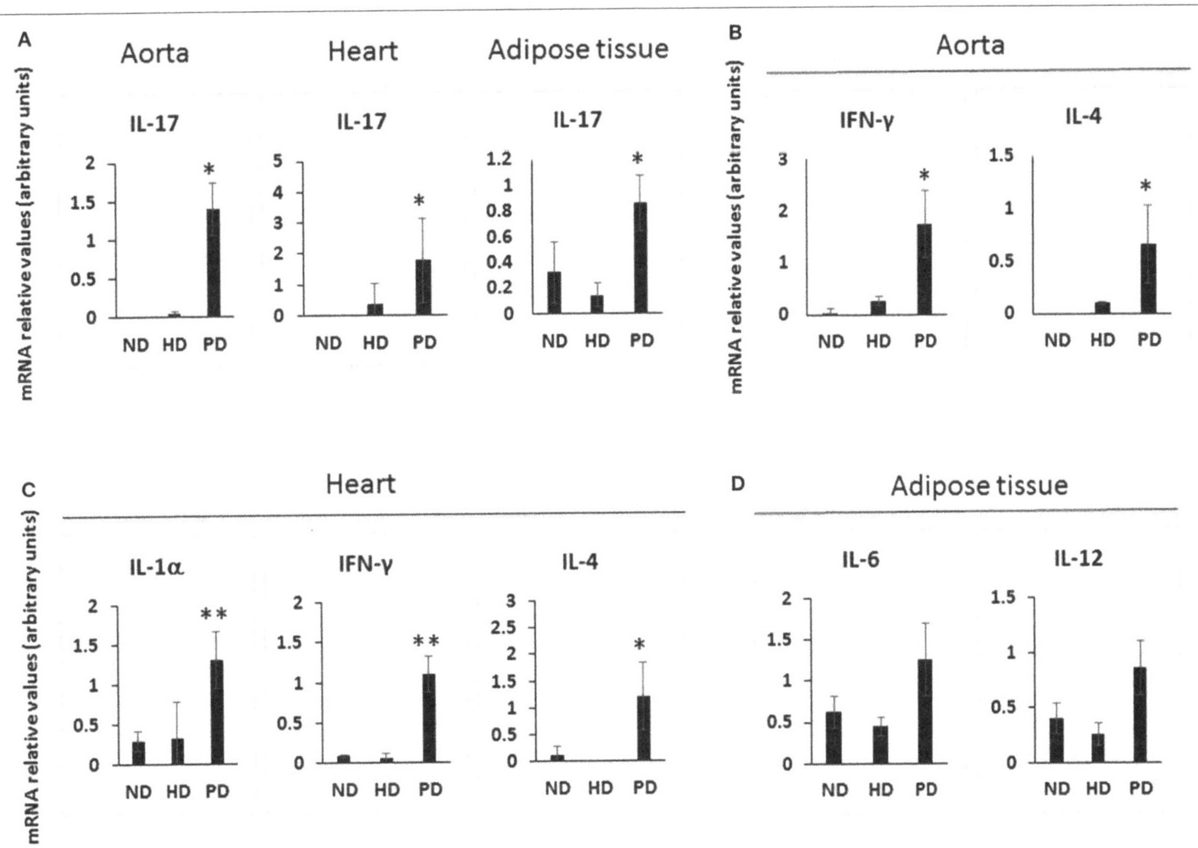

FIGURE 5 | Cytokine gene expression in the tissues of Normal diet (ND)-, High fat diet (HD)-, and Paigen diet (PD)-fed mice. Single cell suspensions were prepared from solid tissues (aorta, heart, and abdominal fat), and used for total RNA extraction and for qPCR. Relative quantification of IL-17A, IFN-γ, IL-4, TGF-β, IL-1α, IL-12, and IL-6 mRNA levels were performed using the comparative CT method with normalization to GAPDH; results were expressed as fold difference relative to a relevant control sample. **(A)** IL-17 mRNA levels in the aorta, heart and adipose tissue. **(B)** IFN-γ and IL-4 mRNA levels in the aorta. **(C)** IL-1α, IFN-γ, and IL-4 mRNA levels in the heart. **(D)** IL-6 and IL-12 mRNA levels in the adipose tissue. $N = 3–4$. $^{*}p < 0.05$; $^{**}p < 0.01$.

PCR amplification was performed using 16S universal primers targeting the V3–V4 region of the bacterial 16S ribosomal gene (Vaiomer universal 16S primers). The joint pair length was set to encompass 476 base pairs amplicon thanks to 2 × 300 paired-end MiSeq kit V3. For each sample, a sequencing library was generated by addition of sequencing adapters. The detection of the sequencing fragments was performed using MiSeq Illumina® technology; (iii) Bioinformatics pipeline, The targeted metagenomic sequences from microbiota were analyzed using the bioinformatics pipeline established by Vaiomer from the FROGS v1.3.0 guidelines. Briefly, after demultiplexing of the bar coded Illumina paired reads, single read sequences are cleaned and paired for each sample independently into longer fragments. Operational taxonomic units (OTU) are produced via single-linkage clustering and taxonomic assignment is performed in order to determine community profiles. PhyloSeq v1.14.0 R package was used to provide a set of classes and tools to facilitate the import, storage, analysis, and graphical display of microbiome census data. The samples with <5,000 sequences after FROGS processing were not included in the statistics (rarefaction analysis, alpha diversity, beta diversity-multidimensional scaling). The raw sequencing data are available upon request.

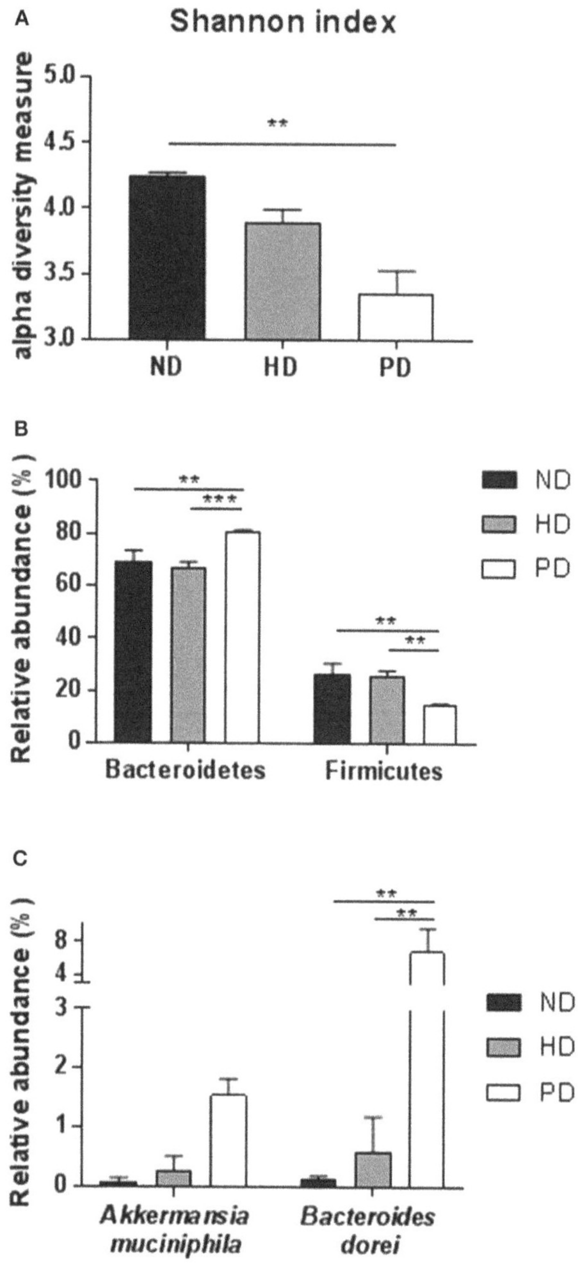

FIGURE 6 | (A) Alpha diversity using Shannon index of the fecal microbiota for each groups. **(B)** Relative abundance of major Phylum (Bacteroidetes and Firmicutes) for each group. **(C)** Relative abundance of most significant species, using RDP v11.4 databank in fecal samples of ND, HD, or PD mice. Graphs are displayed as mean ± SEM. $^{**}p < 0.01$; $^{***}p < 0.001$, One-Way Anova followed by Kruskal–Wallis test.

LEfSe Method

The OTU files generated were uploaded and formatted for LEfSe analysis using the per sample normalization of sum values option. The linear discriminant analysis effect size was determined using default values (alpha value of 0.5 for both the factorial Kruskal–Wallis test among classes and the pairwise Wilcoxon test between subclasses, threshold of 2.0 for the logarithmic LDA score for discriminative features) and the strategy for multi-class analysis set to "allagainst-all." LEfSe cladograms from the LDS effect size data were generated with Bacteria as the tree root. Differential features detected as biomarkers from the raw data used to generate the cladograms were plotted as abundance histograms with class and subclass information.

Statistical Methods

The parametric Student's *t*-test (2-sample *t*-test) was used to compare the difference in mean of immune cells by type of diet (HD vs. ND), and difference in mean of cytokines by type of diet (HD vs. ND). The non-parametric Mann-Whitney *U*-test was also used to check if the results were basically similar to the *t*-test using GraphPad Prism Software (version 5.00 for Windows, San Diego, CA, USA): a $p < 0.05$ was considered significant. To explore the association of gut microbiota with immune cells and cytokines levels, analyses were carried out using STATA/SE software. As preliminary analysis, mean and standard deviation (SD) of each gut microbiota type and adaptive immune system parameters measured in the aorta, heart, liver, spleen, and fat were calculated. The Pearson's correlations between each gut microbiota and adaptive immune system parameters were also examined. In the final analysis, associations between gut microbiota and adaptive immune system parameters levels were explored by using linear regression models. In each of the models, the associations between each bacterial taxa and adaptive immune system parameters were reported as absolute difference (β), with 95% Confidence Intervals (CI), in immune system parameters levels by % of increase in the proportion of the bacterial taxa. Coefficient of determination (R^2) was also reported.

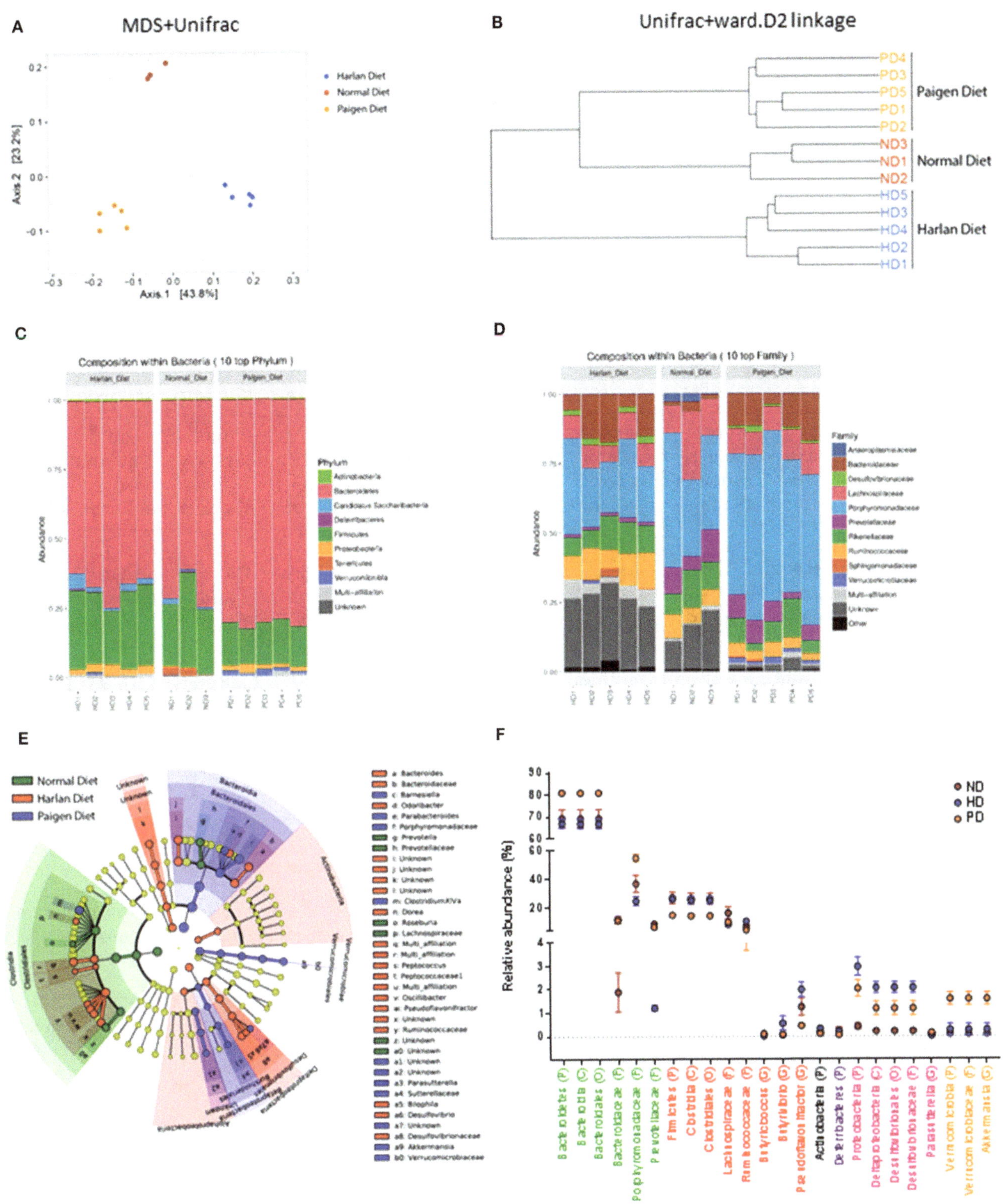

FIGURE 7 | Gut microbiota profiling in Normal diet (ND)-, High fat diet (HD)-, and Paigen diet (PD)-fed mice. **(A)** Multi Dimentional Scaling (MSD) of Unifrac distances of the fecal microbiota for each groups. **(B)** Hierarchical clustering of Unifrac distances of the fecal microbiota for each groups. **(C,D)** Relative abundance of Phylum and Family, respectively for each fecal sample. **(E)** Cladogram representing taxa enriched in fecal samples of ND, HD, or PD mice detected by the LEfSe tool. **(F)** Relative abundance of most significant taxa in fecal samples of ND, HD, or PD mice. Graphs are displayed as mean ± SEM.

TABLE 1 | Associations from linear models between gut microbiota and alterations of adaptive immune system parameters measured in the Aorta.

	IL-17 β (95% CI)	IFNg β (95% CI)	IL-4 β (95% CI)	TGFb β (95% CI)	IL-6 β (95% CI)	Lymphocytes β (95% CI)	CD45+ β (95% CI)	CD4+ β (95% CI)	CD8+ β (95% CI)
Actinobacteria	−2.0 (−6.1, 2.1) p = 0.287 R2 = 0.159	−1.7 (−7.0, 3.5) p = 0.459 R^2 = 0.081	−1.0 (−3.1, 1.0) p = 0.271 R^2 = 0.169	−32.5 (−101.3, 36.3) p = 0.301 R^2 = 0.151	−8.9 (−24.2, 6.5) p = 0.214 R^2 = 0.211	35.7 (−84.2, 155.5) p = 0.526 R^2 = 0.037	25.2 (−85.6, 136.1) p = 0.626 R^2 = 0.022	−30.2 (−63.5, 3.1) p = 0.071 R^2 = 0.290	−16.5 (−42.8, 9.8) p = 0.195 R^2 = 0.147
Alphaproteobacteria	0.1 (−0.6, 0.8) p = 0.815 R^2 = 0.008	0.1 (−0.7, 1.0) p = 0.727 R^2 = 0.018	0.1 (−0.3, 0.4) p = 0.624 R^2 = 0.036	−6.0 (−16.5, 4.5) p = 0.219 R^2 = 0.207	0.4 (−2.3, 3.1) p = 0.725 R^2 = 0.019	7.8 (−11.8, 27.5) p = 0.399 R^2 = 0.066	6.9 (−11.2, 25.0) p = 0.417 R^2 = 0.061	0.6 (−5.1, 6.2) p = 0.833 R^2 = 0.005	0.8 (−3.9, 5.5) p = 0.715 R^2 = 0.013
Bacilli	−0.1 (−0.7, 0.5) p = 0.642 R^2 = 0.033	−0.1 (−0.8, 0.6) p = 0.753 R^2 = 0.015	−0.0 (−0.3, 0.3) p = 0.876 R^2 = 0.004	−1.3 (−11.5, 8.8) p = 0.764 R^2 = 0.014	−0.2 (−2.6, 2.1) p = 0.837 R^2 = 0.006	−2.1 (−19.5, 15.3) p = 0.795 R^2 = 0.006	−2.0 (−18.0, 14.0) p = 0.791 R^2 = 0.007	−1.8 (−6.6, 2.9) p = 0.412 R^2 = 0.068	−1.6 (−5.5, 2.4) p = 0.405 R^2 = 0.064
Bacteroidia	**0.07** **(0.02, 0.12)** **p = 0.012** **R^2 = 0.615**	**0.09** **(0.02, 0.15)** **p = 0.018** **R^2 = 0.576**	**0.03** **(0.00, 0.06)** **p = 0.035** **R^2 = 0.492**	−0.5 (−1.8, 0.8) p = 0.370 R^2 = 0.116	**0.2** **(0.0, 0.5)** **p = 0.043** **R^2 = 0.465**	0.5 (−1.4, 2.5) p = 0.564 R^2 = 0.031	0.3 (−1.5, 2.1) p = 0.684 R^2 = 0.016	0.5 (−0.0, 0.9) p = 0.055 R^2 = 0.321	**0.4** **(0.0, 0.8)** **p = 0.043** **R^2 = 0.323**
Betaproteobacteria	**7.6** **(0.7, 14.6)** **p = 0.036** **R^2 = 0.490**	8.3 (−1.1, 17.6) p = 0.076 R^2 = 0.382	3.2 (−0.8, 7.2) p = 0.103 R^2 = 0.334	9.4 (−154.1, 172.9) p = 0.896 R^2 = 0.003	24.4 (−6.4, 55.2) p = 0.104 R^2 = 0.333	41.4 (−139.0, 221.8) p = 0.623 R^2 = 0.023	30.5 (−135.7, 196.8) p = 0.694 R^2 = 0.015	38.5 (−5.2, 82.3) p = 0.078 R^2 = 0.278	35.1 (−0.6, 70.7) p = 0.053 R^2 = 0.299
Clostridia	**−0.07** **(−0.13, −0.01)** **p = 0.021** **R^2 = 0.554**	**−0.09** **(−0.16, −0.02)** **p = 0.020** **R^2 = 0.563**	**−0.03** **(−0.10, −0.00)** **p = 0.033** **R^2 = 0.500**	1.0 (−0.2, 2.2) p = 0.094 R^2 = 0.349	−0.3 (−0.5, 0.0) p = 0.052 R^2 = 0.440	−1.0 (−3.1, 1.1) p = 0.305 R^2 = 0.095	−0.8 (−2.7, 1.2) p = 0.409 R^2 = 0.063	−0.5 (−1.0, 0.1) p = 0.073 R^2 = 0.286	**−0.4** **(−0.9, −0.0)** **p = 0.044** **R^2 = 0.319**
Deferribacteres	−1.7 (−5.0, 1.7) p = 0.285 R^2 = 0.161	−1.8 (−6.0, 2.4) p = 0.349 R^2 = 0.126	−0.6 (−2.3, 1.2) p = 0.483 R^2 = 0.073	23.0 (−35.6, 81.6) p = 0.384 R^2 = 0.110	−3.9 (−17.8, 10.1) p = 0.533 R^2 = 0.058	−45.0 (−142.6, 52.5) p = 0.332 R^2 = 0.086	−35.1 (−125.7, 55.6) p = 0.413 R^2 = 0.062	−18.8 (−45.1, 7.5) p = 0.142 R^2 = 0.202	−19.2 (−39.3, 1.0) p = 0.060 R^2 = 0.285
Deltaproteobacteria	0.2 (−0.5, 0.9) p = 0.496 R^2 = 0.069	0.4 (−0.4, 1.1) p = 0.298 R^2 = 0.153	0.2 (−0.2, 0.5) p = 0.267 R^2 = 0.172	**−9.0** **(−17.3, −0.7)** **p = 0.037** **R^2 = 0.485**	1.0 (−1.5, 3.5) p = 0.364 R^2 = 0.118	12.0 (−3.6, 27.6) p = 0.120 R^2 = 0.205	9.2 (−5.6, 24.1) p = 0.198 R^2 = 0.146	−1.3 (−6.7, 4.0) p = 0.594 R^2 = 0.029	−0.7 (−4.7, 3.4) p = 0.722 R^2 = 0.012
Erysipelotrichia	−1.0 (−3.4, 1.5) p = 0.377 R^2 = 0.113	−1.0 (−4.1, 2.0) p = 0.460 R^2 = 0.080	−0.3 (−1.6, 0.9) p = 0.557 R^2 = 0.051	−16.5 (−57.5, 24.5) p = 0.373 R^2 = 0.114	−3.2 (−12.8, 6.5) p = 0.465 R^2 = 0.079	32.6 (−39.8, 105.1) p = 0.342 R^2 = 0.082	31.2 (−35.0, 97.4) p = 0.322 R^2 = 0.089	−6.6 (−28.2, 14.9) p = 0.507 R^2 = 0.045	−4.0 (−21.5, 13.4) p = 0.621 R^2 = 0.023
Gammaproteobacteria	3.5 (−11.1, 18.0) p = 0.590 R^2 = 0.044	4.9 (−12.8, 22.6) p = 0.534 R^2 = 0.058	−1.9 (−9.2, 5.4) p = 0.558 R^2 = 0.051	−118.3 (−345.4, 108.7) p = 0.257 R^2 = 0.178	−21.9 (−76.3, 32.4) p = 0.372 R^2 = 0.115	106.9 (−106.6, 320.4) p = 0.294 R^2 = 0.100	71.4 (−129.6, 272.3) p = 0.451 R^2 = 0.053	−28.1 (−88.3, 32.1) p = 0.324 R^2 = 0.097	−4.8 (−57.2, 47.6) p = 0.845 R^2 = 0.004
Mollicutes	−0.2 (−0.7, 0.2) p = 0.298 R^2 = 0.153	−0.3 (−0.9, 0.3) p = 0.269 R^2 = 0.171	−0.1 (−0.4, 0.1) p = 0.276 R^2 = 0.167	5.6 (−1.5, 12.7) p = 0.105 R^2 = 0.331	−0.7 (−2.6, 1.2) p = 0.414 R^2 = 0.097	**−14.9** **(−25.9, −3.9)** **p = 0.013** **R^2 = 0.445**	**−12.5** **(−23.3, −1.7)** **p = 0.027** **R^2 = 0.370**	−1.7 (−5.7, 2.3) p = 0.370 R^2 = 0.081	−2.2 (−5.3, 0.9) p = 0.150 R^2 = 0.179

(Continued)

TABLE 1 | Continued

	IL-17 β (95% CI)	IFNg β (95% CI)	IL-4 β (95% CI)	TGFb β (95% CI)	IL-6 β (95% CI)	Lymphocytes β (95% CI)	CD45+ β (95% CI)	CD4+ β (95% CI)	CD8+ β (95% CI)
Multi-affiliation	−1.4 (−3.5, 0.7) $p = 0.161$ $R^2 = 0.260$	−1.5 (−4.2, 1.2) $p = 0.236$ $R^2 = 0.193$	−0.6 (−1.7, 0.6) $p = 0.270$ $R^2 = 0.170$	−9.2 (−49.7, 31.3) $p = 0.608$ $R^2 = 0.040$	−4.8 (−13.3, 3.7) $p = 0.220$ $R^2 = 0.206$	10.2 (−20.9, 41.3) $p = 0.484$ $R^2 = 0.045$	7.2 (−21.6, 36.0) $p = 0.595$ $R^2 = 0.026$	−0.6 (−9.4, 8.3) $p = 0.891$ $R^2 = 0.002$	0.9 (−6.5, 8.3) $p = 0.799$ $R^2 = 0.006$
Negativicutes	2.1 (−2.6, 6.7) $p = 0.332$ $R^2 = 0.134$	2.7 (−3.0, 8.3) $p = 0.297$ $R^2 = 0.154$	−0.3 (−2.8, 2.2) $p = 0.792$ $R^2 = 0.011$	−32.4 (−111.5, 46.8) $p = 0.366$ $R^2 = 0.118$	−4.2 (−23.2, 14.9) $p = 0.622$ $R^2 = 0.037$	52.8 (−87.0, 192.6) $p = 0.423$ $R^2 = 0.059$	35.8 (−94.3, 165.9) $p = 0.557$ $R^2 = 0.032$	2.3 (−45.7, 50.3) $p = 0.918$ $R^2 = 0.001$	8.4 (−24.7, 41.6) $p = 0.587$ $R^2 = 0.028$
Verrucomicrobiae	**0.5** **(0.1, 1.0)** $\mathbf{p = 0.027}$ $\mathbf{R^2 = 0.526}$	0.6 (−0.0, 1.2) $p = 0.057$ $R^2 = 0.425$	0.2 (0.1, 0.5) $p = 0.100$ $R^2 = 0.338$	−6.4 (−16.2, 3.3) $p = 0.164$ $R^2 = 0.257$	1.5 (−0.7, 3.8) $p = 0.147$ $R^2 = 0.276$	14.9 (−0.3, 30.2) $p = 0.054$ $R^2 = 0.297$	13.8 (−0.2, 27.8) $p = 0.052$ $R^2 = 0.301$	**6.4** **(3.9, 8.9)** $\mathbf{p < 0.001}$ $\mathbf{R^2 = 0.761}$	**5.5** **(3.4, 7.7)** $\mathbf{p < 0.001}$ $\mathbf{R^2 = 0.750}$

In each of the models, the associations are reported as absolute difference (β), with 95% Confidence Intervals (CI), in immune system parameters levels by 1 unit increase in gut microbiota. In bold are reported the statistically significant results ($p < 0.05$). Per each of the models, the Coefficient of determination (R^2) is also reported.

RESULTS

Modeling Healthy Obesity and Metabolic Syndrome during Leanness in Mice

To model diets able to mimic MSL and MHO conditions in humans, three groups ($N = 10$) of 4 weeks old C57/BL6 mice were fed different dietary regimens: (i) a control normal diet (ND, 21.2% kcal from proteins, 58% kcal from carbohydrate, and 17% from fat); (ii) high fat diet, rich in fatty acids (HD, 21.2% kcal from proteins, 24% kcal from carbohydrate, and 58% from fat) and with 0.1% cholesterol, and (iii) atherogenic/inflammatory Paigen diet (PD), containing similar composition of the normal diet with in addition 1.25% cholesterol and 0.5% sodium cholate (**Figure 1A**). C57/BL6 mice had similar baseline weight before starting being fed the diets (mean = ∼21 ± 0.4 g). After 15 weeks of dietary regimens, body weight was unchanged in mice on the control ND or the PD, which both increased body weight during growth by ∼33% (ND = 28.3 ± 0.7 g and PD = 28.8 ± 0.77 g, respectively, **Figure 1B**). In contrast, mice on the HD gained ∼65% in weight (HD = 35.9 ± 0.6 g), compared to their baseline, indicating that only HD diet was obesogenic ($p < 0.001$ vs. ND and vs. PD). We then examined glucose and insulin levels at the end of the dietary treatment. Basal insulin and glucose fasting levels were considerably higher in PD vs. ND and HD (**Figures 2A,B**). A similar trend was observed for serum triglycerides and cholesterol levels, which were highest in the PD group vs. ND and HD (**Figures 2C,D**). Obesogenic HD regimen triggered lipid accumulation in the liver under the form of simple steatosis, whereas atherogenic/inflammatory PD regimen induced NAFLD/NASH at the end of its pathologic spectrum, characterized by lipid accumulation, ballooning, fibrosis, and inflammatory infiltrates, as quantified by NAFLD/NASH score (**Figure 1C** upper panels, **Figure 1D**), consistent with previous finding that the cholesterol and cholate components of Paigen diet induces genes involved in inflammation and fibrosis, respectively, in the liver (Vergnes et al., 2003). Cross-sectional analysis of aortas walls suggested an increased infiltration of inflammatory cells in the PD-fed mice, in comparison to ND or HD fed mice (**Figure 1C**, lower panels). Altogether, these data indicate that PD triggers prominent features of metabolic syndrome and inflammation in mice in absence of weight gain, compared to obesogenic HD.

Dissecting Diet-Dependent Intra-Tissue Adaptive Immune Changes

Cells of the innate immune system, in particular macrophages, mediate chronic inflammation (Sell et al., 2012). Moreover, B and T lymphocytes of the adaptive immune system have been recently recognized as important modulators of glucose homeostasis, indicating that antigen-driven immune responses could influence insulin resistance. Like macrophages, lymphocytes can be divided into populations with primarily proinflammatory functions (including CD8+ cytotoxic T cells, Th1, Th17) or primarily regulatory functions (including Treg or Th2) and the skewing of the adaptive immune milieu toward a proinflammatory phenotype can exacerbate the metabolic disturbances associated to obesity (Nishimura et al., 2009; Winer et al., 2009; Shen et al., 2015). Moreover, it is known since 1980 that T lymphocyte subsets and related cytokines are present in atherosclerotic lesions and affect their development (Lichtman, 2013). Here, to analyze the changes of adaptive immunity between MSL and MHO, we analyzed T cell populations from the blood and the spleen (secondary lymphoid organ), from the heart and the aorta (cardiovascular tissue), from the liver and from the adipose tissue (metabolic and nutrient hubs) of ND, PD, and HD-fed mice, using the flow cytometry gating strategy depicted in **Figure 2**. Briefly, CD4+ and CD8+ T cells were identified from the CD45+ lymphocyte populations, whereas to study the myeloid lineage, CD11b+ subpopulation was further analyzed for Ly6G+ cells (neutrophils), CD11b+CD11c+ cells

TABLE 2 | Associations from linear regression models between gut microbiota and alterations of adaptive immune system parameters measured in the heart.

	IL-17 β (95% CI)	IFNg β (95% CI)	IL-4 β (95% CI)	IL-1α β (95% CI)	IL-6 β (95% CI)	Lymphocytes β (95% CI)	CD45+ β (95% CI)	CD4+ β (95% CI)	CD8+ β (95% CI)
Actinobacteria	−1.6 (−8.4, 5.2) $p = 0.602$ $R^2 = 0.041$	−1.8 (−4.7, 1.1) $p = 0.178$ $R^2 = 0.243$	−3 (−8.6, 2.5) $p = 0.201$ $R^2 = 0.368$	−1.5 (−4.9, 1.9) $p = 0.321$ $R^2 = 0.140$	−6 (−15.0, 3.0) $p = 0.157$ $R^2 = 0.264$	65 (−39.7, 169.7) $p = 0.199$ $R^2 = 0.145$	55.1 (−45.7, 156.0) $p = 0.254$ $R^2 = 0.116$	**−30.9** **(−58.7, −3.1)** $\mathbf{p = 0.032}$ $\mathbf{R^2 = 0.353}$	−7.1 (−35.7, 21.5) $p = 0.597$ $R^2 = 0.026$
Alphaproteobacteria	0.1 (−1.0, 1.2) $p = 0.882$ $R^2 = 0.003$	0 (−0.5, 0.6) $p = 0.900$ $R^2 = 0.002$	−0.1 (−1.1, 0.9) $p = 0.751$ $R^2 = 0.028$	0 (−0.6, 0.5) $p = 0.848$ $R^2 = 0.006$	0.2 (−1.4, 1.9) $p = 0.773$ $R^2 = 0.013$	−1.1 (−20.0, 17.7) $p = 0.896$ $R^2 = 0.002$	3.4 (−14.3, 21.1) $p = 0.680$ $R^2 = 0.016$	0.4 (−5.3, 6.2) $p = 0.879$ $R^2 = 0.002$	1.1 (−3.7, 5.9) $p = 0.625$ $R^2 = 0.022$
Bacilli	−0.1 (−1.1, 0.8) $p = 0.740$ $R^2 = 0.017$	−0.1 (−0.6, 0.3) $p = 0.570$ $R^2 = 0.048$	−0.2 (−1.0, 0.6) $p = 0.485$ $R^2 = 0.129$	−0.2 (−0.7, 0.2) $p = 0.283$ $R^2 = 0.162$	−0.2 (−1.7, 1.2) $p = 0.709$ $R^2 = 0.021$	2.9 (−13.2, 19.0) $p = 0.697$ $R^2 = 0.014$	1.9 (−13.5, 17.2) $p = 0.795$ $R^2 = 0.006$	−1.2 (−6.1, 3.7) $p = 0.597$ $R^2 = 0.026$	−0.3 (−4.4, 3.9) $p = 0.894$ $R^2 = 0.002$
Bacteroidia	0.1 (−0.0, 0.2) $p = 0.094$ $R^2 = 0.349$	**0.1** **(0.0, 0.1)** $\mathbf{p = 0.011}$ $\mathbf{R^2 = 0.628}$	**0.2** **(0.1, 0.3)** $\mathbf{p = 0.014}$ $\mathbf{R^2 = 0.814}$	0 (−0.0, 0.1) $p = 0.053$ $R^2 = 0.437$	**0.2** **(0.0, 0.3)** $\mathbf{p = 0.033}$ $\mathbf{R^2 = 0.501}$	**−1.6** **(−3.1, −0.2)** $\mathbf{p = 0.034}$ $\mathbf{R^2 = 0.349}$	−0.6 (−2.3, 1.1) $p = 0.490$ $R^2 = 0.044$	**0.6** **(0.2, 1.0)** $\mathbf{p = 0.009}$ $\mathbf{R^2 = 0.480}$	0.3 (−0.1, 0.7) $p = 0.119$ $R^2 = 0.207$
Betaproteobacteria	8.1 (−5.3, 21.5) $p = 0.196$ $R^2 = 0.226$	**5.9** **(0.8, 10.9)** $\mathbf{p = 0.029}$ $\mathbf{R^2 = 0.518}$	8.1 (−2.0, 18.1) $p = 0.090$ $R^2 = 0.553$	**6.1** **(0.4, 11.9)** $\mathbf{p = 0.041}$ $\mathbf{R^2 = 0.473}$	16.7 (−0.7, 34.2) $p = 0.058$ $R^2 = 0.423$	−98.3 (−254.5, 57.8) $p = 0.193$ $R^2 = 0.149$	−28.3 (−187.4, 130.9) $p = 0.703$ $R^2 = 0.014$	**58.5** **(24.4, 92.5)** $\mathbf{p = 0.003}$ $\mathbf{R^2 = 0.564}$	12.5 (−30.0, 55.0) $p = 0.531$ $R^2 = 0.037$
Clostridia	−0.1 (−0.2, 0.0) $p = 0.095$ $R^2 = 0.347$	**−0.1** **(−0.1, −0.0)** $\mathbf{p = 0.023}$ $\mathbf{R^2 = 0.547}$	−0.1 (−0.3, 0.0) $p = 0.086$ $R^2 = 0.563$	0 (−0.1, 0.0) $p = 0.083$ $R^2 = 0.369$	**−0.2** **(−0.3, −0.0)** $\mathbf{p = 0.045}$ $\mathbf{R^2 = 0.458}$	**1.7** **(0.1, 3.4)** $\mathbf{p = 0.042}$ $\mathbf{R^2 = 0.324}$	0.5 (−1.4, 2.4) $p = 0.544$ $R^2 = 0.034$	**−0.6** **(−1.1, −0.1)** $\mathbf{p = 0.017}$ $\mathbf{R^2 = 0.417}$	−0.4 (−0.8, 0.1) $p = 0.113$ $R^2 = 0.212$
Deferribacteres	−0.7 (−6.4, 5.1) $p = 0.789$ $R^2 = 0.011$	−1.1 (−3.7, 1.4) $p = 0.323$ $R^2 = 0.139$	4.5 (−9.2, 18.2) $p = 0.411$ $R^2 = 0.174$	−1.2 (−4.1, 1.6) $p = 0.334$ $R^2 = 0.133$	−3 (−11.3, 5.3) $p = 0.424$ $R^2 = 0.093$	34.3 (−57.5, 126.1) $p = 0.428$ $R^2 = 0.058$	−23.7 (−111.9, 64.5) $p = 0.566$ $R^2 = 0.031$	−15.9 (−42.8, 10.9) $p = 0.218$ $R^2 = 0.134$	−9.8 (−33.1, 13.5) $p = 0.375$ $R^2 = 0.072$
Deltaproteobacteria	0.7 (−0.1, 1.6) $p = 0.074$ $R^2 = 0.387$	0.2 (−0.3, 0.6) $p = 0.485$ $R^2 = 0.072$	0.7 (−0.2, 1.5) $p = 0.086$ $R^2 = 0.562$	0.2 (−0.4, 0.7) $p = 0.516$ $R^2 = 0.063$	0.5 (−1.1, 2.0) $p = 0.490$ $R^2 = 0.070$	−2.2 (−18.4, 13.9) $p = 0.767$ $R^2 = 0.008$	−6.5 (−21.2, 8.3) $p = 0.356$ $R^2 = 0.078$	−0.5 (−5.4, 4.4) $p = 0.829$ $R^2 = 0.004$	0.3 (−3.8, 4.5) $p = 0.870$ $R^2 = 0.003$
Erysipelotrichia	−0.8 (−4.8, 3.2) $p = 0.636$ $R^2 = 0.034$	−0.8 (−2.6, 1.1) $p = 0.359$ $R^2 = 0.121$	−66.6 (−257.8, 124.7) $p = 0.389$ $R^2 = 0.189$	−0.7 (−2.7, 1.3) $p = 0.434$ $R^2 = 0.090$	−2 (−7.9, 3.8) $p = 0.436$ $R^2 = 0.089$	26.4 (−41.5, 94.2) $p = 0.411$ $R^2 = 0.062$	3.5 (−62.8, 69.8) $p = 0.910$ $R^2 = 0.001$	−8.8 (−29.4, 11.7) $p = 0.365$ $R^2 = 0.075$	−5.9 (−23.4, 11.7) $p = 0.477$ $R^2 = 0.047$
Gammaproteobacteria	−5 (−27.8, 17.9) $p = 0.624$ $R^2 = 0.036$	−0.4 (−11.5, 10.7) $p = 0.939$ $R^2 = 0.001$	−5.3 (−23.8, 13.2) $p = 0.473$ $R^2 = 0.136$	−2.5 (−14.5, 9.5) $p = 0.639$ $R^2 = 0.033$	−11.9 (−45.4, 21.7) $p = 0.430$ $R^2 = 0.091$	4.1 (−204.5, 212.7) $p = 0.966$ $R^2 = 0.000$	35.4 (−160.7, 231.6) $p = 0.699$ $R^2 = 0.014$	−35.8 (−94.8, 23.3) $p = 0.209$ $R^2 = 0.139$	10.9 (−42.0, 63.8) $p = 0.659$ $R^2 = 0.018$
Mollicutes	−0.3 (−1.1, 0.4) $p = 0.322$ $R^2 = 0.140$	−0.2 (−0.5, 0.2) $p = 0.329$ $R^2 = 0.136$	−0.3 (−1.1, 0.5) $p = 0.373$ $R^2 = 0.201$	−0.2 (−0.6, 0.2) $p = 0.398$ $R^2 = 0.104$	−0.5 (−1.6, 0.7) $p = 0.378$ $R^2 = 0.113$	3.9 (−9.6, 17.4) $p = 0.540$ $R^2 = 0.035$	1 (−12.0, 14.0) $p = 0.868$ $R^2 = 0.003$	−1.5 (−5.6, 2.6) $p = 0.433$ $R^2 = 0.057$	−1.1 (−4.5, 2.4) $p = 0.504$ $R^2 = 0.042$

(Continued)

TABLE 2 | Continued

	IL-17 β (95% CI)	IFNg β (95% CI)	IL-4 β (95% CI)	IL-1α β (95% CI)	IL-6 β (95% CI)	Lymphocytes β (95% CI)	CD45+ β (95% CI)	CD4+ β (95% CI)	CD8+ β (95% CI)
Multi-affiliation	−1.3	−1.1	−4.9	−1.1	−3.2	6.7	5.6	0.4	−2.2
	(−4.9, 2.4)	(−2.6, 0.5)	(−13.7, 3.9)	(−2.8, 0.7)	(−8.3, 1.8)	(−22.5, 35.8)	(−22.0, 33.3)	(−8.6, 9.4)	(−9.6, 5.2)
	$p = 0.443$	$p = 0.139$	$p = 0.196$	$p = 0.192$	$p = 0.177$	$p = 0.625$	$p = 0.662$	$p = 0.922$	$p = 0.527$
	$R^2 = 0.086$	$R^2 = 0.285$	$R^2 = 0.375$	$R^2 = 0.230$	$R^2 = 0.244$	$R^2 = 0.022$	$R^2 = 0.018$	$R^2 = 0.001$	$R^2 = 0.037$
Negativicutes	1.3	0.8	0.1	1.3	−1.8	−68.7	35.8	−19.6	**32.3**
	(−6.5, 9.0)	(−2.9, 4.5)	(−7.5, 7.8)	(−2.7, 5.2)	(−13.5, 10.0)	(−194.3, 57.0)	(−88.6, 160.1)	(−58.3, 19.0)	**(5.7, 59.0)**
	$p = 0.706$	$p = 0.629$	$p = 0.964$	$p = 0.470$	$p = 0.732$	$p = 0.254$	$p = 0.540$	$p = 0.287$	**$p = 0.022$**
	$R^2 = 0.022$	$R^2 = 0.035$	$R^2 = 0.001$	$R^2 = 0.077$	$R^2 = 0.018$	$R^2 = 0.116$	$R^2 = 0.035$	$R^2 = 0.102$	**$R^2 = 0.394$**
Verrucomicrobiae	0.6	**0.4**	0.4	**0.6**	1.2	−10.6	2.9	**4.4**	3.1
	(−0.4, 1.5)	**(0.1, 0.8)**	(−0.5, 1.2)	**(0.4, 0.8)**	(−0.1, 2.4)	(−25.9, 4.8)	(−13.0, 18.8)	**(0.1, 8.6)**	(−0.7, 6.9)
	$p = 0.195$	**$p = 0.025$**	$p = 0.303$	**$p = 0.000$**	$p = 0.058$	$p = 0.158$	$p = 0.696$	**$p = 0.044$**	$p = 0.097$
	$R^2 = 0.227$	**$R^2 = 0.534$**	$R^2 = 0.258$	**$R^2 = 0.850$**	$R^2 = 0.423$	$R^2 = 0.173$	$R^2 = 0.014$	**$R^2 = 0.319$**	R2 = 0.231

In each of the models, the associations are reported as absolute difference (β), with 95% Confidence Intervals (CI), in immune system parameters levels by 1 unit increase in gut microbiota. In bold are reported the statistically significant results ($p < 0.05$). Per each of the models, the Coefficient of determination (R^2) is also reported.

(conventional dendritic cells), and CD11b+CD11c-F4/80+ cells (macrophages; **Figure 3**). In parallel, we measured by qPCR the intra-tissue expression levels of the following panel of cytokines that play a major role in the adaptive immune system being secreted by helper CD4+ T cells (Th1, Th2, Th17, and Treg) and stimulating several cell types: IL-1α, IL-4, IL-6, IL-12, IL-17 and IFN-γ. IL-1α, IL-12, IL 17, and IFN-γ are generally regarded as pro-inflammatory and pro-atherogenic, while IL-4 and IL-6 display pro- and anti-inflammatory properties which are context-dependent (Hunter and Jones, 2015; Zarzycka et al., 2015). Our analyses showed a great enrichment in myeloid cells, CD45+, CD11b+, CD11c, F480+, Ly6G+ upon PD- in the spleen compared to ND- and HD-feeding (**Figure 4A**), a massive lymphocyte infiltration in the aorta and in the liver upon both PD and HD compared to ND diet (**Figure 4B**), a significant increase in CD4+ and CD8+ positive cells percentage exclusively in the aorta and in the hearts of PD-fed animals compared to ND and HD (**Figure 4C**); no changes were observed in abdominal fat tissues (*data not shown*). At the cytokine level, IL-17 was greatly increased in the aorta, heart and fat only in PD-fed mice compared to HD and ND (**Figure 5A**). IL-1α, IFN-γ, and IL-4 levels were augmented in the aorta and/or in the heart only in PD-fed mice compared to HD and ND (**Figures 5B,C**). Finally, we report a trend in increased IL-6 and IL-12 mRNA levels in adipose tissue of PD mice compared to HD- and ND-fed mice (**Figure 5D**). Collectively, our data surprisingly indicate activation of several components of the adaptive immune system in the metabolic syndrome lean PD mouse model compared to an established mouse model of diet-induced obesity.

Gut Microbiota Profiling By Metagenomic Sequencing

The reciprocal interaction between the gut microbiota and the adaptive immunity contributes to the insurgence of metabolic diseases and of inflammation (Kato et al., 2014; Zhang and Luo, 2015; Marchesi et al., 2016). It is however unknown how this interplay adapts to the MSL or MHO clinical features. To this aim we identified bacterial populations contained in fecal samples from ND-, HD-, and PD-fed mice using next generation high throughput sequencing of variable regions (V3–V4) of the 16S rDNA bacterial gene (Lluch et al., 2015; Paisse et al., 2016). Alpha diversity analyses, representing the mean of species diversity in each sample showed that ND-fed mice had a higher taxonomic diversity than the HD-fed mice, which in turn have a higher taxonomic diversity than the PD-fed mice (**Figure 6A**). Feces microbial composition after 20 weeks of different diet is highly different between the three groups, as shown by beta diversity metrics based multi-dimensional scaling Unifrac analysis (**Figure 7A**) and by hierarchical clustering (**Figure 7B**). The community structures observed in the different groups were significantly different. At the phylum level, Firmicutes and Bacteroidetes dominated the fecal microbiota in all groups (**Figure 7C**). No differences of Firmicutes and Bacteroidetes relative abundance were observed between ND and HD groups (**Figure 7C**). However, an increase in Bacteroidetes and a decrease in Firmicutes were observed in PD groups (**Figure 6B**). At the family level, the fecal microbiota was dominated by Porphyromonadaceae in all groups (**Figure 7D**) and are significantly higher in Paigen Diet mice compared to HD and ND groups (**Figure 7F**). Focusing on diet effect between the three groups of mice, broad population changes were seen from phylum to genus level (**Figure 7E**), significantly enriched taxa for all groups are identified using LDA Effect Size (LEfSe) analysis. Clostridia class are significantly enriched in ND and HD mice compared to PD mice (**Figures 7E,F**). Actinobacteria and Deltaproteobacteria are enriched in HD group compared to ND and PD groups (**Figures 7E,F**). Bacteroidia and Verrucomicrobia are enriched in PD group compared to ND and HD groups (**Figures 7E,F**). Interestingly we have identified (with databank

TABLE 3 | Associations from linear regression models between gut microbiota and alterations of adaptive immune system parameters measured in the adipose tissue.

	IL-17 β (95% CI)	IL-12 β (95% CI)	IL-6 β (95% CI)
Actinobacteria	−1.6 (−3.4, 0.1) $p = 0.065$ $R^2 = 0.407$	**−1.6** **(−2.9, −0.4)** $\mathbf{p = 0.020}$ $\mathbf{R^2 = 0.564}$	−1.9 (−4.1, 0.2) $p = 0.071$ $R^2 = 0.393$
Alphaproteobacteria	0 (−0.4, 0.3) $p = 0.761$ $R^2 = 0.014$	0 (−0.3, 0.3) $p = 0.841$ $R^2 = 0.006$	0 (−0.5, 0.4) $p = 0.799$ $R^2 = 0.010$
Bacilli	−0.1 (−0.4, 0.1) $p = 0.294$ $R^2 = 0.155$	−0.1 (−0.3, 0.2) $p = 0.470$ $R^2 = 0.077$	−0.1 (−0.5, 0.3) $p = 0.561$ $R^2 = 0.050$
Bacteroidia	0.02 (−0.01, 0.06) $p = 0.186$ $R^2 = 0.235$	0.02 (−0.01, 0.05) $p = 0.093$ $R^2 = 0.350$	0.04 (−0.00, 0.07) $p = 0.072$ $R^2 = 0.390$
Betaproteobacteria	**5.1** **(3.0, 7.2)** $\mathbf{p = 0.001}$ $\mathbf{R^2 = 0.830}$	**3.7** **(1.0, 6.4)** $\mathbf{p = 0.014}$ $\mathbf{R^2 = 0.599}$	4.4 (−0.2, 9.1) $p = 0.058$ $R^2 = 0.423$
Clostridia	0 (−0.1, 0.0) $p = 0.315$ $R^2 = 0.143$	0 (−0.1, 0.0) $p = 0.185$ $R^2 = 0.236$	0 (−0.1, 0.0) $p = 0.148$ $R^2 = 0.274$
Deferribacteres	−0.4 (−2.3, 1.5) $p = 0.633$ $R^2 = 0.034$	−0.3 (−1.9, 1.3) $p = 0.660$ $R^2 = 0.029$	−0.3 (−2.6, 2.0) $p = 0.739$ $R^2 = 0.017$
Deltaproteobacteria	−0.1 (−0.4, 0.3) $p = 0.685$ $R^2 = 0.025$	0 (−0.3, 0.3) $p = 0.905$ $R^2 = 0.002$	0.1 (−0.3, 0.5) $p = 0.525$ $R^2 = 0.060$
Erysipelotrichia	−0.5 (−1.8, 0.7) $p = 0.367$ $R^2 = 0.117$	−0.4 (−1.5, 0.7) $p = 0.412$ $R^2 = 0.098$	−0.5 (−2.1, 1.0) $p = 0.452$ $R^2 = 0.083$
Gammaproteobacteria	0.4 (−7.3, 8.0) $p = 0.908$ $R^2 = 0.002$	−2.6 (−8.7, 3.5) $p = 0.346$ $R^2 = 0.127$	−2.5 (−11.5, 6.6) $p = 0.540$ $R^2 = 0.056$
Mollicutes	0 (−0.3, 0.2) $p = 0.840$ $R^2 = 0.006$	−0.1 (−0.3, 0.2) $p = 0.580$ $R^2 = 0.046$	−0.1 (−0.4, 0.2) $p = 0.471$ $R^2 = 0.077$

(Continued)

TABLE 3 | Continued

	IL-17 β (95% CI)	IL-12 β (95% CI)	IL-6 β (95% CI)
Multi-affiliation	−0.8 (−1.8, 0.2) $p = 0.111$ $R^2 = 0.321$	−0.6 (−1.5, 0.3) $p = 0.157$ $R^2 = 0.264$	−0.7 (−2.1, 0.7) $p = 0.252$ $R^2 = 0.182$
Negativicutes	0.7 (−1.8, 3.2) $p = 0.550$ $R^2 = 0.053$	−0.4 (−2.6, 1.7) $p = 0.654$ $R^2 = 0.030$	−0.1 (−3.2, 3.1) $p = 0.965$ $R^2 = 0.000$
Verrucomicrobiae	**0.3** **(0.1, 0.5)** $\mathbf{p = 0.022}$ $\mathbf{R^2 = 0.551}$	0.2 (−0.1, 0.4) $p = 0.106$ $R^2 = 0.330$	0.2 (−0.2, 0.6) $p = 0.258$ $R^2 = 0.178$

In each of the models, the associations are reported as absolute difference (β), with 95% Confidence Intervals (CI), in immune system parameters levels by 1 unit increase in gut microbiota. In bold are reported the statistically significant results ($p < 0.05$). Per each of the models, the Coefficient of determination (R^2) is also reported.

RDP v11.4) an increase in *Akkermansia muciniphila* and *Bacteroides dorei* in PD groups compared to HD and ND groups (**Figure 6C**). Therefore, the most striking result of our metagenomic analyses in gut microbiota composition between the MSL and MHO mimicking diets (PD and HD, respectively) is the preponderance of Bacteroidia and Verrucomicrobia in PD compared to HD and control ND.

Association of Gut Microbiota Profile with Adaptive Immune Factors

We then sought to explore correlation between changes in gut microbiota composition with the over-responses of the adaptive immune system in mice, irrespective of the diet administered, using linear regression. The associations from regression analyses between gut microbiota classes and cytokines or immune cell types are shown in full in **Tables 1–5**. Some statistically significant associations were observed in each of the organs analyzed (aorta, heart, adipose tissue, liver, and spleen). For example (1) a linear increase in *Bacteroidia* and a decrease in Clostridiae were associated to an increase in IL-17, IFN-γ, IL-4, and CD8+ cells in the aorta. A decrease in Mollicutes and an increase in Verrucomicrobia was associated to increased infiltration of leukocytes (CD45+) as well as CD4+ and in CD8+ T cells and to an increase in IL-17, in the aorta (**Table 1**); (2) A linear increase in Bacteroidia and a decrease in Clostridiae was associated to an increase in IFN-γ, IL-6, lymphocytes, and CD4+ cells in the heart. An increase in Verrucomicrobia was associated to increased CD45+ cells and lymphocytes and to an increase in IL-1a, IFN-γ, and in CD4+ cells in the heart (**Table 2**). (3) A linear decrease in Actinobacteria and in Betaproteobacteria was associate to an increase in IL-6 and/or in IL-12 in the adipose tissue (**Table 3**). An increase in Verrucomicrobia was associated to increased IL-17 in the adipose tissue (**Table 3**). (4)

TABLE 4 | Associations from linear regression models between gut microbiota and alterations of adaptive immune system parameters measured in the liver.

	Myeloid cells β (95% CI)	Lymphocytes β (95% CI)	CD4+ β (95% CI)	CD8+ β (95% CI)	CD45+ β (95% CI)	CD11b+ β (95% CI)	CD11c+ β (95% CI)	F480+ β (95% CI)	Ly6G+ β (95% CI)
Actinobacteria	−14.9 (−67.9, 38.1) $p = 0.549$ $R^2 = 0.034$	−6.3 (−128.4, 115.7) $p = 0.911$ $R^2 = 0.001$	0.5 (−18.9, 19.9) $p = 0.952$ $R^2 = 0.000$	0.6 (−10.9, 12.1) $p = 0.912$ $R^2 = 0.001$	0.4 (−70.6, 71.4) $p = 0.991$ $R^2 = 0.000$	−25.6 (−55.4, 4.1) $p = 0.085$ $R^2 = 0.246$	10.4 (−32.8, 53.7) $p = 0.606$ $R^2 = 0.025$	−36.5 (−77.9, 4.9) $p = 0.079$ $R^2 = 0.255$	−70.7 (−167.3, 26.0) $p = 0.136$ $R^2 = 0.191$
Alphaproteobacteria	5.7 (−2.4, 13.9) $p = 0.148$ $R^2 = 0.180$	8.8 (−10.7, 28.3) $p = 0.341$ $R^2 = 0.083$	0.9 (−2.3, 4.1) $p = 0.539$ $R^2 = 0.035$	0.7 (−1.2, 2.6) $p = 0.421$ $R^2 = 0.060$	4.1 (−7.4, 15.6) $p = 0.444$ $R^2 = 0.054$	1.4 (−4.3, 7.0) $p = 0.601$ $R^2 = 0.026$	1.8 (−5.4, 9.0) $p = 0.587$ $R^2 = 0.028$	−1.8 (−9.7, 6.1) $p = 0.627$ $R^2 = 0.022$	−12.7 (−28.5, 3.0) $p = 0.103$ $R^2 = 0.223$
Bacilli	2.3 (−5.3, 9.9) $p = 0.516$ $R^2 = 0.039$	−0.8 (−18.3, 16.7) $p = 0.922$ $R^2 = 0.001$	−0.2 (−3.0, 2.6) $p = 0.863$ $R^2 = 0.003$	−0.1 (−1.7, 1.6) $p = 0.901$ $R^2 = 0.002$	−1.4 (−11.5, 8.7) $p = 0.765$ $R^2 = 0.009$	0.5 (−4.4, 5.4) $p = 0.814$ $R^2 = 0.005$	0.4 (−5.8, 6.7) $p = 0.884$ $R^2 = 0.002$	−1.5 (−8.3, 5.3) $p = 0.644$ $R^2 = 0.020$	−6.3 (−21.1, 8.5) $p = 0.367$ $R^2 = 0.074$
Bacteroidia	**1.2** **(0.7, 1.6)** **P<0.001** $\mathbf{R^2 = 0.773}$	1.6 (−0.0, 3.3) $p = 0.054$ $R^2 = 0.297$	0.2 (−0.1, 0.5) $p = 0.172$ $R^2 = 0.163$	0.1 (−0.1, 0.3) $p = 0.264$ $R^2 = 0.112$	0.8 (−0.2, 1.8) $p = 0.115$ $R^2 = 0.210$	**0.6** **(0.2, 1.0)** $\mathbf{p = 0.004}$ $\mathbf{R^2 = 0.551}$	0.2 (−0.5, 0.9) $p = 0.490$ $R^2 = 0.044$	0.5 (−0.3, 1.2) $p = 0.183$ $R^2 = 0.155$	−0.7 (−2.4, 0.9) $p = 0.359$ $R^2 = 0.077$
Betaproteobacteria	51.6 (−21.3, 124.5) $p = 0.148$ $R^2 = 0.180$	115.5 (−50.0, 281.0) $p = 0.153$ $R^2 = 0.177$	14.1 (−13.3, 41.6) $p = 0.281$ $R^2 = 0.105$	5.6 (−11.2, 22.5) $p = 0.478$ $R^2 = 0.047$	55.2 (−44.4, 154.7) $p = 0.248$ $R^2 = 0.119$	38.3 (−6.2, 82.7) $p = 0.085$ $R^2 = 0.246$	40.9 (−18.6, 100.4) $p = 0.159$ $R^2 = 0.172$	11.6 (−59.6, 82.8) $p = 0.727$ $R^2 = 0.012$	−33.2 (−192.2, 125.7) $p = 0.654$ $R^2 = 0.019$
Clostridia	**−1.3** **(−1.8, −0.8)** **p<0.001** $\mathbf{R^2 = 0.755}$	**−1.9** **(−3.7, −0.1)** $\mathbf{p = 0.044}$ $\mathbf{R^2 = 0.319}$	−0.2 (−0.5, 0.1) $p = 0.169$ $R^2 = 0.164$	−0.1 (−0.3, 0.1) $p = 0.234$ $R^2 = 0.126$	−0.9 (−2.0, 0.2) $p = 0.099$ $R^2 = 0.228$	**−0.6** **(−1.1, −0.1)** $\mathbf{p = 0.019}$ $\mathbf{R^2 = 0.406}$	−0.3 (−1.1, 0.4) $p = 0.369$ $R^2 = 0.074$	−0.3 (−1.2, 0.5) $p = 0.379$ $R^2 = 0.071$	1 (−0.8, 2.8) $p = 0.234$ $R^2 = 0.126$
Deferribacteres	**−50.6** **(−80.6, −20.6)** $\mathbf{p = 0.003}$ $\mathbf{R^2 = 0.555}$	−66.7 (−158.6, 25.1) $p = 0.138$ $R^2 = 0.189$	−10.1 (−24.9, 4.6) $p = 0.159$ $R^2 = 0.172$	−6.6 (−15.2, 2.0) $p = 0.120$ $R^2 = 0.205$	−37.3 (−91.2, 16.6) $p = 0.156$ $R^2 = 0.174$	**−29.3** **(−50.3, −8.4)** $\mathbf{p = 0.011}$ $\mathbf{R^2 = 0.463}$	−5.6 (−42.0, 30.8) $p = 0.741$ $R^2 = 0.010$	−20 (−57.8, 17.8) $p = 0.269$ $R^2 = 0.110$	44 (−40.9, 128.8) $p = 0.278$ $R^2 = 0.106$
Deltaproteobacteria	0.9 (−6.9, 8.6) $p = 0.812$ $R^2 = 0.005$	10.6 (−5.4, 26.6) $p = 0.173$ $R^2 = 0.162$	1.7 (−0.8, 4.3) $p = 0.165$ $R^2 = 0.168$	0.9 (−0.6, 2.5) $p = 0.201$ $R^2 = 0.144$	6.3 (−3.0, 15.6) $p = 0.165$ $R^2 = 0.167$	−2.8 (−7.4, 1.7) $p = 0.201$ $R^2 = 0.144$	1.2 (−5.0, 7.5) $p = 0.672$ $R^2 = 0.017$	−3.8 (−10.2, 2.6) $p = 0.219$ $R^2 = 0.134$	−10.1 (−24.0, 3.8) $p = 0.137$ $R^2 = 0.190$
Erysipelotrichia	−23.4 (−52.9, 6.1) $p = 0.109$ $R^2 = 0.216$	−48.7 (−117.0, 19.6) $p = 0.145$ $R^2 = 0.183$	−7.2 (−18.2, 3.9) $p = 0.181$ $R^2 = 0.157$	−3.6 (−10.3, 3.2) $p = 0.267$ $R^2 = 0.111$	−26.3 (−66.6, 14.0) $p = 0.179$ $R^2 = 0.158$	−11.8 (−31.5, 7.9) $p = 0.215$ $R^2 = 0.136$	−0.1 (−27.2, 27.0) $p = 0.996$ $R^2 = 0.000$	−11.1 (−39.9, 17.6) $p = 0.412$ $R^2 = 0.062$	28.4 (−35.3, 92.1) $p = 0.348$ $R^2 = 0.080$
Gammaproteobacteria	13.6 (−85.3, 112.6) $p = 0.767$ $R^2 = 0.008$	123.7 (−85.7, 333.0) $p = 0.220$ $R^2 = 0.133$	**30.8** **(1.5, 60.1)** $\mathbf{p = 0.041}$ $\mathbf{R^2 = 0.327}$	16.7 (−1.5, 34.8) $p = 0.068$ $R^2 = 0.271$	86.8 (−30.6, 204.2) $p = 0.132$ $R^2 = 0.194$	−11.7 (−74.4, 50.9) $p = 0.688$ $R^2 = 0.015$	−0.3 (−81.0, 80.3) $p = 0.993$ $R^2 = 0.000$	−27.4 (−113.8, 59.1) $p = 0.501$ $R^2 = 0.042$	−100.9 (−287.0, 85.3) $p = 0.258$ $R^2 = 0.115$
Mollicutes	**−6** **(−11.2, −0.8)** $\mathbf{p = 0.028}$ $\mathbf{R^2 = 0.370}$	−10.7 (−23.7, 2.3) $p = 0.098$ $R^2 = 0.229$	−1.7 (−3.8, 0.4) $p = 0.098$ $R^2 = 0.229$	**−1.2** **(−2.3, −0.0)** $\mathbf{p = 0.049}$ $\mathbf{R^2 = 0.308}$	−6.2 (−13.8, 1.4) $p = 0.099$ $R^2 = 0.228$	−2.9 (−6.6, 0.7) $p = 0.107$ $R^2 = 0.219$	−0.5 (−5.8, 4.8) $p = 0.838$ $R^2 = 0.004$	−1.4 (−7.1, 4.4) $p = 0.610$ $R^2 = 0.024$	8 (−3.9, 19.9) $p = 0.169$ $R^2 = 0.165$

(Continued)

TABLE 4 | Continued

	Myeloid cells β (95% CI)	Lymphocytes β (95% CI)	CD4+ β (95% CI)	CD8+ β (95% CI)	CD45+ β (95% CI)	CD11b+ β (95% CI)	CD11c+ β (95% CI)	F480+ β (95% CI)	Ly6G+ β (95% CI)
Multi–affiliation	−2.6 (−16.5, 11.4) $p = 0.693$ $R^2 = 0.015$	9.6 (−21.6, 40.7) $p = 0.513$ $R^2 = 0.040$	2.1 (−2.7, 7.0) $p = 0.355$ $R^2 = 0.078$	1.3 (−1.6, 4.2) $p = 0.333$ $R^2 = 0.085$	8.3 (−9.3, 26.0) $p = 0.321$ $R^2 = 0.089$	0.7 (−8.2, 9.6) $p = 0.869$ $R^2 = 0.003$	−1.4 (−12.8, 9.9) $p = 0.788$ $R^2 = 0.007$	−1.2 (−13.7, 11.2) $p = 0.831$ $R^2 = 0.004$	−4 (−31.8, 23.9) $p = 0.758$ $R^2 = 0.009$
Negativicutes	23.9 (−37.8, 85.5) $p = 0.412$ $R^2 = 0.062$	35.5 (−106.6, 177.6) $p = 0.593$ $R^2 = 0.027$	6.8 (−15.7, 29.3) $p = 0.519$ $R^2 = 0.039$	−2.2 (−15.8, 11.3) $p = 0.723$ $R^2 = 0.012$	25.8 (−56.2, 107.8) $p = 0.503$ $R^2 = 0.042$	10.6 (−29.2, 50.4) $p = 0.568$ $R^2 = 0.030$	−11.8 (−62.9, 39.2) $p = 0.621$ $R^2 = 0.023$	31.1 (−21.6, 83.8) $p = 0.221$ $R^2 = 0.133$	8.6 (−118.0, 135.2) $p = 0.884$ $R^2 = 0.002$
Verrucomicrobiae	**7.9** **(1.9, 14.0)** $\mathbf{p = 0.015}$ $\mathbf{R^2 = 0.429}$	15 (−0.3, 30.2) $p = 0.053$ $R^2 = 0.299$	1.6 (−1.1, 4.3) $p = 0.214$ $R^2 = 0.137$	1 (−0.5, 2.6) $p = 0.178$ $R^2 = 0.159$	8.4 (−0.6, 17.4) $p = 0.065$ $R^2 = 0.276$	4.1 (−0.3, 8.4) $p = 0.063$ $R^2 = 0.281$	1.8 (−4.6, 8.2) $p = 0.551$ $R^2 = 0.033$	3.8 (−2.9, 10.5) $p = 0.241$ $R^2 = 0.123$	−6.1 (−21.6, 9.3) $p = 0.401$ $R^2 = 0.065$

In each of the models, the associations are reported as absolute difference (β), with 95% Confidence Intervals (CI), in immune system parameters levels by 1 unit increase in gut microbiota. In bold are reported the statistically significant results ($p < 0.05$). Per each of the models, the Coefficient of determination (R^2) is also reported.

A linear increase in Bacteroidia and a decrease in Clostridiae were associated to increased myeloid cells and CD11b+ cells in the liver. Also a decrease in Mollicutes and an increase in Verrucomicrobia was associated to increased myeloid cells in the liver (**Table 4**). (5) A linear increase in Bacteroidia and in Verrucomicrobia, and a decrease in Clostridiae, were associated to increased myeloid cell markers CD11b+, CD11c+, F4/90+, and Ly6G+ cells in the spleen (**Table 5**).

DISCUSSION

The results of our study in mice suggest that diet composition might have a pervasive role in co-regulating adaptive immunity and gut microbiota's profile in healthy obese subjects and in atherogenesis/inflammation in subjects with normal BMI. There has been recently a great focus on a particular subset of overweight and obese individuals having normal metabolic profile despite highly increased adipose mass (MHO = metabolic healthy obese; Karelis, 2008; Flegal et al., 2013). Individuals with adverse metabolic status despite a normal BMI have also been described (MSL = metabolic syndrome lean; Karelis, 2008; Flegal et al., 2013). It is currently unclear whether metabolic dysfunctions affects the higher morbidity and mortality observed in individuals with higher BMI: the concept of "benign obesity" has been challenged by some meta-analyses (Kramer et al., 2013) but not by others (Dhana et al., 2016), suggesting that MetS and not elevated BMI is an unequivocal risk factor for cardiovascular diseases (CVD). As it was previously reported, we confirmed that mice in a C57/BL6 genetic background fed a Paigen diet (PD) developed features of MetS, including hyperinsulinemia, hyperglycaemia, steatohepatitis, and inflammatory infiltration into the aorta, without increase in body weight (Getz and Reardon, 2006). Although, atherosclerosis is not observed without ApoE$^{-/-}$ mutation in mice, this study reports for the first time a systemic activation of the immune system upon an atherogenic diet, with high tissue infiltration of myeloid cell subsets CD45+CD11b+CD11c, CD45+ F4/80+, CD45+ CD11b+Ly6G+ in the spleen, a massive lymphocyte infiltration in the aorta and in the liver, a significant increase in CD4+ and CD8+ positive cells in the aorta and in the hearts, paralleled by increased IL-17, IL-1, IFN-γ, and IL-4 levels in the aorta and heart. The elevated level of gene expression for IL-1α detected in the heart might indicate the activation of myeloid cell types, probably macrophages, which have been described as the main proinflammatory cell population in atherosclerotic plaques (Jonasson et al., 1986), and also play a crucial role in the development of heart failure (Heidt et al., 2014). In general, IL-1 critically orchestrates the inflammatory events that are considered building blocks for the formation atherosclerotic plaques, precursors and risk factor for CVD such as myocardial infarction (Van Tassell et al., 2013; Gallego-Colon et al., 2015; Taleb et al., 2015). In this study, mice in a C57/BL6 genetic background fed a high fat diet (HD) developed obesity, increased body weight and fatty liver without systemic inflammation and activation of the adaptive immune system. We took advantage of these two phenotypically characterized mice models of MSL and MHO, to scrutinize the composition of gut microbiota in the stool of these metabolic exceptions. High-throughput 16S targeted sequencing showed a dominion of Bacteroidia, Deltaproteobacteria and Verrucomicrobia and under-representation of Clostridia in MSL PD-fed mice. Generally, Proteobacteria and Verrucomicrobia are not abundant in the healthy gut, but abundant in the gut dysbiosis of patients with type 2 diabetes or with inflammatory bowel disease (IBD) (Larsen et al., 2010; Qin et al., 2012; Shin et al., 2015). More abundant bacteria such as Bacteroidiales and Clostridiales are more and less represented, respectively, in type 2 diabetes compared to obesity (Larsen et al., 2010; Qin et al., 2012). Bacteroidiales are associated to weight loss (Million et al., 2013). Our results are completely in line with the above reports

TABLE 5 | Associations from linear regression models between gut microbiota and alterations of adaptive immune system parameters measured in the spleen.

	IL-17 β (95% CI)	IFNg β (95% CI)	Myeloid cells β (95% CI)	CD45+ β (95% CI)	CD11b+ β (95% CI)	CD11c+ β (95% CI)	F480+ β (95% CI)	Ly6G β (95% CI)
Actinobacteria	−0.4 (−14.5, 13.7) $p = 0.947$ $R^2 = 0.001$	−2.5 (−18.6, 13.6) $p = 0.726$ $R^2 = 0.019$	−7.3 (−21.0, 6.4) $p = 0.267$ $R^2 = 0.111$	−6.4 (−17.1, 4.4) $p = 0.220$ $R^2 = 0.134$	−5.2 (−13.9, 3.6) $p = 0.220$ $R^2 = 0.133$	−1.1 (−2.6, 0.5) $p = 0.155$ $R^2 = 0.175$	−1.8 (−4.9, 1.4) $p = 0.240$ $R^2 = 0.123$	−3.9 (−9.7, 2.0) $p = 0.171$ $R^2 = 0.163$
Alphaproteobacteria	−0.9 (−3.0, 1.2) $p = 0.349$ $R^2 = 0.126$	−0.8 (−3.3, 1.6) $p = 0.454$ $R^2 = 0.082$	0.3 (−2.1, 2.7) $p = 0.769$ $R^2 = 0.008$	0.3 (−1.7, 2.2) $p = 0.771$ $R^2 = 0.008$	0.2 (−1.4, 1.7) $p = 0.826$ $R^2 = 0.005$	0.1 (−0.2, 0.3) $p = 0.671$ $R^2 = 0.017$	0 (−0.5, 0.6) $p = 0.877$ $R^2 = 0.002$	0.1 (−0.9, 1.2) $p = 0.807$ $R^2 = 0.006$
Bacilli	0.1 (−1.8, 2.0) $p = 0.912$ $R^2 = 0.002$	−0.6 (−2.7, 1.6) $p = 0.547$ $R^2 = 0.054$	−0.5 (−2.5, 1.6) $p = 0.615$ $R^2 = 0.024$	−0.4 (−2.0, 1.2) $p = 0.602$ $R^2 = 0.026$	−0.3 (−1.7, 1.0) $p = 0.598$ $R^2 = 0.026$	0 (−0.3, 0.2) $p = 0.688$ $R^2 = 0.015$	−0.1 (−0.6, 0.3) $p = 0.570$ $R^2 = 0.030$	−0.2 (−1.1, 0.7) $p = 0.588$ $R^2 = 0.028$
Bacteroidia	−0.1 (−0.3, 0.1) $p = 0.362$ $R^2 = 0.120$	−0.2 (−0.4, 0.1) $p = 0.217$ $R^2 = 0.208$	**0.2** **(0.0, 0.4)** $\mathbf{p = 0.020}$ $\mathbf{R^2 = 0.402}$	**0.2** **(0.0, 0.3)** $\mathbf{p = 0.015}$ $\mathbf{R^2 = 0.432}$	**0.1** **(0.0, 0.3)** $\mathbf{p = 0.015}$ $\mathbf{R^2 = 0.429}$	**0** **(0.0, 0.0)** $\mathbf{p = 0.005}$ $\mathbf{R^2 = 0.519}$	**0.1** **(0.0, 0.1)** $\mathbf{p = 0.021}$ $\mathbf{R^2 = 0.399}$	**0.1** **(0.0, 0.2)** $\mathbf{p = 0.011}$ $\mathbf{R^2 = 0.459}$
Betaproteobacteria	−16.2 (−43.6, 11.2) $p = 0.204$ $R^2 = 0.219$	−18.6 (−50.1, 12.9) $p = 0.206$ $R^2 = 0.217$	14 (−5.7, 33.6) $p = 0.146$ $R^2 = 0.182$	11.8 (−3.5, 27.2) $p = 0.118$ $R^2 = 0.207$	9.5 (−3.1, 22.0) $p = 0.125$ $R^2 = 0.200$	1.9 (−0.3, 4.1) $p = 0.082$ $R^2 = 0.249$	3.1 (−1.4, 7.7) $p = 0.159$ $R^2 = 0.172$	6.2 (−2.4, 14.8) $p = 0.140$ $R^2 = 0.187$
Clostridia	0.2 (−0.1, 0.4) $p = 0.157$ $R^2 = 0.264$	0.1 (−0.2, 0.4) $p = 0.410$ $R^2 = 0.099$	**−0.2** **(−0.4, −0.0)** $\mathbf{p = 0.025}$ $\mathbf{R^2 = 0.379}$	**−0.2** **(−0.4, −0.0)** $\mathbf{p = 0.019}$ $\mathbf{R^2 = 0.405}$	**−0.2** **(−0.3, −0.0)** $\mathbf{p = 0.021}$ $\mathbf{R^2 = 0.396}$	**0** **(−0.1, −0.0)** $\mathbf{p = 0.007}$ $\mathbf{R^2 = 0.493}$	**−0.1** **(−0.1, −0.0)** $\mathbf{p = 0.029}$ $\mathbf{R^2 = 0.363}$	**−0.1** **(−0.2, −0.0)** $\mathbf{p = 0.015}$ $\mathbf{R^2 = 0.429}$
Deferribacteres	1.3 (−10.4, 13.0) $p = 0.802$ $R^2 = 0.010$	4.9 (−7.9, 17.7) $p = 0.396$ $R^2 = 0.105$	−6.6 (−17.9, 4.8) $p = 0.228$ $R^2 = 0.129$	−5.2 (−14.2, 3.7) $p = 0.226$ $R^2 = 0.130$	−4.5 (−11.7, 2.8) $p = 0.204$ $R^2 = 0.142$	−0.8 (−2.1, 0.5) $p = 0.199$ $R^2 = 0.145$	−1.6 (−4.2, 1.0) $p = 0.204$ $R^2 = 0.142$	−3 (−7.9, 2.0) $p = 0.213$ $R^2 = 0.137$
Deltaproteobacteria	−1.5 (−3.2, 0.2) $p = 0.083$ $R^2 = 0.369$	0.5 (−2.0, 3.0) $p = 0.641$ $R^2 = 0.033$	0.1 (−2.0, 2.1) $p = 0.945$ $R^2 = 0.001$	0 (−1.6, 1.7) $p = 0.950$ $R^2 = 0.000$	−0.1 (−1.4, 1.3) $p = 0.933$ $R^2 = 0.001$	0 (−0.2, 0.3) $p = 0.918$ $R^2 = 0.001$	0 (−0.5, 0.4) $p = 0.879$ $R^2 = 0.002$	0 (−0.9, 0.9) $p = 0.962$ $R^2 = 0.000$
Erysipelotrichia	−1.8 (−9.9, 6.3) $p = 0.612$ $R^2 = 0.039$	**9** **(4.0, 14.0)** $\mathbf{p = 0.004}$ $\mathbf{R^2 = 0.723}$	−3.9 (−12.5, 4.7) $p = 0.336$ $R^2 = 0.084$	−3.2 (−10.0, 3.6) $p = 0.320$ $R^2 = 0.090$	−2.6 (−8.2, 2.9) $p = 0.321$ $R^2 = 0.089$	−0.5 (−1.5, 0.5) $p = 0.321$ $R^2 = 0.089$	−1 (−2.9, 1.0) $p = 0.301$ $R^2 = 0.097$	−1.8 (−5.6, 2.0) $p = 0.323$ $R^2 = 0.089$
Gammaproteobacteria	−15.7 (−60.9, 29.6) $p = 0.440$ $R^2 = 0.087$	−7.6 (−61.7, 46.4) $p = 0.749$ $R^2 = 0.016$	−0.1 (−26.9, 26.6) $p = 0.991$ $R^2 = 0.000$	−1.1 (−22.4, 20.1) $p = 0.909$ $R^2 = 0.001$	−0.8 (−18.0, 16.5) $p = 0.926$ $R^2 = 0.001$	−0.5 (−3.6, 2.6) $p = 0.745$ R2 = 0.010	−0.1 (−6.3, 6.1) $p = 0.975$ $R^2 = 0.000$	−1.7 (−13.4, 10.0) $p = 0.755$ $R^2 = 0.009$
Mollicutes	0.9 (−0.5, 2.3) $p = 0.168$ $R^2 = 0.252$	−0.1 (−2.0, 1.8) $p = 0.908$ $R^2 = 0.002$	−0.6 (−2.3, 1.1) $p = 0.440$ $R^2 = 0.055$	−0.5 (−1.9, 0.9) $p = 0.442$ $R^2 = 0.055$	−0.3 (−1.5, 0.8) $p = 0.509$ $R^2 = 0.041$	−0.1 (−0.3, 0.1) $p = 0.349$ $R^2 = 0.080$	−0.1 (−0.5, 0.3) $p = 0.573$ $R^2 = 0.030$	−0.2 (−1.0, 0.5) $p = 0.505$ $R^2 = 0.042$

(Continued)

TABLE 5 | Continued

	IL-17 β (95% CI)	IFNg β (95% CI)	Myeloid cells β (95% CI)	CD45+ β (95% CI)	CD11b+ β (95% CI)	CD11c+ β (95% CI)	F480+ β (95% CI)	Ly6G β (95% CI)
Multi−affiliation	0.3 (−7.5, 8.1) $p = 0.921$ $R^2 = 0.002$	**8** **(2.5, 13.5)** $\mathbf{p = 0.011}$ $\mathbf{R^2 = 0.629}$	−0.9 (−4.7, 2.8) $p = 0.599$ $R^2 = 0.026$	−0.7 (−3.7, 2.2) $p = 0.593$ $R^2 = 0.027$	−0.7 (−3.1, 1.7) $p = 0.515$ $R^2 = 0.039$	−0.1 (−0.6, 0.3) $p = 0.469$ $R^2 = 0.049$	−0.2 (−1.1, 0.7) $p = 0.614$ $R^2 = 0.024$	−0.4 (−2.0, 1.3) $p = 0.614$ $R^2 = 0.024$
Negativicutes	−5.5 (−20.7, 9.6) $p = 0.418$ $R^2 = 0.096$	−5.8 (−23.4, 11.8) $p = 0.464$ $R^2 = 0.079$	**14.5** **(0.3, 28.7)** $\mathbf{p = 0.045}$ $\mathbf{R^2 = 0.316}$	10.8 (−0.8, 22.4) $p = 0.064$ $R^2 = 0.278$	9.1 (−0.1, 18.4) $p = 0.053$ $R^2 = 0.300$	1.3 (−0.4, 3.1) $p = 0.128$ $R^2 = 0.198$	**3.3** **(0.0, 6.6)** $\mathbf{p = 0.048}$ $\mathbf{R^2 = 0.310}$	5.5 (−1.1, 12.1) $p = 0.094$ $R^2 = 0.234$
Verrucomicrobiae	**−1.6** **(−3.2, −0.0)** $\mathbf{p = 0.048}$ $\mathbf{R^2 = 0.451}$	−1.1 (−3.4, 1.1) $p = 0.274$ $R^2 = 0.167$	**2.1** **(0.5, 3.8)** $\mathbf{p = 0.015}$ $\mathbf{R^2 = 0.431}$	**1.7** **(0.5, 3.0)** $\mathbf{p = 0.012}$ $\mathbf{R^2 = 0.449}$	**1.4** **(0.3, 2.4)** $\mathbf{p = 0.016}$ $\mathbf{R^2 = 0.422}$	**0.3** **(0.1, 0.4)** $\mathbf{p = 0.008}$ $\mathbf{R^2 = 0.488}$	**0.5** **(0.1, 0.9)** $\mathbf{p = 0.024}$ $\mathbf{R^2 = 0.385}$	**0.9** **(0.2, 1.7)** $\mathbf{p = 0.015}$ $\mathbf{R^2 = 0.429}$

In each of the models, the associations are reported as absolute difference (β), with 95% Confidence Intervals (CI), in immune system parameters levels by 1 unit increase in gut microbiota. In bold are reported the statistically significant results ($p < 0.05$). Per each of the models, the Coefficient of determination (R^2) is also reported.

and with the strong pro-inflammatory and pro-MetS role of PD compared to ND and HD. To our knowledge, a limited number of studies described clearly a role for gut microbiota in the onset of the MHO phenotype. It has been shown that separate cohorts of mice belonging to the same genetic background (C57/BL6) became either diabetic or resistant to diabetes and related metabolic dysfunctions despite being eating the same high-fat diet triggering obesity (Serino et al., 2012). The gut microbiota of the diabetes-resistant mice displayed a 20% decrease in the abundance of Firmicutes that were replaced by a parallel increase in Bacteriodetes (Serino et al., 2012). Moreover, the microbiota of diabetes-resistant mice presented with less bacteria of the *helicobacter* genus compared to the diabetic mice; instead, actinobacteria levels were unchanged (Serino et al., 2012). Our and these published studies suggest that the gut microbiota might reflect faithfully the metabolic phenotype irrespective of variability in the genetic background and diets of the host. Results of a recent study performed in the brown bear (*Ursus arctos*) are consistent with this (Sommer et al., 2016). The bear is a mammal accumulating enormous quantities of adipose fat in a seasonal manner (summer); by doing so, bears develop hyperlipidemia while maintaining metabolic health and being resistant to the development of atherosclerosis (Arinell et al., 2012). In fact, during summer season, the gut of bears harbored a different composition of microbiota than during winter season. In summer it was shown that gut microbiota was richer in Actinobacteria, Firmicutes, Proteobacteria, and poorer in Bacteroidetes (Sommer et al., 2016).

Several groups have provided data supporting a role for gut microbiota in the establishment of the MSL. If intestinal microbiota is suppressed in atherosclerosis-prone mice, an inhibition of dietary-choline-dependent atherosclerosis is observed (Wang et al., 2011). Patients with symptomatic atherosclerosis and normal body weight showed enrichment of the genus *Collinsella* of Actinobacteria in the gut (Karlsson et al., 2012). Generally, gut microbiota can affect atherosclerosis even in absence obesity or high fat feeding by different pathways: (i) infection activating the immune system and causing an inflammatory and proatherogenic response at distant sites; (ii) alteration of the levels of serum triglycerides and cholesterol, and of the metabolism of bile acids; (iii) dietary components (such as choline) and microbial metabolites [such as trimethylamine N-oxide (TMAO) generated from microbial metabolism of phosphatidylcholine, which is common in red meat and shellfish] lead to the production of both beneficial and harmful molecules (Jonsson and Backhed, 2017). For this reasons, gut microbiome is sometimes described as "endocrine" organ contributing to organism homeostasis [47].

Here, observed pro-inflammatory cytokines levels and tissue infiltrates correlating with decreased numbers of Clostridia corroborate previous findings on their regulatory functions. Clostridia strains presented in colon environment synergise to induce Tregs development [48, 49]. Tregs are fundamental to maintain mucosal homeostasis; therefore their insufficient development has pathological potential. Atherosclerosis develops upon stimulation of dendritic cells with oxidized low-density lipoproteins, the pathology is orchestrated by Th17 produced IL-17 [50], pro-autoimmune role of Th17 in atherosclerosis as well as association to HD induced chronic inflammation is well-described. Bacteroidetes has been associated to "healthy" non-obese homeostatic microbiome and with immunomodulation [51]. Interestingly addition of short chain fatty acids to the diet can result in Bacteroidetes abundance also during HD [52]. *Bacteroides fragilis* polysaccharide A (PSA) promotes T cells development [53], furthermore dysbiosis is frequently described as reduced Firmicutes/Bacteroidetes ratio, and this change was associated with IL-17 production and Th17 responses [54, 55].

Our result shows that increase proportion of Verrucomicrobiae correlates with higher percentage of myeloid cells markers. Interestingly, Roopchand et al. has shown that presence of *A. muciniphila* from Verrucomicrobiae together with presence of Bacteroidetes has significant role in protection to diet-induced obesity and metabolic dysbiosis in mice fed with HD [56]. Furthermore, in support to our data Ganesh et al. showed that presence of *A. muciniphila* increased levels of IL-17 in Salmonella infected mice [57].

It has been already demonstrated that diet shapes gut microbiome composition (De Filippo et al., 2010), and it is also now recognized that commensal microorganisms impact host gene expression not only in the gastrointestinal tract but also in other systems (Levy et al., 2015). Moreover, microbial cell components and secreted intermediate metabolites appear to be implicated in the response of the host to microbial colonization at the level of gene expression, which in turn reciprocally influence the disease progression. Noteworthy, both immunosuppressive drugs and probiotics affect the balance between microbiota and the immune system (Bartman et al., 2015). Particularly, probiotics supplementation have been shown to be effective in restoring and/or renovating the microbiota changes stimulating a number of health benefits, nevertheless whether modulation of gastrointestinal microbiota composition could have an effect on the amelioration of metabolic syndrome in obese or lean subjects, remains to be further investigated.

Supporting the link between metagenomics and immunogenomics, our data underline that understanding the reciprocal cross-talk between host immunity and microbiota will pave the way to the development of new therapeutic strategies against microbiome-driven common diseases, such as the metabolic syndrome.

AUTHOR CONTRIBUTIONS

All authors made substantial contributions to the conception of the work; to the acquisition, analysis, or interpretation of data for the work; to the drafting the work and revising it critically for important intellectual content; and they finally approved the version to be published. All authors are accountable for all aspects of the work in ensuring that questions related to the accuracy or integrity of the work.

FUNDING

This work was supported by the European Social Fund and European Regional Development Fund—Project MAGNET (No. CZ.02.1.01/0.0/0.0/15_003/0000492) to MV, and by "Italian Ministry of Health" from grant RC1603GA31 (to VP).

ACKNOWLEDGMENTS

We thank all the members of CTM-ICRC, St'Agata, and the technical personnel of the University of Veterinary and Pharmaceutical Sciences (Brno, Czech Republic) for help and assistance.

REFERENCES

Alberti, K. G., Zimmet, P., and Shaw, J. (2005). Group IDFETFC. The metabolic syndrome-a new worldwide definition. *Lancet* 366, 1059–1062. doi: 10.1016/S0140-6736(05)67402-8

Arinell, K., Sahdo, B., Evans, A. L., Arnemo, J. M., Baandrup, U., and Frobert, O. (2012). Brown bears (*Ursus arctos*) seem resistant to atherosclerosis despite highly elevated plasma lipids during hibernation and active state. *Clin. Transl. Sci.* 5, 269–272. doi: 10.1111/j.1752-8062.2011.00370.x

Bartman, C., Chong, A. S., and Alegre, M. L. (2015). The influence of the microbiota on the immune response to transplantation. *Curr. Opin. Organ Transplant.* 20, 1–7. doi: 10.1097/MOT.0000000000000150

Belkaid, Y., and Hand, T. W. (2014). Role of the microbiota in immunity and inflammation. *Cell* 157, 121–141. doi: 10.1016/j.cell.2014.03.011

Benegiamo, G., Mazzoccoli, G., Cappello, F., Rappa, F., Scibetta, N., Oben, J., et al. (2013). Mutual antagonism between circadian protein period 2 and hepatitis C virus replication in hepatocytes. *PLoS ONE* 8:e60527. doi: 10.1371/journal.pone.0060527

Cederroth, C. R., Vinciguerra, M., Gjinovci, A., Kuhne, F., Klein, M., Cederroth, M., et al. (2008). Dietary phytoestrogens activate AMP-activated protein kinase with improvement in lipid and glucose metabolism. *Diabetes* 57, 1176–1185. doi: 10.2337/db07-0630

Clarke, G., Stilling, R. M., Kennedy, P. J., Stanton, C., Cryan, J. F., and Dinan, T. G. (2014). Minireview: gut microbiota: the neglected endocrine organ. *Mol. Endocrinol.* 28, 1221–1238. doi: 10.1210/me.2014-1108

Cox, A. J., West, N. P., and Cripps, A. W. (2015). Obesity, inflammation, and the gut microbiota. *Lancet Diabetes Endocrinol.* 3, 207–215. doi: 10.1016/S2213-8587(14)70134-2

David, L. A., Maurice, C. F., Carmody, R. N., Gootenberg, D. B., Button, J. E., Wolfe, B. E., et al. (2014). Diet rapidly and reproducibly alters the human gut microbiome. *Nature* 505, 559–563. doi: 10.1038/nature12820

De Filippo, C., Cavalieri, D., Di Paola, M., Ramazzotti, M., Poullet, J. B., Massart, S., et al. (2010). Impact of diet in shaping gut microbiota revealed by a comparative study in children from Europe and rural Africa. *Proc. Natl. Acad. Sci. U.S.A.* 107, 14691–14696. doi: 10.1073/pnas.1005963107

Despres, J. P., Lemieux, I., Bergeron, J., Pibarot, P., Mathieu, P., Larose, E., et al. (2008). Abdominal obesity and the metabolic syndrome: contribution to global cardiometabolic risk. *Arterioscler. Thromb. Vasc. Biol.* 28, 1039–1049. doi: 10.1161/ATVBAHA.107.159228

Dhana, K., Koolhaas, C. M., van Rossum, E. F., Ikram, M. A., Hofman, A., Kavousi, M., et al. (2016). Metabolically healthy obesity and the risk of cardiovascular disease in the elderly population. *PLoS ONE* 11:e0154273. doi: 10.1371/journal.pone.0154273

Flegal, K. M., Kit, B. K., Orpana, H., and Graubard, B. I. (2013). Association of all-cause mortality with overweight and obesity using standard body mass index categories: a systematic review and meta-analysis. *JAMA* 309, 71–82. doi: 10.1001/jama.2012.113905

Gaboriau-Routhiau, V., Rakotobe, S., Lecuyer, E., Mulder, I., Lan, A., Bridonneau, C., et al. (2009). The key role of segmented filamentous bacteria in the coordinated maturation of gut helper T cell responses. *Immunity* 31, 677–689. doi: 10.1016/j.immuni.2009.08.020

Gallego-Colon, E., Sampson, R. D., Sattler, S., Schneider, M. D., Rosenthal, N., and Tonkin, J. (2015). Cardiac-restricted IGF-1Ea overexpression reduces the early accumulation of inflammatory myeloid cells and mediates expression of extracellular matrix remodelling genes after myocardial infarction. *Mediators Inflamm.* 2015:484357. doi: 10.1155/2015/484357

Getz, G. S., and Reardon, C. A. (2006). Diet and murine atherosclerosis. *Arterioscler. Thromb. Vasc. Biol.* 26, 242–249. doi: 10.1161/01.ATV.0000201071.49029.17

Heidt, T., Courties, G., Dutta, P., Sager, H. B., Sebas, M., Iwamoto, Y., et al. (2014). Differential contribution of monocytes to heart macrophages in steady-state and after myocardial infarction. *Circ. Res.* 115, 284–295. doi: 10.1161/CIRCRESAHA.115.303567

Honda, K., and Littman, D. R. (2016). The microbiota in adaptive immune homeostasis and disease. *Nature* 535, 75–84. doi: 10.1038/nature18848

Hunter, C. A., and Jones, S. A. (2015). IL-6 as a keystone cytokine in health and disease. *Nat. Immunol.* 16, 448–457. doi: 10.1038/ni.3153

Ivanov, I. I., Frutos Rde, L., Manel, N., Yoshinaga, K., Rifkin, D. B., Sartor, R. B., et al. (2008). Specific microbiota direct the differentiation of IL-17-producing T-helper cells in the mucosa of the small intestine. *Cell Host Microbe* 4, 337–349. doi: 10.1016/j.chom.2008.09.009

Jonasson, L., Holm, J., Skalli, O., Bondjers, G., and Hansson, G. K. (1986). Regional accumulations of T cells, macrophages, and smooth muscle cells in the human atherosclerotic plaque. *Arteriosclerosis* 6, 131–138. doi: 10.1161/01.ATV.6.2.131

Jonsson, A. L., and Backhed, F. (2017). Role of gut microbiota in atherosclerosis. *Nat. Rev. Cardiol.* 14, 79–87. doi: 10.1038/nrcardio.2016.183

Karelis, A. D. (2008). Metabolically healthy but obese individuals. *Lancet* 372, 1281–1283. doi: 10.1016/S0140-6736(08)61531-7

Karlsson, F. H., Fak, F., Nookaew, I., Tremaroli, V., Fagerberg, B., Petranovic, D., et al. (2012). Symptomatic atherosclerosis is associated with an altered gut metagenome. *Nat. Commun.* 3:1245. doi: 10.1038/ncomms2266

Kato, L. M., Kawamoto, S., Maruya, M., and Fagarasan, S. (2014). The role of the adaptive immune system in regulation of gut microbiota. *Immunol. Rev.* 260, 67–75. doi: 10.1111/imr.12185

Kleiner, D. E., Brunt, E. M., Van Natta, M., Behling, C., Contos, M. J., Cummings, O. W., et al. (2005). Design and validation of a histological scoring system for nonalcoholic fatty liver disease. *Hepatology* 41, 1313–1321. doi: 10.1002/hep.20701

Kramer, C. K., Zinman, B., and Retnakaran, R. (2013). Are metabolically healthy overweight and obesity benign conditions?: a systematic review and meta-analysis. *Ann. Intern. Med.* 159, 758–769. doi: 10.7326/0003-4819-159-11-201312030-00008

Larsen, N., Vogensen, F. K., van den Berg, F. W., Nielsen, D. S., Andreasen, A. S., Pedersen, B. K., et al. (2010). Gut microbiota in human adults with type 2 diabetes differs from non-diabetic adults. *PLoS ONE* 5:e9085. doi: 10.1371/journal.pone.0009085

Levy, M., Thaiss, C. A., and Elinav, E. (2015). Metagenomic cross-talk: the regulatory interplay between immunogenomics and the microbiome. *Genome Med.* 7:120. doi: 10.1186/s13073-015-0249-9

Lichtman, A. H. (2013). Adaptive immunity and atherosclerosis: mouse tales in the AJP. *Am. J. Pathol.* 182, 5–9. doi: 10.1016/j.ajpath.2012.10.006

Lluch, J., Servant, F., Paisse, S., Valle, C., Valiere, S., Kuchly, C., et al. (2015). The Characterization of novel tissue microbiota using an optimized 16S metagenomic sequencing pipeline. *PLoS ONE* 10:e0142334. doi: 10.1371/journal.pone.0142334

Marchesi, J. R., Adams, D. H., Fava, F., Hermes, G. D., Hirschfield, G. M., Hold, G., et al. (2016). The gut microbiota and host health: a new clinical frontier. *Gut* 65, 330–339. doi: 10.1136/gutjnl-2015-309990

Million, M., Lagier, J. C., Yahav, D., and Paul, M. (2013). Gut bacterial microbiota and obesity. *Clin. Microbiol. Infect.* 19, 305–313. doi: 10.1111/1469-0691.12172

Munoz-Garach, A., Cornejo-Pareja, I., and Tinahones, F. J. (2016). Does metabolically healthy obesity exist? *Nutrients* 8:E320. doi: 10.3390/nu8060320

Nishimura, S., Manabe, I., Nagasaki, M., Eto, K., Yamashita, H., Ohsugi, M., et al. (2009). CD8+ effector T cells contribute to macrophage recruitment and adipose tissue inflammation in obesity. *Nat. Med.* 15, 914–920. doi: 10.1038/nm.1964

Paisse, S., Valle, C., Servant, F., Courtney, M., Burcelin, R., Amar, J., et al. (2016). Comprehensive description of blood microbiome from healthy donors assessed by 16S targeted metagenomic sequencing. *Transfusion* 56, 1138–1147. doi: 10.1111/trf.13477

Pazienza, V., Panebianco, C., Rappa, F., Memoli, D., Borghesan, M., Cannito, S., et al. (2016). Histone macroH2A1.2 promotes metabolic health and leanness by inhibiting adipogenesis. *Epigenetics Chromatin* 9:45. doi: 10.1186/s13072-016-0098-9

Qin, J., Li, Y., Cai, Z., Li, S., Zhu, J., Zhang, F., et al. (2012). A metagenome-wide association study of gut microbiota in type 2 diabetes. *Nature* 490, 55–60. doi: 10.1038/nature11450

Sell, H., Habich, C., and Eckel, J. (2012). Adaptive immunity in obesity and insulin resistance. *Nat. Rev. Endocrinol.* 8, 709–716. doi: 10.1038/nrendo.2012.114

Serino, M., Luche, E., Gres, S., Baylac, A., Berge, M., Cenac, C., et al. (2012). Metabolic adaptation to a high-fat diet is associated with a change in the gut microbiota. *Gut* 61, 543–553. doi: 10.1136/gutjnl-2011-301012

Shen, L., Chng, M. H., Alonso, M. N., Yuan, R., Winer, D. A., and Engleman, E. G. (2015). B-1a lymphocytes attenuate insulin resistance. *Diabetes* 64, 593–603. doi: 10.2337/db14-0554

Shin, N. R., Whon, T. W., and Bae, J. W. (2015). Proteobacteria: microbial signature of dysbiosis in gut microbiota. *Trends Biotechnol.* 33, 496–503. doi: 10.1016/j.tibtech.2015.06.011

Sommer, F., Stahlman, M., Ilkayeva, O., Arnemo, J. M., Kindberg, J., Josefsson, J., et al. (2016). The gut microbiota modulates energy metabolism in the hibernating brown bear *Ursus arctos*. *Cell Rep.* 14, 1655–1661. doi: 10.1016/j.celrep.2016.01.026

Taleb, S., Tedgui, A., and Mallat, Z. (2015). IL-17 and Th17 cells in atherosclerosis: subtle and contextual roles. *Arterioscler. Thromb. Vasc. Biol.* 35, 258–264. doi: 10.1161/ATVBAHA.114.303567

Thaiss, C. A., Levy, M., Suez, J., and Elinav, E. (2014). The interplay between the innate immune system and the microbiota. *Curr. Opin. Immunol.* 26, 41–48. doi: 10.1016/j.coi.2013.10.016

Van Tassell, B. W., Toldo, S., Mezzaroma, E., and Abbate, A. (2013). Targeting interleukin-1 in heart disease. *Circulation* 128, 1910–1923. doi: 10.1161/CIRCULATIONAHA.113.003199

Vergnes, L., Phan, J., Strauss, M., Tafuri, S., and Reue, K. (2003). Cholesterol and cholate components of an atherogenic diet induce distinct stages of hepatic inflammatory gene expression. *J. Biol. Chem.* 278, 42774–42784. doi: 10.1074/jbc.M306022200

Wang, Z., Klipfell, E., Bennett, B. J., Koeth, R., Levison, B. S., Dugar, B., et al. (2011). Gut flora metabolism of phosphatidylcholine promotes cardiovascular disease. *Nature* 472, 57–63. doi: 10.1038/nature09922

Winer, S., Paltser, G., Chan, Y., Tsui, H., Engleman, E., Winer, D., et al. (2009). Obesity predisposes to Th17 bias. *Eur. J. Immunol.* 39, 2629–2635. doi: 10.1002/eji.200838893

Zarzycka, B., Nicolaes, G. A., and Lutgens, E. (2015). Targeting the adaptive immune system: new strategies in the treatment of atherosclerosis. *Expert Rev. Clin. Pharmacol.* 8, 297–313. doi: 10.1586/17512433.2015.1025052

Zhang, H., and Luo, X. M. (2015). Control of commensal microbiota by the adaptive immune system. *Gut Microbes* 6, 156–160. doi: 10.1080/19490976.2015.1031946

Zupancic, M. L., Cantarel, B. L., Liu, Z., Drabek, E. F., Ryan, K. A., Cirimotich, S., et al. (2012). Analysis of the gut microbiota in the old order Amish and its relation to the metabolic syndrome. *PLoS ONE* 7:e43052. doi: 10.1371/journal.pone.0043052

13

Prophylactic Supplementation of *Bifidobacterium longum* 5^{1A} Protects Mice from Ovariectomy-Induced Exacerbated Allergic Airway Inflammation and Airway Hyperresponsiveness

*Eduardo Mendes[1†], Beatriz G. Acetturi[2†], Andrew M. Thomas[3,4,5], Flaviano dos S. Martins[6], Amanda R. Crisma[7], Gilson Murata[7], Tárcio T. Braga[8], Niels O. S. Câmara[8], Adriana L. dos S. Franco[9], João C. Setubal[4], Willian R. Ribeiro[1], Claudete J. Valduga[10], Rui Curi[7], Emmanuel Dias-Neto[3,11], Wothan Tavares-de-Lima[2] and Caroline M. Ferreira[1]**

[1] Department of Pharmaceutics Sciences, Institute of Environmental, Chemistry and Pharmaceutical Sciences, Universidade Federal de São Paulo, Diadema, Brazil, [2] Department of Pharmacology, Institute of Biomedical Sciences I, University of São Paulo, São Paulo, Brazil, [3] Medical Genomics Laboratory, CIPE/A.C.Camargo Cancer Center, São Paulo, Brazil, [4] Department of Biochemistry, Institute of Chemistry, University of São Paulo, São Paulo, Brazil, [5] Bioinformatics Graduate Program, University of São Paulo, São Paulo, Brazil, [6] Department of Microbiology, Institute of Biological Sciences, Federal University of Minas Gerais, Belo Horizonte, Brazil, [7] Department of Physiology and Biophysics, Institute of Biomedical Sciences, University of São Paulo, São Paulo, Brazil, [8] Department of Immunology, Institute of Biomedical Sciences IV, University of São Paulo, São Paulo, Brazil, [9] Post Graduate Program in Biophotonics Applied to Health Sciences, Universidade Nove de Julho, São Paulo, Brazil, [10] Department of Pharmacy and Biotechnology, Universidade de Anhanguera de São Paulo, São Paulo, Brazil, [11] Laboratory of Neurosciences (LIM-27), Institute of Psychiatry, Medical School University of São Paulo, São Paulo, Brazil

***Correspondence:**
Caroline M. Ferreira
caroline.nu.ferreira@gmail.com

†These authors are co-first authors.

Asthma is a chronic inflammatory disease that affects more females than males after puberty, and its symptoms and severity in women change during menstruation and menopause. Recently, evidence has demonstrated that interactions among the microbiota, female sex hormones, and immunity are associated with the development of autoimmune diseases. However, no studies have investigated if therapeutic gut microbiota modulation strategies could affect asthma exacerbation during menstruation and menopause. Here we aimed to examine the preventive effects of a probiotic, *Bifidobacterium longum* 5^{1A}, on airway inflammation exacerbation in allergic ovariectomized mice. We first evaluated the gut microbiota composition and diversity in mice 10 days after ovariectomy. Next, we examined whether re-exposure of ovariectomized allergic mice to antigen (ovalbumin) would lead to exacerbation of lung inflammation. Finally, we evaluated the preventive and treatment effect of *B. longum* 5^{1A} on lung inflammation and airway hyperresponsiveness. Our results showed that whereas ovariectomy caused no alterations in the gut microbiota composition and diversity in this animal model, 10 days after ovariectomy, preventive use administration of *B. longum* 5^{1A}, rather than its use after surgery was capable of attenuate the exacerbated lung inflammation and hyperresponsiveness in ovariectomized allergic mice. This prophylactic effect of *B. longum* 5^{1A} involves acetate production, which led to increased fecal acetate levels and, consequently, increased Treg cells in ovariectomized allergic mice.

Keywords: probiotic, *Bifidobacterium longum*, airway inflammation, ovariectomy, microbiota

INTRODUCTION

Asthma is a chronic inflammatory lung disease and a serious health concern (Cohn et al., 2004; Leynaert et al., 2012). The number of people with asthma worldwide increased from 235 to 334 million between 2011 and 2014 (Ellwood et al., 2017). At age 11, the prevalence of asthma is greater in males than in females; however, after puberty, this trend reverses. Furthermore, in adulthood, the mean duration of hospital stay is longer for women than for men, suggesting not only that the prevalence is greater in women after puberty but also that the disease is more severe (Hanley, 1981; Gibbs et al., 1984; Eliasson et al., 1986). Clinical evidence shows that a significant percentage of women with asthma exhibit worsening of symptoms during the perimenstrual phase (shortly before and during the first few days of the menstrual period). Terms such as (pre)menstrual, perimenstrual or circamenstrual asthma have been used to describe this phenomenon. It has been suggested that hormonal fluctuations during the menstrual cycle play a significant role in the periodic worsening of asthma severity in adult females. The hormonal fluctuations that occur in menopause can also trigger or exacerbate adult-onset asthma (Troisi et al., 1995; Bellia and Augugliaro, 2007; Zemp et al., 2012; Triebner et al., 2016). The roles of gender and sex hormones in asthma are very complex. Recently, experimental findings have demonstrated that interactions among the microbiota, female sex hormones, and immunity are associated with the development of autoimmune diseases (Markle et al., 2013; Yurkovetskiy et al., 2013). In this scenario, it has been clearly recognized that germ-free NOD female mice lack the commonly observed gender bias of diabetes, with enhanced type 1 diabetes development found in these females, showing a pivotal role of the gut microbiota in disease development. On the other hand, after castration, male mice exhibit a microbiota composition that is more similar to that found in female mice. Overall, these data demonstrate that female sex hormones, rather than X chromosome-associated factors, are involved in the modulation of microbiota composition (Markle et al., 2013; Yurkovetskiy et al., 2013). Thus, it is strongly suggested that hormones and the microbiota cooperate to modify the course of disease progression. Given the recognized role of the gut microbiota in regulating the immune response via hormone interactions, it is not surprising that the oscillating hormone levels observed during the menstrual cycle and in menopausal women could interfere with the gut microbiota profile, which in turn may affect female asthma symptoms.

The most popular probiotics are lactobacillus and bifidobacteria. Probiotic strains such as *Lactobacillus reuteri* (Miraglia Del Giudice et al., 2012) and *L. casei* (Yu et al., 2010) have been studied for their amelioration of allergic disease. Moreover, experimental studies have demonstrated the immunomodulatory role of probiotic bacteria, notably *Bifidobacterium*, in reducing the Th2 inflammation profile induced in mice (Abrahamsson et al., 2007; Iwabuchi et al., 2009; MacSharry et al., 2012). In general, the strategy has been to maintain or restore a healthy gut microbiota by regular supplementation with the abovementioned probiotics. Recently, studies have demonstrated that oral administration of probiotics protects female mice from bone density loss caused by ovary removal (Sjogren et al., 2012; Britton et al., 2014; Ohlsson et al., 2014; Parvaneh et al., 2015). Despite the role of probiotics in the Th2 inflammatory response, there are no experimental studies investigating the preventive action of probiotics on the exacerbation of asthma by low levels of sex hormones, which occurs in asthmatic women during the menstrual cycle and menopause. Considering that life expectancy has increased and that most women now undergo menopause, strategies to prevent the initiation or exacerbation of asthma in this life stage are highly relevant (Troisi et al., 1995; Gong et al., 2016). Thus, the purpose of this study was to determine whether *Bifidobacterium longum* 5^{1A} exerts a modulatory effect on the exacerbated lung inflammatory response induced in ovariectomized allergic mice. Here, we show for the first time that *B. longum* 5^{1A} administered to ovariectomized allergic mice prevented the exacerbation of lung inflammation and airway hyperresponsiveness.

MATERIALS AND METHODS

Animals

Female Balb/c mice (18–20 g) were obtained from the animal facility of the Institute of Biomedical Sciences, University of Sao Paulo. Animals were housed in groups of five per cage in a light- and temperature-controlled room (12 h light/dark cycles, 21 $\pm$ 2°C) with free access to food (AIN93-M) (Reeves et al., 1993) and water. The local Animal Care Committee of the University of Sao Paulo Institute of Biomedical Sciences approved the experiments.

Ovariectomy

Mice were anesthetized by an intraperitoneal (i.p.) injection of ketamine/xylazine (100 and 20 mg/kg, respectively). After an incision was made in the lower part of the abdomen, the ovaries were identified and removed from the adherent tissue. The effectiveness of the OVx procedure was assessed by analyzing the morphologic features of cells in vaginal smears and by quantifying the uterine weight. Mice subjected to similar manipulations except for the ovary removal were used as the sham-operated controls and labeled 'sham' animals. The same surgeon performed all surgical procedures.

Microbial Community Profiling

Fecal samples were collected 1 day before and 10 days after surgery and fecal pellets were frozen in 2 mL tubes at −80°C until DNA extraction. Pellets were placed in MoBio PowerSoil bead tubes and incubated at 70°C for 10 min before proceeding with the protocol recommended by the manufacturer. Extracted DNA was quantified using a Qubit spectrophotometer (Thermo Scientific Technologies) and visualized in 2% agarose gels stained with ethidium bromide to evaluate DNA integrity. Microbiote analysis was performed essentially as described by Thomas et al. (2016). In summary, for PCR amplification and amplicon sequencing, the V4–V5 region of the 16S rRNA gene was amplified using the forward 5′-AYTGGGYDTAAAGNG-3′ and reverse primer 5′-CCGTCAATTCNTTTRAGTTT-3′, corresponding to the positions 562 and 906, respectively, of the *Escherichia coli* 16S rRNA gene. Three 20 μl amplification reactions were performed per sample, each containing: 2.5 μM of each primer; 10 μl of Kapa Hotstart High Fidelity Master Mix (Kapa Technologies); and 25 ng of genomic DNA (gDNA). Thermocycling conditions were: 95°C, 3 min; 98°C, 15 s; and 40°C, 30 s for 35 cycles. This was followed by a last extension step at 72°C for 5 min. Amplicons of the three reactions of each sample were pooled and purified using a MinElute PCR Purification Kit (Qiagen). The purified products were run on 1.5% agarose gels and bands within the expected amplicon range were excised using sterile and disposable scalpels and purified using the Qiaquick gel extraction kit (Qiagen) to remove artifacts, primer-dimers, and non-specific bands. Amplicons were end-repaired and Ion Torrent adaptors with barcodes were ligated using the Ion Plus Fragment Library Kit (Thermo Scientific). Equimolar amounts of barcoded-amplicons from each sample were pooled, using the Ion Torrent qPCR quantitation kit (Thermo Scientific), and used for emulsion PCR using the Ion PGM Template OT2 400 Kit (Thermo Scientific). All samples were sequenced on the Ion torrent PGM platform using a v2 chip and the Ion PGM Sequencing 400 Kit (Thermo Scientific). Sequences processed by the latest version of the Ion Torrent server (v3.6.2) were used as input into the *Qiime* (*Quantitative insights into microbial ecology*) software package (Version 1.6.0) (Caporaso et al., 2010). We removed sequences with an average quality score <20 using a 50 nt sliding window. Then, we identified barcodes used for fecal sample, allowing a maximum of two mismatches, and discarded sequences with no barcodes, and <200 nt or >500 nt after barcode removal. PCR primers identified at the start or at the end of the reads, allowing a maximum of 4 nt mismatches, were trimmed and sequences with no identifiable primers were discarded. After primer trimming, we removed all sequences below 200 nt and the remaining sequences were used as input for downstream analysis. Filtered sequences were clustered with 97% identity using UPARSE (implemented in USEARCH v7 – Edgar, 2013) and the seed sequence of each cluster was picked as a representative. Chimeric sequences (and clusters) were identified using UCHIME (Edgar et al., 2011) and the Broad Institute's chimera slayer database (version microbiomeutil-r20110519) and excluded from further analysis. With the *Qiime* interface (default parameters), the RDP classifier (Wang et al., 2007) was used to assign a taxonomic rank to each sequence using a minimum confidence value of 80% and, subsequently, to each operational taxonomic unit (OTU). Unless otherwise stated, OTUs that occurred in fewer than 25% of all samples and with less than 3 reads were not considered. Using *Qiime*, we rarefied the OTU table to a depth of 13,851 sequences in order to calculate species richness and phylogenetic diversity, using the total number of observed OTUs and Faith's phylogenetic diversity (Faith et al., 2009), respectively. Rarefaction analysis was performed using *Qiime* and a cutoff of 13,851 for species richness. For beta-diversity analysis, OTU-representative sequences were aligned using PyNAST (Caporaso et al., 2010) against the aligned green genes core set (DeSantis et al., 2006) using *Qiime* default parameters, and the alignments were lane-mask filtered to build a phylogenetic tree using FastTree (Price et al., 2009). Distance matrices were generated for four metrics, unweighted and weighted UniFrac (Lozupone and Knight, 2005) Bray–Curtis and Euclidean, to compare pairwise distances between the four groups using ADONIS (Oksanen et al., 2016). Due to unequal sequence sampling depth across samples, we normalized the raw number of reads for each OTU using metagenome Seq's (Paulson et al., 2013) cumulative sum scaling function. We then used normalized counts to investigate differences between the groups at the OTU, genera, and family level.

Probiotic Supplementation

The species of bifidobacteria (*B. longum* 5^{1A}) used in this study was isolated and characterized at the Laboratory of Ecology and Physiology of Microorganisms, Institute of Biological Sciences, Federal University of Minas Gerais (Souza et al., 2013). The bifidobacteria were isolated from the feces of healthy children up to 5 years old in the city of Salvador (Bahia, Brazil) and identified by morfotintorial, respiratory, and biochemical tests, followed by multiplex PCR (Kwon et al., 2005). The bacteria were replicated in MRS broth medium (Difco) and grown under anaerobic conditions in an anaerobic jar at 37°C without stirring for 48 h. For the administration of probiotic bacteria, the mice received a daily inoculum by gavage of 0.1 mL containing 10^8 bacterial cells, beginning 15 days before the first sensitization (when animals were 4 weeks old) and until ovariectomy for prophylactic administration and 1 day after ovariectomy for the treatment protocol.

Induction of Allergic Lung Inflammation

Mice were sensitized intraperitoneally with 10 μg of chicken egg OVALBUMIN (OVA) grade V (Sigma Chemical Co., Saint Louis, MO, United States) dissolved in 0.2 mL of Imject alum suspension (1 mg). At days 14, 15, and 16, the mice were exposed to aerosolized OVA (1% in phosphate-buffered saline PBS) for 15 min using an ultrasonic nebulizer device (Respira Max®, SP, Brazil) coupled to a plastic inhalation chamber (18.5 cm × 18.5 cm × 13.5 cm). Ten days after the last challenge, the animals were subjected to ovariectomy (OVx), and 10 days later, they were re-challenged over 3 days as described above.

The experimental asthma protocols were started when mice were 6 weeks old. All measurements of inflammatory parameters were performed 24 h after the last aerosol re-challenge.

Short-Chain Fatty Acid (SCFA) Measurements

Acetic acid (99.7%) and citric acid were purchased from Sigma-Aldrich (St. Louis, MO, United States), butanol from Carlo Erba (Cornaredo, Italy), acetonitrile from Merck (Darmstadt, Germany), and tetrahydrofuran from Acros Organics (Fair Lawn, NJ, United States). Chromatographic analyses were performed using an Agilent 6850 system with EzChrom software, equipped with a 7683B automatic liquid sampler, a flame ionization detector (FID) (Agilent Technologies, United States), and a fused-silica capillary DB-23 column (Agilent Technologies, United States) with dimensions of 60 m × 0.25 mm internal diameter (i.d.) coated with a 0.15 μm thick layer of 80.2% 1-methylnaphatalene. The initial oven temperature was 100°C (hold 7 min), which was then increased to 200°C at a rate of 25°C/min (hold 5 min). The FID temperature was maintained at 260°C, and the flow rates of H2, air, and the make-up gas N2 were 30, 350, and 25 mL/min, respectively. Sample volumes of 5 μL were injected at 250°C using a split ratio of approximately 25:1. Nitrogen was used as the carrier gas at 1 mL/min (hold 4 min), reduced to 0.8 mL/min (hold 1 min) and then 0.6 mL/min (hold 1 min), and finally increased to 1 mL/min. The runtime for each analysis was 16.5 min. Acetic acid (HAc) was diluted to 1.0 mg/mL in butanol:tetrahydrofuran:acetonitrile (5:3:2), and further dilutions were made using the same solvent to generate a series of standard solutions. Blank human plasma was spiked with 1.0 mg/mL HAc. This solution was further diluted with blank plasma to prepare plasma standards of 0.015–1 mg/mL. To each tube, 40 mg of sodium chloride, 20 mg of citric acid, 40 μL of 0.1 M hydrochloric acid, and 200 μL of butanol:tetrahydrofuran:acetonitrile (5:3:2) were added. To quantify the acids, a calibration curve for the concentration range of 0.015–1 mg/mL was constructed. Probiotic culture medium (100 μL) was used to measure the acetate concentration. The concentration of plasma acetate was expressed in mM. Fecal samples were weighed into 1.5 mL tubes, crushed and homogenized in 100 mL of distilled water. Subsequently, 40 mg of sodium chloride, 20 mg of citric acid, 40 μL of 0.1 M hydrochloric acid, and 200 μL of butanol: tetrahydrofuran: acetonitrile (5:3:2) were added. The tubes were vortexed for 1 min and centrifuged at 10,000 rpm for 10 min. The supernatant was transferred to microtubes, and 5 μL was injected in triplicate into the gas chromatograph. The retention time was 7.2 min. The precision and accuracy of the assay were evaluated by analyzing samples (0.62, 0.25, and 0.75 mg/mL) in five replicates. The precision, expressed as relative standard deviation (RSD), was less than 14.34%, and the accuracy was between 87.51 and 113.56%. The standard acids, HAc, HPr, and HBu, were successfully separated in the gas-liquid chromatogram and eluted between 7 and 10 min in the temperature and gas flow program used here. The retention time was 7.2, 8.2, and 9.2 min for HAc, HPr, and HBu, respectively. The standard calibration curves showed linear relationships for all acids ($r = 0.999$). There was no interference present in the blanks at the retention time of the acids analyzed, and the analyte peaks were identifiable, discrete, and reproducible. The precision and accuracy of the assay were evaluated by analyzing samples (0.62, 0.25, and 0.75 mg/mL) in five replicates. The precision, expressed as RSD, was less than 14.34, 13.93, and 12.68%, for HAc, HPr, and HBu, respectively. The accuracy was between 87.51 and 113.56% for HAc, 91.44 and 111.60% for HPr, and 86.71 and 98.56% for HBu. The limit of quantification (LOQ) was 0.031 mg/mL for both acids analyzed, with a precision lower than 15% and accuracy within ±15%. The limit of detection (LOD) for both acids was 0.015 mg/mL, where the mean coefficient of variation (CV) value was under 20% for precision and under ±20% for accuracy. The feces extraction efficiency was 97.35 ± 5.23%. Therefore, the developed methods were shown to be reliable (Shah et al., 1991) for quantifying the SCFAs HAc, HPr, and HBu in mouse feces.

Bronchoalveolar Lavage (BAL)

Female mice were anesthetized with ketamine/xylazine (100 and 20 mg/kg, respectively), the trachea was exposed, and a cannula was inserted. The lungs were washed three times with aliquots (each 0.8 mL) of saline injected through the cannula. From the BAL fluid (BALF), the total number of cells was counted microscopically using a Neubauer chamber. Differential cell counts were performed by cytospin analysis and prepared from aliquots of BALF (200 μL) centrifuged at 300 g for 1 min using a Citospin® (Fanem). The cells were stained with Instant Prov (Newprov@, São Paulo, Brazil), and a total of 300 cells were counted to determine the proportion of neutrophils, eosinophils, and mononuclear cells using standard morphological criteria.

Lung Function Analysis

All animals were anesthetized with ketamine (100 mg/kg, i.p.) and xylazine (20 mg/kg) and paralyzed with pancuronium bromide, and a stable depth of anesthesia was maintained (Ferreira et al., 2012). After tracheostomy, the trachea was cannulated with a blunt 18-gauge metal tube, and the mouse was ventilated with a computer-controlled small-animal ventilator (flexiVent; Scireq, Montreal, QC, Canada) using a tidal volume of 10 mL/kg and a respiratory frequency of 150 breaths/min. A positive end-expiratory pressure (PEEP) of 2 cm H_2O was applied throughout. An external jugular vein was isolated for an intravenous (i.v.) infusion of methacholine (MCh). At the outset, 6 μg of MCh was provided intravenously to ensure that the animal was indeed responsive to MCh and that airway resistance returned to the baseline value after its MCh-induced rise, which indicated that the mouse was in stable physiological condition. To obtain a dose-response curve, a bolus of MCh was then injected starting at a dose of 4 μg (200 μg/mL solution in PBS; i.v. boluses of 10–40 μL). Prior to each MCh dose, the expiratory path was obstructed for 15 s to produce a deep inflation, after which exhalation was immediately allowed. Ventilation was continued for approximately 2 min between consecutive MCh doses. Airway responsiveness was equal to the Newtonian resistance (Rn) (Ferreira et al., 2012).

Analysis of Histological Changes to Lung Tissue

Lungs were removed from mice after BAL and fixed by immersion in 4% paraformaldehyde. The lobes were sagittally sectioned, embedded in paraffin, cut into 5-μm sections, and stained with periodic acid-Schiff (PAS); mucus production was measured as previously described (Tong et al., 2006).

Flow Cytometry

Mouse Treg cells were collected from the BALF and analyzed for $CD4^+$ $CD25^+$ $Foxp3^+$ expression using a mouse Treg cell staining kit containing APC-labeled anti-CD4, PE-labeled anti-CD25, and FITC-labeled anti-Foxp3 (eBioscience) according to the manufacturer's instructions. Briefly, prepared cells (1×10^6) were washed by centrifugation with cold PBS, resuspended in 1 mL of fixation/permeabilization solution, and incubated in the dark at 4°C for 30–60 min. The cells were washed once with 2 mL of permeabilization buffer, collected by centrifugation, resuspended in 20 mL of blocking agent with 2% (2 mL) normal rat serum in permeabilization buffer, and incubated at 4°C for 15 min. Next, 20 mL of a fluorochrome-conjugated antibody or isotype control in permeabilization buffer was added, followed by incubation in the dark at 4°C for 30 min. Finally, the cells were washed with 2 mL of permeabilization buffer, resuspended in flow cytometry buffer (PBS with 2% FBS), and analyzed using a FACSCanto II cytometer (BD Bioscience, San Diego, CA, United States). The data were analyzed using FlowJo® software.

Quantification of Cytokine Levels in BAL and of Female Sex Hormones in Serum

Commercial preparations of paired antibodies and protein standards for measurements of mouse IL-4, IL-5, IL-10, and IFN-γ (BD Bioscience) in the BAL were used to develop ELISAs according to the manufacturer's instructions. The determinations were performed in duplicate. Serum estradiol and progesterone concentrations were determined using an enzyme immunoassay kit according to the manufacturer's instructions (Cayman Chemical, Ann Arbor, MI, United States).

Statistical Analysis

The data are presented as the mean ± standard error of mean, Student's *t*-test and ANOVA followed by a Bonferroni post-test were used for comparisons between 2 and 3 or more groups, respectively. Values of $p \leq 0.05$ were considered significant.

RESULTS

Ovariectomy Efficacy

Ten days after ovariectomy, we measured the body and uterus weight of female mice and analyzed the vaginal cell morphology. The ovariectomized (OVx) animals had significantly higher body weights and lower uterus weights than animals subjected to false surgery (Sham). In addition, the vaginal cell morphological changes observed after ovariectomy were representative of diestrus phase and were corroborated by decreased plasma concentrations of estrogen and progesterone (**Table 1**). **Table 1** shows the parameters measured to analyze ovariectomy efficacy of animals studied in the **Figure 1**.

Effect of Ovary Removal on the Gut Microbial Profile

To analyze the effect of ovariectomy on gut microbial diversity and composition, we performed 16S rRNA next-generation sequencing. We obtained a total of 1,246,075 QC-passed sequences with an average length of 329 ± 2.9 nt and an average of 56,639 sequences/sample. A total of 258 operational taxonomic units (OTUs) were obtained, which was reduced to 248 after filtering to include only those OTUs present in at least 25% of samples and with at least three reads. When analyzing species richness, we found no significant differences between groups for any of the comparisons (**Figure 1A**) but did find increased phylogenetic diversity when comparing OVx POS (post-ovariectomy) mice with Sham PRE (pre-ovariectomy) mice and OVx PRE mice with Sham PRE mice. We found significant differences in pairwise distances using the weighted UniFrac metric when we compared OVx POS mice with Sham POS mice and all groups simultaneously (**Table 2**). Multidimensional scaling (MDS) revealed that the OVx POS samples clustered farther away from the other samples (**Figure 1B**). Bacterial community composition was also investigated, revealing that the most abundant bacterial phyla were (in decreasing order of abundance) *Bacteroidetes*, *Firmicutes*, and *Proteobacteria*. Despite seeing increases in *Bacteroidetes* abundance and decreases in *Firmicutes* abundance in OVx POS mice, these were non-significant. At the family level, the most abundant bacterial families among the groups were *Porphyromonadaceae*, unclassified *Clostridiales*, *Bacteroidaceae*, *Lachnospiraceae*, and *Ruminococcaceae*. Hierarchical clustering of rarefied OTU abundances clustered all samples from the OVx POS group together in one main tree branch, whereas samples from the other groups were scattered across various branches (**Figure 1C**). When we evaluated differences between the groups at different taxonomic levels, we found a significant increase of *Bifidobacteriaceae*, but not any other bacterial taxon, in OVx POS samples (**Figure 1D**).

Ovariectomy Exacerbates Lung Inflammation and Airway Hyperresponsiveness in Re-challenged Allergic Mice

We next investigated whether re-exposure of OVx allergic mice to antigen (OVA) exacerbates lung inflammation (**Figure 2A**). We found a significant increase in total cells recovered in the BALF from Sham and OVx allergic mice that was exacerbated by re-exposure of OVx allergic mice to OVA (**Figure 2C**). Moreover, the number of eosinophils in the BAL from re-challenged OVx allergic mice significantly increased compared with Sham allergic mice. The total cells in the BAL recovered from non-sensitized or OVx mice did not differ.

Next, considering that airway hyperresponsiveness is a hallmark of asthma and that its evolution is often associated

TABLE 1 | Animal characteristics, body and tissue weights, and hormone measures

Group	Number animals	Average body weight (g)	Uterus weight (g)	17 Beta estradiol (pg/mL)	Progesterone (ng/mL)	Diestro phase
Ovx	7	24.5 ± 1.0*	0.015 ± 0.004*	21.0 ± 9.9*	0.78 ± 1.1*	Positive
Sham	4	22.7 ± 1.0	0.028 ± 0.006	41.5 ± 3.3*	1.7 ± 0.6*	Negative

*Values are mean ± SD. *p =< 0.05 Sham vs. OVX.*

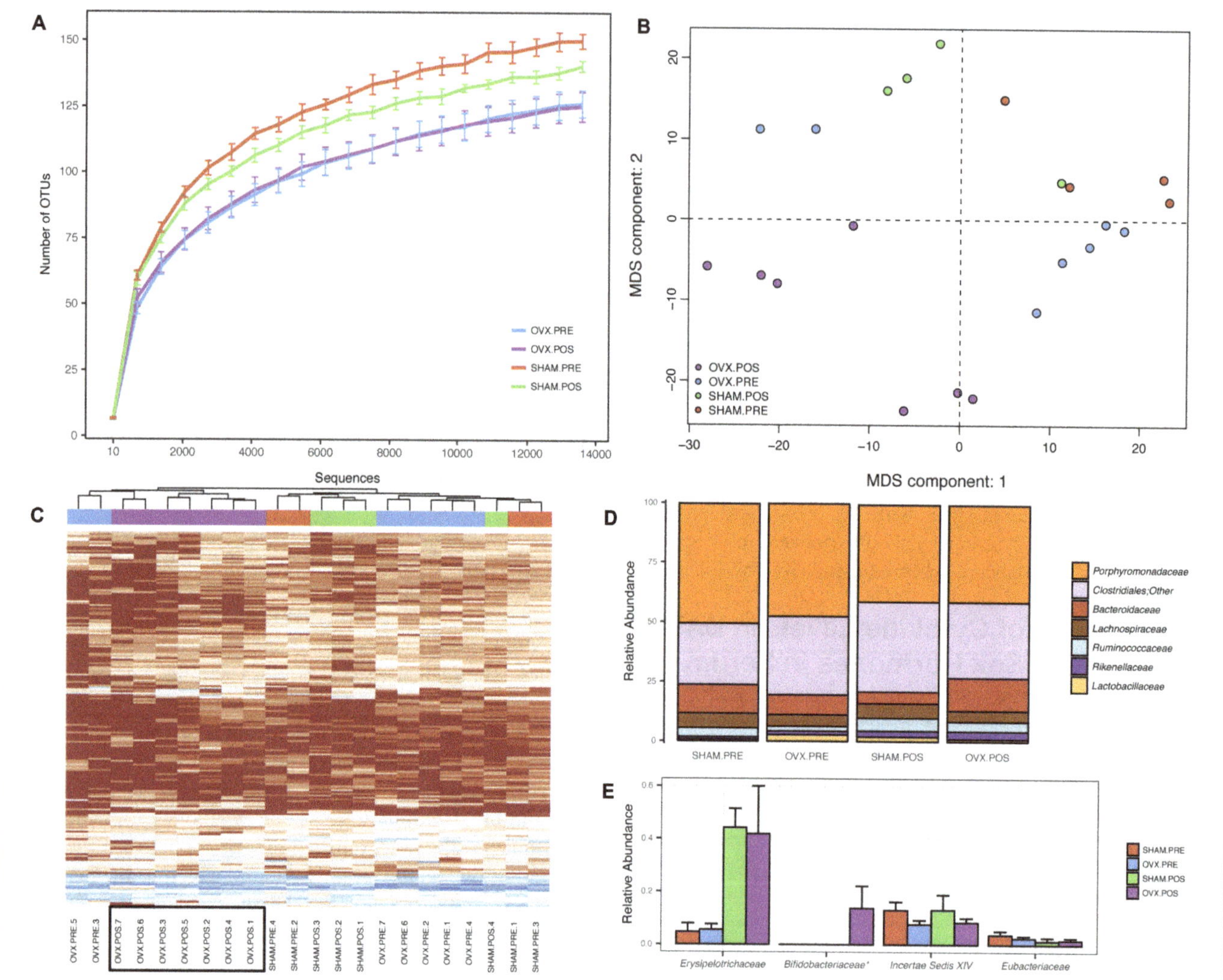

FIGURE 1 | Bacterial community profiling of fecal samples from Balb/c before and after ovariectomy. **(A)** Rarefaction analysis indicating the average number of OTUs per sequence sampling depth for each of the groups. Error bars represent the standard error of the mean. **(B)** Multidimensional scaling of Euclidean distances between mouse fecal samples. **(C)** Heatmap and hierarchical clustering of mouse fecal samples using rarefied OTU abundances. **(D)** Mean relative abundances of the most abundant bacterial families identified in the samples. **(E)** Mean relative abundances of the least abundant bacterial families identified in the samples. Error bars represent the standard error of the mean and * indicates a *p*-value < 0.05.

with lung inflammation (Maddox and Schwartz, 2002; Tong et al., 2006), we investigated whether the ovariectomy of allergic mice would also lead to exacerbated hyperresponsiveness. We quantified the respiratory Newtonian resistance (Rn) changes in response to intravenous administration of a cholinergic agent, methacholine (MCh), after the last re-exposure to antigen challenge. Re-challenged OVx allergic mice exhibited significantly increased airway hyperresponsiveness to MCh compared with Sham OVx allergic mice (**Figure 2B**).

We also determined the effect of ovariectomy on the Th2 cytokine profile. Our data revealed a significant increase in IL-5 levels in the BAL recovered from OVx allergic mice re-exposed to antigen challenge compared with that of Sham OVx allergic mice (**Figure 2D**). Although a low level of IL-4 was found in the BALF, no significant difference between

TABLE 2 | Alpha and beta diversity *p*-values for various group comparisons.

Comparison	Metrics					
	Bray–Curtis	Euclidean	Unweighted unifrac	Weighted unifrac	Observed species	Phylogenetic diversity
All	0.18	0.638	**0.047**	0.517	NA	NA
OVX POS vs. SHAM POS	0.055	0.164	**0.045**	0.351	0.492	1
OVX POS vs. SHAM PRE	0.212	0.339	0.089	0.433	0.138	**0.006**
OVX PRE vs. OVX POS	0.095	0.085	0.063	0.283	1	1
OVX PRE vs. SHAM POS	0.679	0.917	0.385	0.688	0.594	1
OVX PRE vs. SHAM PRE	0.953	0.995	0.373	0.682	0.096	**0.018**
SHAM PRE vs. SHAM POS	0.164	0.589	0.056	0.358	0.168	0.312

Bold values = P < 0.05.

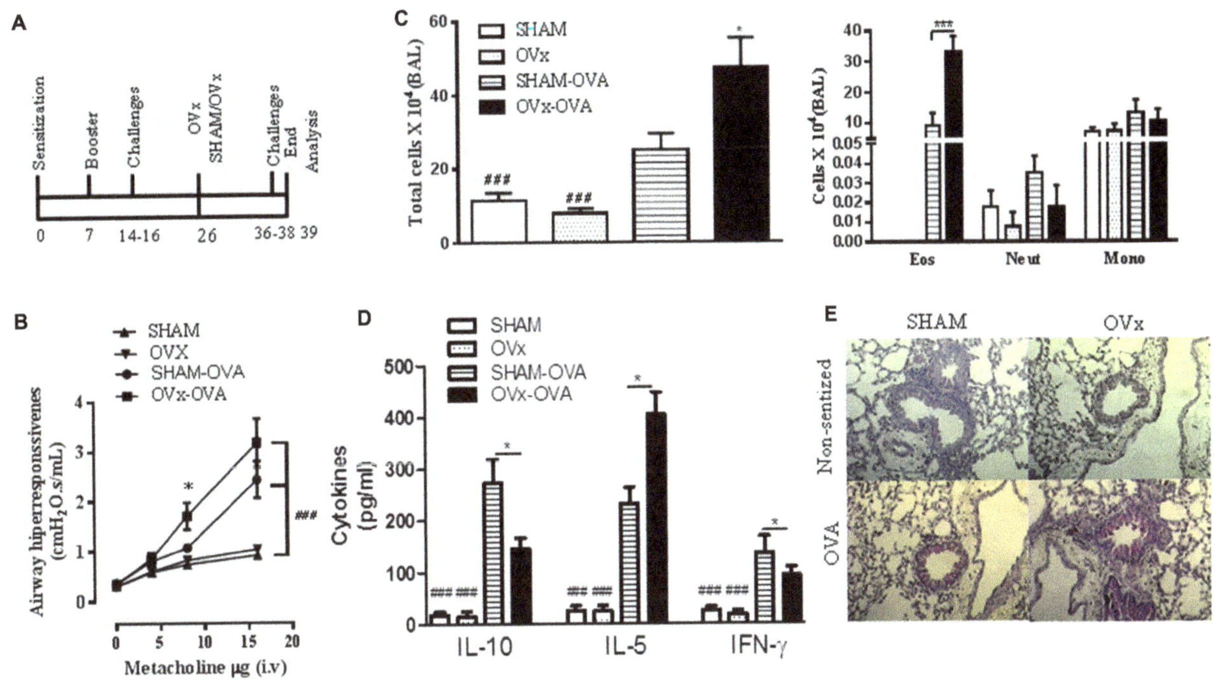

FIGURE 2 | Ovariectomy exacerbates the lung inflammation and airway hyperresponsiveness of re-challenged allergic mice. **(A)** Ten days before being ovariectomized (OVx) or not (Sham), the animals were sensitized and challenged. Ten days after ovariectomy, the animals were re-challenged. All parameters were analyzed 24 h after the last re-challenge. **(B)** Measurement of AHR, as assessed by Newtonian airway resistance to increasing doses of methacholine. **(C)** Quantification of the total number of cells in the bronchoalveolar lavage (BAL). **(D)** Concentration of IL-10, IL-5, and INF-γ in the BAL. **(E)** Representative periodic acid–Schiff (PAS)-stained lung tissue from mice in the SHAM, OVx, SHAM OVA, and OVx OVA groups. Scale bars, 200 μm. All results are representative of data generated in two different experiments and are expressed as the mean ± SEM (n = 5 in all groups). Statistical significance was determined by a one-way analysis of variance (ANOVA), except in **(B)**, in which a two-way ANOVA test was used. Hash symbol: non-allergic (sham and OVx) groups vs. respective allergic group (sham Ova and OVx OVA), $^{###}P < 0.001$; asterisk: Sham OVA vs. OVx OVA. $^{*}P < 0.05$, $^{**}P < 0.01$, $^{***}P < 0.001$.

these two groups was observed (unpublished data). In contrast, IFN-γ and IL-10 were reduced in the BAL of re-challenged OVx allergic mice compared with Sham OVx allergic mice (**Figure 2D**).

Excessive mucus production is a characteristic of asthmatic airways; therefore, we evaluated the presence of PAS-stained cells in the lungs of re-challenged mice. As seen in **Figure 2E**, a significant increase in PAS-stained cells was observed in the lungs of re-challenged OVx allergic mice compared with re-challenged Sham OVx allergic mice. The lungs of non-sensitized mice did not show PAS-stained cells (**Figure 2E**).

Preventive Oral Probiotic Supplementation Attenuates the Exacerbation of Lung Inflammation and Airway Hyperresponsiveness in Re-challenged OVx Allergic Mice

The role of probiotics in regulating the immune system and allergic diseases has been extensively debated (Abrahamsson et al., 2007). An oral probiotic (*B. longum* 5^{1A}) was administered daily by gavage for 15 days before the first OVA sensitization of mice and continued until 4 h before the mouse ovaries

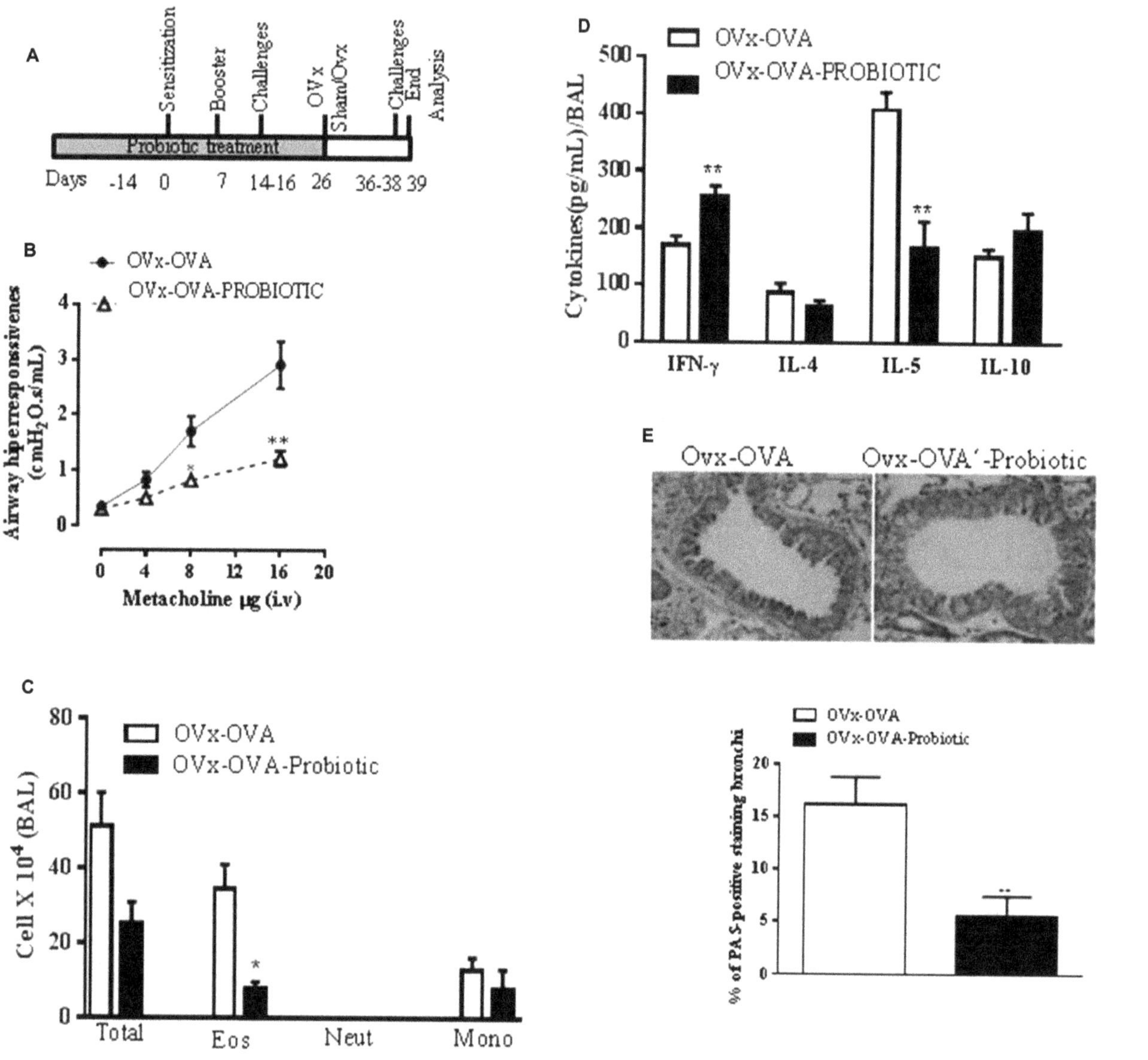

FIGURE 3 | Preventive oral probiotic supplementation decreased the allergic airway inflammation and airway hyperresponsiveness of re-challenged ovariectomized allergic mice. **(A)** An oral probiotic (*B. longum* 5^{1A}) was administered by gavage daily for 15 days before the first OVA sensitization of mice and continued until 4 h before the ovaries of the mice were removed. **(B)** AHR in mice supplemented with the probiotic or saline. **(C)** Differential cell counts in the BAL. Total number of cells infiltrating the airways in the BAL. **(D)** Concentration of INF-γ, IL-4, IL-5, and IL-10 expression levels in the BAL. **(E)** Representative periodic acid–Schiff (PAS)-stained lung tissue from mice on either a control or probiotic on day 16. Scale bars, 200 μm. All results are representative of data generated in two different experiments and are expressed as the mean ± SEM (n = 4 control mice, and n = 5 mice given the probiotic supplementation). Statistical significance was determined with Student's t-test, except in **(B)**, in which a two-way ANOVA test was used. $^{*}P < 0.05$, $^{**}P < 0.01$, $^{***}P < 0.001$, $^{****}P < 0.0001$.

were removed (**Figure 3A**). The preventive effect of *B. longum* 5^{1A} supplementation on the exacerbation of lung inflammation and airway hyperresponsiveness in re-challenged OVx allergic mice was investigated. Oral supplementation with *B. longum* 5^{1A} attenuated the exacerbation of the MCh-induced airway hyperreactivity of re-challenged OVx allergic mice. The airway hyperresponsiveness of supplemented OVx-OVA mice was significantly reduced compared to the OVx-OVA group. Additionally, *B. longum* 5^{1A} treatment significantly reduced the number of eosinophils recovered from the BAL of re-challenged OVx allergic mice (**Figure 3B**). *B. longum* 5^{1A} administration also resulted in a significant reduction of IL-5 levels in the BAL of re-challenged OVx allergic mice relative to non-treated mice (**Figure 3C**). By contrast, *B. longum* 5^{1A} treatment significantly increased the levels of IFN-γ in re-challenged OVx allergic mice. The BAL levels of IL-4 and IL-10 were not changed (**Figure 3D**). The probiotic treatment also significantly reduced the mucus production in the lungs of re-challenged OVx allergic mice compared with non-treated re-challenged OVx allergic mice (**Figure 3E**).

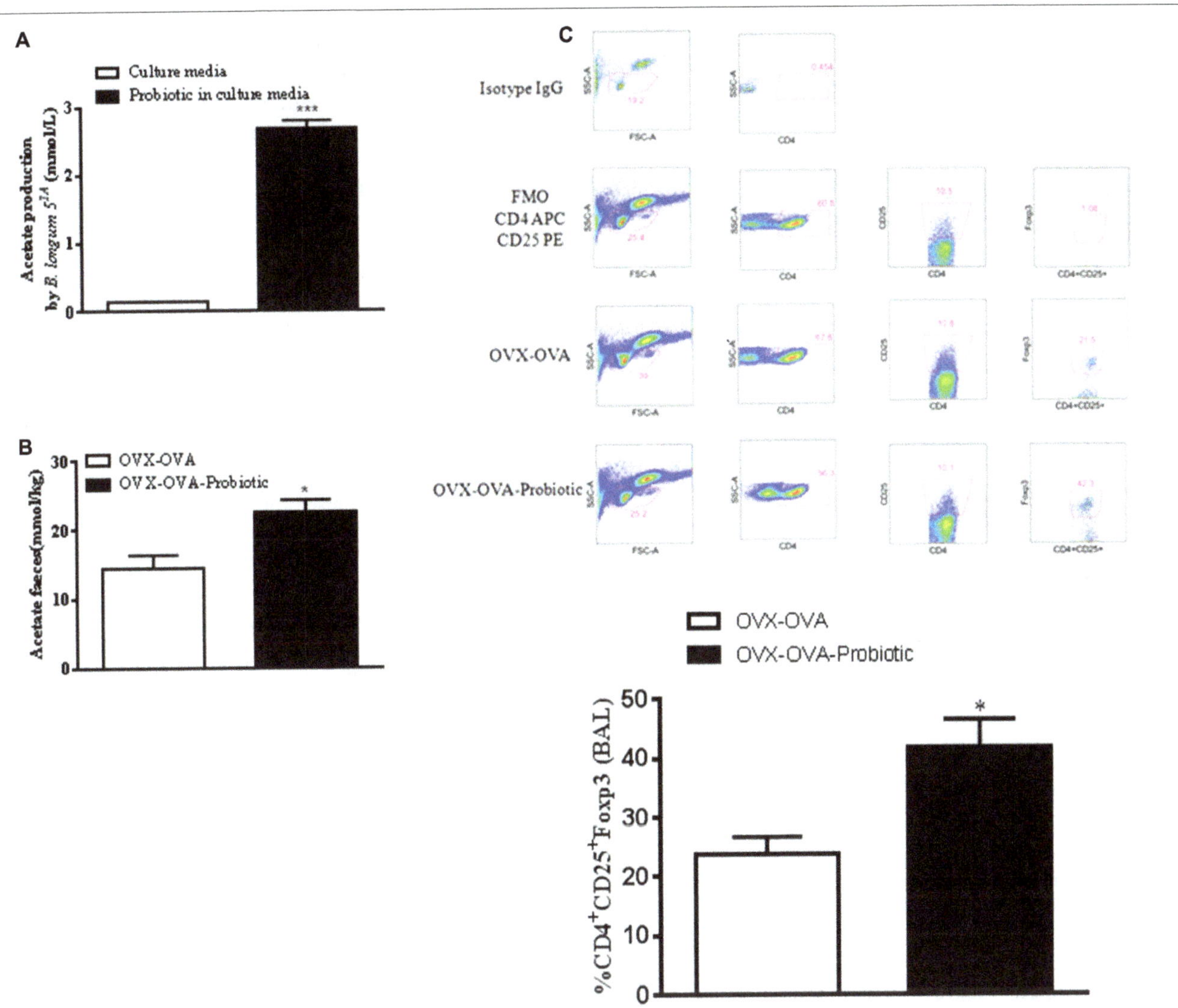

FIGURE 4 | Preventive supplementation with *B. longum* 5^{1A} increases the production of short-chain fatty acids (SCFAs) and the number of lung Treg cells of re-challenged OVx allergic mice. **(A)** Sterile bacterial culture medium and *B. longum* in culture medium. Fecal SCFA concentrations from the mice depicted in **(B)**. **(C)** An oral probiotic (*B. longum* 5^{1A}) was administered by gavage daily for 15 days before the first OVA sensitization of mice and continued until 24 h before the mouse ovaries were removed. After the last re-challenge, cells from the BALF were subjected to flow cytometry and stained for CD4-APC, CD25-PE, and FoxP3-FITC. The dot plot demonstrates the gate strategy of Treg (Isotype control, Fluorescence Minus One Control-FMO, OVA-OVx, and OVA-OVx-probiotic) and the percentage of positive Treg cells. The graph is representative of two independent experiments. All results are representative of data generated in two different experiments and are expressed as the mean ± SEM [$n = 3$ for all groups in **(A)**, $n = 4$ in **(B,C)**]. Statistical significance was determined by a one-way ANOVA. $^{*}P < 0.05$, $^{***}P < 0.001$.

Preventive Supplementation with *B. longum* 5^{1A} Increases the Production of SCFAs and the Number of Lung Treg Cells in Re-challenged OVx Allergic Mice

Because SCFAs, especially acetate, have anti-inflammatory properties, we hypothesized that SCFA production by *B. longum* 5^{1A} could modulate allergic lung inflammation. Thus, we measured SCFAs in the probiotic culture medium and in mouse feces. Our data indicated that acetate was the SCFA quantified in the bacterial medium (**Figure 4A**), whereas we did not find measurable levels of propionate or butyrate. In addition, *B. longum* 5^{1A} treatment significantly increased the levels of acetate in the feces of re-challenged OVA allergic mice compared to non-treated mice (**Figure 4B**). Butyrate was also measured but did not differ between groups (unpublished data). Since Treg cells play a role in the control of asthma, and SCFAs interfere with the functional activity of Tregs, we examined the levels of Tregs in the BALF of the re-challenged OVx allergic mice previously treated with *B. longum*. The re-challenged OVx allergic mice supplemented with the probiotic exhibited a significant increased percentage of Tregs in BALF compared with non-treated mice (**Figure 4C**).

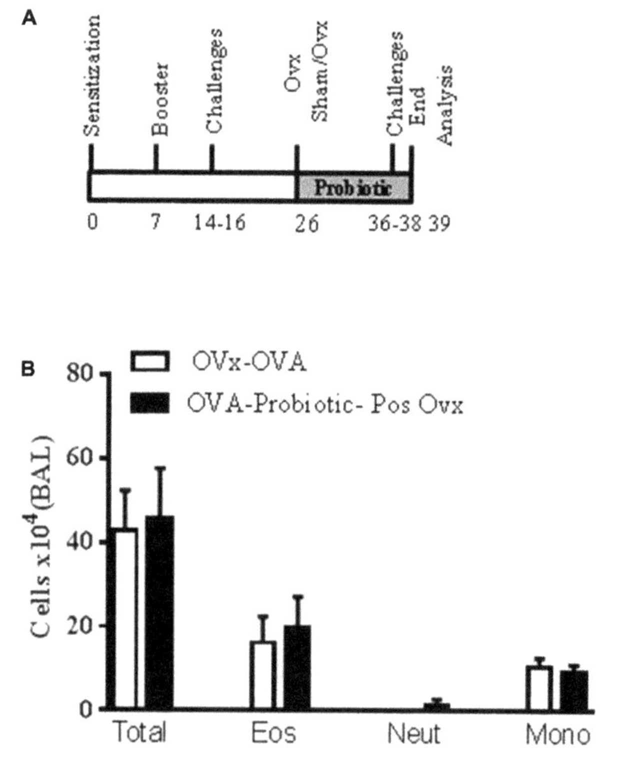

FIGURE 5 | Oral probiotic supplementation after ovariectomy does not alter airway inflammation. An oral probiotic (*B. longum* 5^{1A}) was administered by gavage 24 h after ovariectomy until the last re-challenge **(A)**. All parameters were analyzed 24 h after the last re-challenge. **(B)** Quantification of the total cells number in the BAL. All results are representative of data generated in one experiment and are expressed as the mean ± SEM (*n* = 4–5 mice in all groups).

Oral Probiotic Supplementation after Ovariectomy Does Not Attenuate the Exacerbated Lung Inflammation and Airway Hyperresponsiveness of Re-challenged Allergic Mice

In this set of experiments, we investigated the effect of probiotic supplementation on exacerbated lung inflammation and airway hyperresponsiveness after ovariectomy, when lung inflammation is established. The mice were supplemented with *B. longum* 5^{1A} after ovary removal. As shown in **Figure 5**, when the probiotic was given after ovary removal, the profile of total inflammatory cells and eosinophils recovered in the BAL was not altered in the re-challenged allergic mice relative to the non-treated re-challenged OVx allergic mice (**Figure 5**).

DISCUSSION

Clinical evidence shows that after puberty, asthma is more frequent in females than in males, which indicates that the oscillation of female sex hormones during the menstrual cycle is involved (Leynaert et al., 2012). In addition, asthma symptoms worsen in menopausal women (Keselman and Heller, 2015). Previous studies have investigated the beneficial effects of probiotics on allergic lung disease (Abrahamsson et al., 2007, 2009, 2011). However, the effect of probiotics on asthma symptoms or exacerbation during the perimenstrual and menopausal phases in women remains clinically debated. Many studies have shown that some Bifidobacterium levels are decreased in the presence of allergic disease (MacSharry et al., 2012). Menopause precedes senescence (Kirkwood and Shanley, 2010), and a negative correlation between senescence and Bifidobacterium use has been described in clinical studies (Arboleya et al., 2016). Additionally, *B. longum* has been associated with protection against asthma in clinical and experimental studies (Iwabuchi et al., 2009; Akay et al., 2014). The effects of *B. longum* 5^{1A} on allergic disease in particular have not been investigated yet. However, it has been demonstrated that oral *B. longum* 5^{1A} treatment resolved the inflammation due to lung infection caused by *Klebsiella pneumoniae* in mice (Vieira et al., 2016) and reduced the inflammatory response in an experimental murine model of gout (Vieira et al., 2015). Additionally, clinical studies have shown that *B. longum* 5^{1A} has an effect on pediatric functional constipation (Guerra et al., 2011).

In this study, we investigated the role of probiotic treatment of ovariectomized re-challenged allergic mice. The study was performed to evaluate the role of probiotics in asthma exacerbation during menopause. First, we confirmed that re-challenging ovariectomized allergic mice exacerbated Th2-mediated airway inflammation and airway reactivity, strongly suggesting that sex hormone deficiency after ovary removal modulates the severity of the asthma phenotype. Accordingly, after re-exposure to the antigen challenge, ovariectomized allergic mice showed exacerbated allergic inflammation, airway hyperresponsiveness, and excess secretion of mucus and the cytokine IL-5. Next, we treated the mice with *B. longum* 5^{1A} before or after the induction of allergic reaction and ovariectomy to evaluate the preventive and therapeutic effect of the probiotic in this model of allergic lung inflammation. Our data demonstrated that *B. longum* 5^{1A} prevented the exacerbation of Th2-mediated airway inflammation induced in re-challenged ovariectomized allergic mice. As the probiotic treatment began 15 days before the antigen sensitization and continued until the day of ovariectomy, we suggest that the probiotic *B. longum* 5^{1A} has a preventive effect on the exacerbation of allergic lung inflammation. In fact, our data revealed a significantly decreased eosinophil influx into the airways. In addition, reduced airway hyperresponsiveness, IL-5 levels, and mucus production were also observed. This is the first study investigating the effect of *B. longum* 5^{1A} on asthma exacerbation during menopause. Since allergic asthma is mediated by Th2 cytokines, and our data revealed an effective involvement of *B. longum* 5^{1A} in the reduction of airway hyperreactivity and eosinophil recruitment into the lungs, we hypothesized that the treatment of mice with the probiotic shifted the Th1/Th2 balance toward a Th1 profile. Indeed, in the present study, we found an association between *B. longum* 5^{1A} intake and an augmented release of the classical Th1 cytokine IFN-γ as well as decreased release

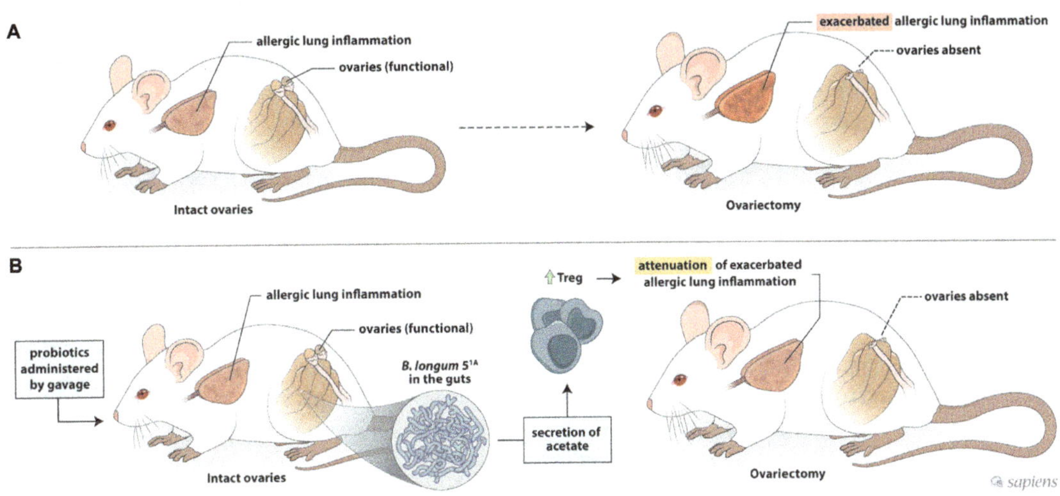

FIGURE 6 | Schematic representation of mechanism underlying the effect of probiotic intake on the asthma exacerbation after ovariectomy. Ovariectomy exacerbates the lung inflammation of re-challenge allergic mice **(A)**. Preventive supplementation with *B. longum* 5^{1A} decreases exarcebation of lung inflammation and increases the production of acetate and Treg cells in re-challenge OVx allergic mice **(B)**.

of the Th2 cytokine IL-5 by the lungs of re-challenged allergic mice. Considering that *B. longum* 5^{1A} treatment increased the number of regulatory T cells recovered in the BALF of re-challenged allergic mice, we note a possible role of *B. longum* in the induction of allergen-specific tolerance or immune suppression by regulatory T cells. Our data are in line with studies (Kwon et al., 2010) showing a suppressive effect of some probiotics on Th2 cytokines with a concomitant increased stimulation of Th1 cytokines. In this context, probiotic strains such as *Lactobacilli* and *Bifidobacteria* recognizably affect regulatory T cell development, modulating the Th1/Th2 balance. Experimental and clinical evidence has shown that fermentation of fiber by microbiota or probiotics mediates the production of SCFAs, such as acetate (De Filippo et al., 2010; Tan et al., 2014; Trompette et al., 2014). To verify the interaction between probiotic intake and the generation of SCFAs in our model of re-challenged allergic mice, we measured SCFAs in the feces of these mice. We found that *B. longum* 5^{1A} intake was positively correlated with the levels of acetate in feces from re-challenged ovariectomized allergic mice. Interestingly, acetate produced by the gut microbiota has been associated with an increased number of regulatory T cells in the lungs in a murine model (Thorburn et al., 2015). It already know that mice deficient in the short chain fatty acid receptor, G-protein coupled receptor 43 (GPR43) show exacerbated asthma response. In addition, acetate can regulate regulatory T cells by interfering with gene transcription, resulting in inhibition of histone deacetylases (Tao et al., 2007; Thorburn et al., 2015). Recently, it was also described that propionate, a SCFA, promotes the development of tolerogenic DCs to the draining mesenteric lymph nodes inducing the development of Treg cells (Trompette et al., 2014). This interaction between distal organ, as lung, and gut microbiota is currently named such as the lung-gut axis (Marsland et al., 2015). Besides this interaction between pulmonary and gut immunity happen due to the production of SCFAs by the gut microbiota, the oral microbiota serves as an inoculum for the intestine (Arimatsu et al., 2014), and possible lungs (Venkataraman et al., 2015; Wu and Segal, 2017). It has suggested that lung microbiota might be transiently recolonized through microaspiration and breathing (Venkataraman et al., 2015). Thus, gut microbiota modulation can be an important strategy to treat lung diseases.

Our data show that probiotic treatment of allergic mice started 1 day after ovariectomy and maintained until the last antigen challenge did not alter the profile of inflammatory cells recruited into the lungs. Thus, protection is not given when therapies are initiated after the disease has been established. Recently, it was demonstrated that preventive rather than therapeutic treatment with a high-fiber diet attenuates clinical and inflammatory markers of acute and chronic DSS-induced colitis in mice (Silveira et al., 2017). These results suggest that any therapy aimed at modifying the gut environment (e.g., prebiotic or probiotic strategies) should be given early in the course of disease. It is also possible that the effectiveness of the probiotic *B. longum* on the control of allergic lung inflammation may involve the activity of sex hormones. There are some bacteria affected by sex hormones; for example, *Prevotella intermedia* takes up estradiol and progesterone, which enhance its growth (Kornman and Loesche, 1982). These findings deserve further investigation.

We have not investigated the specific roles of estradiol in this study, but data from the literature show that the role of estradiol in allergic disease is very complex. Data from our group show that removal of the ovaries 7 days before sensitization to OVA significantly inhibited lung eosinophilia and IL-5 levels in lung lavage fluid (de Oliveira et al., 2007). However, if ovaries are removed 1 day before sensitization to OVA, lung eosinophilia and IL-5 levels are increased (Riffo-Vasquez et al., 2007). These data suggest that sex hormone levels during sensitization are relevant to asthma. Considering that the worsening of pulmonary function observed in clinical studies during the perimenstrual and menopausal phases is a consequence of asthma, we investigated the repercussions of re-exposure to the antigen after removal of the ovaries from animals with asthma already triggered. The experimental model proposed here is novel and important for studying therapeutic alternatives to treat asthma exacerbation during the perimenstrual and menopausal phases.

We examined microbiota composition and diversity 10 days after ovariectomy and, after this period we observed no differences in the microbiota diversity between the sham and ovariectomized groups or between the pre- and post-surgery groups. However, hierarchical clustering of rarefied OTU abundances clustered all samples from the ovariectomized group together in one main tree branch, while samples from the other groups were scattered across various branches. These results suggest that the microbiota in the ovariectomized animals may have a similar composition that would cluster them separately from the other groups. Importantly, the fecal microbiome was evaluated here is a single point, and this could maybe a too short period to observe significant differences in microbiota composition.

We also observed that mice in the same experimental group showed clear variations in gut microbiota composition, though they were housed in the same facilities and treated under the same conditions. Mice with the same maternal origin but from different litters do show some differences in gut microbiota composition (Ubeda et al., 2012). The mice analyzed in our experiments were not from the same litter or mothers and maybe this could explain some of the intragroup discrepancies observed here. It is also known that male and female- derived microbiota exhibit distinct circadian rhythmicity, with females showing a more obvious oscillation than males (Liang et al., 2015). In this study, we always collected feces at the same time, in the morning, to attenuate a possible circadian influence. Another important finding was that the ovariectomized group showed increased levels of bifidobacteria. Clinical studies have shown some differences in bifidobacteria species between atopic and healthy children (Stsepetova et al., 2007). *B. adolescentis* was isolated from allergic infants, and *B. infants* and *B. bifidum* were isolated from healthy infants (He et al., 2001; Stsepetova et al., 2007; Melli et al., 2016). Studies *in vitro* and *in vivo* have shown that the ability of Bifidobacterium to stimulate the immune system is species specific (Menard et al., 2008). *B. adolescentis* is an example of a bacteria that may not regulate the immune system in some situations, and it is not an important acetate producer (Menard et al., 2008). Due to the limitations of our microbiota analyses, we did not evaluate which specific strain of bifidobacteria was increased in ovariectomized mice.

In summary, our data show that the preventive supplementation of the probiotic *B. longum* 5^{1A} clearly attenuated the exacerbated airway inflammation and hyperresponsiveness in re-challenged ovariectomized allergic mice (**Figure 6**). However, the probiotic protection was lost when treatment was initiated after ovariectomy and disease was already established. These results suggest that therapeutic strategies to modulate the gut microbiota have the potential to prevent asthma exacerbation in the perimenstrual and menopausal phases. However, these strategies should be implemented before sex hormone levels decline.

AVAILABILITY OF SUPPORTING DATA

Nucleotide sequences used for this study have been deposited in the SRA under accession, SRP105204.

AUTHOR CONTRIBUTIONS

Conceived and designed the experiments: CF, WT-L, ED-N, RC, and NC. Performed the experiments: EM, BA, AT, AF, AC, GM, and CF. Analyzed the data: EM, CF, TB, JS, and AT. Contributed reagents/materials/analysis tools: CV, WR, RC, and FM. Wrote the paper: CF, WT-L, ED-N, and RC.

ACKNOWLEDGMENTS

This study was funded by São Paulo Research Foundation (FAPESP), project number 2012/50410-8 to CF, 2012, and CNPq (The National Council for Scientific and Technological Development), project number 486037/2012-6 to CF.

REFERENCES

Abrahamsson, T. R., Jakobsson, T., Bottcher, M. F., Fredrikson, M., Jenmalm, M. C., Bjorksten, B., et al. (2007). Probiotics in prevention of IgE-associated eczema: a double-blind, randomized, placebo-controlled trial. *J. Allergy Clin. Immunol.* 119, 1174–1180. doi: 10.1016/j.jaci.2007.01.007

Abrahamsson, T. R., Sandberg Abelius, M., Forsberg, A., Bjorksten, B., and Jenmalm, M. C. (2011). A Th1/Th2-associated chemokine imbalance during infancy in children developing eczema, wheeze and sensitization. *Clin. Exp. Allergy* 41, 1729–1739. doi: 10.1111/j.1365-2222.2011.03827.x

Abrahamsson, T. R., Sinkiewicz, G., Jakobsson, T., Fredrikson, M., and Bjorksten, B. (2009). Probiotic lactobacilli in breast milk and infant stool in relation to oral intake during the first year of life. *J. Pediatr. Gastroenterol. Nutr.* 49, 349–354. doi: 10.1097/MPG.0b013e31818f091b

Akay, H. K., Bahar Tokman, H., Hatipoglu, N., Hatipoglu, H., Siraneci, R., Demirci, M., et al. (2014). The relationship between bifidobacteria and allergic asthma and/or allergic dermatitis: a prospective study of 0-3 years-old children in Turkey. *Anaerobe* 28, 98–103. doi: 10.1016/j.anaerobe.2014.05.006

Arboleya, S., Watkins, C., Stanton, C., and Ross, R. P. (2016). Gut bifidobacteria populations in human health and aging. *Front. Microbiol.* 7:1204. doi: 10.3389/fmicb.2016.01204

Arimatsu, K., Yamada, H., Miyazawa, H., Minagawa, T., Nakajima, M., Ryder, M. I., et al. (2014). Oral pathobiont induces systemic inflammation and metabolic changes associated with alteration of gut microbiota. *Sci. Rep.* 4:4828. doi: 10.1038/srep04828

Bellia, V., and Augugliaro, G. (2007). Asthma and menopause. *Monaldi Arch. Chest Dis.* 67, 125–127. doi: 10.4081/monaldi.2007.482

Britton, R. A., Irwin, R., Quach, D., Schaefer, L., Zhang, J., Lee, T., et al. (2014). Probiotic *L. reuteri* treatment prevents bone loss in a menopausal ovariectomized mouse model. *J. Cell Physiol.* 229, 1822–1830. doi: 10.1002/jcp.24636

Caporaso, J. G., Kuczynski, J., Stombaugh, J., Bittinger, K., Bushman, F. D., Costello, E. K., et al. (2010). QIIME allows analysis of high-throughput community sequencing data. *Nat. Methods* 7, 335–336. doi: 10.1038/nmeth.f.303

Cohn, L., Elias, J. A., and Chupp, G. L. (2004). Asthma: mechanisms of disease persistence and progression. *Annu. Rev. Immunol.* 22, 789–815. doi: 10.1146/annurev.immunol.22.012703.104716

De Filippo, C., Cavalieri, D., Di Paola, M., Ramazzotti, M., Poullet, J. B., Massart, S., et al. (2010). Impact of diet in shaping gut microbiota revealed by a comparative study in children from Europe and rural Africa. *Proc. Natl. Acad. Sci. U.S.A.* 107, 14691–14696. doi: 10.1073/pnas.1005963107

de Oliveira, A. P., Domingos, H. V., Cavriani, G., Damazo, A. S., Dos Santos Franco, A. L., Oliani, S. M., et al. (2007). Cellular recruitment and cytokine generation in a rat model of allergic lung inflammation are differentially modulated by progesterone and estradiol. *Am. J. Physiol. Cell Physiol.* 293, C1120–C1128. doi: 10.1152/ajpcell.00286.2006

DeSantis, T. Z., Hugenholtz, P., Larsen, N., Rojas, M., Brodie, E. L., Keller, K., et al. (2006). Greengenes, a chimera-checked 16S rRNA gene database and workbench compatible with ARB. *Appl. Environ. Microbiol.* 72, 5069–5072. doi: 10.1128/AEM.03006-05

Edgar, R. C. (2013). UPARSE: highly accurate OTU sequences from microbial amplicon reads. *Nat. Methods* 10, 996–998. doi: 10.1038/nmeth.2604

Edgar, R. C., Haas, B. J., Clemente, J. C., Quince, C., and Knight, R. (2011). UCHIME improves sensitivity and speed of chimera detection. *Bioinformatics* 27, 2194–2200. doi: 10.1093/bioinformatics/btr381

Eliasson, O., Scherzer, H. H., and DeGraff, A. C. Jr. (1986). Morbidity in asthma in relation to the menstrual cycle. *J. Allergy Clin. Immunol.* 77(1 Pt 1), 87–94. doi: 10.1016/0091-6749(86)90328-3

Ellwood, P., Asher, M. I., Billo, N. E., Bissell, K., Chiang, C. Y., Ellwood, E. M., et al. (2017). The global asthma network rationale and methods for phase I global surveillance: prevalence, severity, management and risk factors. *Eur. Respir. J.* 49:1601605. doi: 10.1183/13993003.01605-2016

Faith, D. P., Lozupone, C. A., Nipperess, D., and Knight, R. (2009). The cladistic basis for the phylogenetic diversity (PD) measure links evolutionary features to environmental gradients and supports broad applications of microbial ecology's "phylogenetic beta diversity" framework. *Int. J. Mol. Sci.* 10, 4723–4741. doi: 10.3390/ijms10114723

Ferreira, C. M., Chen, J. L., Li, J., Shimomura, K., Yang, X., Lussier, Y. A., et al. (2012). Genetic interactions between chromosomes 11 and 18 contribute to airway hyperresponsiveness in mice. *PLOS ONE* 7:e29579. doi: 10.1371/journal.pone.0029579

Gibbs, C. J., Coutts, I. I., Lock, R., Finnegan, O. C., and White, R. J. (1984). Premenstrual exacerbation of asthma. *Thorax* 39, 833–836. doi: 10.1136/thx.39.11.833

Gong, D., Sun, J., Zhou, Y., Zou, C., and Fan, Y. (2016). Early age at natural menopause and risk of cardiovascular and all-cause mortality: a meta-analysis of prospective observational studies. *Int. J. Cardiol.* 203, 115–119. doi: 10.1016/j.ijcard.2015.10.092

Guerra, P. V., Lima, L. N., Souza, T. C., Mazochi, V., Penna, F. J., Silva, A. M., et al. (2011). Pediatric functional constipation treatment with *Bifidobacterium*-containing yogurt: a crossover, double-blind, controlled trial. *World J. Gastroenterol.* 17, 3916–3921. doi: 10.3748/wjg.v17.i34.3916

Hanley, S. P. (1981). Asthma variation with menstruation. *Br. J. Dis. Chest* 75, 306–308. doi: 10.1016/0007-0971(81)90010-3

He, F., Ouwehand, A. C., Isolauri, E., Hashimoto, H., Benno, Y., and Salminen, S. (2001). Comparison of mucosal adhesion and species identification of bifidobacteria isolated from healthy and allergic infants. *FEMS Immunol. Med. Microbiol.* 30, 43–47. doi: 10.1111/j.1574-695X.2001.tb01548.x

Iwabuchi, N., Takahashi, N., Xiao, J. Z., Yonezawa, S., Yaeshima, T., Iwatsuki, K., et al. (2009). Suppressive effects of *Bifidobacterium longum* on the production of Th2-attracting chemokines induced with T cell-antigen-presenting cell interactions. *FEMS Immunol. Med. Microbiol.* 55, 324–334. doi: 10.1111/j.1574-695X.2008.00510.x

Keselman, A., and Heller, N. (2015). Estrogen signaling modulates allergic inflammation and contributes to sex differences in asthma. *Front. Immunol.* 6:568. doi: 10.3389/fimmu.2015.00568

Kirkwood, T. B., and Shanley, D. P. (2010). The connections between general and reproductive senescence and the evolutionary basis of menopause. *Ann. N. Y. Acad. Sci.* 1204, 21–29. doi: 10.1111/j.1749-6632.2010.05520.x

Kornman, K. S., and Loesche, W. J. (1982). Effects of estradiol and progesterone on *Bacteroides melaninogenicus* and *Bacteroides gingivalis*. *Infect. Immun.* 35, 256–263.

Kwon, H. K., Lee, C. G., So, J. S., Chae, C. S., Hwang, J. S., Sahoo, A., et al. (2010). Generation of regulatory dendritic cells and CD4+Foxp3+ T cells by probiotics administration suppresses immune disorders. *Proc. Natl. Acad. Sci. U.S.A.* 107, 2159–2164. doi: 10.1073/pnas.0904055107

Kwon, H. S., Yang, E. H., Lee, S. H., Yeon, S. W., Kang, B. H., and Kim, T. Y. (2005). Rapid identification of potentially probiotic *Bifidobacterium* species by multiplex PCR using species-specific primers based on the region extending from 16S rRNA through 23S rRNA. *FEMS Microbiol. Lett.* 250, 55–62. doi: 10.1016/j.femsle.2005.06.041

Leynaert, B., Sunyer, J., Garcia-Esteban, R., Svanes, C., Jarvis, D., Cerveri, I., et al. (2012). Gender differences in prevalence, diagnosis and incidence of allergic and non-allergic asthma: a population-based cohort. *Thorax* 67, 625–631. doi: 10.1136/thoraxjnl-2011-201249

Liang, X., Bushman, F. D., and FitzGerald, G. A. (2015). Rhythmicity of the intestinal microbiota is regulated by gender and the host circadian clock. *Proc. Natl. Acad. Sci. U.S.A.* 112, 10479–10484. doi: 10.1073/pnas.1501305112

Lozupone, C., and Knight, R. (2005). UniFrac: a new phylogenetic method for comparing microbial communities. *Appl. Environ. Microbiol.* 71, 8228–8235. doi: 10.1128/AEM.71.12.8228-8235.2005

MacSharry, J., O'Mahony, C., Shalaby, K. H., Sheil, B., Karmouty-Quintana, H., Shanahan, F., et al. (2012). Immunomodulatory effects of feeding with *Bifidobacterium longum* on allergen-induced lung inflammation in the mouse. *Pulm. Pharmacol. Ther.* 25, 325–334. doi: 10.1016/j.pupt.2012.05.011

Maddox, L., and Schwartz, D. A. (2002). The pathophysiology of asthma. *Annu. Rev. Med.* 53, 477–498. doi: 10.1146/annurev.med.53.082901.103921

Markle, J. G., Frank, D. N., Mortin-Toth, S., Robertson, C. E., Feazel, L. M., Rolle-Kampczyk, U., et al. (2013). Sex differences in the gut microbiome drive hormone-dependent regulation of autoimmunity. *Science* 339, 1084–1088. doi: 10.1126/science.1233521

Marsland, B. J., Trompette, A., and Gollwitzer, E. S. (2015). The gut-lung axis in respiratory disease. *Ann. Am. Thorac. Soc.* 12(Suppl. 2), S150–S156. doi: 10.1513/AnnalsATS.201503-133AW

Melli, L. C., do Carmo-Rodrigues, M. S., Araujo-Filho, H. B., Sole, D., and de Morais, M. B. (2016). Intestinal microbiota and allergic diseases: a systematic review. *Allergol. Immunopathol.* 44, 177–188. doi: 10.1016/j.aller.2015.01.013

Menard, O., Butel, M. J., Gaboriau-Routhiau, V., and Waligora-Dupriet, A. J. (2008). Gnotobiotic mouse immune response induced by *Bifidobacterium* sp. strains isolated from infants. *Appl. Environ. Microbiol.* 74, 660–666. doi: 10.1128/AEM.01261-07

Miraglia Del Giudice, M., Maiello, N., Decimo, F., Fusco, N., D' Agostino, B., Sullo, N., et al. (2012). Airways allergic inflammation and *L. reuterii* treatment in asthmatic children. *J. Biol. Regul. Homeost. Agents* 26(1 Suppl.), S35–S40.

Ohlsson, C., Engdahl, C., Fak, F., Andersson, A., Windahl, S. H., Farman, H. H., et al. (2014). Probiotics protect mice from ovariectomy-induced cortical bone loss. *PLOS ONE* 9:e92368. doi: 10.1371/journal.pone.0092368

Oksanen, J., Guillaume, B. F., Friendly, M., Kindt, R., Legendre, P., McGlinn, D., et al. (2016). *vegan: Community Ecology Package. R Package Version* 2.4-1. Available at: https://CRAN.R-project.org/package=vegan

Parvaneh, K., Ebrahimi, M., Sabran, M. R., Karimi, G., Hwei, A. N., Abdul-Majeed, S., et al. (2015). Probiotics (*Bifidobacterium longum*) increase bone mass density and upregulate Sparc and Bmp-2 genes in rats with bone loss resulting from ovariectomy. *Biomed. Res. Int.* 2015:897639. doi: 10.1155/2015/897639

Paulson, J. N., Stine, O. C., Bravo, H. C., and Pop, M. (2013). Differential abundance analysis for microbial marker-gene surveys. *Nat. Methods* 10, 1200–1202. doi: 10.1038/nmeth.2658

Price, A. L., Tandon, A., Patterson, N., Barnes, K. C., Rafaels, N., Ruczinski, I., et al. (2009). Sensitive detection of chromosomal segments of distinct ancestry in admixed populations. *PLOS Genet.* 5:e1000519. doi: 10.1371/journal.pgen.1000519

Reeves, P. G., Nielsen, F. H., and Fahey, G. C. Jr. (1993). AIN-93 purified diets for laboratory rodents: final report of the American Institute of Nutrition ad hoc writing committee on the reformulation of the AIN-76A rodent diet. *J. Nutr.* 123, 1939–1951.

Riffo-Vasquez, Y., Ligeiro de Oliveira, A. P., Page, C. P., Spina, D., and Tavares-de-Lima, W. (2007). Role of sex hormones in allergic inflammation in mice. *Clin. Exp. Allergy* 37, 459–470. doi: 10.1111/j.1365-2222.2007.02670.x

Shah, V. P., Midha, K. K., Dighe, S., McGilveray, I. J., Skelly, J. P., Yacobi, A., et al. (1991). Analytical methods validation: bioavailability, bioequivalence and pharmacokinetic studies. Conference report. *Eur. J. Drug Metab. Pharmacokinet.* 16, 249–255. doi: 10.1007/BF03189968

Silveira, A. L., Ferreira, A. V., de Oliveira, M. C., Rachid, M. A., da Cunha Sousa, L. F., Dos Santos, et al. (2017). Preventive rather than therapeutic treatment with high fiber diet attenuates clinical and inflammatory markers of acute and chronic DSS-induced colitis in mice. *Eur. J. Nutr.* 56, 179–191. doi: 10.1007/s00394-015-1068-x

Sjogren, K., Engdahl, C., Henning, P., Lerner, U. H., Tremaroli, V., Lagerquist, M. K., et al. (2012). The gut microbiota regulates bone mass in mice. *J. Bone. Miner. Res.* 27, 1357–1367. doi: 10.1002/jbmr.1588

Souza, T. C., Silva, A. M., Drews, J. R., Gomes, D. A., Vinderola, C. G., and Nicoli, J. R. (2013). In vitro evaluation of *Bifidobacterium* strains of human origin for potential use in probiotic functional foods. *Benef. Microbes* 4, 179–186. doi: 10.3920/BM2012.0052

Stsepetova, J., Sepp, E., Julge, K., Vaughan, E., Mikelsaar, M., and de Vos, W. M. (2007). Molecularly assessed shifts of *Bifidobacterium* ssp. and less diverse microbial communities are characteristic of 5-year-old allergic children. *FEMS Immunol. Med. Microbiol.* 51, 260–269. doi: 10.1111/j.1574-695X.2007.00306.x

Tan, J., McKenzie, C., Potamitis, M., Thorburn, A. N., Mackay, C. R., and Macia, L. (2014). The role of short-chain fatty acids in health and disease. *Adv. Immunol.* 121, 91–119. doi: 10.1016/B978-0-12-800100-4.00003-9

Tao, R., de Zoeten, E. F., Ozkaynak, E., Chen, C., Wang, L., Porrett, P. M., et al. (2007). Deacetylase inhibition promotes the generation and function of regulatory T cells. *Nat. Med.* 13, 1299–1307. doi: 10.1038/nm1652

Thomas, A. M., Jesus, E. C., Lopes, A., Aguiar, S. Jr., Begnami, M. D., Rocha, R. M., et al. (2016). Tissue-associated bacterial alterations in rectal carcinoma patients revealed by 16S rRNA community profiling. *Front. Cell Infect. Microbiol.* 6:179. doi: 10.3389/fcimb.2016.00179

Thorburn, A. N., McKenzie, C. I., Shen, S., Stanley, D., Macia, L., Mason, L. J., et al. (2015). Evidence that asthma is a developmental origin disease influenced by maternal diet and bacterial metabolites. *Nat. Commun.* 6:7320. doi: 10.1038/ncomms8320

Tong, J., Bandulwala, H. S., Clay, B. S., Anders, R. A., Shilling, R. A., Balachandran, D. D., et al. (2006). Fas-positive T cells regulate the resolution of airway inflammation in a murine model of asthma. *J. Exp. Med.* 203, 1173–1184. doi: 10.1084/jem.20051680

Triebner, K., Johannessen, A., Puggini, L., Benediktsdottir, B., Bertelsen, R. J., Bifulco, E., et al. (2016). Menopause as a predictor of new-onset asthma: a longitudinal Northern European population study. *J. Allergy Clin. Immunol.* 137, 50–57.e56. doi: 10.1016/j.jaci.2015.08.019

Troisi, R. J., Speizer, F. E., Willett, W. C., Trichopoulos, D., and Rosner, B. (1995). Menopause, postmenopausal estrogen preparations, and the risk of adult-onset asthma. A prospective cohort study. *Am. J. Respir. Crit. Care Med.* 152(4Pt 1), 1183–1188. doi: 10.1164/ajrccm.152.4.7551368

Trompette, A., Gollwitzer, E. S., Yadava, K., Sichelstiel, A. K., Sprenger, N., Ngom-Bru, C., et al. (2014). Gut microbiota metabolism of dietary fiber influences allergic airway disease and hematopoiesis. *Nat. Med.* 20, 159–166. doi: 10.1038/nm.3444

Ubeda, C., Lipuma, L., Gobourne, A., Viale, A., Leiner, I., Equinda, M., et al. (2012). Familial transmission rather than defective innate immunity shapes the distinct intestinal microbiota of TLR-deficient mice. *J. Exp. Med.* 209, 1445–1456. doi: 10.1084/jem.20120504

Venkataraman, A., Bassis, C. M., Beck, J. M., Young, V. B., Curtis, J. L., Huffnagle, G. B., et al. (2015). Application of a neutral community model to assess structuring of the human lung microbiome. *mBio* 6:e02284-14. doi: 10.1128/mBio.02284-14

Vieira, A. T., Macia, L., Galvao, I., Martins, F. S., Canesso, M. C., Amaral, F. A., et al. (2015). A role for gut microbiota and the metabolite-sensing receptor GPR43 in a murine model of gout. *Arthritis Rheumatol.* 67, 1646–1656. doi: 10.1002/art.39107

Vieira, A. T., Rocha, V. M., Tavares, L., Garcia, C. C., Teixeira, M. M., Oliveira, S. C., et al. (2016). Control of *Klebsiella pneumoniae* pulmonary infection and immunomodulation by oral treatment with the commensal probiotic *Bifidobacterium longum* 5(1A). *Microbes Infect.* 18, 180–189. doi: 10.1016/j.micinf.2015.10.008

Wang, Q., Garrity, G. M., Tiedje, J. M., and Cole, J. R. (2007). Naive Bayesian classifier for rapid assignment of rRNA sequences into the new bacterial taxonomy. *Appl. Environ. Microbiol.* 73, 5261–5267. doi: 10.1128/AEM.00062-07

Wu, B. G., and Segal, L. N. (2017). Lung microbiota and its impact on the mucosal immune phenotype. *Microbiol. Spectr.* 5:BAD-0005-2016. doi: 10.1128/microbiolspec.BAD-0005-2016

Yu, J., Jang, S. O., Kim, B. J., Song, Y. H., Kwon, J. W., Kang, M. J., et al. (2010). The effects of *Lactobacillus rhamnosus* on the prevention of asthma in a murine model. *Allergy Asthma Immunol. Res.* 2, 199–205. doi: 10.4168/aair.2010.2.3.199

Yurkovetskiy, L., Burrows, M., Khan, A. A., Graham, L., Volchkov, P., Becker, L., et al. (2013). Gender bias in autoimmunity is influenced by microbiota. *Immunity* 39, 400–412. doi: 10.1016/j.immuni.2013.08.013

Zemp, E., Schikowski, T., Dratva, J., Schindler, C., and Probst-Hensch, N. (2012). Asthma and the menopause: a systematic review and meta-analysis. *Maturitas* 73, 212–217. doi: 10.1016/j.maturitas.2012.08.010

14

The Virome and its Major Component, Anellovirus, a Convoluted System Molding Human Immune Defenses and Possibly Affecting the Development of Asthma and Respiratory Diseases in Childhood

Giulia Freer[1]*, Fabrizio Maggi*[2]*, Massimo Pifferi*[3]*, Maria E. Di Cicco*[3]*, Diego G. Peroni*[3*†] *and Mauro Pistello*[1,2†]

[1] Retrovirus Center, Department of Translational Research, University of Pisa, Pisa, Italy, [2] Virology Unit, University Hospital of Pisa, Pisa, Italy, [3] Department of Clinical and Experimental Medicine, Section of Pediatrics, University of Pisa, Pisa, Italy

***Correspondence:**
Diego G. Peroni
diego.peroni@unipi.it

† These authors have contributed equally to this work.

The microbiome, a thriving and complex microbial community colonizing the human body, has a broad impact on human health. Colonization is a continuous process that starts very early in life and occurs thanks to shrewd strategies microbes have evolved to tackle a convoluted array of anatomical, physiological, and functional barriers of the human body. Cumulative evidence shows that viruses are part of the microbiome. This part, called virome, has a dynamic composition that reflects what we eat, how and where we live, what we do, our genetic background, and other unpredictable variables. Thus, the virome plays a chief role in shaping innate and adaptive host immune defenses. Imbalance of normal microbial flora is thought to trigger or exacerbate many acute and chronic disorders. A compelling example can be found in the respiratory apparatus, where early-life viral infections are major determinants for the development of allergic diseases, like asthma, and other non-transmissible diseases. In this review, we focus on the virome and, particularly, on *Anelloviridae*, a recently discovered virus family. Anelloviruses are major components of the virome, present in most, if not all, human beings, where they are acquired early in life and replicate persistently without causing apparent disease. We will discuss how modulation of innate and adaptive immune systems by Anelloviruses can influence the development of respiratory diseases in childhood and provide evidence for the use of Anelloviruses as useful and practical molecular markers to monitor inflammatory processes and immune system competence.

Keywords: virome, microbiome, anelloviruses, torque teno virus, asthma, respiratory diseases, wheezing

INTRODUCTION

At birth, both the digestive system and the airways are immediately exploited as portals of entry by a number of microbes, most of which are likely to persist and become part of the so-called "microbiome." This is a community of microorganisms that live on the human body without apparently affecting health (Whipps and Karen Lewis, 1988; Hooper et al., 2012; Tremaroli and Bäckhed, 2012). It has long been known that the microbiome is beneficial to hosts in a number of ways, and, in recent years, its interaction with the immune system has even been recognized as fundamental for immune system maturation, reactivity to specific antigens and development of tolerance (Scharschmidt et al., 2015; Ignacio et al., 2016; Kim et al., 2016). The microbiome, from this point of view, tunes immunity by acting as a constant source of stimuli (Belkaid and Hand, 2014; Belkaid and Segre, 2014).

Recently, with the advent of high throughput sequencing methods, the diversity of the microbiome inhabiting gut, lung, skin, and even blood in physiological conditions has been found to be much larger than first thought. In particular, a constantly fluctuating population of viruses have joined the list of infectious agents that are now considered part of the microbiome in several body sites (Blaser and Valentine, 2008; Shulman and Davidson, 2017). Very recent work has estimated that roughly 45% of mammalian viruses can be detected in healthy humans (Olival et al., 2017).

Most initial interactions between hosts and viruses are governed by the innate immune system, that prevents colonizing infectious agents from spreading systemically and maintains mucosal homeostasis (Medzhitov and Janeway, 2002; Lamkanfi and Dixit, 2011). Activation of the innate immune responses triggers a cascade reaction that results in secretion of cytokines and chemokines, and often engages different cells to control invasion (Freer et al., 2017). Following recognition of specific microbial, viral and damage stimuli, intracellular multiprotein complexes called inflammasomes assemble and induce downstream immune responses to specific pathogens. The effects of turning on immunity generally protects against pathogen invasion, but reactions to harmless antigens may lead to the establishment of disease in predisposed individuals. In this review, we discuss the multiple effects of the virome on host health, with special reference to Anelloviruses.

THE HUMAN VIROME

Although viruses have long been considered "bad news in a protein coat" (Medawar and Medawar, 1983), many novel viruses are found to replicate in healthy individuals. So far, roughly 220 viruses are known to infect humans and only about half are pathogens (Parker, 2016). Truly apathogenic viruses can be grossly divided in viruses infecting bacteria, integrating into human chromosomes as endogenous retroelements, and persisting indefinitely. They are referred to as "commensal" viruses that are part of the virome without an apparent clinical outcome (Rascovan et al., 2016). Many viruses that infect humans may even have a beneficial role (Phan et al., 2016): in animal models, resident intestinal viruses were shown to reduce intestinal inflammation by inducing interferon (IFN)-β, secreted mainly by plasmacytoid dendritic cells (DCs) (Yang et al., 2016), or by providing resistance to infection by bacterial pathogens (Barton et al., 2007).

The number of apathogenic viruses includes many genera detected in various tissues of healthy people, especially infants (Allander et al., 2005; Wang et al., 2016; Moustafa et al., 2017). What role they play in human physiology is still unknown, although they are currently hypothesized to alter disease susceptibility. This is suggested by many epidemiological observations and findings in animal models (Roossinck, 2011; Virgin, 2014).

Resident viruses influence the immune system helping it to develop properly, similarly to bacterial microbiome. Indeed, Cadwell demonstrated that mouse norovirus, a commensal relative of a human pathogen, restored intestinal morphology and immunological functions in germ-free newborn mice, where it is normally perturbed (Cadwell, 2015). On the other hand, the immune system has been recently demonstrated to control virome expansion, similarly to bacteria: HIV-infected patients exhibited low peripheral $CD4^{+}$ T cell counts and dramatic expansion of enteric virome adenovirus titers, possibly contributing to AIDS-associated enteropathy and disease progression. These findings suggest that virome expansion is linked to the pathogenesis of AIDS and highlights the role of the immune system in controlling viral populations in the intestine (Monaco et al., 2016). In addition, enteric viral communities have been found to change during HIV infection and raises in Anelloviridae and other virus titers have been associated to increased pathology (Gootenberg et al., 2017).

Anelloviruses and TTV

A group of viruses discovered in 1997 (Nishizawa et al., 1997; Okamoto et al., 1998), now called Anelloviruses (AV), represents about 70% of total viruses detected in blood and in most tissues and organs (De Vlaminck et al., 2013). Their prototype, presently named torquetenovirus (TTV), is one of a vast spectrum of viral agents with similar genomes, like torquetenominivirus (Takahashi et al., 2000) and torquetenomidivirus (Ninomiya et al., 2007), both of which have smaller genomes than TTV. All these viruses are classified in the newly established family Anelloviridae (from *anellus*, Latin for ring, for their circular genome). AV are characterized by a small (2.2 to 3.7 kb), single stranded DNA (ssDNA) circular genome, which makes AV the genetically simplest of all known replication-competent animal viruses. In addition, they are extremely diverse genetically, more than any other viral family. They all lead to persistent, possibly life-long infections and they can be detected at very high levels in blood and in practically all tissues of almost 100% of people worldwide. Different genetic forms are found in a large proportion of individuals regardless of age, socio-economical standing and health conditions, being acquired very soon after birth or even prenatally (Maggi and Bendinelli, 2010).

No specific pathogenic effect has so far been pinpointed to any AV, although similarity of human *Anelloviridae* to avian ones suggests that their pathogenicity might be underestimated (Davidson and Shulman, 2008). Increased viremia levels of AV have been found in immune suppressed individuals and in subjects with inflammatory diseases, suggesting that they are normally kept under immunological control, but may contribute to maintain the background level of inflammation chronically elevated in the body (Maggi et al., 2004; Li et al., 2013; Young et al., 2015; Abbas et al., 2016).

How TTV Interacts and Modulates Host Defenses

TTV interacts with many pathogen-associated molecular pattern (PAMP) receptors (PRR) that fuel immune and inflammatory responses (Zheng et al., 2007; Rocchi et al., 2009; Kincaid et al., 2013). *In vitro* studies show that TTV ORF2 protein suppressed the activity of NFκB, crucial for the expression of many genes connected to inflammation. ORF2 protein of TTV is able to influence the activity of NFκB by inhibiting its translocation to the cell nucleus and, consequently, its ability to activate transcription of genes, such as IL-6, -8, and cyclo-oxygenase-2 (Zheng et al., 2007).

In addition, the genome of TTV and its replication intermediates may stimulate TLRs in infected cells and consequently synthesis of pro-inflammatory molecules. Unmethylated heterodimers of guanosine and cytosine (CpGs) in bacterial and viral DNA are absent in mammalian DNA and therefore seen as molecular signatures of foreign DNA. The importance of these molecules as PAMPs is demonstrated by the fact that one PPR, namely toll-like receptor (TLR)-9, is specialized to detect CpGs. Depending on the number or nucleotides flanking CpGs, it triggers production of inflammatory cytokines, such as IFN-α, Interleukin (IL)-6, and IL-12, or, alternatively, it may generate an inhibitory signal (Krieg, 2002). Both stimulatory and inhibitory CpGs are present in DNA of TTV and in most microbes, and their relative frequency may differ considerably, even within strains of the same species, thus probably influencing the way they interact and stimulate TLR-9. For instance, we have found that TTV genogroup 4, detected at higher levels in pediatric patients with bronchopneumonia compared to those with milder acute respiratory diseases (ARDs) (Maggi et al., 2003), was rich in stimulatory CpGs and activated TLR-9 in mouse spleen cells *in vitro*, causing abundant production of pro-inflammatory cytokines (Zheng et al., 2007; Rocchi et al., 2009).

MicroRNAs (miRNA) are ~22 nt small, single-stranded, non-coding RNAs produced by hosts and pathogens. They are potent modulators of pathogen recognition and host defense in a vast array of cellular metabolic pathways. As regards microbe-host interaction, cellular miRNAs seem to modulate immune responses and inflammation and to play a direct antiviral role by blocking translation of viral genes, counteracting block of apoptosis and persistent replication. Very recent work shows that miRNA can polarize macrophages toward allergic reactions in animal models (Zhou et al., 2017). Their role in inflammation is probably very complex, since they may both up- and down-regulate inflammation in several diseases, including asthma (Dissanayake and Inoue, 2016). Viruses, including small ones like TTV, encode their own miRNAs that cooperate with viral proteins to regulate the expression of viral genes, replication, pathogenesis and immune evasion, and the whole process of virus-related inflammation (Kincaid and Sullivan, 2012; Cullen, 2013; Sorel and Dewals, 2016). Of note, both cellular and viral miRNAs have been found to transmit information to distant cells by circulating within plasma exosomes.

Interestingly, TTV was also found to encode *in vivo* miRNAs possibly involved in viral immune evasion and that could be involved in the regulation of IFN signaling (Kincaid et al., 2013). Different TTV species have been shown to encode miRNAs and cause these molecules to be found as plasma exosomes in many infected individuals. Production and release was not correlated with virus replication, as monitored by measuring TTV viremia levels. Notably, TTV miRNA profiles differed depending on patients' health status; the type of miRNAs produced also differed within sick patients (Vignolini et al., 2016). Role and significance of TTV miRNAs are not yet understood and warrant further studies. An overview of the mechanisms exploited by TTV to stimulate or soothe host innate and adaptive defenses is shown in **Figure 1**.

Role of Microbial Exposure and Viral Infections in Wheezing and Asthma Development

Asthma is a multifactorial inflammatory disease of the lower airways, caused by environmental and genetic factors. The disease incidence seems to be increasing especially in industrialized countries (Ellwood et al., 2017). A long-standing theory, the hygiene hypothesis, suggests that insufficient interaction with microbes in early life leads to the development of allergic reactions (Liu, 2015). Significant differences in the prevalence of asthma were found between Amish and Hutterite schoolchildren, despite similar genetic ancestries and lifestyles. As compared with the Hutterites, the Amish practice traditional farming and are exposed to an environment rich in microbes. The significantly lower rates of asthma and the distinct immune profiles in the Amish suggest that environment and sustained microbial exposure have profound effects on innate immunity (Stein et al., 2016). Further data generated in an experimental model of asthma support this notion by showing that the protective effect of the Amish environment requires the activation of innate immune signaling.

On the other hand, there is a consensus on the notion that early respiratory viral and bacterial infections are potent triggers of wheezing-related disorders and development of asthma later in life (Lemanske, 2004; Gern et al., 2005). Growing evidence indicates that respiratory viral infections, especially when acquired in early life may provide the stimulus to inflammasomes assembly, and prime immature DCs toward a Th2 response that, eventually, may sensitize genetically predisposed individuals to local allergens (Holgate, 2011; Lee et al., 2014).

Virus and microorganisms in general may act through several PRRs including TLRs (TLRs and TLR-9 in particular) on DCs. Virus infections have been shown to modulate the responses

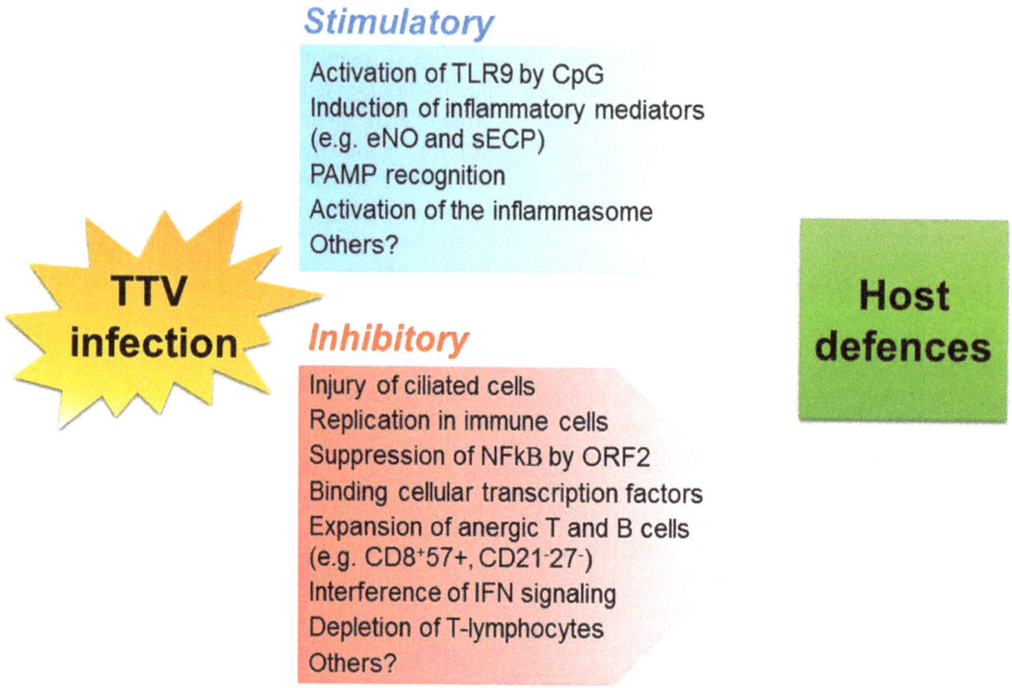

FIGURE 1 | Possible mechanisms whereby TTV infection may modulate host defenses. TLR, toll-like receptor; CpG, unmethylated heterodimers of guanosine and cytosine; eNO, exhaled nitric oxide; sECP, secreted eosinophil cationic protein; PAMP, pathogen-associated molecular pattern.

of TLRs and miRNAs on the balance of T cells toward Th1, Th2, Th17, or T-regulatory (Treg) subtypes in respiratory airways (Durrani et al., 2012; Holt and Sly, 2012). Microbial products may in turn bind TLRs on airway epithelial cells, leading to the release of the IL-7-like cytokines and thymic stromal lymphopoietin. They may also interact with TLRs on DCs and upregulate the expression of costimulatory molecules to enhance Th2 polarization, also activating mast cells for Th2 cytokine production (de Heer et al., 2004; Troy and Bosco, 2016). Recently, the role of respiratory syncytial virus (RSV) and its impact on bronchiolitis at the time of infection and respiratory morbidity later in life has been revisited (Rossi and Colin, 2017). It has been shown, although controversially, that patients with RSV infection receiving hospital-based care have a higher incidence of asthma and reduced pulmonary function in childhood and in adolescence (Sigurs et al., 2010). In addition, large-scale use of molecular diagnostic techniques pinpointed human rhinovirus (HRV) to infant wheezing and asthma development (Song, 2016). Indeed, HRV has been isolated in 90% of children with asthma exacerbations and found closely connected to hospitalization risk in cohort studies (Bizzintino et al., 2010; Foxman and Iwasaki, 2011). Further evidence on the role of HRV infections during infancy in asthma development has been found: the Childhood Origin of Asthma (COAST) cohort study showed that at least one HRV infection during infancy was the most significant risk factor for persistent wheezing at the age of 3 years (Lemanske et al., 2005). Also, having an HRV wheezing episode in the first 3 years of life was a strong risk factor for asthma not only in childhood (Hyvärinen et al., 2005; Jackson et al., 2015), but also in adolescence (Rubner et al., 2017). In fact, in a high-risk birth cohort, HRV wheezing, associated with early life aeroallergen sensitization, had additive effects on asthma risk at adolescence (Rubner et al., 2017). Other detrimental effects have been associated to various respiratory viruses, such as metapneumovirus and bocavirus (Camargo et al., 2008; Söderlund-Venermo et al., 2009; Rudd et al., 2017). Indeed, atopy predisposition may be the individual driving factor involved in promoting asthma development via interaction with HRV, and possibly other respiratory viral infections, in infancy (Song, 2016). Allergic sensitizations and viral infections may in turn skew immune responses to produce Th2 cytokines that may at the same time amplify allergic inflammation and reduce the host antiviral responses, resulting in increased viral replication and cellular damage (Xatzipsalti et al., 2008).

AV and Respiratory Allergy

Although TTV has been investigated to a reasonable extent, its role on asthma is far from clear. Previous studies of our group have shown that presence or viremia levels of TTV were significantly associated with ARDs in pediatric patients and that children with bronchopneumonia (BP) have considerably higher TTV loads than do children with milder respiratory disease. Further, high TTV loads correlate with a decrease in circulating $CD3^{+}$ and $CD4^{+}$ T cells, an increment in B cells, and increased activity of eosinophils, again emphasizing the immunomodulatory activity of TTV (Maggi et al., 2004; Pifferi et al., 2005). In another study, a positive association was found between nasal TTV loads and levels of eosinophil cationic protein, a marker of bronchial inflammation. These markers were found particularly elevated in the children with asthma who had moderately to severely compromised spirometric indices. This study was the first performed in children with asthma and suggested that TTV might be a contributing factor in lung impairment (Pifferi et al., 2005).

Concerning a mechanistic role of TTV in respiratory dysfunction, it has been postulated that this virus, either alone or synergistically with other viruses, may act as an enhancer of inflammation systemically or at specific body sites such as upper and lower airways (Maggi and Bendinelli, 2009). One possible way can be envisioned via high amounts of immune complexes that form following TTV replication in blood. In infants with ARD, the airways were shown to be the sites of primary infection and continual replication by TTV, with higher viral loads in patients with more severe lower respiratory tract infections (Maggi et al., 2003). Furthermore, TTV may worsen the extent and the severity of the inflammatory response due to allergens, if sensitization is present in the subject. This hypothesis is supported, in children with ARD, by the positive correlation between TTV loads and serum concentration of eosinophil cationic protein (Maggi et al., 2004), and of exhaled nitric oxide, a sensitive marker of airway inflammation in asthmatic children (Li et al., 2013). In another study, we were able to demonstrate a high prevalence of TTV infections in children with bronchiectasis, a chronic respiratory disorder associated with several invalidating airway diseases: indeed, strong correlation between TTV loads and airflow limitation within the more peripheral airways was found, as well as between severity of the disorder and limitation of the lung function (Pifferi et al., 2006).

CONCLUSION

Most viral infections elicit robust immune responses but viral clearance is not always obtained. Consequently, there must be unidentified factors/conditions that determine a tolerogenic status toward non-pathogenic viruses, and strong immune opposition against pathogenic ones. Tolerance may depend on host genetic, life-style and environmental factors, or alternatively on the ability of "commensal" viruses not to stir up inflammasomes and innate immune effectors.

Increasing evidence shows that the virome is actually beneficial to the host, who seems to tolerate "commensal" viruses, although they replicate and circulate among individuals. AV infect and persist in nearly all mammals and represent a large body of the human virome. They continuously replicate with no overt damage to the host and, therefore, are a good example of commensal viruses in this respect. Several clinical studies suggest that TTV plays a role in the development and/or exacerbation of respiratory diseases in childhood. Although further studies are warranted to draw firm conclusions, the virome and AV are one the best examples of a virus-host relationship. Its understanding will help clarify the role of viruses in shaping human immune defenses and perhaps contribute to their derangement.

AUTHOR CONTRIBUTIONS

GF, FM, DP, and MauP contributed to the elaboration of this mini review. MasP and MDC performed TTV studies in infants and made some unpublished results available. All authors read and approved the final manuscript.

FUNDING

This work was supported by Progetti di Ricerca di Ateneo 2017–2018 of University of Pisa, Project No. PRA_2017_38, DR n. 83/2017.

REFERENCES

Abbas, A. A., Diamond, J. M., Chehoud, C., Chang, B., Kotzin, J. J., Young, J. C., et al. (2016). The perioperative lung transplant virome: torque teno viruses are elevated in donor lungs and show divergent dynamics in primary graft dysfunction. *Am. J. Transplant.* 17, 1313–1324. doi: 10.1111/ajt.14076

Allander, T., Tammi, M. T., Eriksson, M., Bjerkner, A., Tiveljung-Lindell, A., and Andersson, B. (2005). Cloning of a human parvovirus by molecular screening of respiratory tract samples. *Proc. Natl. Acad. Sci. U.S.A.* 102, 12891–12896. doi: 10.1073/pnas.0504666102

Barton, E. S., White, D. W., Cathelyn, J. S., Brett-McClellan, K. A., Engle, M., Diamond, M. S., et al. (2007). Herpesvirus latency confers symbiotic protection from bacterial infection. *Nature* 447, 326–329. doi: 10.1038/nature05762

Belkaid, Y., and Hand, T. W. (2014). Role of the microbiota in immunity and inflammation. *Cell* 157, 121 141. doi: 10.1016/j.cell.2014.03.011

Belkaid, Y., and Segre, J. A. (2014). Dialogue between skin microbiota and immunity. *Science* 346, 954–959. doi: 10.1126/science.1260144

Bizzintino, J., Lee, W. M., Laing, I. A., Vang, F., Pappas, T., Zhang, G., et al. (2010). Association between human rhinovirus C and severity of acute asthma in children. *Eur. Respir. J.* 37, 1037–1042. doi: 10.1183/09031936.00092410

Blaser, M. J., and Valentine, F. T. (2008). Viral commensalism in humans? *J. Infect. Dis.* 198, 1–3. doi: 10.1086/588705

Cadwell, K. (2015). Expanding the role of the virome: commensalism in the gut. *J. Virol.* 89, 1951–1953. doi: 10.1128/JVI.02966-14

Camargo, C. A. Jr, Ginde, A. A., Clark, S., Cartwright, C. P., Falsey, A. R., and Niewoehner, D. E. (2008). Viral pathogens in acute exacerbations of chronic obstructive pulmonary disease. *Intern. Emerg. Med.* 3, 355–359. doi: 10.1007/s11739-008-0197-0

Cullen, B. R. (2013). MicroRNAs as mediators of viral evasion of the immune system. *Nat. Immunol.* 14, 205–210. doi: 10.1038/ni.2537

Davidson, I., and Shulman, L. M. (2008). Unravelling the puzzle of human anellovirus infections by comparison with avian circovirus infections. *Virus Res.* 137, 1–15. doi: 10.1016/j.virusres.2008.06.014

de Heer, H. J., Hammad, H., Soullié, T., Hijdra, D., Vos, N., Willart, M. A., et al. (2004). Essential role of lung plasmacytoid dendritic cells in preventing asthmatic reactions to harmless inhaled antigen. *J. Exp. Med.* 5, 89–98. doi: 10.1084/Jem.20040035

De Vlaminck, I., Khush, K. K., Strehl, C., Kohli, B., Luikart, H., Neff, N. F., et al. (2013). Temporal response of the human virome to immunosuppression and antiviral therapy. *Cell* 55, 1178–1187. doi: 10.1016/j.cell.2013.10.034

Dissanayake, E., and Inoue, Y. (2016). MicroRNAs in allergic disease. *Curr. Allergy Asthma Rep.* 16:67. doi: 10.1007/s11882-016-0648-z

Durrani, S. R., Montville, D. J., Pratt, A. S., Sahu, S., Devries, M. K., Rajamanickam, V., et al. (2012). Innate immune responses to rhinovirus are reduced by the high-affinity IgE receptor in allergic asthmatic children. *J. Allergy Clin. Immunol.* 130, 489–495. doi: 10.1016/j.jaci.2012.05.023

Ellwood, P., Asher, M. I., Billo, N. E., Bissell, K., Chiang, C. Y., Ellwood, E. M., et al. (2017). The Global Asthma Network rationale and methods for Phase I global surveillance: prevalence, severity, management and risk factors. *Eur. Respir. J.* 49:1601605. doi: 10.1183/13993003.01605-2016

Foxman, E. F., and Iwasaki, A. (2011). Genome-virome interactions: examining the role of common viral infections in complex disease. *Nat. Rev.* 9, 254–264. doi: 10.1038/nrmicro2541

Freer, G., Maggi, F., and Pistello, M. (2017). Virome and inflammasomes, a finely tuned balance with important consequences for the host health. *Curr. Med. Chem.* doi: 10.2174/0929867324666171005112921 [Epub ahead of print].

Gern, J. E., Rosenthal, L. A., Sorkness, R. L., and Lemanske, R. F. Jr. (2005). Effects of viral respiratory infections on lung development and childhood asthma. *J. Allergy Clin. Immunol.* 115, 668–674. doi: 10.1016/j.jaci.2005.01.057

Gootenberg, D. B., Paer, J. M., Luevano, J. M., and Kwon, D. S. (2017). HIV-associated changes in the enteric microbial community: potential role in loss of homeostasis and development of systemic inflammation. *Curr. Opin. Infect. Dis.* 30, 31–34. doi: 10.1097/QCO.0000000000000341

Holgate, S. T. (2011). The sentinel role of the airway epithelium in asthma pathogenesis. *Immunol. Rev.* 242, 205–219. doi: 10.1111/j.1600-065X.2011.01030

Holt, P. G., and Sly, P. D. (2012). Viral infections and atopy in asthma pathogenesis: new rationales for asthma prevention and treatment. *Nat. Med.* 18, 726–735. doi: 10.1038/nm.2768

Hooper, L. V., Littman, D. R., and Macpherson, A. J. (2012). Interactions between the microbiota and the immune system. *Science* 336, 1268–1273. doi: 10.1126/science.1223490

Hyvärinen, M. K., Kotaniemi-Syrjänen, A., Reijonen, T. M., Korhonen, K., and Korppi, M. O. (2005). Teenage asthma after severe early childhood wheezing: an 11-year prospective follow-up. *Pediatr. Pulmonol.* 40, 316–323. doi: 10.1002/ppul.20273

Ignacio, A., Morales, C. I., Câmara, N. O. S., and Almeida, R. R. (2016). Innate sensing of the gut microbiota: modulation of inflammatory and autoimmune diseases. *Front. Immunol.* 7:54. doi: 10.3389/fimmu.2016.00054

Jackson, D. J., Glanville, N., Trujillo-Torralbo, M. B., Shamji, B. W., Del-Rosario, J., Mallia, P., et al. (2015). Interleukin-18 is associated with protection against rhinovirus-induced colds and asthma exacerbations. *Clin. Infect. Dis.* 15, 1528–1531. doi: 10.1093/cid/civ062

Kim, K. S., Hong, S. W., Han, D., Yi, J., Jung, J., Yang, B. G., et al. (2016). Dietary antigens limit mucosal immunity by inducing regulatory T cells in the small intestine. *Science* 351, 858–863. doi: 10.1126/science.aac5560

Kincaid, R. P., Burke, J. M., Cox, J. C., de Villiers, E. M., and Sullivan, C. S. (2013). A human torque teno virus encodes a microRNA that inhibits interferon signaling. *PLoS Pathog.* 9:e1003818. doi: 10.1371/journal.ppat.1003818

Kincaid, R. P., and Sullivan, C. S. (2012). Virus-encoded microRNAs: an overview and a look to the future. *PLoS Pathog.* 8:e1003018. doi: 10.1371/journal.ppat.1003018

Krieg, A. M. (2002). CpG motifs in bacterial DNA and their immune effects. *Annu. Rev. Immunol.* 20, 709–760. doi: 10.1146/annurev.immunol.20.100301.064842

Lamkanfi, M., and Dixit, V. M. (2011). Modulation of inflammasome pathways by bacterial and viral pathogens. *J. Immunol.* 187, 597–602. doi: 10.4049/jimmunol.1100229

Lee, T. H., Song, H. J., and Park, C. S. (2014). Role of inflammasome activation in development and exacerbation of asthma. *Asia Pac. Allergy* 4, 187–196. doi: 10.5415/apallergy.2014.4.4.187

Lemanske, R. F. Jr. (2004). Viral infections and asthma inception. *J. Allergy Clin. Immunol.* 114, 1023–1026. doi: 10.1016/j.jaci.2004.08.031

Lemanske, R. F. Jr, Jackson, D. J., Gangnon, R. E., Evans, M. D., Li, Z., Shult, P. A., et al. (2005). Rhinovirus illnesses during infancy predict subsequent childhood wheezing. *J. Allergy Clin. Immunol.* 116, 571–577. doi: 10.1016/j.jaci.2005.06.024

Li, L., Deng, X., Linsuwanon, P., Bangsberg, D., Bwana, M. B., Hunt, P., et al. (2013). AIDS alters the commensal plasma virome. *J. Virol.* 87, 10912–10915. doi: 10.1371/journal.pone.0135573

Liu, A. H. (2015). Revisiting the hygiene hypothesis for allergy and asthma. *J. Allergy Clin. Immunol.* 136, 860–865. doi: 10.1016/j.jaci.2015.08.012

Maggi, F., and Bendinelli, M. (2009). Immunobiology of the Torque teno viruses and other anelloviruses. *Curr. Top. Microbiol. Immunol.* 331, 65–90. doi: 10.1007/978-3-540-70972-5_5

Maggi, F., and Bendinelli, M. (2010). Human anelloviruses and the central nervous system. *Rev. Med. Virol.* 20, 392–407. doi: 10.1002/rmv.668

Maggi, F., Pifferi, M., Tempestini, E., Fornai, C., Lanini, L., Andreoli, E., et al. (2003). TT virus loads and lymphocyte subpopulations in children with acute respiratory diseases. *J. Virol.* 77, 9081–9083. doi: 10.1128/JVI.77.16.9081-9083.2003

Maggi, F., Pifferi, M., Tempestini, E., Lanini, L., De Marco, E., Fornai, C., et al. (2004). Correlation between Torque tenovirus infection and serum levels of eosinophil cationic protein in children hospitalized for acute respiratory diseases. *J. Infect. Dis.* 19, 971–974. doi: 10.1086/423143

Medawar, P. B., and Medawar, J. S. (1983). *Aristotle to Zeus, a Philosophical Dictionary of Biology*. Cambridge, MA: Harvard University Press, 27.

Medzhitov, R., and Janeway, C. A. Jr. (2002). Decoding the patterns of self, and nonself by the innate immune system. *Science* 296, 298–300. doi: 10.1126/science.1068883

Monaco, C. L., Gootenberg, D. B., Zhao, G., Handley, S. A., Ghebremichael, M. S., Lim, E. S., et al. (2016). Altered virome and bacterial microbiome in human immunodeficiency virus-associated acquired immunodeficiency syndrome. *Cell Host Microbe* 19, 311–322. doi: 10.1016/j.chom.2016.02.011

Moustafa, A., Xie, C., Kirkness, E., Biggs, W., Wong, E., Turpaz, Y., et al. (2017). The blood DNA virome in 8,000 humans. *PLoS Pathog.* 13:e1006292. doi: 10.1371/journal.ppat.1006292

Ninomiya, M., Nishizawa, T., Takahashi, M., Lorenzo, F. R., Shimosegawa, T., and Okamoto, H. (2007). Identification and genomic characterization of a novel human Torque teno virus of 3.2 kilobases. *J. Gen. Virol.* 88, 1939–1944. doi: 10.1099/vir.0.82895-0

Nishizawa, T., Okamoto, H., Konishi, K., Yoshizawa, H., Miyakawa, Y., and Mayumi, M. (1997). A novel DNA virus (TTV) associated with elevated transaminase levels in posttransfusion hepatitis of unknown etiology. *Biochem. Biophys. Res. Commun.* 241, 92–97. doi: 10.1006/bbrc.1997.7765

Okamoto, H., Nishizawa, T., Kato, N., Ukita, M., Ikeda, H., Iizuka, H., et al. (1998). Molecular cloning and characterization of a novel DNA virus (TTV) associated with posttransfusion hepatitis of unknown etiology. *Hepatol. Res.* 10, 1–16. doi: 10.1016/S1386-6346(97)00123-X

Olival, K. J., Hosseini, P. R., Zambrana-Torrelio, C., Ross, N., Bogich, T. L., and Daszak, P. (2017). Host and viral traits predict zoonotic spillover from mammals. *Nature* 546, 646–650. doi: 10.1038/nature22975

Parker, M. T. (2016). An ecological framework of the human virome provides classification of current knowledge and identifies areas of forthcoming discovery. *Yale J. Biol. Med.* 89, 339–351.

Phan, T. G., da, Costa AC, Del, Valle Mendoza J, Bucardo-Rivera, F., Nordgren, J., O'Ryan, M., et al. (2016). The fecal virome of South and Central American children with diarrhea includes small circular DNA viral genomes of unknown origin. *Arch. Virol.* 161, 959–966. doi: 10.1007/s00705-016-2756-4

Pifferi, M., Maggi, F., Andreoli, E., Lanini, L., Marco, E. D., Fornai, C., et al. (2005). Associations between nasal torquetenovirus load and spirometric indices in children with asthma. *J. Infect. Dis.* 192, 1141–1148. doi: 10.1086/444389

Pifferi, M., Maggi, F., Caramella, D., De Marco, E., Andreoli, E., Meschi, S., et al. (2006). High torquetenovirus loads are correlated with bronchiectasis and peripheral airflow limitation in children. *Pediatr. Infect. Dis. J.* 25, 804–808. doi: 10.1097/01.inf.0000232723.58355.f4

Rascovan, N., Duraisamy, R., and Desnues, C. (2016). Metagenomics and the human virome in asymptomatic individuals. *Annu. Rev. Microbiol.* 70, 125–141. doi: 10.1086/444389

Rocchi, J., Ricci, V., Albani, M., Lanini, L., Andreoli, E., Macera, L., et al. (2009). Torquetenovirus DNA drives proinflammatory cytokines production and secretion by immune cells via toll-like receptor 9. *Virology* 394, 235–242. doi: 10.1016/j.virol.2009.08.036

Roossinck, M. J. (2011). The good viruses: viral mutualistic symbioses. *Nat. Rev. Microbiol.* 9, 99–108. doi: 10.1038/nrmicro2491

Rossi, G. A., and Colin, A. A. (2017). Respiratory syncytial virus-Host interaction in the pathogenesis of bronchiolitis and its impact on respiratory morbidity in later life. *Pediatr. Allergy Immunol.* 28, 320–331. doi: 10.1111/pai.12716

Rubner, F. J., Jackson, D. J., Evans, M. D., Gangnon, R. E., Tisler, C. J., Pappas, T. E., et al. (2017). Early life rhinovirus wheezing, allergic sensitization, and asthma risk at adolescence. *J. Allergy Clin. Immunol.* 139, 501–507. doi: 10.1016/j.jaci.2016.03.049

Rudd, P. A., Thomas, B. J., Zaid, A., MacDonald, M., Kan-O, K., Rolph, M. S., et al. (2017). Role of human metapneumovirus and respiratory syncytial virus in asthma exacerbations: where are we now? *Clin. Sci. (Lond.)* 131, 1713–1721. doi: 10.1042/CS20160011

Scharschmidt, T. C., Vasquez, K. S., Truong, H. A., Gearty, S. V., Pauli, M. L., Nosbaum, A., et al. (2015). A wave of regulatory T cells into neonatal skin mediates tolerance to commensal microbes. *Immunity* 43, 1011–1021. doi: 10.1016/j.immuni.2015.10.016

Shulman, L. M., and Davidson, I. (2017). Viruses with Circular Single-Stranded Genomes Are Everywhere! *Annu. Rev. Virol.* 4, 155–180. doi: 10.1146/annurev-virology-101416-041953

Sigurs, N., Aljassim, F., Kjellman, B., Robinson, P. D., Sigurbergsson, F., Bjarnason, R., et al. (2010). Asthma and allergy patterns over 18 years after severe RSV bronchiolitis in the first year of life. *Thorax* 65, 1045–1052. doi: 10.1136/thx.2009.121582

Söderlund-Venermo, M., Lahtinen, A., Jartti, T., Hedman, L., Kemppainen, K., Lehtinen, P., et al. (2009). Clinical assessment and improved diagnosis of bocavirus-induced wheezing in children, Finland. *Emerg. Infect. Dis.* 15, 1423–1430. doi: 10.3201/eid1509.090204

Song, D. J. (2016). Rhinovirus and childhood asthma: an update. *Korean J. Pediatr.* 59, 432–439. doi: 10.3345/kjp.2016.59.11.432

Sorel, O., and Dewals, B. G. (2016). MicroRNAs in large herpesvirus DNA genomes: recent advances. *Biomol. Concepts* 7, 229–239. doi: 10.1099/jgv.0.000272

Stein, M. M., Hrusch, C. L., Gozdz, J., Igartua, C., Pivniouk, V., Murray, S. E., et al. (2016). Innate immunity and asthma risk in Amish and Hutterite farm children. *N. Engl. J. Med.* 375, 411–421. doi: 10.1056/NEJMoa1508749

Takahashi, K., Iwasa, Y., Hijikata, M., and Mishiro, S. (2000). Identification of a new human DNA virus (TTV-like mini virus, TLMV) intermediately related to TT virus and chicken anemia virus. *Arch. Virol.* 145, 979–993. doi: 10.1007/s007050050689

Tremaroli, V., and Bäckhed, F. (2012). Functional interactions between the gut microbiota and host metabolism. *Nature* 489, 242–249. doi: 10.1038/nature11552

Troy, N. M., and Bosco, A. (2016). Respiratory viral infections and host responses; insights from genomics. *Respir. Res.* 17:156. doi: 10.1186/s12931-016-0474-9

Vignolini, T., Macera, L., Antonelli, G., Pistello, M., Maggi, F., and Giannecchini, S. (2016). Investigation on torquetenovirus (TTV) microRNA transcriptome in vivo. *Virus Res.* 217, 18–22. doi: 10.1016/j.virusres.2016.03.003

Virgin, H. W. (2014). The virome in mammalian physiology and disease. *Cell* 157, 142–150. doi: 10.1016/j.cell.2014.02.032

Wang, Y., Zhu, N., Li, Y., and Lu, R. (2016). Metagenomic analysis of viral genetic diversity in respiratory samples from children with severe acute respiratory infection in China. *Clin. Microbiol. Infect.* 22, .e1–.e9. doi: 10.1016/j.cmi.2016.01.006

Whipps, J. M., and Karen Lewis, R. C. (1988). "Fungi biol control syst," in *Mycoparasitism and Plant Disease Control*, ed. N. Burge (Manchester: Manchester University Press), 161–187.

Xatzipsalti, M., Psarros, F., Konstantinou, G., Gaga, M., Gourgiotis, D., Saxoni-Papageorgiou, P., et al. (2008). Modulation of the epithelial inflammatory response to rhinovirus in an atopic environment. *Clin. Exp. Allergy* 38, 466–472. doi: 10.1111/j.1365-2222.2007.02906.x

Yang, J. Y., Kim, M. S., Kim, E., Cheon, J. H., Lee, Y. S., Kim, Y., et al. (2016). Enteric viruses ameliorate gut inflammation via Toll-like receptor 3 and toll-like receptor 7-mediated interferon-β production. *Immunity* 44, 889–900. doi: 10.1016/j.immuni.2016.03.009

Young, J. C., Chehoud, C., Bittinger, K., Bailey, A., Diamond, J. M., Cantu, E., et al. (2015). Viral metagenomics reveal blooms of anelloviruses in the respiratory tract of lung transplant recipients. *Am. J. Transplant.* 15, 200–209. doi: 10.1111/ajt.13031

Zheng, H., Ye, L., Fang, X., Li, B., Wang, Y., Xiang, X., et al. (2007). Torque teno virus (SANBAN isolate) ORF2 protein suppresses NF-kappaB pathways via interaction with ikappaB kinases. *J. Virol.* 81, 11917–11924. doi: 10.1128/JVI.01101-07

Zhou, Y., Do, D. C., Ishmael, F. T., Squadrito, M. L., Tang, H. M., Tang, H. L., et al. (2017). Mannose receptor modulates macrophage polarization and allergic inflammation through miR-511-3p. *J. Allergy Clin. Immunol.* 141, 350–364.e8. doi: 10.1016/j.jaci.2017.04.049

15

Oral Bacterial and Fungal Microbiome Impacts Colorectal Carcinogenesis

Klara Klimesova, Zuzana Jiraskova Zakostelska and Helena Tlaskalova-Hogenova*

Laboratory of Cellular and Molecular Immunology, Institute of Microbiology of the CAS, Prague, Czechia

***Correspondence:**
Klara Klimesova
klimesov@biomed.cas.cz

Host's physiology is significantly influenced by microbiota colonizing the epithelial surfaces. Complex microbial communities contribute to proper mucosal barrier function, immune response, and prevention of pathogen invasion and have many other crucial functions. The oral cavity and large intestine are distant parts of the digestive tract, both heavily colonized by commensal microbiota. Nevertheless, they feature different proportions of major bacterial and fungal phyla, mostly due to distinct epithelial layers organization and different oxygen levels. A few obligate anaerobic strains inhabiting the oral cavity are involved in the pathogenesis of oral diseases. Interestingly, these microbiota components are also enriched in gut inflammatory and tumor tissue. An altered microbiota composition – dysbiosis – and formation of polymicrobial biofilms seem to play important roles in the development of oral diseases and colorectal cancer. In this review, we describe the differences in composition of commensal microbiota in the oral cavity and large intestine and the mechanisms by which microbiota affect the inflammatory and carcinogenic response of the host.

Keywords: microbiome, mycobiome, pathobiont, dysbiosis, biofilm, *Fusobacterium*, oral diseases

INTRODUCTION

Both the upper and lower parts of the human digestive tract harbor a complex ecosystem of bacteria, fungi, protozoa, and viruses, referred to as the microbiome. It begins to form even before birth, in the uterus, developing for another 2–3 years after birth to become a stable, fully functioning microbiome, until the physiological changes associated with senescence lead again to substantial shifts in its composition (Adlerberth and Wold, 2009; Aagaard et al., 2014; Maffei et al., 2017). The lower part of the digestive tract gets "inoculated" every day by about 10^{11} bacteria from the oral cavity and microbial species detected in the oral and fecal microbiota overlap in about 45% of tested individuals (Socransky and Haffajee, 2002; Segata et al., 2012). Moreover, via the blood stream, these oral bacteria can disseminate all over the body. Fungal microbiota can colonize the gut perorally as well, with some strains detected in the gut likely to be contaminants from the environment or food, rather than commensals (Trojanowska et al., 2010). The composition and function of the microbiome change along the digestive tract, from the oral cavity to the rectum. These differences have been previously described in detail (Arumugam et al., 2011; Human Microbiome Project Consortium, 2012) and will be briefly outlined below.

Collectively, the genes encoded by the microbial genomes outnumber the genes in the human genome about 100-fold and this variation enables the commensal microbiota to use substrates indigestible by humans (Qin et al., 2010). Products of microbial metabolic activity include vitamins, short-chain fatty acids (SCFAs), and other compounds important for host cell metabolism and survival. Moreover, the host's physical interaction with or sensing of the microbial components is important for proper mucosal barrier function and mucosal immune system development and homeostasis. On the other hand, recent studies have shown that some commensal microbes can under certain conditions become pathogenic – so called pathobionts. Mechanisms include expression of virulence factors, such as adhesion molecules or proteases, or formation of a biofilm, and such activity can lead to disease initiation or progression. One such example is *Escherichia coli*, a large and diverse group of various bacterial serotypes. *E. coli* strains differ in their activities and biological roles: some of them are gut commensals and commercially available probiotics, others can be pathogens causing gastrointestinal and urinary infections or pathobionts associated with inflammatory bowel disease (IBD) and colorectal cancer (CRC).

The jury is still out on what triggers this transformation of commensals into pathobionts; it might be that a change in the gut microenvironment simply allows the microbes to interact with the host in an aberrant way. The gut microbiota composition and function can be influenced by various factors (**Figure 1**). For instance, many substances produced by the host and secreted into gut lumen, such as antibacterial peptides, secretory IgA, mucins, cytokines, or neuromediators, can shape the microbial community. Their production depends on host gene polymorphisms and their expression in host cells is often driven by microbial stimulation, creating a positive feedback loop. Mechanisms responsible for cancer development include some of these factors but others are still under scientific investigation.

Colorectal cancer is the most prevalent type of cancer in developed and developing countries (Ferlay et al., 2015).

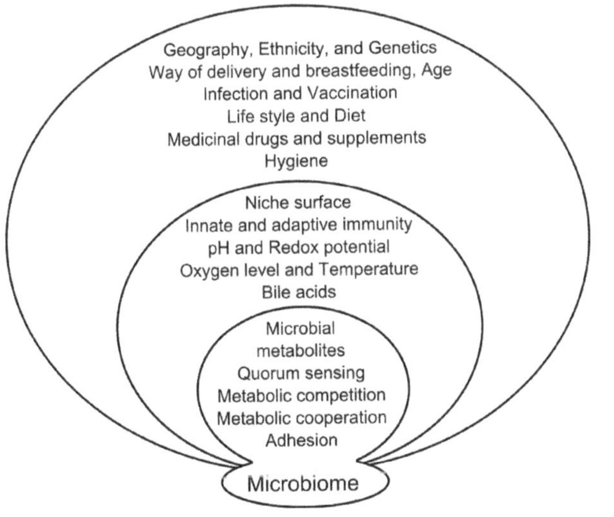

FIGURE 1 | Factors influencing microbiome composition. Microbiome composition is influenced on several levels by factors from external environment, factors resulting from the interaction of microbiota with the host and mutual interaction of the microbiome components.

Only a small percentage of colorectal cancers is hereditary or associated with certain predisposing conditions, such as chronic intestinal inflammation in IBD patients. The majority of cases thus represents sporadic cancers (85–95%) and can be, to some extent, influenced by environmental factors. The composition and metabolic activity of gut microbiota may be therefore a crucial component of CRC pathogenesis (Arthur and Jobin, 2011).

Findings of significant colonization of cancer tissue by microbes usually found in the oral cavity have sparked a debate about a possible involvement of oral microbiota in CRC development process. Many experimental studies have provided evidence for a significant role of microbiota in carcinogenesis. However, due to the complexity of microbial cooperation and interaction with the host, all the underlying mechanisms are yet to be elucidated. Here, we review the properties of bacterial and fungal populations inhabiting the oral cavity and gut, with emphasis on their association with CRC pathogenesis.

ORAL MICROBIOTA

The microorganisms found in the human oral cavity are referred to as the human oral microbiome and play a crucial role in maintenance of homeostasis in the mouth. Each individual's oral microbiome consists of a distinct set of microorganisms. The mouth supports one of the most diverse microbial communities compared with other body sites, such as the skin and vagina, due to its heterogeneity and the interrelationships between the different anatomic structures (Wade, 2013). The constantly humid environment of the oral cavity is maintained at a relatively stable temperature (34–36°C), while the varying pH levels and different types of diet contribute to the substantial microbiome variability (Marcotte and Lavoie, 1998). Habitats of the oral cavity are represented by both hard (teeth) and soft tissues (cheek, tongue, lip, gingival sulcus, attached gingiva, hard and soft palate) and their interface (subgingival and supragingival margins, and gingival crevices around teeth). The contiguous extensions of the oral cavity, including the tonsils, pharynx, esophagus, Eustachian tube, middle ear, trachea, lungs, nasal passages, and sinuses, are also colonized by the oral microbiome but the majority of studies describing the oral microbiome composition include only samples from the oral cavity (Mager et al., 2003; Aas et al., 2005). Moreover, all these structures are constantly moistened by two physiological fluids, saliva and the gingival crevicular fluid, which help to maintain the oral microbiome homeostasis by providing water, nutrients, antibodies, and antimicrobial and adherence factors (Marcotte and Lavoie, 1998).

The National Institute of Health's Human Microbiome Project identified the most dominant phyla that account for over 95% of the entire oral microbiome: *Firmicutes*, with the *Streptococcus* as a dominant genus, *Bacteroidetes*, strongly represented by *Prevotella* and *Proteobacteria*, with highly abundant *Haemophilus*, *Fusobacteria*, and *Actinobacteria* (Human Microbiome Project Consortium, 2012; Huse et al., 2012; Zhou et al., 2013). The oral cavity displays greater alpha-diversity (species richness) than either the skin or vagina, characterized by uniform abundance of the major species (Huse et al., 2012). On the other hand, beta-diversity, i.e., differences in microbiome composition in oral sites among various subjects, is the lowest compared to the other body sites (Huse et al., 2012). Within the oral cavity, the highest microbiota richness has been found in the gingival plaque and in saliva, whereas the lowest richness has been described in keratinized gingiva (Huse et al., 2012; Zhou et al., 2013). It seems that saliva contributes unevenly to the microbial composition of different sites in the oral cavity. Due to its rapid turnover and low levels of nutrients, saliva itself does not contain a stable indigenous biota and owes its high alpha-diversity primarily to bacteria shed from other oral tissues (Mager et al., 2003). In general, species like *Streptococcus, Gemmella, Granulicatella, Veillonella,* and *Fusobacterium* can be detected across almost all oral sites, while others are represented only at one or two oral sites, e.g., *Prevotella, Bacteroides, Corynebacterium, Pasteurella,* and *Neisseria* (Huse et al., 2012). Bacterial species in the oral cavity find the most stable environment at the supragingival or subgingival tooth surfaces. These non-shedding surfaces are covered by persisting biofilms composed mainly by *Streptococcus* and *Actinomyces*, representing the earliest colonizers of teeth, and *Veillonella* (Socransky and Haffajee, 2005; Teles et al., 2013). Taken together, although most microbial species found in the oral cavity differ in their abundance, their representation and activity is more important.

ORAL MICROBIOME AND ORAL DISEASES

A considerable number of oral conditions, including caries and periodontal diseases, endodontic infections, alveolar osteitis, and tonsillitis is connected to detrimental alteration in microbiota composition – a dysbiosis (Costalonga and Herzberg, 2014; Proctor and Relman, 2017). For instance, periodontal inflammation is directly induced by microbes colonizing the biofilm in the gingival sulcus and, at later stages, in the periodontal pockets. These oral biofilms contain 100s of different bacterial species in one periodontal lesion, with composition different from that in healthy periodontium (Socransky and Haffajee, 2005; Teles et al., 2013). Initially, the plaque forms only supragingivally but if it is not removed properly, after a few days it spreads below the gingival margin and into the sulcus. There, after the depletion of oxygen, a new environment is established, where anaerobic bacteria can flourish. Three most destructive anaerobic bacteria involved in severe periodontal disease, the so called "red complex," include *Treponema denticola, Tannerella forsythia* and *Porphyromonas gingivalis* (Socransky et al., 1998). Aggressive form of periodontitis is further associated with *Aggregatibacter actinomycetemcomitans* (Slots, 1976). The immunopathological mechanisms in periodontal disease development and course have been recently thoroughly reviewed by Hajishengallis and Korostoff (2017). Recurrent aphthous stomatitis is also connected to changes in microbiota composition; decreased abundance of *Streptococcus salivarius* and increased *Acinetobacter johnsonii* have been linked to the disease incidence (Bankvall et al., 2014; Kim et al., 2016).

As mentioned previously, the human microbiome diversity is not limited only to bacteria but also includes fungal species. However, this oral mycobiome have been only recently characterized and despite its potential great scientific importance, we found only few studies where its composition was analyzed using high throughput sequencing. Ghannoum et al. (2010) reported that healthy oral mycobiota contained 74 culturable and 11 non-culturable fungal genera. They have revealed great inter-individual variation and proposed that the presence of certain fungal isolates (e.g., *Candida, Aspergillus, Cryptococcus*) probably predisposes the host to opportunistic infections. *Malassezia* species, previously described as commensals and pathogens of the skin and lungs, have been recently found as predominant commensals in saliva (Saunders et al., 2012; Dupuy et al., 2014). Many other species are likely still waiting to be discovered and were not detected earlier because of their special growth requirements (Nagano et al., 2010). The first evidence of interactions among members of the oral mycobiome community and their association with specific disease came from a study characterizing the oral mycobiome in HIV patients (Mukherjee et al., 2014). The authors found that a decrease in abundance of an indigenous fungus *Pichia* in uninfected individuals went hand in hand with an increase in abundance of *Candida*, suggesting an antagonistic relationship. *Pichia* inhibits *Candida* by different mechanisms, including competition for nutrients and secretion of factors that disrupt the latter's ability to adhere, germinate, and form biofilms. Moreover, they found a negative correlation between *Candida* and *Campylobacter* in HIV-infected subjects, whereas in healthy subjects, no correlation between *Candida* and bacterial species was detected (Mukherjee et al., 2014). Recently, Peters et al. (2017) published a pilot study describing oral mycobiome in healthy subjects and those with periodontal disease. In diseased subjects, they found a slightly increased abundance of *Candida* genera which is in agreement with previous culture-based studies (Urzúa et al., 2008; Canabarro et al., 2013). Despite those first studies aiming for a deeper understanding of the factors affecting the oral mycobiota composition, information about their direct and indirect effects on human health and the interactions between the fungi and bacteria is still lacking.

The involvement of microbiota in the pathogenesis of oral diseases has been documented using gnotobiotic rat and mouse models of human diseases. Germ-free animals can be obtained by delivering the young by sterile Cesarean section and raising them aseptically in isolators for germ-free rearing. Such animals made it possible to study the effects of commensal bacteria in the oral cavity, including the effects on periodontal tissues. In germ-free mice and rats, it was demonstrated that periodontal disease and caries, similarly to other human inflammatory diseases, cannot be experimentally induced in the absence of microbiota (Heijl et al., 1980; Tlaskalova-Hogenova et al., 2004). Experimental animal models (e.g., the gavage model of periodontal disease) and *in vitro* studies revealed that certain components of oral microbiota, mainly *P. gingivalis*, play a crucial role in the innate host defense of periodontium and that dysregulation of the immune response in the presence of oral microbiota leads to inflammation and alveolar bone loss (Ivanyi et al., 1991; Darveau et al., 2012; Papadopoulos et al., 2013). The mechanisms by which microbiota triggers the pathological changes are not yet fully understood, however, new approaches promise to shed light on the role of oral microbiota (Kinane et al., 2017; Pitts et al., 2017).

ORAL MICROBIOME AND EXTRA-ORAL DISEASES

Dysbiosis of the oral microbiome is not only connected with the incidence and maintenance of oral diseases, but has been also implicated in the pathogenesis of autoimmune, inflammatory, and neoplastic diseases (e.g., heart disease, respiratory illnesses, psoriasis, psoriatic arthritis, and carcinogenesis at various sites) (He et al., 2015; Roberts and Darveau, 2015; Egeberg et al., 2017; Ungprasert et al., 2017). Moreover, oral microbiota seems to affect the outcome of pathological pregnancy (preterm birth, abortions, etc.); reviewed by Cobb et al. (2017). Periodontal bacterial DNA has been found in atherosclerotic plaques of patients suffering from ischemic heart disease and atherosclerosis (Ford et al., 2005, 2006). Bacteria may initiate or exacerbate atherosclerotic processes through activation of innate immunity, direct involvement of mediators activated by dental plaque antigens in atheroma processes, or involvement of cytokines and heat shock proteins from dental plaque bacteria. There might be also genetic predisposing factors influencing both diseases (Bartova et al., 2014). Furthermore, patients with rheumatoid arthritis have a higher prevalence of periodontal disease and vice versa (Kasser et al., 1997; Greenwald and Kirkwood, 1999). Bacterial DNA has been detected in the synovial fluid of patients with rheumatoid arthritis or with failed prosthetic joints, suggesting the possibility of infection translocating from the periodontal tissue to the synovium (Temoin et al., 2012). The oral microbiome is not confined to spreading to contiguous epithelial surfaces, but can also be carried by the bloodstream to distant body sites, such as the heart, skin, and joints. Oral microbiota enters the bloodstream during routine daily activities like tooth brushing or through inflamed tissue in the course of oral diseases (Tomas et al., 2012). The mechanisms of dissemination of potentially pathogenic microbes from the oral cavity through bloodstream are still not clear. Potential connection with systemic low-grade inflammation has been also discussed (Potgieter et al., 2015).

In most conditions discussed so far, no particular microbe or microbes have been described as a causative agent. However, thanks to advances in molecular methods, presence of *Fusobacteria* and other oral bacteria has been recently demonstrated in various systemic pathological conditions, including digestive diseases, such as appendicitis, IBD and CRC. Moreover, a correlation of the presence of oral bacteria *P. gingivalis* and *A. actinomycetemcomitans* with an increased risk of developing pancreatic cancer has been observed in a large group of subjects with incident primary pancreatic adenocarcinoma (Fan et al., 2016). Several recent studies have repeatedly confirmed the presence of oral bacteria in the gut, especially in association with CRC mucosa. For instance, Nakatsu et al. (2015) have shown that a substantial part of gut microbiome associated with CRC is composed of oral bacteria and *Fusobacterium* in particular. Momen-Heravi et al. (2017) also proposed a role of oral bacteria in CRC development. They conducted a retrospective study in a huge cohort of women and discovered an association of periodontal disease and tooth loss with CRC morbidity and found that women with less than 17 teeth may be at a greater risk of incident CRC (Momen-Heravi et al., 2017).

ORAL MICROBIOTA AND COLORECTAL CARCINOGENESIS

It is generally accepted that the gut microbiome plays a role in CRC development. Experimental proof of gut microbiota involvement in CRC development came from gnotobiotic animal models (Reddy et al., 1975; Vannucci et al., 2008; Arthur and Jobin, 2011; Klimesova et al., 2013; Tlaskalova-Hogenova et al., 2014). Recent studies using next generation sequencing and polymerase chain reaction have shown that *Fusobacterium nucleatum* is frequently detected in stool and biopsy samples from CRC patients (Castellarin et al., 2012; Kostic et al., 2012; Flanagan et al., 2014). These adhesive, anaerobic Gram-negative bacteria attract considerable attention in search for possible mechanisms behind their inflammatory and tumorigenic activity. Some of the features of *F. nucleatum* and the host responses are already known: *F. nucleatum* modulates E-cadherin/β-catenin signaling via its FadA adhesin/invasin – a key virulence factor, and alters macrophage infiltration and methylation of the CDKN2A promoter in CRC lesions (Rubinstein et al., 2013; Park et al., 2017). It seems that Fap2 Gal-GalNAc lectin of *F. nucleatum* could be responsible for its tendency to bind to tumor cells displaying Gal-GalNAc moieties (Abed et al., 2016). Moreover, several other virulence proteins that might participate in inflammatory and neoplastic processes have been described in *F. nucleatum*, using proteomic approaches (Zanzoni et al., 2017). In the host, *F. nucleatum* activates numerous immune responses including human β-defensin production, lymphocyte apoptosis, and production of proinflammatory cytokines interleukin (IL)-6, IL-8, and TNF-α (Han, 2015).

The fact that *Fusobacterium* is highly abundant in patients with CRC led to various efforts to apply this finding for clinical purposes. For instance, a highly sensitive DNA test for *F. nucleatum* has been developed for screening and prognosis of CRC in Japan (Yamaoka et al., 2017). *Fusobacterium* has been recently shown to predict the aggressiveness and recurrence of CRC and its resistance to chemotherapy. It seems to be modifying the innate immune signaling and regulating specific microRNAs that activate the autophagy pathway (Yu et al., 2017). In connection with this finding, an argument has been made to use anti-*F. nucleatum* therapy together with chemotherapy.

The dietary patterns leading to CRC development have been studied for several decades. Recently, it was shown that individuals consuming a western-type diet have a higher incidence of *Fusobacterium*-associated CRC and that diets rich in whole grains and dietary fiber are associated with a lower risk of *F. nucleatum*-positive CRC (Mehta et al., 2017).

Despite the clinical observation of increased abundance of *Fusobacterium* in patients with CRC (especially in chemoresistant forms of CRC), direct clinical evidence of a causal relationship is still lacking. A recent study revealed that fusobacterial abundance is not significantly increased in fecal samples of patients with adenomas, implying that the relationship between *Fusobacterium* and CRC might not be causal after all. Amitay et al. (2017) hypothesize that *Fusobacterium* is more likely just a passenger colonizing the favorable niche in a gut with CRC, rather than the driver of cancer development. Experimental evidence of its potential causal role is based on *in vitro* and animal models of CRC. For instance, it has been shown that *F. nucleatum* potentiates tumorigenesis in monoassociated $Apc^{min/+}$ mice (Kostic et al., 2013).

While *Fusobacterium* is the most studied periodontal microbe in connection to CRC, other components of the oral microbiome may also be implicated in CRC pathogenesis and will be discussed later (**Table 1**).

TABLE 1 | Oral microbiota and its possible mechanisms related to tumorigenesis.

Microbial genera	Activity	Reference
Streptococcus	Adhesion, co-aggregation Biofilm formation Protease activity Hemolytic activity	da Silva et al., 2014 Diaz et al., 2012 Kilian et al., 1988 Wong et al., 2016
Peptostreptococcus	Biofilm formation Antiapoptotic effect Hydrogen sulfide production	Tsoi et al., 2017 Persson et al., 1990
Parvimonas	Biofilm formation Hemolytic activity Proinflammatory stimulation Hydrogen sulfide production	Wong et al., 2016 Marchesan et al., 2016 Carlsson et al., 1993
Dialister	Biofilm formation Proinflammatory stimulation	da Silva et al., 2014 Sousa et al., 2014
Mogibacterium	Biofilm formation	Casarin et al., 2012
Fusobacterium	Adhesion Proinflammatory stimulation Immune evasion Hemolytic activity Hydrogen sulfide production	Kostic et al., 2013 Rubinstein et al., 2013 Wong et al., 2016 Claesson et al., 1990
Porphyromonas	Biofilm formation Immune evasion Antiapoptotic effect Protease activity Hemolytic activity Hydrogen sulfide production Proinflammatory stimulation	Inaba et al., 2013 Mao et al., 2007 Potempa et al., 2003 Wong et al., 2016 Persson et al., 1990 Sousa et al., 2014
Campylobacter	Hemolytic activity Proinflammatory stimulation	Wong et al., 2016 Marchesan et al., 2016
Candida	Adhesion Biofilm formation Protease activity Hemolytic activity	Diaz et al., 2012 Gomes et al., 2017

GUT MICROBIOME, METABOLIC ACTIVITY, AND COLON CARCINOGENESIS

Thanks to advances in high-throughput sequencing and metabolomic approaches, we have a growing understanding of the composition and metabolic activity of the microbiome associated with colorectal carcinogenesis. Studies have shown that gut microbiome differs between healthy individuals and adenoma/carcinoma patients and that microbial diversity in cancer is reduced (Peters et al., 2016). The adenoma-carcinoma sequence in CRC development suggests an associated continuous alteration of the resident microbiome, which is supported by recent research. Analyses of fecal microbiome composition in patients with adenoma have shown increased normalized abundance of genera such as *Actinomyces*, *Corynebacterium*, *Porphyromonas*, *Mogibacterium*, and *Haemophilus* when compared with healthy individuals (Peters et al., 2016; Hale et al., 2017). Cancer patients have shown further differences in fecal microbiota composition, with a marked enrichment of *Ruminococcus*, *Oscillibacter*, and *Roseburia*, and *Porphyromonas*, *Fusobacterium*, and *Peptostreptococcus*, i.e., strains associated with periodontal disease (**Table 1**) (Shen et al., 2010; Flemer et al., 2017; Liang et al., 2017).

Moreover, fecal samples reflect the microbial colonization of tissues, as biopsies from adenomas and carcinomas have been similarly different from healthy mucosa (Flemer et al., 2017). The findings that there is very little difference in microbiota composition between diseased and adjacent unaffected tissue suggest that the microbiome undergoes a systemic change, affecting the whole community (Lu et al., 2016; Flemer et al., 2017). Such results support the driver/passenger model, the idea that certain strains disturb the microbial community and the mucosal microenvironment (drivers) and such changes lead to subsequent colonization by pathobionts and pathogens (passengers) (Tjalsma et al., 2012). Both the drivers and the passengers modulate the local microenvironment through different means, such as virulence factors or metabolic activity. Drivers thus promote cancer initiation at the very beginning by their involvement in DNA damage, cell cycle regulation, apoptosis and epithelium proliferation, whereas passengers more likely promote tumorigenesis via chronic proinflammatory stimulation and direct tissue damage.

Drivers often include microbes that produce genotoxic substances, which damage DNA, or cyclomodulins, which can modulate the epithelial cell cycle – recently thoroughly reviewed by Gagniere et al. (2016) and El-Aouar et al. (2017). *Bacteroides fragilis* and *Enterococcus faecalis* have the potential to damage epithelial cells and initiate cancer formation by producing the enterotoxin fragilysin and reactive oxygen species, such as superoxide, respectively (Huycke et al., 2002; Toprak et al., 2006). Several studies confirmed that *E. coli* strains encoding the genotoxic polyketide synthase (pks) island are associated with inflamed gut mucosa and CRC (Swidsinski et al., 1998; Nougayrede et al., 2006; Arthur et al., 2012; Raisch et al., 2014). Interestingly, members of the family Enterobacteriaceae, including *E. coli*, can produce several types of genotoxins or cyclomodulins. Cytotoxic necrotizing factors and cycle-inhibiting factor modulate the cell cycle and can lead to uncontrolled proliferation or cell cycle arrest, respectively (Taieb et al., 2006; Miraglia et al., 2007). Cytolethal distending toxins, similarly to pks, induce DNA double-strand breaks and apoptosis, but can also promote proinflammatory cytokine production in the host (Blazkova et al., 2010). In summary, the interplay of these factors with gut epithelium and immune cells can promote low-grade inflammation and cancer initiation. Moreover, we can assume that these molecules represent just the tip of the iceberg of as yet unknown microbial products of gut commensals with the potential to harm the gut epithelium.

Mycobiome, i.e., the fungal microbiome, forms an integral part of the gut microbial community, although it is much less investigated then the bacterial part. The most common genera residing in a healthy gut are *Candida*, *Saccharomyces*, and *Cladosporium* (Hoffmann et al., 2013). However, some non-commensal transient fungi, acquired with food or from the environment, can be also found in fecal samples and may comprise potentially pathogenic species. Trojanowska et al. (2010) have shown that the gut is colonized also by the oral mycobiome, as they found a genetically identical *Candida albicans* strain in the mouth and colon of patients with IBD. Unfortunately, data about fungal colonization of the digestive tract in relation to neoplastic diseases are still sparse. A disruption of the bacterial and fungal community – dysbiosis, has been observed in individuals with IBD (Sokol et al., 2017), who are known to be at increased risk of CRC development. Interestingly, reduced richness and diversity has been detected not only in bacterial, but also in fungal microbiome (Chehoud et al., 2015; Liguori et al., 2016; Sokol et al., 2017). For instance, the Cystofilobasidiaceae family, *Dioszegia* genus and *Candida glabrata* have been found to be enriched in Crohn's disease compared with healthy mucosa (Liguori et al., 2016). The only published study on fungal microbiota in CRC deals with comparison of adenomas and adjacent tissues. Luan et al. (2015) have observed an increased abundance of *Phoma* and *Candida* genera and *Candida tropicalis* in adenomas. As pathobionts, these genera may be involved in cancer initiation, but further studies are needed to investigate whether they work as drivers or passengers.

Microbiome in the colon makes use of various catabolic and anabolic pathways, which enable it to utilize a broad spectrum of substrates that are not absorbed in the small intestine. These pathways interact with the metabolism of xenobiotics and influence micronutrient bioavailability, lead to the production of essential vitamins and degradation of fibers, and regulate the secretion of various molecules (Arthur and Jobin, 2011). Different dietary components can shift the microbiome composition. For instance, a diet high in resistant starch increases the abundance of bacteria metabolizing non-digestible polysaccharides (Walker et al., 2011). Indeed, increased abundance of *Prevotella* and *Bacteroides* has been observed in individuals preferring high sugar and high protein diet, respectively (Wu et al., 2011). Our digestion pathways lack the enzymes for the degradation of resistant starch and dietary fiber but the distal gut microbiome encodes about 81 different families of glycoside hydrolases (bacterial polysaccharidases, glycosidases), which are not present in the human genome (Gill et al., 2006). The microbiome thus significantly contributes to the utilization of starch, primary fiber, host-derived secretions (mucus glycans), sucrose, and monosaccharides.

Subsequent fermentation of depolymerized molecules leads to the production of SCFAs, mainly acetate, propionate, and butyrate. Compared with other microbiomes in gene libraries, the human gut microbiome is enriched with genes involved in the pathways generating SCFAs (Gill et al., 2006). Main producers of butyrate within the human gut microbiome are *Faecalibacterium prausnitzii* and *Eubacterium rectale/Roseburia* group (Louis et al., 2010). SCFAs provide one of the most important sources of energy, not only for intestinal epithelial cells but also for muscles, kidneys, heart, and brain. Their physiologic production impacts the metabolism and transport through the epithelium, as well as epithelial cell renewal and differentiation. Moreover, SCFAs greatly influence the immune system, colonic functions, and carcinogenesis. Butyrate production, for example, improves gut barrier integrity and reduces local oxidative stress and inflammation (Macfarlane and Macfarlane, 2012). Recently, Kaiko et al. (2016) came with an interesting finding that butyrate levels are much lower at the intestinal crypt base than in the lumen. Differentiated enterocytes use butyrate as an energy source and thus reduce its concentration along the way to the lamina propria, where a low concentration of butyrate keeps the epithelial progenitors proliferating and stimulates tolerogenic immune response (Kaiko et al., 2016). The role of SCFAs in cancerogenesis is not fully understood but their concentration could be an important factor.

On the other hand, degradation and fermentation of dietary proteins, peptides, and amino acids by bacteria generates by-products, such as phenols, indoles, ammonia, amines, and hydrogen sulfite, all of which are to some extent harmful to the host, being co-carcinogens, mutagens, and cellular toxins (Macfarlane and Macfarlane, 2012). Moreover, hydrogen released as the end-product of fermentation is processed by methanogenic species of Archaea (e.g., *Methanobrevibacter*) to methane, which changes local conditions (redox potential and pH) and thus regulates biochemical pathways (Gill et al., 2006).

Fungal metabolic activity includes the digestion of polysaccharides and fat residuals from the diet and host residuals, leading to the synthesis of a variety of secondary metabolites, which can substantially influence the surrounding prokaryotic and eukaryotic cells. An investigation of the relationship between fungal diversity and diet revealed a positive correlation of *Candida* with diet rich in saccharides and a negative correlation of *Aspergillus* with SCFAs (Hoffmann et al., 2013). Thus, close relationships between bacterial and fungal metabolic requirements can help structure the microbial community in the gut. For instance, antimicrobial treatment can significantly disrupt the ecological balance of microbiota throughout the digestive tract. Antibiotics eradicate some sensitive bacteria and their niche can be subsequently invaded by other bacteria or fungi (Huffnagle and Noverr, 2013). Interestingly, a nested case-control study has shown that bacterial or fungal outgrowth after multiple penicillin treatments slightly increases the risk of CRC development (Boursi et al., 2015). And, last but not least, consumption of food-associated mycotoxins – secondary metabolites of fungi, has been linked to carcinogenesis throughout the digestive tract (De Ruyck et al., 2015). Several *in vitro* studies have shown that exposure to mycotoxins affects apoptosis, intestinal barrier integrity and mucus production and causes DNA damage, suggesting a possible role of mycotoxins in CRC development; reviewed by Maresca and Fantini (2010).

HOST–MICROBIOME INTERACTION AND DISEASE DEVELOPMENT

Host derived proteoglycans, forming the mucus layer, are an important part of the mucosal immune system. They protect the epithelium from an extensive contact with the microbiome and reduce the risk of microbial invasion. The oral cavity and esophagus harbor several layers of tight and largely inert squamous epithelium, whereas the remaining parts of the digestive tract are covered with a single layer of intensely active cells (Johansson et al., 2013). The structure of the mucus layers and types of mucin (MUC) vary widely along the digestive tract. The salivary glands in the oral cavity produce mainly MUC5B and MUC7, glands in the stomach and duodenum secrete gel-forming mucins MUC5AC and MUC6, and goblet cells in the gut specialize in MUC2 production (Khan et al., 1998; Wickstrom et al., 1998; Nordman et al., 2002). While in the small intestine, MUC2 forms a loose unattached mucus layer, in the colon it has two parts with different functions, an inner, attached layer and an outer, unattached one (Johansson et al., 2013). The inner layer, which is about 50–100 μm thick, is dense and impenetrable to most microbes, while the outer layer flows with the gut content. Mucus contains distinct products of epithelial cells, such as antimicrobial peptides and secretory IgA, which play an important role in the protection of gut mucosa against pathogen invasion or excessive inflammatory response to commensals (Johansson et al., 2011).

Interestingly, some members of the oral and gut microbiome can form a multilayer structure, composed of microbes and a polymeric matrix, termed a biofilm. Biofilm formation is one example of the mechanisms microorganisms use to evade antimicrobial defenses in the hostile environment of the host. Most biofilms are of polymicrobial nature and members of the biofilm community are distinct from the planktonic microbiota colonizing the mucosal surfaces throughout the body. Polymeric matrix formation and subsequent microbial colonization is the consequence of adhesion processes mediated by a wide spectrum of glycoproteins. Caries and periodontal disease are associated with biofilm formation by well-known periodontopathic bacteria. Biofilm in dental caries contains mainly streptococci, *L. acidophilus*, and *Actinomyces* and is secondarily colonized by anaerobic species, such as *F. nucleatum* and *P. gingivalis* (Chenicheri et al., 2017). In periodontal disease, early biofilm colonizers are mainly represented by streptococci and *Actinomyces*. Later on, more pathogenic bacteria such as *F. nucleatum*, *P. gingivalis*, *T. forsythia*, *T. denticola*, and *A. actinomycetemcomitans* appear (Socransky and Haffajee, 2005; Teles et al., 2013). The tendency of some microscopic fungi to form biofilms is also well-established in the literature. Recently, cooperation between *Candida* and oral commensal streptococci has been described as a significant factor in biofilm formation. Such cohabitation supports *Candida* growth and survival by providing it with an adhesive surface and the ability to invade tissue by promoting hyphae formation (Diaz et al., 2012).

Current research has confirmed the presence of polymicrobial biofilms on gut mucosa of CRC patients, suggesting their possible role in CRC pathogenesis. Even in healthy mucosa, biofilm formation is associated with oncogenic potential and might be used to predict susceptibility to cancer development (Dejea et al., 2014). These biofilms consist of periodontopathic bacteria – *F. nucleatum* and *P. gingivalis*, as well as oral commensals, such as *Peptostreptococcus*, *Prevotella*, and *Parvimonas*, and their metabolic products, which may contribute to CRC progression (Li et al., 2017). Microbial biofilms disrupt mucus layers, enabling potentially harmful microbes to attach to or even invade the mucosa and directly affect the epithelial cells by cytotoxic or genotoxic metabolites. Indeed, a recent study by Johnson et al. (2015) has provided evidence that the presence of biofilm increases polyamine metabolites in cancer tissues. Interestingly, fungal genera *Phoma* and *Candida* have been detected in higher quantities in adenoma biopsies (Luan et al., 2015). However, to date, the connection of these mixed-species biofilms with CRC has not been thoroughly studied.

When passing from the upper to the lower digestive tract, some previously mentioned bacteria change their oxygen requirements from facultative anaerobic to strict anaerobic, thereby switching to asaccharolytic and proteolytic metabolism (Eley and Cox, 2003). Microbial proteolytic enzymes break down the host's extracellular matrix and soluble factors to get nutrients and invade the tissue. Periodontopathic bacteria produce a wide spectrum of enzymes, including collagenases, elastases, peptidases, etc. For instance, gingipains are cysteine proteases secreted by *P. gingivalis*, classified as either arginine (Rgp) or lysine (Kgp) specific (Potempa et al., 2003). They play a key role in biofilm formation, consequent host tissue destruction and vascular permeability induction (Kadowaki et al., 2000; Eley and Cox, 2003). Some of the *P. gingivalis* proteases can degrade immunologically active molecules, such as immunoglobulins, cytokines and components of the complement, and thus modulate the antibacterial immune response. Similarly, oral streptococci produce proteases which have been shown to cleave IgA1 (Kilian et al., 1988). Interestingly, 88% of the streptococci that initiate plaque formation on dental enamel possess IgA1 protease activity. Moreover, oral streptococci attack human

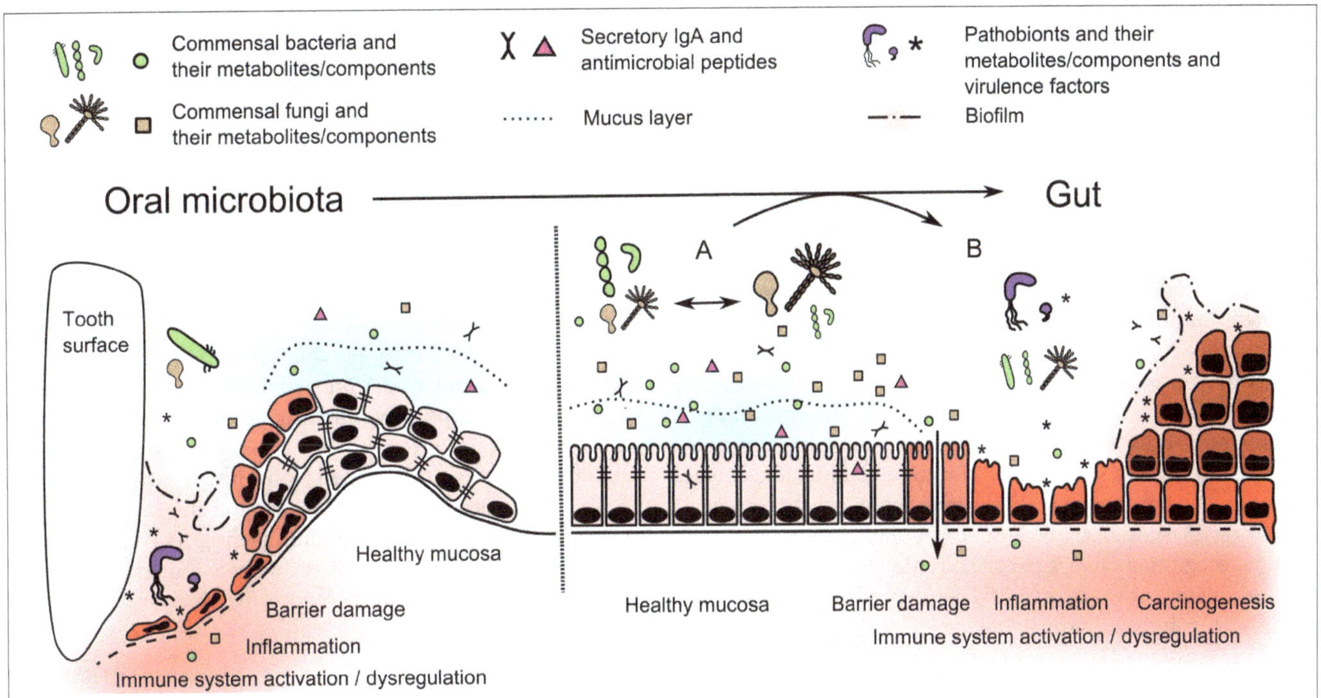

FIGURE 2 | Oral microbiota moves to the gut and alter local microenvironment. In oral cavity, periodontal pathogens use several mechanisms, such as adhesion, biofilm formation and protease activity (see **Table 1**), to disrupt the barrier and trigger the inflammatory changes in periodontium. In the gut, healthy stable microbiome can undergo temporary dynamic perturbations promoting growth of bacterial or fungal part of the microbiome **(A)**. These shifts are mostly reversible, do not disrupt mucosal barrier function, nor induce proinflammatory immune response. Nevertheless, microbes associated with periodontal disease can further disseminate into the gut becoming a part of altered gut microbiome with pathogenic potential. They can use similar mechanisms as in oral cavity and produce virulence and growth-promoting factors or substitute missing beneficial commensals. This can affect the stability of resident microbiome and promote their selective outgrowth leading to a dysbiosis **(B)**. Subsequent adhesion and biofilm formation, proteolytic activity or accumulation of harmful metabolites and soluble components can damage the integrity of gut barrier. These pathogenic mechanisms, together with dysregulated host immune response, can lead to inflammation and/or colorectal cancer initiation.

immunoglobulin IgA1 not only by protease production but also by glycosidases (neuraminidase and beta-galactosidase). Oral streptococci thus cleave the alpha chains and also the carbohydrate moiety of IgA1. This finding suggests that the ability of streptococci to evade secretory immune mechanisms is one of the factors that enable them to colonize the oral cavity (Kilian et al., 1989).

Another important feature of the microbiota that protects the host against pathogens is resistance to outsider invasion. Microbiota presents a competitive barrier to pathogenic microbes by active struggle for existence, fighting for nutrients and niche occupation. Moreover, commensals express antimicrobial effector molecules (bacteriocins) that serve as an effective tool for community shaping by endogenous microbiota. The third mechanism is indirect through constitutive stimulation of the mucosal immune system by commensal microbes, which strengthens the mucosal barrier, thus reducing pathogen translocation (Robinson et al., 2010; Stecher and Hardt, 2011; Backhed et al., 2012).

Mucosal surface of the gut is in continuous contact with foreign compounds derived from diet as well as from commensal or pathogenic microorganisms. Therefore, maintaining balance between the inner and outer milieu is the hallmark of the whole mucosal immune system. Many different cell types and their products are involved in this complex dialog, including epithelial and immune cells, cells of supporting tissues, antimicrobial peptides, growth factors, cytokines, and other mediators. Various components of microbiota can differentially trigger cellular pathways that shape local as well as systemic immune response and physiological functions. Recognition of these microbe-associated molecular patterns (MAMPs) is one of the most important features of the mucosal immune system. Receptors facilitating this are known as pattern-recognition receptors and can be divided into several families, such as retinoic acid inducible gene I-like receptors, nod-like receptors, toll-like receptors (TLR), and lectin receptors. Proinflammatory processes that are mediated by MAMPs, such as lipopolysaccharide, polysaccharides, peptidoglycan, flagella, and microbial DNA/RNA, activate pattern-recognition receptors on various host cells. These cells elicit local pro-inflammatory response and/or drive the differentiation of adaptive immune response (Sartor, 2008; Underhill and Iliev, 2014). Therefore, a persistent inflammatory reaction of the host, constantly challenging the mucosal immune system, can lead to disease initiation (Tlaskalova-Hogenova et al., 2004). Appropriate immune response requires that recognition of commensals on the apical side of the epithelium induces tolerance, while recognition of pathogens on the basolateral membrane or inside the cell induces inflammation. Moreover, TLRs are important for stimulation of gut epithelium growth and barrier integrity as well as production of mucus, secretory IgA, antimicrobial peptides, and chemokines (Abreu, 2010). Generally, the expression of *TLR*s in the epithelium is low in the steady state but increases during inflammation. Indeed, recent studies suggested the association of *TLR* polymorphisms with the progression of IBD into CRC, as *TLR*s expression is changed during gut inflammation (Bank et al., 2015).

Chronic inflammation leads to massive accumulation of activated immune cells and their mediators (cytokines and chemokines), residues of damaged cells, and large amounts of oxygen and nitrogen reactive species. Isolated dysplastic cells are further modified by the local microenvironment, as pro-inflammatory cells and cytokines promote the progression of dysplasia into carcinoma. During chronic inflammation, innate immune cells produce excessive quantities of reactive oxygen and nitrogen species that cause DNA and cellular damage. Pattern-recognition receptors signalization in the milieu of chronic inflammation activates MyD88-dependent pathways that promote pro-inflammatory cytokine release and subsequent tumor progression (Tlaskalova-Hogenova et al., 2014).

CONCLUSION

There are two fundamental links between microbes and diseases. The first involves the host's recognition and immune response mechanisms and the second involves the microbiota itself, its presence and metabolic activity. Impaired barrier function, inadequate activation of the innate immune system and dysregulation of the appropriate mucosal immune response to gut microbiota (tolerance) are the primary elements of disease development. Low microbiome diversity seems to be a common feature in the pathogenesis of diseases of the digestive tract, suggesting that high microbial richness, both bacterial and fungal, is crucial for physiological homeostasis. Normally, a dynamic balance is maintained, where reduction of the bacterial community leads to outgrowth of the fungal one and vice versa. Disruption of this balance is associated with outgrowth of certain pathobionts at the expense of a complex community and may lead to disease initiation (**Figure 2**). Established dysbiosis is supported by local proinflammatory and tumor microenvironment which creates distinct nutritional conditions. A growing body of literature dealing with microbiome metabolic activities gradually unravels the complex host–microbe interactions. Nevertheless, collecting data about these interactions at the time of disease development is especially challenging in humans. In this respect, we still have to rely on retrospective clinical studies and animal models to generate helpful insights. Elucidation of the underlying mechanisms involving the interactions of the immune system with the microbiome, pathogens, or pathobionts can lead to the development of early screening and preventive interventions and, ultimately, reduce the risk of severe colon cancer.

AUTHOR CONTRIBUTIONS

KK, ZJZ, and HT-H wrote the manuscript and approved its final version.

FUNDING

The authors are supported by Czech Science Foundation (17-06632Y and 16-06326S), Ministry of Health of the Czech Republic (15-27580A, 15-29336A, 15-28064A, and 15-30782A), and Institutional Research Concept (RVO: 61388971).

REFERENCES

Aagaard, K., Ma, J., Antony, K. M., Ganu, R., Petrosino, J., and Versalovic, J. (2014). The placenta harbors a unique microbiome. *Sci. Transl. Med.* 6:237ra65. doi: 10.1126/scitranslmed.3008599

Aas, J. A., Paster, B. J., Stokes, L. N., Olsen, I., and Dewhirst, F. E. (2005). Defining the normal bacterial flora of the oral cavity. *J. Clin. Microbiol.* 43, 5721–5732. doi: 10.1128/Jcm.43.11.5721-5732.2005

Abed, J., Emgard, J. E. M., Zamir, G., Faroja, M., Almogy, G., Grenov, A., et al. (2016). Fap2 mediates *Fusobacterium nucleatum* colorectal adenocarcinoma enrichment by binding to tumor-expressed Gal-GalNAc. *Cell Host Microbe* 20, 215–225. doi: 10.1016/j.chom.2016.07.006

Abreu, M. T. (2010). Toll-like receptor signalling in the intestinal epithelium: how bacterial recognition shapes intestinal function. *Nat. Rev. Immunol.* 10, 131–144. doi: 10.1038/nri2707

Adlerberth, I., and Wold, A. E. (2009). Establishment of the gut microbiota in Western infants. *Acta Paediatr.* 98, 229–238. doi: 10.1111/j.1651-2227.2008.01060.x

Amitay, E. L., Werner, S., Vital, M., Pieper, D. H., Hofler, D., Gierse, I. J., et al. (2017). Fusobacterium and colorectal cancer: causal factor or passenger? Results from a large colorectal cancer screening study. *Carcinogenesis* 38, 781–788. doi: 10.1093/carcin/bgx053

Arthur, J. C., and Jobin, C. (2011). The struggle within: microbial influences on colorectal cancer. *Inflamm. Bowel Dis.* 17, 396–409. doi: 10.1002/ibd.21354

Arthur, J. C., Perez-Chanona, E., Muhlbauer, M., Tomkovich, S., Uronis, J. M., Fan, T. J., et al. (2012). Intestinal inflammation targets cancer-inducing activity of the microbiota. *Science* 338, 120–123. doi: 10.1126/science.1224820

Arumugam, M., Raes, J., Pelletier, E., Le Paslier, D., Yamada, T., Mende, D. R., et al. (2011). Enterotypes of the human gut microbiome. *Nature* 473, 174–180. doi: 10.1038/nature09944

Backhed, F., Fraser, C. M., Ringel, Y., Sanders, M. E., Sartor, R. B., Sherman, P. M., et al. (2012). Defining a healthy human gut microbiome: current concepts, future directions, and clinical applications. *Cell Host Microbe* 12, 611–622. doi: 10.1016/j.chom.2012.10.012

Bank, S., Andersen, P. S., Burisch, J., Pedersen, N., Roug, S., Galsgaard, J., et al. (2015). Polymorphisms in the toll-like receptor and the IL-23/IL-17 pathways were associated with susceptibility to inflammatory bowel disease in a danish cohort. *PLoS One* 10:e0145302. doi: 10.1371/journal.pone.0145302

Bankvall, M., Sjoberg, F., Gale, G., Wold, A., Jontell, M., and Ostman, S. (2014). The oral microbiota of patients with recurrent aphthous stomatitis. *J. Oral Microbiol.* 6:25739. doi: 10.3402/Jom.V6.25739

Bartova, J., Sommerova, P., Lyuya-Mi, Y., Mysak, J., Prochazkova, J., Duskova, J., et al. (2014). Periodontitis as a risk factor of atherosclerosis. *J. Immunol. Res.* 2014:636893. doi: 10.1155/2014/636893

Blazkova, H., Krejcikova, K., Moudry, P., Frisan, T., Hodny, Z., and Bartek, J. (2010). Bacterial intoxication evokes cellular senescence with persistent DNA damage and cytokine signalling. *J. Cell Mol. Med.* 14, 357–367. doi: 10.1111/j.1582-4934.2009.00862.x

Boursi, B., Haynes, K., Mamtani, R., and Yang, Y. X. (2015). Impact of antibiotic exposure on the risk of colorectal cancer. *Pharmacoepidemiol. Drug Saf.* 24, 534–542. doi: 10.1002/pds.3765

Canabarro, A., Valle, C., Farias, M. R., Santos, F. B., Lazera, M., and Wanke, B. (2013). Association of subgingival colonization of *Candida albicans* and other yeasts with severity of chronic periodontitis. *J. Periodontal Res.* 48, 428–432. doi: 10.1111/jre.12022

Carlsson, J., Larsen, J. T., and Edlund, M. B. (1993). *Peptostreptococcus micros* has a uniquely high capacity to form hydrogen sulfide from glutathione. *Oral Microbiol. Immunol.* 8, 42–45. doi: 10.1111/j.1399-302X.1993.tb00541.x

Casarin, R. C., Saito, D., Santos, V. R., Pimentel, S. P., Duarte, P. M., Casati, M. Z., et al. (2012). Detection of *Mogibacterium timidum* in subgingival biofilm of aggressive and non-diabetic and diabetic chronic periodontitis patients. *Braz. J. Microbiol.* 43, 931–937. doi: 10.1590/S1517-838220120003000012

Castellarin, M., Warren, R. L., Freeman, J. D., Dreolini, L., Krzywinski, M., Strauss, J., et al. (2012). *Fusobacterium nucleatum* infection is prevalent in human colorectal carcinoma. *Genome Res.* 22, 299–306. doi: 10.1101/gr.1265 16.111

Chehoud, C., Albenberg, L. G., Judge, C., Hoffmann, C., Grunberg, S., Bittinger, K., et al. (2015). Fungal signature in the gut microbiota of pediatric patients with inflammatory bowel disease. *Inflamm. Bowel Dis.* 21, 1948–1956. doi: 10.1097/ MIB.0000000000000454

Chenicheri, S., Usha, R., Ramachandran, R., Thomas, V., and Wood, A. (2017). Insight into oral biofilm: primary, secondary and residual caries and phyto-challenged solutions. *Open Dent J.* 11, 312–333. doi: 10.2174/ 1874210601711010312

Claesson, R., Edlund, M. B., Persson, S., and Carlsson, J. (1990). Production of volatile sulfur compounds by various Fusobacterium species. *Oral Microbiol. Immunol.* 5, 137–142. doi: 10.1111/j.1399-302X.1990.tb00411.x

Cobb, C. M., Kelly, P. J., Williams, K. B., Babbar, S., Angolkar, M., and Derman, R. J. (2017). The oral microbiome and adverse pregnancy outcomes. *Int. J. Womens Health* 9, 551–559. doi: 10.2147/Ijwh.S142730

Costalonga, M., and Herzberg, M. C. (2014). The oral microbiome and the immunobiology of periodontal disease and caries. *Immunol. Lett.* 162, 22–38. doi: 10.1016/j.imlet.2014.08.017

da Silva, E. S., Feres, M., Figueiredo, L. C., Shibli, J. A., Ramiro, F. S., and Faveri, M. (2014). Microbiological diversity of peri-implantitis biofilm by Sanger sequencing. *Clin. Oral Implants Res.* 25, 1192–1199. doi: 10.1111/clr. 12231

Darveau, R. P., Hajishengallis, G., and Curtis, M. A. (2012). *Porphyromonas gingivalis* as a potential community activist for disease. *J. Dent. Res.* 91, 816–820. doi: 10.1177/0022034512453589

De Ruyck, K., De Boevre, M., Huybrechts, I., and De Saeger, S. (2015). Dietary mycotoxins, co-exposure, and carcinogenesis in humans: short review. *Mutat. Res. Rev. Mutat. Res.* 766, 32–41. doi: 10.1016/j.mrrev.2015.07.003

Dejea, C. M., Wick, E. C., Hechenbleikner, E. M., White, J. R., Mark Welch, J. L., Rossetti, B. J., et al. (2014). Microbiota organization is a distinct feature of proximal colorectal cancers. *Proc. Natl. Acad. Sci. U.S.A.* 111, 18321–18326. doi: 10.1073/pnas.1406199111

Diaz, P. I., Xie, Z. H., Sobue, T., Thompson, A., Biyikoglu, B., Ricker, A., et al. (2012). Synergistic interaction between *Candida albicans* and commensal oral streptococci in a novel *in vitro* mucosal model. *Infect. Immun.* 80, 620–632. doi: 10.1128/Iai.05896-11

Dupuy, A. K., David, M. S., Li, L., Heider, T. N., Peterson, J. D., Montano, E. A., et al. (2014). Redefining the human oral mycobiome with improved practices in amplicon-based taxonomy: discovery of malassezia as a prominent commensal. *PLoS One* 9:e90899. doi: 10.1371/journal.pone.0090899

Egeberg, A., Mallbris, L., Gislason, G., Hansen, P. R., and Mrowietz, U. (2017). Risk of periodontitis in patients with psoriasis and psoriatic arthritis. *J. Eur. Acad. Dermatol. Venereol.* 31, 288–293. doi: 10.1111/jdv.13814

El-Aouar, R. A., Nicolas, A., Castro, T. L. D., Deplanche, M., Azevedo, V. A. D., Goossens, P. L., et al. (2017). Heterogeneous family of cyclomodulins: smart weapons that allow bacteria to hijack the eukaryotic cell cycle and promote infections. *Front. Cell Infect. Microbiol.* 7:208. doi: 10.3389/Fcimb.2017.00364

Eley, B. M., and Cox, S. W. (2003). Proteolytic and hydrolytic enzymes from putative periodontal pathogens: characterization, molecular genetics, effects on host defenses and tissues and detection in gingival crevice fluid. *Periodontol* 31, 105–124. doi: 10.1034/j.1600-0757.2003.03107.x

Fan, X., Alekseyenko, A. V., Wu, J., Jacobs, E. J., Gapstur, S. M., Purdue, M. P., et al. (2016). Human oral microbiome and prospective risk for pancreatic cancer: a population based, nested case control study. *Cancer Res.* 76:4350. doi: 10.1158/1538-7445.AM2016-4350

Ferlay, J., Soerjomataram, I., Dikshit, R., Eser, S., Mathers, C., Rebelo, M., et al. (2015). Cancer incidence and mortality worldwide: sources, methods and major patterns in GLOBOCAN 2012. *Int. J. Cancer* 136, E359–E386. doi: 10.1002/ijc. 29210

Flanagan, L., Schmid, J., Ebert, M., Soucek, P., Kunicka, T., Liska, V., et al. (2014). *Fusobacterium nucleatum* associates with stages of colorectal neoplasia development, colorectal cancer and disease outcome. *Eur. J. Clin. Microbiol. Infect. Dis.* 33, 1381–1390. doi: 10.1007/s10096-014-2081-3

Flemer, B., Lynch, D. B., Brown, J. M., Jeffery, I. B., Ryan, F. J., Claesson, M. J., et al. (2017). Tumour-associated and non-tumour-associated microbiota in colorectal cancer. *Gut* 66, 633–643. doi: 10.1136/gutjnl-2015-309595

Ford, P. J., Gemmell, E., Chan, A., Carter, C. L., Walker, P. J., Bird, P. S., et al. (2006). Inflammation, heat shock proteins and periodontal pathogens in atherosclerosis: an immunohistologic study. *Oral Microbiol. Immunol.* 21, 206–211. doi: 10.1111/j.1399-302X.2006.00276.x

Ford, P. J., Gemmell, E., Hamlet, S. M., Hasan, A., Walker, P. J., West, M. J., et al. (2005). Cross-reactivity of GroEL antibodies with human heat shock protein 60 and quantification of pathogens in atherosclerosis. *Oral Microbiol. Immunol.* 20, 296–302. doi: 10.1111/j.1399-302X.2005.00230.x

Gagniere, J., Raisch, J., Veziant, J., Barnich, N., Bonnet, R., Buc, E., et al. (2016). Gut microbiota imbalance and colorectal cancer. *World J. Gastroenterol.* 22, 501–518. doi: 10.3748/wjg.v22.i2.501

Ghannoum, M. A., Jurevic, R. J., Mukherjee, P. K., Cui, F., Sikaroodi, M., Naqvi, A., et al. (2010). Characterization of the oral fungal microbiome (Mycobiome) in healthy individuals. *PLoS Pathog.* 6:e1000713. doi: 10.1371/journal.ppat. 1000713

Gill, S. R., Pop, M., DeBoy, R. T., Eckburg, P. B., Turnbaugh, P. J., Samuel, B. S., et al. (2006). Metagenomic analysis of the human distal gut microbiome. *Science* 312, 1355–1359. doi: 10.1126/science.1124234

Gomes, C. C., Guimarães, L. S., Pinto, L. C. C., Camargo, G. A. D. C. G., Valente, M. I. B., and Sarquis, M. I. M. (2017). Investigations of the prevalence and virulence of *Candida albicans* in periodontal and endodontic lesions in diabetic and normoglycemic patients. *J. Appl. Oral Sci.* 25, 274–281. doi: 10.1590/1678-7757-2016-0432

Greenwald, R. A., and Kirkwood, K. (1999). Adult periodontitis as a model for rheumatoid arthritis (with emphasis on treatment strategies). *J. Rheumatol.* 26, 1650–1653.

Hajishengallis, G., and Korostoff, J. M. (2017). Revisiting the page & schroeder model: the good, the bad and the unknowns in the periodontal host response 40 years later. *Periodontol* 75, 116–151. doi: 10.1111/prd.12181

Hale, V. L., Chen, J., Johnson, S., Harrington, S. C., Yab, T. C., Smyrk, T. C., et al. (2017). Shifts in the fecal microbiota associated with adenomatous polyps. *Cancer Epidemiol. Biomarkers Prev.* 26, 85–94. doi: 10.1158/1055-9965.EPI-16-0337

Han, Y. W. (2015). *Fusobacterium nucleatum*: a commensal-turned pathogen. *Curr. Opin. Microbiol.* 23, 141–147. doi: 10.1016/j.mib.2014.11.013

He, J. Z., Li, Y., Cao, Y. P., Xue, J., and Zhou, X. D. (2015). The oral microbiome diversity and its relation to human diseases. *Folia Microbiol.* 60, 69–80. doi: 10.1007/s12223-014-0342-2

Heijl, L., Wennstrom, J., Lindhe, J., and Socransky, S. S. (1980). Periodontal-disease in gnotobiotic-rats. *J. Periodontal Res.* 15, 405–419. doi: 10.1111/j.1600-0765. 1980.tb00298.x

Hoffmann, C., Dollive, S., Grunberg, S., Chen, J., Li, H., Wu, G. D., et al. (2013). Archaea and fungi of the human gut microbiome: correlations with diet and bacterial residents. *PLoS One* 8:e66019. doi: 10.1371/journal.pone.00 66019

Huffnagle, G. B., and Noverr, M. C. (2013). The emerging world of the fungal microbiome. *Trends Microbiol.* 21, 334–341. doi: 10.1016/j.tim.2013.04.002

Human Microbiome Project Consortium (2012). Structure, function and diversity of the healthy human microbiome. *Nature* 486, 207–214. doi: 10.1038/ nature11234

Huse, S. M., Ye, Y. Z., Zhou, Y. J., and Fodor, A. A. (2012). A core human microbiome as viewed through 16S rRNA sequence clusters. *PLoS One* 7:e34242. doi: 10.1371/journal.pone.0034242

Huycke, M. M., Abrams, V., and Moore, D. R. (2002). Enterococcus faecalis produces extracellular superoxide and hydrogen peroxide that damages colonic epithelial cell DNA. *Carcinogenesis* 23, 529–536. doi: 10.1093/carcin/23.3.529

Inaba, H., Sugita, H., Kuboniwa, M., Iwai, S., Hamada, M., Noda, T., et al. (2013). *Porphyromonas gingivalis* promotes invasion of oral squamous cell carcinoma through induction of proMMP9 and its activation. *Cell Microbiol.* 16, 131–145. doi: 10.1111/cmi.12211

Ivanyi, L., Newman, H. N., and Marsh, P. D. (1991). T-cell proliferative responses to molecular fractions of periodontopathic bacteria. *Clin. Exp. Immunol.* 83, 108–111. doi: 10.1111/j.1365-2249.1991.tb05597.x

Johansson, M. E., Larsson, J. M., and Hansson, G. C. (2011). The two mucus layers of colon are organized by the MUC2 mucin, whereas the outer layer is a legislator of host-microbial interactions. *Proc. Natl. Acad. Sci. U.S.A.* 108, 4659–4665. doi: 10.1073/pnas.1006451107

Johansson, M. E., Sjovall, H., and Hansson, G. C. (2013). The gastrointestinal mucus system in health and disease. *Nat. Rev. Gastroenterol. Hepatol.* 10, 352–361. doi: 10.1038/nrgastro.2013.35

Johnson, C. H., Dejea, C. M., Edler, D., Hoang, L. T., Santidrian, A. F., Felding, B. H., et al. (2015). Metabolism links bacterial biofilms and colon carcinogenesis. *Cell Metab.* 21, 891–897. doi: 10.1016/j.cmet.2015.04.011

Kadowaki, T., Nakayama, K., Okamoto, K., Abe, N., Baba, A., Shi, Y. X., et al. (2000). *Porphyromonas gingivalis* proteinases as virulence determinants in progression of periodontal diseases. *J. Biochem.* 128, 153–159. doi: 10.1093/oxfordjournals.jbchem.a022735

Kaiko, G. E., Ryu, S. H., Koues, O. I., Collins, P. L., Solnica-Krezel, L., Pearce, E. J., et al. (2016). The colonic crypt protects stem cells from microbiota-derived metabolites. *Cell* 165, 1708–1720. doi: 10.1016/j.cell.2016.10.034

Kasser, U. R., Gleissner, C., Dehne, F., Michel, A., Willershausen-Zonnchen, B., and Bolten, W. W. (1997). Risk for periodontal disease in patients with longstanding rheumatoid arthritis. *Arthritis Rheum.* 40, 2248–2251. doi: 10.1002/art.1780401221

Khan, S. H., Aguirre, A., and Bobek, L. A. (1998). In-situ hybridization localized MUC7 mucin gene expression to the mucous acinar cells of human and MUC7-transgenic mouse salivary glands. *Glycoconj. J.* 15, 1125–1132. doi: 10.1023/A:1006955604501

Kilian, M., Mestecky, J., and Russell, M. W. (1988). Defense mechanisms involving Fc-dependent functions of immunoglobulin A and their subversion by bacterial immunoglobulin A proteases. *Microbiol. Rev.* 52, 296–303.

Kilian, M., Reinholdt, J., Nyvad, B., Frandsen, E. V., and Mikkelsen, L. (1989). IgA1 proteases of oral streptococci: ecological aspects. *Immunol. Invest.* 18, 161–170. doi: 10.3109/08820138909112235

Kim, Y. J., Choi, Y. S., Baek, K. J., Yoon, S. H., Park, H. K., and Choi, Y. (2016). Mucosal and salivary microbiota associated with recurrent aphthous stomatitis. *BMC Microbiol.* 16:57. doi: 10.1186/s12866-016-0673-z

Kinane, D. F., Stathopoulou, P. G., and Papapanou, P. N. (2017). Periodontal diseases. *Nat. Rev. Dis. Primers* 3:17038. doi: 10.1038/Nrdp.2017.38

Klimesova, K., Kverka, M., Zakostelska, Z., Hudcovic, T., Hrncir, T., Stepankova, R., et al. (2013). Altered gut microbiota promotes colitis-associated cancer in IL-1 receptor-associated kinase M-deficient mice. *Inflamm. Bowel Dis.* 19, 1266–1277. doi: 10.1097/MIB.0b013e318281330a

Kostic, A. D., Chun, E. Y., Robertson, L., Glickman, J. N., Gallini, C. A., Michaud, M., et al. (2013). *Fusobacterium nucleatum* potentiates intestinal tumorigenesis and modulates the tumor-immune microenvironment. *Cell Host Microbe* 14, 207–215. doi: 10.1016/j.chom.2013.07.007

Kostic, A. D., Gevers, D., Pedamallu, C. S., Michaud, M., Duke, F., Earl, A. M., et al. (2012). Genomic analysis identifies association of Fusobacterium with colorectal carcinoma. *Genome Res.* 22, 292–298. doi: 10.1101/gr.126573.111

Li, S., Konstantinov, S. R., Smits, R., and Peppelenbosch, M. P. (2017). Bacterial biofilms in colorectal cancer initiation and progression. *Trends Mol. Med.* 23, 18–30. doi: 10.1016/j.molmed.2016.11.004

Liang, Q., Chiu, J., Chen, Y., Huang, Y., Higashimori, A., Fang, J., et al. (2017). Fecal bacteria act as novel biomarkers for noninvasive diagnosis of colorectal cancer. *Clin. Cancer Res.* 23, 2061–2070. doi: 10.1158/1078-0432.CCR-16-1599

Liguori, G., Lamas, B., Richard, M. L., Brandi, G., da Costa, G., Hoffmann, T. W., et al. (2016). Fungal dysbiosis in mucosa-associated microbiota of crohn's disease patients. *J. Crohns Colitis* 10, 296–305. doi: 10.1093/ecco-jcc/jjv209

Louis, P., Young, P., Holtrop, G., and Flint, H. J. (2010). Diversity of human colonic butyrate-producing bacteria revealed by analysis of the butyryl-CoA: acetate CoA-transferase gene. *Environ. Microbiol.* 12, 304–314. doi: 10.1111/j.1462-2920.2009.02066.x

Lu, Y., Chen, J., Zheng, J., Hu, G., Wang, J., Huang, C., et al. (2016). Mucosal adherent bacterial dysbiosis in patients with colorectal adenomas. *Sci. Rep.* 6:26337. doi: 10.1038/srep26337

Luan, C., Xie, L., Yang, X., Miao, H., Lv, N., Zhang, R., et al. (2015). Dysbiosis of fungal microbiota in the intestinal mucosa of patients with colorectal adenomas. *Sci. Rep.* 5:7980. doi: 10.1038/srep07980

Macfarlane, G. T., and Macfarlane, S. (2012). Bacteria, colonic fermentation, and gastrointestinal health. *J. AOAC Int.* 95, 50–60. doi: 10.5740/jaoacint.SGE_Macfarlane

Maffei, V. J., Kim, S., Blanchard, E., Luo, M., Jazwinski, S. M., Taylor, C. M., et al. (2017). Biological aging and the human gut microbiota. *J. Gerontol. A Biol. Sci. Med. Sci.* 72, 1474–1482. doi: 10.1093/gerona/glx042

Mager, D. L., Ximenez-Fyvie, L. A., Haffajee, A. D., and Socransky, S. S. (2003). Distribution of selected bacterial species on intraoral surfaces. *J. Clin. Periodontol.* 30, 644–654. doi: 10.1034/j.1600-051X.2003.00376.x

Mao, S., Park, Y., Hasegawa, Y., Tribble, G. D., James, C. E., Handfield, M., et al. (2007). Intrinsic apoptotic pathways of gingival epithelial cells modulated by *Porphyromonas gingivalis*. *Cell Microbiol.* 9, 1997–2007. doi: 10.1111/j.1462-5822.2007.00931.x

Marchesan, J., Jiao, Y., Schaff, R. A., Hao, J., Morelli, T., Kinney, J. S., et al. (2016). TLR4, NOD1 and NOD2 mediate immune recognition of putative newly identified periodontal pathogens. *Mol. Oral Microbiol.* 31, 243–258. doi: 10.1111/omi.12116

Marcotte, H., and Lavoie, M. C. (1998). Oral microbial ecology and the role of salivary immunoglobulin A. *Microbiol. Mol. Biol. Rev.* 62, 71–109.

Maresca, M., and Fantini, J. (2010). Some food-associated mycotoxins as potential risk factors in humans predisposed to chronic intestinal inflammatory diseases. *Toxicon* 56, 282–294. doi: 10.1016/j.toxicon.2010.04.016

Mehta, R. S., Nishihara, R., Cao, Y., Song, M., Mima, K., Qian, Z. R., et al. (2017). Association of dietary patterns with risk of colorectal cancer subtypes classified by *Fusobacterium nucleatum* in tumor tissue. *JAMA Oncol.* 3, 921–927. doi: 10.1001/jamaoncol.2016.6374

Miraglia, A. G., Travaglione, S., Meschini, S., Falzano, L., Matarrese, P., Quaranta, M. G., et al. (2007). Cytotoxic necrotizing factor 1 prevents apoptosis via the Akt/IkappaB kinase pathway: role of nuclear factor-kappaB and Bcl-2. *Mol. Biol. Cell* 18, 2735–2744. doi: 10.1091/mbc.E06-10-0910

Momen-Heravi, F., Babic, A., Tworoger, S. S., Zhang, L., Wu, K., Smith-Warner, S. A., et al. (2017). Periodontal disease, tooth loss and colorectal cancer risk: results from the Nurses' Health Study. *Int. J. Cancer* 140, 646–652. doi: 10.1002/ijc.30486

Mukherjee, P. K., Chandra, J., Retuerto, M., Sikaroodi, M., Brown, R. E., Jurevic, R., et al. (2014). Oral mycobiome analysis of HIV-infected patients: identification of Pichia as an antagonist of opportunistic fungi. *PLoS Pathog.* 10:e1003996. doi: 10.1371/journal.ppat.1003996

Nagano, Y., Elborn, J. S., Miller, B. C., Walker, J. M., Goldsmith, C. E., Rendall, J., et al. (2010). Comparison of techniques to examine the diversity of fungi in adult patients with cystic fibrosis. *Med. Mycol.* 48, 166–176. doi: 10.3109/13693780903127506

Nakatsu, G., Li, X. C., Zhou, H. K., Sheng, J. Q., Wong, S. H., Wu, W. K. K., et al. (2015). Gut mucosal microbiome across stages of colorectal carcinogenesis. *Nat. Commun.* 6:8727. doi: 10.1038/Ncomms9727

Nordman, H., Davies, J. R., Lindell, G., de Bolos, C., Real, F., and Carlstedt, I. (2002). Gastric MUC5AC and MUC6 are large oligomeric mucins that differ in size, glycosylation and tissue distribution. *Biochem. J.* 364, 191–200. doi: 10.1042/bj3640191

Nougayrede, J. P., Homburg, S., Taieb, F., Boury, M., Brzuszkiewicz, E., Gottschalk, G., et al. (2006). *Escherichia coli* induces DNA double-strand breaks in eukaryotic cells. *Science* 313, 848–851. doi: 10.1126/science.1127059

Papadopoulos, G., Weinberg, E. O., Massari, P., Gibson, F. C. III, Wetzler, L. M., Morgan, E. F., et al. (2013). Macrophage-specific TLR2 signaling mediates pathogen-induced TNF-dependent inflammatory oral bone loss. *J. Immunol.* 190, 1148–1157. doi: 10.4049/jimmunol.1202511

Park, H. E., Kim, J. H., Cho, N. Y., Lee, H. S., and Kang, G. H. (2017). Intratumoral *Fusobacterium nucleatum* abundance correlates with macrophage infiltration and CDKN2A methylation in microsatellite-unstable colorectal carcinoma. *Virchows Arch.* 471, 329–336. doi: 10.1007/s00428-017-2171-6

Persson, S., Edlund, M. B., Claesson, R., and Carlsson, J. (1990). The formation of hydrogen sulfide and methyl mercaptan by oral bacteria. *Oral Microbiol. Immunol.* 5, 195–201. doi: 10.1111/j.1399-302X.1990.tb00645.x

Peters, B. A., Dominianni, C., Shapiro, J. A., Church, T. R., Wu, J., Miller, G., et al. (2016). The gut microbiota in conventional and serrated precursors of colorectal cancer. *Microbiome* 4:69. doi: 10.1186/s40168-016-0218-6

Peters, B. A., Wu, J., Hayes, R. B., and Ahn, J. (2017). The oral fungal mycobiome: characteristics and relation to periodontitis in a pilot study. *BMC Microbiol.* 17:157. doi: 10.1186/s12866-017-1064-9

Pitts, N. B., Zero, D. T., Marsh, P. D., Ekstrand, K., Weintraub, J. A., Ramos-Gomez, F., et al. (2017). Dental caries. *Nat. Rev. Dis. Primers* 3:17030. doi: 10.1038/nrdp.2017.30

Potempa, J., Sroka, A., Imamura, T., and Travis, J. (2003). Gingipains, the major cysteine proteinases and virulence factors of *Porphyromonas gingivalis*: structure, function and assembly of multidomain protein complexes. *Curr. Protein Pept. Sci.* 4, 397–407. doi: 10.2174/1389203033487036

Potgieter, M., Bester, J., Kell, D. B., and Pretorius, E. (2015). The dormant blood microbiome in chronic, inflammatory diseases. *FEMS Microbiol. Rev.* 39, 567–591. doi: 10.1093/femsre/fuv013

Proctor, D. M., and Relman, D. A. (2017). The landscape ecology and microbiota of the human nose, mouth, and throat. *Cell Host Microbe* 21, 421–432. doi: 10.1016/j.chom.2017.03.011

Qin, J., Li, R., Raes, J., Arumugam, M., Burgdorf, K. S., Manichanh, C., et al. (2010). A human gut microbial gene catalogue established by metagenomic sequencing. *Nature* 464, 59–65. doi: 10.1038/nature08821

Raisch, J., Buc, E., Bonnet, M., Sauvanet, P., Vazeille, E., de Vallee, A., et al. (2014). Colon cancer-associated B2 *Escherichia coli* colonize gut mucosa and promote cell proliferation. *World J. Gastroenterol.* 20, 6560–6572. doi: 10.3748/wjg.v20.i21.6560

Reddy, B. S., Narisawa, T., Maronpot, R., Weisburger, J. H., and Wynder, E. L. (1975). Animal models for the study of dietary factors and cancer of the large bowel. *Cancer Res.* 35, 3421–3426.

Roberts, F. A., and Darveau, R. P. (2015). Microbial protection and virulence in periodontal tissue as a function of polymicrobial communities: symbiosis and dysbiosis. *Periodontol* 69, 18–27. doi: 10.1111/prd.12087

Robinson, C. J., Bohannan, B. J. M., and Young, V. B. (2010). From structure to function: the ecology of host-associated microbial communities. *Microbiol. Mol. Biol. R* 74, 453–476. doi: 10.1128/Mmbr.00014-10

Rubinstein, M. R., Wang, X., Liu, W., Hao, Y., Cai, G., and Han, Y. W. (2013). *Fusobacterium nucleatum* promotes colorectal carcinogenesis by modulating E-cadherin/beta-catenin signaling via its FadA adhesin. *Cell Host Microbe* 14, 195–206. doi: 10.1016/j.chom.2013.07.012

Sartor, R. B. (2008). Microbial influences in inflammatory bowel diseases. *Gastroenterology* 134, 577–594. doi: 10.1053/j.gastro.2007.11.059

Saunders, C. W., Scheynius, A., and Heitman, J. (2012). Malassezia fungi are specialized to live on skin and associated with dandruff, eczema, and other skin diseases. *PLoS Pathog.* 8:e1002701. doi: 10.1371/journal.ppat.1002701

Segata, N., Haake, S. K., Mannon, P., Lemon, K. P., Waldron, L., Gevers, D., et al. (2012). Composition of the adult digestive tract bacterial microbiome based on seven mouth surfaces, tonsils, throat and stool samples. *Genome Biol.* 13:R42. doi: 10.1186/gb-2012-13-6-r42

Shen, X. J., Rawls, J. F., Randall, T., Burcal, L., Mpande, C. N., Jenkins, N., et al. (2010). Molecular characterization of mucosal adherent bacteria and associations with colorectal adenomas. *Gut Microbes* 1, 138–147. doi: 10.4161/gmic.1.3.12360

Slots, J. (1976). Predominant cultivable organisms in juvenile periodontitis. *Scand. J. Dent. Res.* 84, 1–10. doi: 10.1111/j.1600-0722.1976.tb00454.x

Socransky, S. S., and Haffajee, A. D. (2002). Dental biofilms: difficult therapeutic targets. *Periodontol* 28, 12–55. doi: 10.1034/j.1600-0757.2002.280102.x

Socransky, S. S., and Haffajee, A. D. (2005). Periodontal microbial ecology. *Periodontol* 38, 135–187. doi: 10.1111/j.1600-0757.2005.00107.x

Socransky, S. S., Haffajee, A. D., Cugini, M. A., Smith, C., and Kent, R. L. (1998). Microbial complexes in subgingival plaque. *J. Clin. Periodontol.* 25, 134–144. doi: 10.1111/j.1600-051X.1998.tb02419.x

Sokol, H., Leducq, V., Aschard, H., Pham, H. P., Jegou, S., Landman, C., et al. (2017). Fungal microbiota dysbiosis in IBD. *Gut* 66, 1039–1048. doi: 10.1136/gutjnl-2015-310746

Sousa, E. L., Martinho, F. C., Leite, F. R., Nascimento, G. G., and Gomes, B. P. (2014). Macrophage cell activation with acute apical abscess contents determined by interleukin-1 Beta and tumor necrosis factor alpha production. *J. Endod.* 40, 1752–1757. doi: 10.1016/j.joen.2014.06.019

Stecher, B., and Hardt, W. D. (2011). Mechanisms controlling pathogen colonization of the gut. *Curr. Opin. Microbiol.* 14, 82–91. doi: 10.1016/j.mib.2010.10.003

Swidsinski, A., Khilkin, M., Kerjaschki, D., Schreiber, S., Ortner, M., Weber, J., et al. (1998). Association between intraepithelial *Escherichia coli* and colorectal cancer. *Gastroenterology* 115, 281–286. doi: 10.1016/S0016-5085(98)70194-5

Taieb, F., Nougayrede, J. P., Watrin, C., Samba-Louaka, A., and Oswald, E. (2006). *Escherichia coli* cyclomodulin Cif induces G2 arrest of the host cell cycle without activation of the DNA-damage checkpoint-signalling pathway. *Cell Microbiol.* 8, 1910–1921. doi: 10.1111/j.1462-5822.2006.00757.x

Teles, R., Teles, F., Frias-Lopez, J., Paster, B., and Haffajee, A. (2013). Lessons learned and unlearned in periodontal microbiology. *Periodontol* 62, 95–162. doi: 10.1111/prd.12010

Temoin, S., Chakaki, A., Askari, A., El-Halaby, A., Fitzgerald, S., Marcus, R. E., et al. (2012). Identification of oral bacterial DNA in synovial fluid of patients with arthritis with native and failed prosthetic joints. *J. Clin. Rheumatol.* 18, 117–121. doi: 10.1097/RHU.0b013e3182500c95

Tjalsma, H., Boleij, A., Marchesi, J. R., and Dutilh, B. E. (2012). A bacterial driver-passenger model for colorectal cancer: beyond the usual suspects. *Nat. Rev. Microbiol.* 10, 575–582. doi: 10.1038/nrmicro2819

Tlaskalova-Hogenova, H., Stepankova, R., Hudcovic, T., Tuckova, L., Cukrowska, B., Lodinova-Zadnikova, R., et al. (2004). Commensal bacteria (normal microflora), mucosal immunity and chronic inflammatory and autoimmune diseases. *Immunol. Lett.* 93, 97–108. doi: 10.1016/j.imlet.2004.02.005

Tlaskalova-Hogenova, H., Vannucci, L., Klimesova, K., Stepankova, R., Krizan, J., and Kverka, M. (2014). Microbiome and colorectal carcinoma: insights from germ-free and conventional animal models. *Cancer J.* 20, 217–224. doi: 10.1097/PPO.0000000000000052

Tomas, I., Diz, P., Tobias, A., Scully, C., and Donos, N. (2012). Periodontal health status and bacteraemia from daily oral activities: systematic review/meta-analysis. *J. Clin. Periodontol.* 39, 213–228. doi: 10.1111/j.1600-051X.2011.01784.x

Toprak, N. U., Yagci, A., Gulluoglu, B. M., Akin, M. L., Demirkalem, P., Celenk, T., et al. (2006). A possible role of *Bacteroides fragilis* enterotoxin in the aetiology of colorectal cancer. *Clin. Microbiol. Infect.* 12, 782–786. doi: 10.1111/j.1469-0691.2006.01494.x

Trojanowska, D., Zwolinska-Wcislo, M., Tokarczyk, M., Kosowski, K., Mach, T., and Budak, A. (2010). The role of Candida in inflammatory bowel disease. Estimation of transmission of *C. albicans* fungi in gastrointestinal tract based on genetic affinity between strains. *Med. Sci. Monit.* 16, Cr451–Cr457.

Tsoi, H., Chu, E. S. H., Zhang, X., Sheng, J., Nakatsu, G., Ng, S. C., et al. (2017). *Peptostreptococcus anaerobius* induces intracellular cholesterol biosynthesis in colon cells to induce proliferation and causes dysplasia in mice. *Gastroenterology* 152, 1419–1433. doi: 10.1053/j.gastro.2017.01.009

Underhill, D. M., and Iliev, I. D. (2014). The mycobiota: interactions between commensal fungi and the host immune system. *Nat. Rev. Immunol.* 14, 405–416. doi: 10.1038/nri3684

Ungprasert, P., Wijarnpreecha, K., and Wetter, D. A. (2017). Periodontitis and risk of psoriasis: a systematic review and meta-analysis. *J. Eur. Acad. Dermatol. Venereol.* 31, 857–862. doi: 10.1111/jdv.14051

Urzúa, B., Hermosilla, G., Gamonal, J., Morales-Bozo, I., Canals, M., Barahona, S., et al. (2008). Yeast diversity in the oral microbiota of subjects with periodontitis: *Candida albicans* and *Candida dubliniensis* colonize the periodontal pockets. *Med. Mycol.* 46, 783–793. doi: 10.1080/13693780802060899

Vannucci, L., Stepankova, R., Kozakova, H., Fiserova, A., Rossmann, P., and Tlaskalova-Hogenova, H. (2008). Colorectal carcinogenesis in germ-free and conventionally reared rats: different intestinal environments affect the systemic immunity. *Int. J. Oncol.* 32, 609–617. doi: 10.3892/ijo.32.3.609

Wade, W. G. (2013). The oral microbiome in health and disease. *Pharmacol. Res.* 69, 137–143. doi: 10.1016/j.phrs.2012.11.006

Walker, A. W., Ince, J., Duncan, S. H., Webster, L. M., Holtrop, G., Ze, X., et al. (2011). Dominant and diet-responsive groups of bacteria within the human colonic microbiota. *ISME J.* 5, 220–230. doi: 10.1038/ismej.2010.118

Wickstrom, C., Davies, J. R., Eriksen, G. V., Veerman, E. C., and Carlstedt, I. (1998). MUC5B is a major gel-forming, oligomeric mucin from human salivary gland, respiratory tract and endocervix: identification of glycoforms and C-terminal cleavage. *Biochem. J.* 334(Pt 3), 685–693. doi: 10.1042/bj3340685

Wong, B. K., McGregor, N. R., Butt, H. L., Knight, R., Liu, L. Y., and Darby, I. B. (2016). Association of clinical parameters with periodontal bacterial haemolytic activity. *J. Clin. Periodontol.* 43, 503–511. doi: 10.1111/jcpe.12554

Wu, G. D., Chen, J., Hoffmann, C., Bittinger, K., Chen, Y. Y., Keilbaugh, S. A., et al. (2011). Linking long-term dietary patterns with gut microbial enterotypes. *Science* 334, 105–108. doi: 10.1126/science.1208344

Yamaoka, Y., Suehiro, Y., Hashimoto, S., Hoshida, T., Fujimoto, M., Watanabe, M., et al. (2017). *Fusobacterium nucleatum* as a prognostic marker of colorectal cancer in a Japanese population. *J. Gastroenterol.* 53, 517–524. doi: 10.1007/s00535-017-1382-6

Yu, T. C., Guo, F. F., Yu, Y. N., Sun, T. T., Ma, D., Han, J. X., et al. (2017). *Fusobacterium nucleatum* promotes chemoresistance to colorectal cancer by modulating autophagy. *Cell* 170, 548–563. doi: 10.1016/j.cell.2017.07.008 e16, doi: 10.1016/j.cell.2017.07.008

Zanzoni, A., Spinelli, L., Braham, S., and Brun, C. (2017). Perturbed human sub-networks by *Fusobacterium nucleatum* candidate virulence proteins. *Microbiome* 5:89. doi: 10.1186/s40168-017-0307-1

Zhou, Y. J., Gao, H. Y., Mihindukulasuriya, K. A., La Rosa, P. S., Wylie, K. M., Vishnivetskaya, T., et al. (2013). Biogeography of the ecosystems of the healthy human body. *Genome Biol.* 14:R1. doi: 10.1186/Gb-2013-14-1-R1

16

Reduced Mass and Diversity of the Colonic Microbiome in Patients with Multiple Sclerosis and their Improvement with Ketogenic Diet

Alexander Swidsinski [1,2], Yvonne Dörffel [3], Vera Loening-Baucke [1], Christoph Gille [1], Önder Göktas [1], Anne Reißhauer [1], Jürgen Neuhaus [4], Karsten-Henrich Weylandt [5], Alexander Guschin [6] and Markus Bock [7]*

[1] *Laboratory for Molecular Genetics, Polymicrobial Infections and Biofilms, Section of Gastroenterology and Hepatology, Department of Medicine, Charité Universitätsmedizin Berlin, Berlin, Germany,* [2] *Institute of Molecular Medicine, Sechenov First Moscow State Medical University, Moscow, Russia,* [3] *Outpatient Clinic, Charité Universitätsmedizin Berlin, Berlin, Germany,* [4] *Faculty of Veterinary Medicine, Centre for Infectious Diseases, University of Leipzig, Leipzig, Germany,* [5] *Charité Universitätsmedizin Berlin, Campus Virchow, Gastroenterology Berlin, Berlin, Germany,* [6] *Laboratory of Molecular Diagnostics, Russian Research Center for Molecular Diagnostics and Therapy, Central Research Institute, Moscow, Russia,* [7] *Experimental and Clinical Research Center, A Joint Cooperation between the Charité Medical Faculty and the Max-Delbrueck Center for Molecular Medicine, Berlin, Germany*

***Correspondence:**
Alexander Swidsinski
alexander.swidsinski@charite.de

Background: Colonic microbiome is thought to be involved in auto-immune multiple sclerosis (MS). Interactions between diet and the colonic microbiome in MS are unknown.

Methods: We compared the composition of the colonic microbiota quantitatively in 25 MS patients and 14 healthy controls.Fluorescence in situ hybridization (FISH) with 162 ribosomal RNA derived bacterial FISH probes was used. Ten of the MS patients received a ketogenic diet for 6 months. Changes in concentrations of 35 numerically substantial bacterial groups were monitored at baseline and at 2, 12, and 23/24 weeks.

Results: No MS typical microbiome pattern was apparent.The total concentrations and diversity of substantial bacterial groups were reduced in MS patients ($P < 0.001$). Bacterial groups detected with EREC (mainly *Roseburia*), Bac303 (*Bacteroides*), and Fprau (*Faecalibacterium prausnitzii*) probes were diminished the most. The individual changes were multidirectional and inconsistent. The effects of a ketogenic diet were biphasic. In the short term, bacterial concentrations and diversity were further reduced. They started to recover at week 12 and exceeded significantly the baseline values after 23–24 weeks on the ketogenic diet.

Conclusions: Colonic biofermentative function is markedly impaired in MS patients.The ketogenic diet normalized concentrations of the colonic microbiome after 6 months.

Keywords: FISH, colonic microbiota, multiple sclerosis, biofermentation, ketogenic diet

INTRODUCTION

There is a growing awareness of the significance of the human microbiome in health and disease. Microbial colonization of the skin and epithelial surfaces protects from pathogens. The biofermentation in the colon delivers energy from digestive leftovers and synthesizes a broad spectrum of vitamins and hormone-like substances, which regulate metabolism and neuronal activity (Galland, 2014). The enormous variety of the healthy microbiome conveys antigenic diversity to the host shaping its immunity and autoimmunity (Berer and Krishnamoorthy, 2014).

An ever growing number of studies demonstrates the involvement of the colonic microbiome in obesity, digestive, endocrine, inflammatory, and auto-immune disorders including multiple sclerosis (MS) (Berer and Krishnamoorthy, 2014; Galland, 2014; Glenn and Mowry, 2016).

Topics, methods and results of these studies are well presented and should not be repeated here. However, the previous studies of the colonic microbiome in MS were restricted to identification of microbial patterns associated with disease (Miyake et al., 2015; Jangi et al., 2016; Tremlett et al., 2016). We found no literature on the quantitative evaluation of the colonic microbiome in MS patients. Microbial concentrations, however, are an important feature, which directly measures their functional contribution to colonic fermentation. The aim of this study was to compare the concentrations of different microbial groups in MS patients and healthy controls and to follow up changes in the colonic microbiome taking place during ketogenic diet.

The option of ketogenic diet was important for the following reasons: as long as complex microbiomes cannot be reliably transferred, maintained and tested *in vitro*, all data raised *in vivo* must remain observational. Therefore, interventions simultaneously affecting the microbiome and disease are necessary to unravel possible causality.

Ketogenic diet influences brain function, inflammation, immunity and the colonic microbiome. It is increasingly applied in clinical studies (Piccio et al., 2008; Kim et al., 2012; Choi et al., 2016). Different to fasting or mono-diets, ketogenic diet can be maintained over months and is well tolerated. Diet prescriptions are often circumvented in real life. The compliance of the ketogenic diet can be reliably verified through measurement of ketone bodies in blood and urine and cannot be falsified.

MATERIALS AND METHODS

Patients/Samples

Fourteen healthy volunteers from the Laboratories of Centre for Infectious Diseases, Faculty of Veterinary Medicine, University of Leipzig and 25 patients with relapsing-remitting multiple sclerosis cared for at the Charité hospital were investigated for the composition of their colonic microbiome using fluorescence *in situ* hybridization ribosomal RNA based FISH probes available in public resources (Loy et al., 2016).

The study was reviewed and approved by institutional review board: Ethikkomission Ethikausschuss 1 an Campus Charite Mitte EA1/130/07.

After the baseline investigation, MS patients received a ketogenic diet for 6 months. The ketogenic diet was designed (1) to achieve a modest ketosis ($\geq$500 μmol/L ß-hydroxybutyrate) in the blood, self-measured after dinner twice a week (FreeStyle Precision, Abbott Diabetes Care Ltd.), (2) to achieve a modest ketosis ($\geq$500 μmol/L acetoacetate) in the urine, self-measured after dinner once a week (Ketostix, Bayer Consumer Care AG), and (3) to maintain compliance. Patients received a booklet with meal suggestions over 28 balanced days and were encouraged to ingest fat. An average daily intake of $<$50 g carbohydrates, $>$160 g fat, and $<$100 g protein was recommended. Patients received detailed information about nutritional facts, glycemic load and learned how to handle carbohydrates by an experienced nutritional coach during group based workshops on 3 weekends.

Ten of the MS patients who were recruited for the ketogenic diet were randomly selected for accompanying microbiome investigations. Stools samples were collected at baseline, week 2, 12, and after 6 months (week 23–25). The evaluation of the clinical effects on MS was not performed because of the low number of patients.

None of the enclosed probands received antibiotics or probiotics in the last 6 month preceding the study.

Fish

Colonic microbiota were investigated using FISH with ribosomal RNA derived probes. Hybridizations were performed on sections of Carnoy fixated, paraffin embedded and otherwise not manipulated stool cylinders (Swidsinski et al., 2010). Four micrometers thick sections were placed on SuperFrost plus slides.

A Nikon e600 fluorescence microscope was used. The images were photo-documented with a Nikon DXM 1200F color camera and software (Nikon, Tokyo, Japan).

Bacterial concentrations of homogeneous populations were enumerated visually in one of the 10 × 10 fields of the ocular raster corresponding to 10 × 10 μm of the section surface at magnification of 1,000. This number was assigned to a concentration of × 10^9 bacteria/ml, which was most equivalent to the calculation formula, that we had used previously (Swidsinski et al., 2010).

In case of uneven distribution of bacteria over the microscopic field, the positive signals were enumerated in 10 fields of the ocular raster along the gradient of distribution and divided by 10.

Bacteria were quantified using group specific C3 probes. The FITC marked universal probe was used in each hybridization to evaluate the number of all bacteria, C5 marked probes with a different specificity to C3 probes were used to determine the spatial relation of different bacterial groups to each other.

Only signals that hybridized with a specific FISH probe and the universal FISH probe, but did not hybridize with specific FISH probes from unrelated bacterial groups, were enumerated (Swidsinski, 2006).

FISH Probes

One hundred sixty-two bacterial FISH probes available from public resources were applied for the comparative analysis of the colonic microbiome in healthy controls and MS patients (**Tables 1A,B**). The names of the FISH probes are listed according to abbreviations of the probeBase resource (http://probebase.csb.univie.ac.at/node/8) (Loy et al., 2016) and the details to FISH probe specificity and hybridization conditions are given. The Fprau probe is described in reference (Suau et al., 2001).

Probes in **Table 1** are alphabetically ordered to subgroups according to abundancy and specificity as described in the result section.

TABLE 1 | Applied FISH-probes.

Part A
Substantial groups
Essential (*N* = 3)
Erec482 (*Eubacterium rectale, Clostridium coccoides* group)
Bac303 (most *Bacteroidaceae*)
Fprau (*Faecalibacterium prausnitzii*)
Individual pioneer (*N* = 4)
Bif153 Genus *Bifidobacterium*
Cdif198 *Clostridium difficile*
Clit135 *Clostridium lituseburense* group including *C. difficile*
Ebac1790 *Enterobacteriaceae*
Individual substantial (*N* = 28)
ACI623 *Acidaminococcaceae* sp. (not the Selenomonas species)
AKK406 *Akkermansia*
Ato291 *Atopobium* cluster
Bbif186 *B. bifidum*
Blon1004 *B. longum*
Bputre698 *Bacteroides putredinis*
Burkho Burkholderia spp.
Ceut705 *C. eutactus*, *Coprococcus* sp.
Chis150 *Clostridium histolyticum*
Cor653 *Coriobacterium* group
Cvir1414 *Clostridium viride* group
Ecyl387 *Eubacterium cylindroides*
Ehal1469 *Eubacterium hallii*
Eram997 *Eubacterium ramulus*
Lab158 *Lactobacillus* sp., *Enterococcus* sp.
Muc1437 *Akkermansia muciniphila*
Myc657 *Mycobacterium* subdivision (mycolic acid-containing *actinomycetes*)
Phasco741 *Phascolarctobacterium faecium*
Pnig657 *Prevotella nigrescens*
ProCo1264 *Ruminococcus productus*
Rbro730 *Clostridium sporosphaeroides*, *Ruminococcus bromii*, *Clostridium leptum*
Rfla729 *Ruminococcus albus*
SFB1 Segmented filamentous bacteria
SNA *Sphaerotilus natans*
Strc493 most *Streptococcus* spp.
SUBU1237 *Burkholderia* spp., *Sutterella* spp.
Urobe63a *Ruminococcus obeum*-like
Veil 223 *Veillonella*
Ver620 *Verrucomicrobium*
Part B
Includes probes with extremely low occurrence and concentrations and probes with uncharacteristic signals:
Accidental groups (*N* = 88)
To low in occurrence and concentrations for statistical analysis
MIB661 mouse intestinal bacteria
AER66 *Aeromonas* spp.
Alac1438 *Anaerococcus lactolyticus*
ARC1430 *Arcobacter*
Avag1280 *Anaerococcus vaginalis*
Bbrel198 *B. breve*
Bden82 *B. dentium*
BFV530 *Bacteroides forsythus*
Bif1278 *Bifidobacterium* spp.
Burcep *Burkholderia cepacia*
CAP365 *Capnoytophaga* sp.
Capno *Capnocytophaga sputigena*
Cj490 *Campylobacter jejuni*
CLOBU1022 *Clostridium butyricum*,
Cperf 191 *Clostridium perfringens*
Cra757 *Clostridium ramosum* assemblage
Csac67 *Clostridium saccharogumia*
CST440 Group 1 clones closely related to *Clostridium stercorarium*
DSV1292 some *Desulfovibrio* and *Bilophila wadsworthia*
DSV687 most *Desulfovibrionales*
E.bar1237 *Eubacterium barkeri*
E.bif462 *Eubacterium biforme*
E.con1122 *Eubacterium contortum*
E.cyl461 *Eubacterium cylindroides*
E.cyl466 *Eubacterium cylindroides*
E.dol183 *Eubacterium dolichum*
E.had579 *Eubacterium hadrum*
E.len194 *Eubacterium lentum*
E.lim1433 *Eubacterium limosum*
E.mon84 *Eubacterium moniliforme*
E.mul *Eubacterium multiforme*
E.sab *Eubacterium saburreum*
E.ven66 *Eubacterium ventriosum*
Enfl84 *Enterococcus faecalis*
Enfm 93 *Enterococcus faecium*
Fnec996 *Fusobacterium necrophorum*
Fnuc133 *Fusobacterium nucleatum*
GAN1237 *Helicobacter ganmani*
Haeinf *Haemophilus influenzae*
HEP642 *Helicobacter hepaticus*
Hpy-1 *Helicobacter pylori*
Hyo1210 *Brachyspira hyodysenteriae*
Lbuc668 *Leptotrichia buccalis*
Lis1255 Genera Listeria, *Brochothrix*
Lis637 Genus *Listeria*,
Lpara *Lactobacillus casei*
Lzeae *Lactobacillus zeae*
Pae997 *Pseudomonas* spp.
Pamic1435 *Parvimonas micra*
Pana134 *Peptostreptococcus anaerobius*
Pden654 *Prevotella denticola*
Pilosi1405 *Brachyspira pilosicoli*
Pilosi209 *Brachyspira pilosicoli*
Pint649 *Prevotella intermedia*
Pint657 *Prevotella intermedia*
Pnasa1254 *Peptoniphilus asaccharolyticus*
Pnhar1466 *Peptoniphilus harei*
Pnivo731 *Peptoniphilus ivorii*
POGI *Porphyromonas gingivalis*

(Continued)

TABLE 1 | Continued

Ppu *Pseudomonas* spp.
Ppu56a *Pseudomonas putida*
Ppu646 *Pseudomonas* spp.
PRIN *Prevotella intermedia*
Saga *Streptococcus agalactiae*
SAL3 Genus *Salmonella*
Sau *Staphylococcus aureus*
Saur327 *Staphylococcus*
Saur72 *Staphylococcus aureus*
Ser1410 Genus *Brachyspira*
SGD229 Genus *Desulfotomaculum*
Sita649 *Candidatus Sphaeronema italicum*
Spn *Streptococcus pneumoniae*
Spy *Streptococcus pyogenes*
Staaur *Staphylococcus aureus*
Staph747 *Staphylococcus* spp.
STEBA1426 *Sterolibacterium* lineage
Stemal *Stenotrophomonas maltophilia*
Strpyo (Streppyo) *Streptococcus pyogenes*
Sval428 Some *Desulfobulbaceae*
TM7305 subdivision 1 of candidate division TM7
Trep-D3-4 32 PT1 *Treponema refringens*
Trep-D4-4 32 PT3 clone DDKL-20 *Treponema refringens*
Trep-HW 170 PT6 clone DDKL-4 *Treponema phagedenis*
Trep-T5-4 32 PT2 *Treponema refringens*
Urobe63b *Ruminococcus obeum*-like
VEPA *Veillonella parvula*
VIB572a Genus *Vibrio*
Y *Yersinia*
FISH probes with signals which could not be definitively assigned to a specific group of bacteria ($N = 31$)
Alf 1b (Alpha) *Alphaproteobacteria*, some *Deltaproteobacteria*, *Spirochaetes*
Arch 915 *Archaea*
B for *Bacteroides forsythus*
B(T)AFO *Tannerella forsythensis*
Bact for *Bacteroides forsythus*
Bang198 *B. angulatum*
Bfra602 most *Flavobacteria*, some *Bacteroidetes*
Bmy843 *Bacillus*
BORR4 Genus *Borrelia*
Bvulg1017 *Bacteroides vulgatus*
CF319a most *Flavobacteria*, some *Bacteroidetes*
CFB560 subgroup of *Bacteroidetes*, *CFB* division
Clept1240 *Clostridium leptum*
Efaec *Enterococcus faecalis*, *Enterococcus sulfuricus*
Enc131 *Enterococcus* spp and other
Ent *Enterobacteriaceae* except *Proteus* spp.
FUS664 most *Fusobacterium* sp
FUSO *Fusobacterium* sp.
MIB724 mouse intestinal bacteria
PBR2 *Bifidobacterium breve*
PseaerA *Pseudomonas aeruginosa*
PseaerB *Pseudomonas aeruginosa*

(Continued)

TABLE 1 | Continued

Rint623 *Roseburia cecicola*, *Roseburia intestinalis*
Rrec584 *Roseburia genus*
SRB385Db *Desulfobacterales*
ssp F suc *Fibrobacter succinogenes* subsp. *Succinogenes*
STA *Staphylococcus* spp.
Str(STR2) *Streptococcus* spp
TRE308 *Treponema* sp.
TrepGen 725 S-S-*Trep* Genus725 (202)
TW652 *Tropheryma whippelii*
FISH probes which delivered identical results to other probes ($N = 8$)
EC1531 *E. coli*
ECO1167 (ECO 45A) *Escherichia coli*
ENT183 *Enterobacteriaceae*
GAM42a *Gamma-proteobacteria*
HGC69a *Actinobacteria* (high G+C Gram-positive bacteria)
Bif164 *Bifidobacteriaceae*, *Bifidobacterium* spp.
EubII *Phylum Planctomycetes*
EubIII *Phylum Verrucomicrobia*

We performed hybridizations with all probes but excluded from analysis 31 of these probes, because they showed multiple uncharacteristic signals, in form and distribution not resembling bacteria or cross-reacting with non-related bacterial groups and eight FISH probes that were identical to related probes for the same species.

To reduce the number of unnecessary investigations, while following the impact of the ketogenic diet on the colonic microbiome, only 35 bacterial groups which were found to have substantial occurrence (in at least 20% of individuals) and concentrations ($>10^9$ in at least one of the stool samples of one individual) were applied.

Statistical Analysis

Differences between groups were evaluated using the two sided *t*-Student *U*-test. Data are presented as means $\pm$ *SD*, $P < 0.05$ was considered statistically significant.

RESULTS

Eligibility of the FISH Probes for Analysis of the Stool Microbiome

Three bacteria detected with EREC (mainly *Roseburia*), Bac303 (*Bacteroides*), and Fprau (*Faecalibacterium prausnitzii*) probes were always present in healthy human controls and MS patients and contributed to about half of the colonic microbiome in each subject. We called these groups **essential bacteria**.

All other investigated bacterial groups were individual, detectable only in a subset of patients. We called them **individual bacterial** groups.

Twenty-eight of the individual bacterial groups were found in at least 30% of the probands (mostly 50–70%) in concentrations of higher than 10^9 bacteria/ml. They contributed substantially to the colonic microbial mass. We called them **individual substantial groups**.

Four of the **individual** bacterial groups including Bif (*Bifidobacteriacae*), Ebac (*Enterobacteriaceae*), Clit (*Clostridium lituseburense*), and Cdif (*Clostridium difficile*) are often found prevalent in newborns, after antibiotic treatment and convalescence patients and thus represent bacterial groups with pioneer function. We evaluated these groups separately.

Individual bacterial groups detected with 88 FISH probes (**Table 1B**) were observed in one, maximal two individuals in marginal concentrations of $\leq 0.1 \times 10^9$ ml. We called these **individual marginal** bacterial groups. Because of the uneven distribution of such bacteria over the stool cylinder, their quantification was highly unreliable.

Thirty-one of investigated FISH probes showed multiple uncharacteristic signals, in form and distribution, cross-reacting with unrelated bacterial groups. The appearance of these signals was not visually different in MS and healthy controls. Because of the uncertainty of what exactly is measured, we did not perform the quantitative analysis of the results detected with these probes.

Eight FISH probes, showed identical results with related probes for the same species/bacterial group, were also not quantitatively evaluated.

Microbiome in Healthy Controls and MS Patients Prior to Diet Intervention

The morphologic appearance of single bacteria detected with corresponding FISH probes was the same in MS patients and healthy controls. The distribution of bacteria over the stool cylinder surface was not noticeably different. None of the investigated bacterial groups, including groups with unspecific signals, demonstrated prevalence or absence in MS patients, which could be interpreted in terms of Koch's postulates.

As long as bacterial groups were compared pairwise, the differences between MS and healthy patients were discordant, gradual and moderate, reaching only in 9 groups statistical significance (**Table 2**). The concentrations of most investigated groups in MS were decreased. Six groups were slightly increased and included Cor653 (*Coriobacterium group*), Cvir1414 (*Clostridium viride* group) Ehal (*Eubacterium hallii*), Ecyl387 (*Eubacterium cylindroides),* Lab158 (*Lactobacillus* sp., *Enterococcus* sp.), Rfla729 (*Ruminococcus albus)* bacterial groups. Seven substantial individual bacterial groups had similar high concentrations in MS and healthy controls.

Due to uncertain occurrence and low concentrations, which was difficult to quantify, we did not compare the single marginal bacterial groups in MS patients and controls quantitatively. No rise of single marginal groups in MS patients was observed.

The difference in the microbiome of MS patients and healthy controls became striking, when concentrations of numerically substantial groups were summarized and considered as a whole (**Table 2**, marked in bold). The diversity of all substantial groups in MS patients was reduced by 36% ($P < 0.001$), the mean sum concentrations of all substantial bacterial groups were reduced by 24% (65 vs. 85.4 $\times 10^9$/bacteria/ml., $P < 0.001$) compared to healthy controls. The decrease in concentrations was most profound in the essential bacteria group (32%) and less impressive in individual substantial (19%) and pioneer groups (14%).

Changes of the Colonic Microbiome with the Ketogenic Diet in 10 MS Patients

The changes in the microbiome during the ketogenic diet were univocal. Except for *Akkermansia*, all groups of bacteria demonstrated consistently more or less marked decreases, leading to a reduction of the total bacterial concentrations of the substantial bacteria from 65 to 25 $\times$ 10^9 bacteria per ml at week 2. Some of the bacterial groups fell below detection level, resulting in further decline of the bacterial diversity from 48 to 36%.

However these tendencies were temporary.

The total bacterial concentrations in MS patients started to increase at week 12, reaching values typical for healthy controls at week 23/24, being then significantly higher than bacterial concentrations in MS patients prior to diet and statistically not different to mean bacterial concentrations in healthy controls ($P = 0.7$). This increase was consistent for all but the pioneer bacterial groups and *Akkermansia*. The concentrations of pioneer bacterial groups fell and remained low, the concentrations of *Akkermansia* increased initially but then declined during the ketogenic diet.

DISCUSSION

Previous investigation, using high throughput DNA sequencing technologies in large scale 16S rRNA or shotgun metagenomic sequencing, demonstrated miscellaneous changes in the composition of the colonic microbiome, which correlated with MS, MS-onset, -therapy or -relapse (Kim et al., 2012; Berer and Krishnamoorthy, 2014; Galland, 2014; Miyake et al., 2015; Glenn and Mowry, 2016; Jangi et al., 2016; Tremlett et al., 2016). Both single bacterial groups were found differently represented and also the whole microbiome was aberrantly composed. While the alpha diversity of MS and the healthy microbiome was similar, the beta diversity differed significantly. In ecology, alpha diversity expresses the mean species diversity in sites or habitat at a local scale, while beta diversity is the ratio between regional and local diversity. The differences indicated shifts in composition of the MS microbiome. The meaning of these observations is unclear. The pure occurrence of bacteria does not automatically mean that they are relevant or biochemically active. The vacant niches may be occupied by chance.

Although we applied publically available FISH probes as broadly as possible and included all groups covering numerically substantial components of the colonic microbiome, no conclusions to the entire biodiversity are possible, since FISH reliably detects only bacteria in concentrations of higher than 10^5 per ml.

However, while sequence analysis is perfect for identification of specific occurrence patterns, its information on physical abundance and contribution of bacteria to biofermentation is poor. Abundance of bacteria within the fecal mass however directly expresses their biofermenting power.

TABLE 2 | Colonic microbiome in healthy and MS patients prior to and during the ketogenic diet.

Week	Healthy	MS				*t*-test
	A	B	C	D	E	
		Initial	2	12	23/24	
	Mean ± *SD* concentrations	Mean ± *SD* concentrations	Mean ± *SD* concentrations	Mean ± *SD* concentrations	Mean ± *SD* concentrations	
Diversity of microbiome as % of substantial bacterial groups (35) positive in each patient	75 ± 15	48 ± 19	35 ± 13	38 ± 6.9	51 ± 10.6	A/B,C,D,E $P < 0.001$; B/C $P = 0.03$–0.05; E/B $P = 0.07$; E/C $P < 0.001$; E/D $P = 0.05$
All bacterial groups x10^9 bacteria/ml	**85.4 ± 25.6**	**65 ± 23.1**	**25.1 ± 17.2**	**36.4 ± 16.8**	**83 ± 25.8**	A/B,C,D $P < 0.001$; A/E $P = 0.7$; B/C,D $P < 0.001$; E/B $P = 0.02$; E/C,D $P < 0.0001$
ESSENTIAL						
All Essential bacteria ($N = 3$)	**36.2 ± 14.7**	**24.6 ± 9.5**	**10.7 ± 8.4**	**16.1 ± 7.4**	**34.4 ± 10**	A/B,C,D $P < 0.001$; A/E $P = 0.4$; B/C $P = 0.001$; B/D $P = 0.7$; E/B $P = 0.05$; E/C,D $P < 0.001$
Erec482 (*Eubacterium rectale*, *Clostridium coccoides* group)	11.7 ± 6.9	6.7 ± 5.8	6.1 ± 2.8	6.4 ± 5.3	10.7 ± 7.3	A/B,C,D $P = 0.02$–0.002; A/E $P = 0.6$; B/C $P = 0.2$; B/D $P = 0.9$; E/B,C,D $P = 0.03$–0.02
Bac303 (*Bacteroides*)	12.9 ± 5.3	9.1 ± 4.9	3.4 ± 3.1	4.2 ± 2.7	11.4 ± 6.2	A/B,C,D P<0.001–0.006; A/E P=0.3; B/C,D P=0.001-0.002; E/B P=0.09; E/C,D P<0.001
Fprau (*Faecalibacterium prausnitzii*)	11.6 ± 5.9	8.8 ± 5.1	2.7 ± 4.2	5.7 ± 4	12.2 ± 7.9	A/B $P < 0.05$; A/E $P = 0.8$; B/C,D $P = 0.001$; B/D $P = 0.08$; E/B $P = 0.05$; E/C,D $P < 0.001$–0.007
INDIVIDUAL PIONEER						
All Individual pioneer bacteria ($N = 4$)	**7.8 ± 5**	**6.7 ± 5.3**	**2.5 ± 3.2**	**1.9 ± 3**	**2.7 ± 4.3**	A/B $P = 0.4$: A/C,D $P = 0.001$–0.005; A/E $P = 0.004$; B/C $P = 0.03$; B/D $P = 0.008$; E/B $P = 0.03$; E/C,D P=0.5-0.2
Ebac1790 (*Enterobacteriaceae*)	0.25 ± 0.8	0.5 ± 1.4	0.4 ± 1.2	0.05 ± 0.2	0.15 ± 0.8	All $P > 0.25$
Bif153 (Genus *Bifidobacterium*)	7.1 ± 5.5	5.7 ± 4.9	2.1 ± 2..4	1.8 ± 3	2.1 ± 3	A/B $P = 0.3$; E/C,D $P > 0.85$; A/C,D $P < 0.001$; B/C,D $P = 0.02$–0.03; B/E $P = 0.008$; E/A $P < 0.001$
Clit135 (*Clostridium lituseburense* group including *C. difficile*)	0.5 ± 0.86	0.4 ± 1.2	0	0.03 ± 0.09	0.2 ± 0.6	All $P > 0.1$
Cdif198 (*Clostridium difficile*)	0.04 ± 0.09	0.04 ± 0.2	0	0.001 ± 0.003	0.2 ± 0.6	All $P > 0.3$
INDIVIDUAL SUBSTANTIAL						
All Individual substantial bacteria ($N = 28$)	**41.7 ± 17.3**	**33.8 ± 16.8**	**11.8 ± 9**	**18.3 ± 11.6**	**46.9 ± 18.9**	A/B $P = 0.08$; A/C,D $P < 0.001$; A/E $P = 0$×.3: B/C $P < 0.001$; B/D $P = 0.006$; E/B $P = 0.02$; E/C,D $P < 0.001$
ACI623 (*Acidaminococcaceae* sp. not the Selenomonas species)	1.4 ± 1.9	0.6 ± 1.4	0.4 ± 1.3	0.2 ± 0.4	0.5 ± 0.7	A/B, $P = 0.0.1$; A/C $P = 0.2$; A/D $P = 0.08$; A/E $P = 0.01$; B/C $P = 0.8$; B/D $P = 0.4$; E/B $P = 0.7$; E/C,D $P = 0.5$–0.7
AKK406 (*Akkermansia*)	2.3 ± 3.7	1.1 ± 2.7	2.1 ± 3.8	0.7 ± 2.2	1 ± 1.7	A/B $P = 0.2$; A/C $P = 0.7$; A/D $P = 0.3$; A/E $P = 0.2$; B/C $P = 0.2$; B/D $P = 0.9$; E/B $P = 0.7$; E/C,D $P = 0.4$–0.9
Ato291 (*Atopobium* cluster)	3.8 ± 2.9	2.9 ± 3.1	0.45 ± 0.5	2.6 ± 2.3	4.1 ± 3.1	A/B $P = 0.3$; A/E $P = 0.7$; B/C $P = 0.02$; E/B $P = 0.2$
Bbif186 (*B. bifidum*)	0.3 ± 0.9	0.1 ± 0.4	0	0	0.05 ± 0.2	A/B $P = 0.3$; A/E $P = 0.2$; B/E $P = 0.6$
Blon1004 (*B. longum*)	0.7 ± 1.2	0.3 ± 0.8	0.2 ± 0.4	0	0.5 ± 0.9	A/B $P = 0.3$; A/E $P = 0.7$; B/C $P = 0.7$; E/B $P = 0.5$
Bputre698 (*Bacteroides putredinis*)	0.8 ± 1.6	0.06 ± 0.2	0.05 ± 0.2	0	0.3 ± 0.8	A/B $P = 0.03$; A/E $P = 0.2$; B/C $P = 0.9$; E/B $P = 0.2$; E/C $P = 0.4$
Burkho (*Burkholderia* spp.)	0.7 ± 0.7	0.7 ± 1.2	0.8 ± 0.7	0.001 ± 0.03	0.9 ± 1.5	A/B $P = 0.98$; B/C $P = 0.5$; E/B $P = 0.7$; E/C $P = 0.4$
Ceut705 (*C. eutactus*, *Coprococcus* sp.)	3.0 ± 4.4	1.7 ± 2.9	0.15 ± 0.3	0.2 ± 0.4	1 ± 2	A/B $P = 0.2$; A/C $P = 0.05$; A/E $P = 0.07$; B/C $P = 0.1$; E/B $P = 0.4$; E/C,D $P = 0.2$

(Continued)

TABLE 2 | Continued

Week	Healthy	MS				*t*-test
	A	B	C	D	E	
		Initial	2	12	23/24	
	Mean ± *SD* concentrations	Mean ± *SD* concentrations	Mean ± *SD* concentrations	Mean ± *SD* concentrations	Mean ± *SD* concentrations	
Chis150 (*Clostridium histolyticum*)	0.6 ± 1.2	0.05 ± 0.2	0.03 ± 0.1	0.04 ± 0.1	1 ± 2.3	A/B $P = 0.03$; A/E $P = 0.5$; B/C,D $P = 0.8$–0.9; E/B $P = 0.08$
Cor653 (*Coriobacterium group*)	0.5 ± 0.8	0.8 ± 1.2	0.5 ± 1.1	0.1 ± 0.3	0.09 ± 0.2	A/B $P = 0.0.3$; A/C, $P = 0.9$; A/E $P = 0.04$; B/C $P = 0.5$; E/B $P = 0.02$; E/C,D $P = 0.1$
Cvir1414 (*Clostridium viride group*)	1.9 ± 2.1	2.2 ± 2.7	0.5 ± 0.4	2 ± 2.6	4.7 ± 3.6	A/B $P = 0.7$; A/C $P = 0.04$; A/E $P = 0.002$; B/C $P = 0.05$; E/B,C,D <0.01
Ecyl387 (*Eubacterium cylindroides*)	0.7 ± 0.5	1 ± 1.2	0.3 ± 0.7	0.3 ± 0.6	0.3 ± 0.8	A/B $P = 0.0.1$; A/E $P = 0.1$; B/C $P = 0.1$; E/B $P = 0.05$
Ehal1469 (*Eubacterium hallii*)	0.6 ± 0.9	1.4 ± 1.9	1.2 ± 1.2	1.7 ± 2.1	2.9 ± 2.1	A/B $P = 0.04$; A/E $P < 0.001$; B/C $P = 0.7$; E/B,C $P < 0.01$
Eram997 (*Eubacterium ramulus*)	0.3 ± 1.3	0.09 ± 0.2	0	0	0.2 ± 0.8	A/B $P = 0.0.4$; A/E $P = 0.8$; B/C $P = 0.2$; E/B $P = 0.5$
Lab158 (*Lactobacillus* sp., *Enterococcus* sp.)	0.1 ± 0.2	1.2 ± 2.9	0.1 ± 0.3	0.02 ± 0.02	0.1 ± 0.4	A/B $P = 0.05$; A/E $P = 0.7$; B/C $P = 0.3$; E/C,D $P = 0.1$
Muc1437 (*Akkermansia muciniphila*)	2.8 ± 3.9	1.7 ± 3.4	1.8 ± 4	0.5 ± 1.5	1 ± 1.2	A/B $P = 0.3$; A/E $P = 0.1$; B/C $P = 0.9$; E/B $P = 0.5$
Myc657 (*Mycobacterium* subdivision, mycolic acid-containing *Actinomycetes*)	3.1 ± 1.5	3 ± 3.1	1.2 ± 1.6	3.3 ± 3	4.2 ± 3.8	A/B $P = 0.9$; A/E $P = 0.2$; B/C $P = 0.09$; E/B $P = 0.3$
Phasco741 (*Phascolarctobacterium faecium*)	0.6 ± 0.9	0.6 ± 2.1	0	0.4 ± 0.8	0.4 ± 0.7	A/B $P = 0.9$; A/E $P = 0.7$; B/C $P = 0.4$; E/B $P = 0.7$
Pnig657 (*Prevotella nigrescens*)	2.2 ± 3.7	0.2 ± 0.6	0	0	1.1 ± 3	A/B $P = 0.01$; A/E $P = 0.4$; B/C $P = 0.3$; E/B $P = 0.3$
ProCo1264 (*Ruminococcus productus*)	0.7 ± 2	0.02 ± 0.08	0	0.09 ± 0.3	0.8 ± 1.8	A/B $P = 0.08$; A/E $P = 0.7$; B/C $P = 0.5$; E/B $P = 0.03$
Rfla729 (*Ruminococcus albus*)	2.2 ± 3.2	5.1 ± 3.2	1.4 ± 2.3	0.6 ± 1.3	6.5 ± 4.4	A/B $P = 0.002$; A/E $P < 0.001$; B/C $P = 0.02$; E/B $P = 0.2$
SFB1 (*Segmented filamentous bacteria*)	2.3 ± 3.3	1.5 ± 3.8	0.4 ± 0.8	1.9 ± 3.5	3.7 ± 4.1	A/B $P = 0.4$; A/E $P = 0.2$; B/C $P = 0.4$; E/B $P = 0.1$
SNA (*Sphaerotilus natans*)	4.3 ± 3.7	3.2 ± 3.7	0.3 ± 0.4	0.001 ± 0.003	5.7 ± 4.8	A/B $P = 0.3$; A/E $P = 0.2$; B/C $P = 0.02$; E/B $P = 0.05$
Strc493 (most *Streptococcus* spp.)	1.3 ± 3.3	0.8 ± 1.5	0.01 ± 0.03	0.4 ± 1.2	1 ± 1.7	A/B $P = 0.4$; A/E $P = 0.8$; B/C $P = 0.1$; E/B $P = 0.6$
SUBU1237 (*Burkholderia* spp., *Sutterella* spp.)	1.7 ± 2.6	0.6 ± 1.2	0.1 ± 0.3	0.1 ± 0.3	1.4 ± 1.6	A/B $P = 0.08$; A/E $P = 0.7$; B/C $P = 0.2$; E/B $P = 0.1$
Urobe63a (*Ruminococcus obeum*-like)	1.6 ± 2.3	1.6 ± 2.8	0.06 ± 0.2	0.7 ± 1.8	2.1 ± 1.9	A/B $P = 0.9$; A/E $P = 0.5$; B/C $P = 0.1$; E/B $P = 0.5$
Veil223 (*Veillonella*)	0.1 ± 0.3	0.04 ± 0.2	0	0.2 ± 0.4	0.16 ± 0.3	A/B $P = 0.2$; A/E $P = 0.8$; B/C $P = 0.5$; E/B $P = 0.2$
Ver620 (*Verrucomicrobium*)	1.7 ± 3.9	1 ± 2.7	0	1.9 ± 3.6	1.2 ± 2.4	A/B $P = 0.5$; A/E $P = 0.6$; B/C $P = 0.2$; E/B $P = 0.9$

Our data quantifying microbial participants clearly demonstrate the impaired colonic function in patients with MS. Both concentrations and biodiversity of numerically substantial bacterial groups were markedly reduced in MS. Essential bacteria were most, individual substantial bacteria less depleted, while pioneer bacteria were nearly unchanged.

This grading of suppression matches well with the proposed role of these groups for colonic function. Essential bacteria are present in every healthy person in large concentrations, contributing roughly to approximately half of the mass of the colonic microbiome. They are obviously important for colonic fermentation and represent main fermentative groups in human. The individual substantial bacterial groups are present only in subsets of healthy persons in varying concentrations, which are each distinctly lower than those of the essential bacterial groups. Their presence is dispensable for colonic fermentation. However, their diversity is high, composition specific for each subject, indicating that they fulfill special tasks not covered by the essential bacterial groups. Despite markedly lower concentrations, when compared to essential bacterial groups, the individual substantial groups constitute together another half of the colonic biomass.

Pioneer bacteria are usually found in low concentration in healthy adults. Their concentrations are high in newborns after antibiotic treatment and in convalescence, while the colonic microbiome is reshaped (Swidsinski et al., 2016).

The fall in concentration in MS patients was gradual, decreasing from essential to individual substantial and further to pioneer bacterial groups. This suggests that the suppression is not due to the loss of responsible microbial groups or reshaping of the microbiome. It presumably results from the general downregulation of the colonic biofermentative function and affects mainly biofermentative active groups, leaving bacterial groups with other specific tasks untouched.

We observed no changes in the microbiome that could be specific for MS.

While mean concentrations of all essential bacteria detected with EREC (mainly *Roseburia*), Bac303 (*Bacteroides*), Fprau (*F. prausnitzii*) probes were consistently reduced in MS, the shifts in individual substantial bacterial groups were multidirectional with concentrations of some bacterial groups unchanged, increased or reduced when compared to healthy controls. Although some of the differences reached the level of statistical significance, the fluctuations in concentrations of individual substantial bacterial groups were moderate and in the range of those, when unmatched groups of subjects are compared with each other. Similar fluctuations are documented while describing microbiome composition in other pathologies such as diarrhea, irritable bowel syndrome, inflammatory bowel disease, and others (Mai et al., 2016; Swidsinski et al., 2016).

Since the microbiome is influenced by a multiplicity of racial, occupational, social, regional, and geographic factors, matching for all of them would be an impossible task. Mean values raised in small cohorts should therefore be critically evaluated, even when they occasionally prove to be statistically highly significant (Mai et al., 2016). Our data allow definitively no conclusions to whether the observed alterations in concentrations of colonic bacteria precede, result, specifically accompany MS or rely on independent coincident processes such as aberrant immunity, impaired digestion or simply changed behavior. However, they clearly demonstrate that the perturbation of the microbiome in MS is not inherent and inevitable but can be definitively corrected with diet, supplementation and other means as assumed previously (Tanca et al., 2015).

After 6 months on the ketogenic diet, the sum concentrations of the substantial microbial groups in MS patients increased significantly when compared to the period prior to intervention (83 vs. 65 $\times$ 10^9 bacteria/ml; P = 0.02) and became indistinguishable from the healthy group (83 vs. 85.4 $\times$ 10^9 bacteria/ml. $P = 0.7$).

Our data also demonstrate that the tracking of the changes in the microbiome should not be restricted to a single time point, but needs surveillance over longer periods of time.

The reduction of microbial concentrations observed 2 weeks after the start of the diet was dramatic, the ranges of suppression were comparable to antibiotics effects (Swidsinski et al., 2016). Concentrations of some individual substantial groups fell under detection limit, leading to further drop in the microbial diversity from mean 48 to 35 percent. However, the processes behind dietetic and antibiotic effects are principally different.

The improvement with antibiotic treatment occurred only after the end of treatment, while with the ketogenic diet, the improvement occurred in succession of the diet and the long-term effects of diet were opposite to the immediate response to the intervention. Although the diversity of the microbiome did not reach the values typical for the healthy population, at the end of the observation period, after 6 months on the ketogenic diet, it completely recovered as compared to basic values prior to treatment.

Obviously the increase in microbial concentrations was mainly due to improvement of colonic function and achieved by preexisting microbial groups. Typical for convalescence after depletion of the colonic microbiome following antibiotic use, stroke or inflammation is a temporary excess of pioneer bacterial groups. Such excess was not observed with the ketogenic diet. In contrast, the pioneer bacterial groups remained reduced over the whole duration of the ketogenic diet (p < 0.05–0.008), indicating an absence of substantial microbiome reshaping.

Although the concentrations and the biodiversity of colonic microbiota are strong markers of the intensity of the microbial metabolism, the shifts in bacterial groups *per se* do not reveal the exact metabolic changes taking place. The role of single substances and metabolites in neurologic disorders is still to be unraveled and follow our preliminary observations.

Summarizing, we state that colonic microbiome and neuropathology are closely interrelated. Concentrations of numerically substantial biofermentative bacteria are significantly reduced in MS patients. The microbial shifts can be reliably quantified and monitored by FISH under ambulatory conditions. The ketogenic diet for 6 months completely restored the microbial biofermentation mass and is an interesting interventional tool for prospective clinical studies.

AUTHOR CONTRIBUTIONS

AS, MB,YD, and AG designed the study, YD, JN, AR, KW, and ÖG conducted the study, ÖG and VL critically revised the manuscript, and AS, AG, CG, and AR. performed FISH, CG, JN statistically analyzed the data. All authors contributed to conception of the work, revising of the data, shaping of the manuscript and approved the final draft submitted.

REFERENCES

Berer, K., and Krishnamoorthy, G. (2014). Microbial view of central nervous system autoimmunity. *FEBS Lett.* 588, 4207–4213. doi: 10.1016/j.febslet.2014.04.007

Choi, I. Y., Piccio, L., Childress, P., Bollman, B., Ghosh, A., Brandhorst, S., et al. (2016). A diet mimicking fasting promotes regeneration and reduces autoimmunity and multiple sclerosis symptoms. *Cell Rep.* 15, 136–146. doi: 10.1016/j.celrep.2016.05.009

Galland, L. (2014). The gut microbiome and the brain. *J. Med. Food* 17, 1261–1272. doi: 10.1089/jmf.2014.7000

Glenn, J. D., and Mowry, E. M. (2016). Emerging concepts on the gut microbiome and multiple sclerosis. *J. Interferon Cytokine Res.* 36, 347–357. doi: 10.1089/jir.2015.0177

Jangi, S., Gandh, R., Cox, L. M., Li, N., von Glehn, F., Yan, R., et al. (2016). Alterations of the human gut microbiome in multiple sclerosis. *Nat. Commun.* 7:12015. doi: 10.1038/ncomms12015

Kim, D. Y., Hao, J., Liu, R., Turner, G., Shi, F. D., and Rho, J. M. (2012). Inflammation-mediated memory dysfunction and effects of a ketogenic diet in a murine model of multiple sclerosis. *PLoS ONE* 7:e35476. doi: 10.1371/journal.pone.0035476

Loy, A., Maixner, F., Wagner, M., and Horn, M. (2016). ProbeBase—an online resource for rRNA-targeted oligonucleotide probes: new features. *Nucleic Acids Res.* 35, 800–804. doi: 10.1093/nar/gkv1232

Mai, V., Prosperi, M., and Yaghjyan, L. (2016). Moving microbiota research toward establishing causal associations that represent viable targets for effective public health interventions. *Ann. Epidemiol.* 26, 306–310. doi: 10.1016/j.annepidem.2016.03.011

Miyake, S., Kim, S., Suda, W., Oshima, K., Nakamura, M., Matsuoka, T., et al. (2015). Dysbiosis in the gut microbiota of patients with multiple sclerosis, with a striking depletion of species belonging to clostridia XIVa and IV clusters. *PLoS ONE* 10:e0137429. doi: 10.1371/journal.pone.0137429.

Piccio, L., Stark, J. L., and Cross, A. H. (2008). Chronic calorie restriction attenuates experimental autoimmune encephalomyelitis. *J. Leukoc. Biol.* 84, 940–948. doi: 10.1189/jlb.0208133

Suau, A., Rochet, V., Sghir, A., Gramet, G., Brewaeys, S., Sutren, M., et al. (2001). *Fusobacterium prausnitzii* and related species represent a dominant group within the human fecal flora. *Syst. Appl. Microbiol.* 24, 139–145. doi: 10.1078/0723-2020-00015

Swidsinski, A. (2006). Standards for bacterial identification by fluorescence *In situ* hybridization within eukaryotic tissue using ribosomal rRNA-based probes. *Inflamm. Bowel Dis.* 12, 824–826.

Swidsinski, A., Loening-Baucke, V., Kirsch, S., and Doerffel, Y. (2010). Functional biostructure of colonic microbiota in healthy subjects and patients with diarrhea treated with *Saccharomyces boulardii*. *Gastroenterol. Clin. Biol.* 34, 79–92. doi: 10.1016/S0399-8320(10)70025-7

Swidsinski, A., Loening-Baucke, V., Schulz, S., Manowsky, J., Verstraelen, H., and Swidsinski, S. (2016). Functional anatomy of the colonic bioreactor: impact of antibiotics and *Saccharomyces boulardii* on bacterial composition in human fecal cylinders. *Syst. Appl. Microbiol.* 39, 67–75. doi: 10.1016/j.syapm.2015.11.002

Tanca, A., Palomba, A., Pisanu, S., Addis, M. F., and Uzzau, S. (2015). Enrichment or depletion? The impact of stool pretreatment on metaproteomic characterization of the human gut microbiota. *Proteomics* 15, 3474–3485. doi: 10.1002/pmic.201400573

Tremlett, H., Fadrosh, D. W., Faruqi, A. A., Zhu, F., Hart, J., Roalstad, S., et al. (2016). Gut microbiota in early pediatric multiple sclerosis: a case-control study. *Eur. J. Neurol.* 23, 1308–1321. doi: 10.1111/ene.13026

17

Unveiling and Characterizing Early Bilateral Interactions between Biofilm and the Mouse Innate Immune System

*Christiane Forestier[1], Elisabeth Billard[2], Geneviève Milon[3] and Pascale Gueirard[1]**

[1] *CNRS UMR 6023, Laboratoire Microorganismes: Génome et Environnement, Université Clermont-Auvergne, Clermont-Ferrand, France,* [2] *INRA USC 2018, Inserm U1071, Laboratoire Microbes Intestin Inflammation et Susceptibilité de l'Hôte, Université Clermont-Auvergne, Clermont-Ferrand, France,* [3] *Institut Pasteur, Paris, France*

***Correspondence:**
Pascale Gueirard
pascale.gueirard@uca.fr

A very substantial progress has been made in our understanding of infectious diseases caused by invasive bacteria. Under their planktonic forms, bacteria transiently reside in the otherwise sterile mammal body tissues, as the physiological inflammation insures both their clearance and repair of any tissue damage. Yet, the bacteria prone to experience planktonic to biofilm developmental transition still need to be studied. Of note, sessile bacteria not only persist but also concur preventing the effectors and regulators of the physiological inflammation to operate. Thus, it is urgent to design biologically sound experimental approaches aimed to extract, at the earliest stage, immune signatures of mono-bacteria planktonic to biofilm developmental transition *in vivo* and *ex vivo*. Indeed, the transition is often the first event to which succeeds the "chronicization" process whereby classical bacteria-targeting therapies are no more efficacious. An *in vivo* model of micro-injection of *Staphylococcus aureus* planktonic or biofilm cells in the ear pinna dermis of laboratory transgenic mice with fluorescent immune cells is proposed. It allows visualizing, in real time, the range of the early interactions between the *S. aureus* and myeloid cell subsets- the resident macrophages and dendritic cells, the recruited neutrophil granulocytes/polymorphonuclear neutrophils, monocytes otherwise known to differentiate as macrophages or dendritic cells. One main objective is to extract contrasting immune signatures of the modulation of the physiological inflammation with respect to the two bacterial lifestyles.

Keywords: bacteria, biofilm, intravital imaging, macrophage/monocyte, mouse, polymorphonuclear neutrophil

INTRODUCTION

Most invasive bacteria display two different lifestyles: whereas the free-floating planktonic bacteria' life style dominates, in some clinical settings, bacteria sensing hostile conditions adhere to biotic or abiotic surfaces and form biofilms (Moormeier and Bayles, 2017). The planktonic to biofilm/sessile lifestyle transition is associated with important metabolic changes and self-production of proteins-lipids-exopolysaccharides-rich as well as extracellular DNA-containing extracellular matrix (Costerton et al., 1999).

According to the National Institutes of Health, biofilms have an enormous impact on human medicine, accounting for over 80% of infectious processes in otherwise sterile tissue (s). Whereas the physiological inflammation is able to both clear invasive planktonic bacteria and to repair tissue damages insuring the return to tissue structural and functional homeostasis, this physiological inflammation does not operate in tissues experiencing sustained colonization by bacterial biofilms. Moreover, contrasting with planktonic bacteria that are cleared by commonly used antibiotics, provided that they do not harbor genetic resistance determinants, the majority of bacteria within the biofilms are resistant to these antibiotics (Lebeaux et al., 2014).

In this review, our present understanding of the professional phagocyte sensors of microbial agonists expected to operate over the *in vivo* planktonic to biofilm lifestyle switch is briefly introduced. Transiently invasive planktonic bacteria are usually cleared by myeloid cells of either the neutrophil granulocyte lineage or/and by mononuclear phagocytes. However, the bilateral interactions engaged or not between sessile bacteria and the myeloid cells are still poorly studied. Until now, most experimentalists have conducted *in vitro* studies with sessile bacteria, exposing them to either one or the other myeloid cell lineage or both (Watters et al., 2016). This review focuses on recent developments obtained in rodent models to characterize inflammatory responses against *Staphylococcus aureus* or *Pseudomonas aeruginosa* sessile bacteria. A new experimental approach combining the mouse ear pinna model and the intravital imaging approach is proposed to analyze these innate immune responses at the dynamic level.

THE PROFESSIONAL PHAGOCYTE SENSORS OF MICROBIAL AGONISTS EXPECTED TO OPERATE OVER THE *IN VIVO* PLANKTONIC TO BIOFILM LIFESTYLE SWITCH

The *in vivo* developmental transition from planktonic to sessile bacteria reflects a range of bilateral cross talks in the fluctuating dynamic tissue milieu colonized by the bacteria under study. At the earliest stage of this developmental transition, communications between key bacterial messengers as well as interactions between bacterial agonists and sensors displayed by the resident and recruited myeloid cells such as the professional phagocytes are initiated and renewed.

The Nucleotide-Based Second Messengers

The cyclic dinucleotides (c-di-NMPs) are recognized as Microbial Associated Molecular Patterns/MAMPs and induce a host type I interferon immune response prolonged by IFNγ production (Valle et al., 2013; Snyder et al., 2017). Moreover, the c-di-NMPs play a central role in many bacterial species during the lifestyle transition (Valle et al., 2013). Using the *P. aeruginosa* model organism, Valentini and Filloux (2016) showed that the bacteria use c-di-GMP as a checkpoint during the different steps of biofilm development. There is indeed a direct correlation between high levels of c-di-GMP in the bacteria and biofilm formation, and between low levels of c-di-GMP and motility (planktonic phenotype). The c-di-GMP second messenger is used by *Escherichia coli* and *Salmonella enterica* serovar Typhimurium over their planktonic to biofilm developmental transition (Allewell, 2016; Valentini and Filloux, 2016) whereas the c-di-AMP is used as a second messenger by other bacteria such as *S. aureus* (Corrigan et al., 2011).

The Guanosine tetraphosphate (ppGpp) and pentaphosphate (pppGpp), also called (p)ppGpp or alarmones are synthetized when bacteria are exposed to cells such as phagocytes in the infected tissue. Considered as bacterial signature of a so called stringent response, these alarmones represent intracellular signaling molecules known to participate to intracellular bacteria survival: Geiger et al. (2012) demonstrated that the stringent response is induced, *in vitro,* after *S. aureus* phagocytosis by neutrophil granulocytes or polymorphonuclears (PMN). The rapid (p)ppGpp synthesis leads to increased *psm* transcription and to participation of synthetized phenol soluble modulins (PSMs) concurring to bacteria survival after phagocytosis (Geiger et al., 2012). Depicted as pro-inflammatory agents, the PSMs also account for the bacteria escape from the transient intracellular niche, followed either by bacteria survival inside the cytosol or by lysis of the cell, all these rapid processes contributing to damages of the *S. aureus*- hosting tissues (Geiger et al., 2012; Peschel and Otto, 2013).

The Quorum Sensing Circuit and Its Additional Regulators

Quorum sensing (QS) is a cell-to-cell signaling process that allows bacteria to sense and process high cell densities. It involves the synthesis, release and accumulation of signaling molecules called auto-inducers (AIs) (Papenfort and Bassler, 2016). At high concentrations, AIs induce cellular signaling cascades that notably control biofilm formation. The QS system of *S. aureus* called accessory gene regulator (Agr) has been extensively studied (Paharik and Horswill, 2016). With other regulators, it constitutes a complex regulatory network that, at any moment, either modifies AGR activity itself, or its downstream signaling or metabolic pathways. At the early stage of *S. aureus* developmental transition from planktonic to biofilm lifestyle, the low Agr concentration allows the production of inter-bacteria/intercellular adhesins whereas toxins' expression is repressed (Balasubramanian et al., 2016). Later, high levels of Agr induce biofilm structuration and dispersion by up-regulating the expression of the pro-inflammatory PSM molecules (Otto, 2008; Periasamy et al., 2012; Kavanaugh and Horswill, 2016; Paharik and Horswill, 2016). Environmental factors also modulate the Agr function in *S. aureus*, with a well-described inhibitory effect of the reactive oxygen species (ROS) produced by innate immune cells (Kavanaugh and Horswill, 2016).

Among other regulators that interact with the *agr* system at later stage of the biofilm development and maturation, the S. *aureus* exoprotein (Sae) two-component system promotes the synthesis and secretion of leucocidins and other virulence determinants that actively participate to *S. aureus* survival after contact with PMN *in vitro* (Paharik and Horswill, 2016). Sae mutants have indeed a decreased capacity to resist to the PMN- clearing functions after contact (Yarwood and Schlievert, 2003; Voyich et al., 2009; Paharik and Horswill, 2016).

RODENT MODELS TO STUDY INFLAMMATORY RESPONSES TO BIOFILMS *IN VIVO*

In rodent laboratory models, the most rapidly recruited cells are phagocytes, namely the PMN. Over any local disruption of mouse tissue homeostasis, PMN stored in the bone marrow egress into the blood vascular bed. Through chemoattractants and cytokines produced by tissue resident mast cells and macrophages (Teng et al., 2017), the PMN rapidly cross the microvessels endothelial cells, reaching the extracellular compartment colonized by invasive bacteria. They represent the first wave of innate immune cells to be recruited from the blood circulation. Most often, PMN efficiently kill and degrade invasive planktonic bacteria by using different antimicrobial strategies: phagocytosis, production of ROS and antimicrobial peptides, as well as cytotoxic components released from their subcellular distinct granules. More recently, neutrophil extracellular traps (NETs) have been observed and included as an additional strategy (Brinkmann et al., 2004). Among the *in vivo* models that allow characterization of the bilateral interactions co-engaged by PMN and sessile bacteria, we selected those relying on either *P. aeruginosa* or *S. aureus* (**Table 1**).

Of note, the features of the biofilm-colonized devices condition the interaction profiles: whereas in devices of hollow type (catheter, silicon splint) bacterial biofilms are protected from the immune cells, on solid devices (K-wire, pin), the bacterial biofilms are directly exposed to the different waves of immune cells. Depending on the model used, many other parameters operate (listed in **Table 1**). In most models, an intense and rapid accumulation of PMN is observed at the proximity of the biofilms (Wagner et al., 2003; Prabhakara et al., 2011a; Torre et al., 2015; Moser et al., 2017; Wang et al., 2017), the PMN representing the most abundant population of recruited cells. Using a non- invasive bioluminescence-based approach, Bernthal et al. (2011) showed that this recruitment is IL-1β dependent, as a 50% decrease in PMNs numbers was observed in the bacteria colonized knee joints of IL-1β deficient mice, as compared to wild-type mice. This PMN infiltration is increased when diabetic mice are treated with insulin in a bacteria-hosting wound, the latter incorporating actin and DNA from lysed PMN, which therefore contributes to the building of biofilms (Watters et al., 2014). Of note, a low PMN recruitment in the target tissues (Thurlow et al., 2011; Scherr et al., 2014; Secor et al., 2017) can be also operating: in particular was noticed an association between the reduced PMN recruitment and the production of Filamentous Pf1-like bacteriophage (Pf phage) by *P. aeruginosa* (Secor et al., 2017). Taken globally, whatever the experimental conditions depicted in **Table 1**, there is a need to capture more comprehensive information documenting, at least at the earliest stages, the *in vivo* dynamic interactions between bacteria and PMN.

Could mature biofilms' matrix components protect bacteria from activated PMN? PMN were indeed shown to be activated, *in vitro*, by bacterial DNA and polysaccharides components such as alginate, the measured outcome being an increase of their respiratory burst (Pedersen et al., 1990; Alvarez et al., 2006; Fuxman Bass et al., 2008; Jensen et al., 2010). *In vivo*, *P. aeruginosa* biofilm interactions with PMN lead to up regulation of the QS-dependent effectors such as rhamnolipids which cause PMN lysis (Alhede et al., 2014). This shielding specific property of rhamnolipids is described in mouse models relying upon the intraperitoneal implant of pre-colonized silicone device (Van Gennip et al., 2012) or on biofilm development in the respiratory tract (Bjarnsholt et al., 2005; Jakobsen et al., 2012). In these models, QS mutants are unable to produce rhamnolipids and are rapidly phagocytosed and cleared by PMN.

Monocytes/macrophages are other key actors recruited and sensing both the other inflammatory cells -e.g., PMN -as well as bacteria agonists. Under homeostatic conditions, circulating macrophage/monocytes qualified as classical/intermediate ones are continuously recruited from the blood and either mature into macrophages or remain as monocytes within tissues (Sprangers et al., 2016; Jakubzick et al., 2017). In the skin, long- lived resident macrophages are also present and maintain their population by self-renewal (Sprangers et al., 2016; Jakubzick et al., 2017). As for PMN, microbe-specific molecules participate to the rapid emigration of classical/intermediate monocytes in the extravascular space which contribute to the resolution of inflammation by recognizing and phagocytosing bacteria and dying cells, and by producing ROS and reactive nitrogen species (RNI) (Sprangers et al., 2016; Jakubzick et al., 2017; Kashem et al., 2017). Once PMNs experience apoptotic death, a second wave of monocytes qualified as non- classical monocytes contribute to the resolution of inflammation and repair of the disrupted tissue (Sprangers et al., 2016).

Only a few studies (Prabhakara et al., 2011a; Thurlow et al., 2011; Hanke et al., 2012, 2013; Scherr et al., 2015; Corrado et al., 2016; Silva-Santana et al., 2016; see **Table 1**) assess the complex recruitment waves and networks of both PMN and monocyte subsets. Of note, an early wave of monocyte recruitment is sometimes predominant, as compared to PMN recruitment (Thurlow et al., 2011). Two main studies were conducted to monitor the abundance and functional features of monocyte/macrophage recruitment in *vivo* at specific time points after contact with biofilms. The biofilms' matrix components clearly modulate the functional properties of recruited cells. In a *S. aureus* pre-colonized catheter-based model, mobilized cells are mainly distant from the catheter and a non-significant proportion of F4/80$^+$ macrophages are able to invade the biofilms. Cells present deeply into the biofilm rapidly die, therefore preventing phagocytosis of biofilm bacteria to be otherwise exerted by

TABLE 1 | Rodent models to study inflammatory responses to biofilms *in vivo*.

Organism	Biomedical device whenever it is implanted	Tissue(s) where are either inoculated bacteria or implanted a bacteria–free or loaded device	Either bacteria inoculation or bacteria-loaded device delivery mode	Inoculum dose (CFU)	Reference
P. aeruginosa	–	Lung (immobilized bacteria in alginate beads)	Intra-tracheal	6×10^6 to $1{,}5 \times 10^7$	Jensen et al., 2004; Bjarnsholt et al., 2005; Alhede et al., 2009; van Gennip et al., 2009; Jakobsen et al., 2012
	–	Oropharyngeal aspiration of a bacterial suspension	Oropharyngeal	$1{,}5 \times 10^7$	Secor et al., 2017
	Biofilm pre-colonized silicone implant	Implant inserted into the peritoneal cavity (hollow tubes)	Intraperitoneal	–	Van Gennip et al., 2012
	Biofilm pre-colonized silicone implant	Implant inserted into the peritoneal cavity (flat implant)	Intraperitoneal	–	Christensen et al., 2007
S. aureus	–	Diabetic mouse-based model allowing systemic invasion outcome	Intraperitoneal	10^8	Hanses et al., 2011
P. aeruginosa and *S. aureus*	–	Chronically wounded diabetic mouse model	Topical application of bacteria onto a peripheral wound	10^4 2×10^5, 2×10^6, 2×10^7	Watters et al., 2013, 2014 Guo et al., 2013
S. aureus	Un-colonized silicon splint	Chronically wounded diabetic mouse model	Dermal application of bacteria onto the wounded surface	10^6	Nguyen et al., 2013
P. aeruginosa	–	Chronic wound model	Subcutaneous injection of bacteria immobilized in alginate beads beneath a thermal skin lesion	10^6	Trøstrup et al., 2013
S. aureus	–	Air pouch model	Inoculation of bacteria in a single pouch	10^7	Torre et al., 2015
S. aureus	–	Hematogenous model of septic arthritis initiated in murine knees	Intravenous	2×10^6 $1{,}5 \times 10^6$, 3×10^7	Corrado et al., 2016 Verdrengh and Tarkowski, 1997
	Un-colonized orthopedic implant (K-wire)	Post-arthroplasty model (K-wire into the right-knee joint)	Inoculation of bacteria into the joint space containing the cut end of the implant	10^3 10^2, 10^3, or 10^4 10^3 10^3 or 10^5	Bernthal et al., 2011; Heim et al., 2014; Scherr et al., 2015 Pribaz et al., 2012 Niska et al., 2012 Vidlak and Kielian, 2016
	Un-colonized catheter inserted in a pouch	Catheter-related model	Intradermal inoculation of bacteria at proximity of the pouch containing the catheter	5×10^5	Silva-Santana et al., 2016
	Un-colonized catheter	Catheter-related model	Intradermal inoculation of bacteria into the catheter lumen	10^3 5×10^5	Hanke et al., 2012, 2013 Thurlow et al., 2011
	Un-colonized orthopedic implant (K-wire)	Hematogenous implant-related bacteria colonization	Intravenous (tail vein) Intravenous (retroorbital sinus)	10^4 to 10^9 10^6, 5×10^6, 10^7	Shiels et al., 2015 Wang et al., 2017
	Pre-colonized flat stainless steel wire	Orthopedic biofilm model	Tibial implant	–	Nishitani et al., 2015
	Pre-colonized pin	Prosthetic implant model	Tibial implant	3×10^5	Prabhakara et al., 2011a,b
P. aeruginosa	Un-colonized polyethylene catheter	Ascending pyelonephritis model	Inoculation of bacteria into the bladder	5×10^6	Mittal et al., 2009

macrophages (Thurlow et al., 2011). A significant reduction of pro-inflammatory cytokines (IL-1β, TNF...) and chemokines (CXCL2, CCL2) production at the boundary of the biofilm-colonized tissue is also observed, associated with a reduced Nitric Oxide synthase (iNOS) induction and an increased arginase-1 expression. The authors conclude to a macrophage polarization toward a counter-inflammatory activated M2 phenotype and to fibrosis with MyD88- signaling as a major effector pathway regulating these two phenomena (Thurlow et al., 2011; Hanke and Kielian, 2012; Hanke et al., 2012). In a lung experiencing colonization with phage Pf- producing *P. aeruginosa*, Secor et al. (2017) also documented a M2 polarization profile. Taken globally, it appears that the macrophage M2 polarization and fibrosis do concur prolonging bacteria biofilm persistence, although the universal character of such responses remains to be assessed.

THE MOUSE EAR PINNA DERMIS IMAGED BY INTRA-VITAL CONFOCAL MICROSCOPY AT STEADY AND NOT STEADY STATE

Intra-vital microscopy is increasingly used in different biomedical research fields to study dynamic processes at the cellular level in their specific tissue environment. Compared to classical methods such as *ex vivo* histology or flow cytometry, intra-vital confocal microscopy live imaging allows dynamic interactions to be captured once fluorescent reporters are expressed by both the microbes and the laboratory mouse cell lineages with which are engaged, more or less durably, dynamic interactions.

Several skin-related models were described in the literature to study the immunobiology of biofilm infections by using classical approaches (**Table 1**). In these models, the biofilm-loaded cutaneous sites were the back or the flank of animals, which represent unsuitable sites for intravital microscopy of cutaneous innate immune responses.

The ear pinnae is one of the most studied appendage in which are delivered microorganisms, enabling the observation of the early and either transient or prolonged dynamic interactions with resident or recruited myeloid cells (Amino et al., 2006, 2007; Peters et al., 2008; Ng et al., 2011; Sumaria et al., 2011; Jain and Weninger, 2013; Tavares et al., 2013; Carneiro et al., 2017). As an imaging site, the ear presents several technical advantages such as the accessibility of the tissue, easy and fast protocols of preparation to perform imaging experiments and obtain reproducible results, and the possibility of imaging for long periods of time in blocks of 20–40 min (Li et al., 2012).

The mouse ear pinna appendage harbors a thin epidermis and an underlying dermis, respectively avascularized and highly vascularized, which contain a broad range of lympho-myeloid cells (Jain and Weninger, 2013). Using a multiphoton microscopy approach and quantitative flow cytometry, Tong et al. (2015) elaborated a 3D immune cell atlas of mouse skin and compared the ear pinnae, dorsal back, footpad, and tail skin. Langerhans cells and dendritic epidermal T cells are present in the epidermis, whereas the dermis mainly harbors in the upper dermis myeloid cells such as dendritic cells, mast cells as well as lymphoid cells (αβT cells, γδT cells, and group 2 Innate Lymphoid Cells), and mainly resident macrophages in the deeper dermis (Tay et al., 2014; Tong et al., 2015). All these dermis-located immune cells are included in a collagen- and elastin- rich and more or less hyaluronan- rich extracellular matrix. In term of cell numbers, the specificities of the ear pinna cutaneous site are the following ones: the total leukocyte density is high, with around 4800 cells per mm^2 and a majority of cells present in the dermis. Macrophages, dermal dendritic cells and mast cells represent the majority of ear dermal leukocytes with respectively around 6000 macrophages per mm^3 and more than 2000 dermal dendritic cells and mast cells per mm^3 (Tong et al., 2015). Of note, the ear pinna dermis presents two specificities regarding the presence of mast cells: their high prevalence and their perivascular localization, in close association to blood vessels, in contrast to dermal dendritic cells (Tong et al., 2015). By using intravital multi-photon microscopy, Ng et al. (2011) showed that PMNs are present in the ear dermis of naive mice, but in small numbers, and patrol, as do dermal dendritic cells. Both cell lineages are likely surveying the presence of either epidermis-restricted microbiota derived agonists that reach the dermis or endogenous agonists through the sensors displayed at the plasma membrane or within the macropinocytosis/endosomal machinery.

THE MOUSE EAR SKIN MODEL TO STUDY THE DYNAMICS OF INNATE IMMUNE RESPONSES AGAINST PLANKTONIC OR SESSILE *Staphylococcus aureus*

By combining intra-vital confocal microscopy approach and the mouse ear pinna infection model, inflammatory responses against biofilms could be analyzed for the first time at the dynamic level in the tissue environment. The **Figure 1** shows the schematic workflow of methods proposed to characterize and compare the innate immune responses against *S. aureus* planktonic and sessile bacteria. Transgenic mice with fluorescent immune cells visible in the skin such as Lysozyme-EGFP (circulating PMNs and monocytes, dermal macrophages), CD11c-EYFP (dermal dendritic cells, epidermal langherans cells) and Mcpt5-Cre+R26Y+ (dermal mast cells) mouse strains have been selected (Faust et al., 2000; Lindquist et al., 2004; Dudeck et al., 2011). The conditions to prepare bacteria inoculum will be set up. The planktonic inoculum will be obtained from an overnight culture of fluorescent *S. aureus* Lyo-S2 strain in Trypticase Soja broth (Marquès et al., 2015). Biofilms will be generated from a planktonic culture incubated at 37°C under static conditions. After 24 h of incubation, biofilms will be gently collected (A). The first series of experiments will be performed

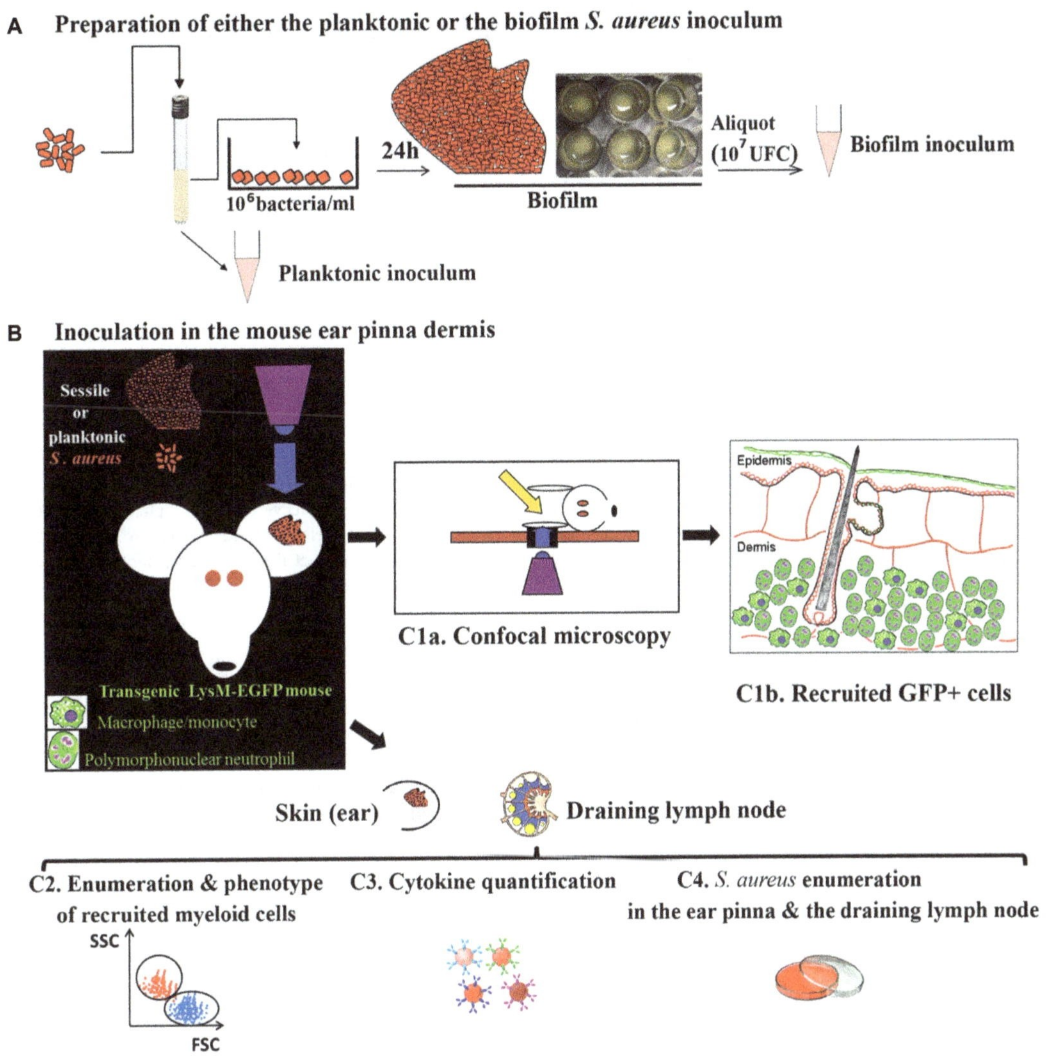

FIGURE 1 | The three steps' workflow proposed for extracting, post either *Staphylococcus aureus* planktonic or biofilm delivery, specific immune signatures displayed by mouse myeloid cells. **(A)** Inoculum preparation *in vitro*. **(B)** Inoculum micro-injection in the ear pinna of mouse (10^7 UFC of either planktonic or sessile bacteria). (C1a) Real time imaging of the ear pinna of a LysM-EGFP transgenic mouse harboring fluorescent phagocytes and fluorescent *S. aureus* bacteria by confocal microscopy. (C1b) Massive recruitment of GFP+ cells post-injection in the upper dermis of the ear pinna of a mouse inoculated with *S. aureus* sessile or planktonic bacteria. (C2), (C3), (C4) Quantitative analyses in the ear pinna and the auricular lymph node to determine (C2) the phenotype of recruited cells, (C3) the cytokine levels and (C4) the bacteria counts.

with Lysozyme-EGFP mice inoculated into the ear tissue with the same number of CFU of either planktonic or sessile bacteria (B). Inoculum will be micro-injected in two injection points in the dermis of the ear pinna tissue with a nanofil syringe (Mac-Daniel et al., 2016). At early time-points, mice will be anesthetized and the cellular recruitment will be analyzed by confocal microscopy at the injection points (C1a and C1b). The behavior of recruited or resident innate immune cells (moving speed, trajectory, distance covered) will be analyzed, as well as their specific interactions with bacteria. In parallel, additional groups of mice will be inoculated with planktonic or biofilm bacteria to perform quantitative analyzes over 14 days in the ear tissue and the cutaneous draining lymph node (auricular lymph node), i.e., determination of the phenotype of recruited cells (C2), of the cytokine levels (C3), and counting of bacteria in the target tissues (C4). The inflammation visible to the eye and macroscopic cutaneous lesions (skin necrosis) will be observed and compared.

CONCLUSION

The objective of the review was to highlight the requirement of developing new *in vivo* models to analyze, at the early stage of infection, the dynamics of innate immune responses against *S. aureus* planktonic or sessile bacteria. A new experimental approach in the field combining the mouse ear pinna model and the intravital imaging approach is proposed. The long term objectives are to use this model as a pre-clinical model to test necessary new therapeutic approaches targeting the host immune system, as proposed initially by Hanke et al. (2013).

AUTHOR CONTRIBUTIONS

CF: intellectual contribution to the work; EB: intellectual contribution to the work; GM: substantial, direct and intellectual contribution to the work; PG: substantial, direct and major intellectual contribution to the work-corresponding author. All authors listed approved the work for publication.

ACKNOWLEDGMENT

The authors wish to acknowledge the contribution of Caroline Vachias at the Confocal Microscopy Facility ICCF (Imagerie Confocale Clermont-Ferrand) at Université Clermont Auvergne.

REFERENCES

Alhede, M., Bjarnsholt, T., Givskov, M., and Alhede, M. (2014). *Pseudomonas aeruginosa* biofilms: mechanisms of immune evasion. *Adv. Appl. Microbiol.* 86, 1–40. doi: 10.1016/B978-0-12-800262-9.00001-9

Alhede, M., Bjarnsholt, T., Jensen, P. Ø., Phipps, R. K., Moser, C., Christophersen, L., et al. (2009). *Pseudomonas aeruginosa* recognizes and responds aggressively to the presence of polymorphonuclear leukocytes. *Microbiol. Read. Engl.* 155, 3500–3508. doi: 10.1099/mic.0.031443-0

Allewell, N. M. (2016). Introduction to biofilms thematic minireview series. *J. Biol. Chem.* 291, 12527–12528. doi: 10.1074/jbc.R116.734103

Alvarez, M. E., Fuxman Bass, J. I., Geffner, J. R., Fernández Calotti, P. X., Costas, M., Coso, O. A., et al. (2006). Neutrophil signaling pathways activated by bacterial DNA stimulation. *J. Immunol.* 1950, 4037–4046. doi: 10.4049/jimmunol.177.6.4037

Amino, R., Thiberge, S., Blazquez, S., Baldacci, P., Renaud, O., Shorte, S., et al. (2007). Imaging malaria sporozoites in the dermis of the mammalian host. *Nat. Protoc.* 2, 1705–1712. doi: 10.1038/nprot.2007.120

Amino, R., Thiberge, S., Martin, B., Celli, S., Shorte, S., Frischknecht, F., et al. (2006). Quantitative imaging of Plasmodium transmission from mosquito to mammal. *Nat. Med.* 12, 220–224. doi: 10.1038/nm1350

Balasubramanian, D., Ohneck, E. A., Chapman, J., Weiss, A., Kim, M. K., Reyes-Robles, T., et al. (2016). *Staphylococcus aureus* coordinates leukocidin expression and pathogenesis by sensing metabolic fluxes via RpiRc. *mBio* 7:e00818-16. doi: 10.1128/mBio.00818-16

Bernthal, N. M., Pribaz, J. R., Stavrakis, A. I., Billi, F., Cho, J. S., Ramos, R. I., et al. (2011). Protective role of IL-1β against post-arthroplasty *Staphylococcus aureus* infection. *J. Orthop. Res.* 29, 1621–1626. doi: 10.1002/jor.21414

Bjarnsholt, T., Jensen, P. Ø., Burmølle, M., Hentzer, M., Haagensen, J. A. J., Hougen, H. P., et al. (2005). *Pseudomonas aeruginosa* tolerance to tobramycin, hydrogen peroxide and polymorphonuclear leukocytes is quorum-sensing dependent. *Microbiol. Read. Engl.* 151, 373–383. doi: 10.1099/mic.0.27463-0

Brinkmann, V., Reichard, U., Goosmann, C., Fauler, B., Uhlemann, Y., Weiss, D. S., et al. (2004). Neutrophil extracellular traps kill bacteria. *Science* 303, 1532–1535. doi: 10.1126/science.1092385

Carneiro, M. B., Hohman, L. S., Egen, J. G., and Peters, N. C. (2017). Use of two-photon microscopy to study Leishmania major infection of the skin. *Methods* 127, 45–52. doi: 10.1016/j.ymeth.2017.04.012

Christensen, L. D., Moser, C., Jensen, P. Ø., Rasmussen, T. B., Christophersen, L., Kjelleberg, S., et al. (2007). Impact of *Pseudomonas aeruginosa* quorum sensing on biofilm persistence in an *in vivo* intraperitoneal foreign-body infection model. *Microbiol. Read. Engl.* 153, 2312–2320. doi: 10.1099/mic.0.2007/006122-0

Corrado, A., Donato, P., Maccari, S., Cecchi, R., Spadafina, T., Arcidiacono, L., et al. (2016). *Staphylococcus aureus*-dependent septic arthritis in murine knee joints: local immune response and beneficial effects of vaccination. *Sci. Rep.* 6:38043. doi: 10.1038/srep38043

Corrigan, R. M., Abbott, J. C., Burhenne, H., Kaever, V., and Gründling, A. (2011). c-di-AMP is a new second messenger in *Staphylococcus aureus* with a role in controlling cell size and envelope stress. *PLOS Pathog.* 7:e1002217. doi: 10.1371/journal.ppat.1002217

Costerton, J. W., Stewart, P. S., and Greenberg, E. P. (1999). Bacterial biofilms: a common cause of persistent infections. *Science* 284, 1318–1322. doi: 10.1126/science.284.5418.1318

Dudeck, A., Dudeck, J., Scholten, J., Petzold, A., Surianarayanan, S., Köhler, A., et al. (2011). Mast cells are key promoters of contact allergy that mediate the adjuvant effects of haptens. *Immunity* 34, 973–984. doi: 10.1016/j.immuni.2011.03.028

Faust, N., Varas, F., Kelly, L. M., Heck, S., and Graf, T. (2000). Insertion of enhanced green fluorescent protein into the lysozyme gene creates mice with green fluorescent granulocytes and macrophages. *Blood* 96, 719–726.

Fuxman Bass, J. I., Gabelloni, M. L., Alvarez, M. E., Vermeulen, M. E., Russo, D. M., Zorreguieta, A., et al. (2008). Characterization of bacterial DNA binding to human neutrophil surface. *Lab. Invest.* 88, 926–937. doi: 10.1038/labinvest.2008.59

Geiger, T., Francois, P., Liebeke, M., Fraunholz, M., Goerke, C., Krismer, B., et al. (2012). The stringent response of *Staphylococcus aureus* and its impact on survival after phagocytosis through the induction of intracellular PSMs expression. *PLOS Pathog.* 8:e1003016. doi: 10.1371/journal.ppat.1003016

Guo, Y., Ramos, R. I., Cho, J. S., Donegan, N. P., Cheung, A. L., and Miller, L. S. (2013). *In vivo* bioluminescence imaging to evaluate systemic and topical antibiotics against community-acquired methicillin-resistant *Staphylococcus aureus*-infected skin wounds in mice. *Antimicrob. Agents Chemother.* 57, 855–863. doi: 10.1128/AAC.01003-12

Hanke, M. L., Angle, A., and Kielian, T. (2012). MyD88-dependent signaling influences fibrosis and alternative macrophage activation during *Staphylococcus aureus* biofilm infection. *PLOS ONE* 7:e42476. doi: 10.1371/journal.pone.0042476

Hanke, M. L., Heim, C. E., Angle, A., Sanderson, S. D., and Kielian, T. (2013). Targeting macrophage activation for the prevention and treatment of *Staphylococcus aureus* biofilm infections. *J. Immunol.* 1950, 2159–2168. doi: 10.4049/jimmunol.1202348

Hanke, M. L., and Kielian, T. (2012). Deciphering mechanisms of staphylococcal biofilm evasion of host immunity. *Front. Cell. Infect. Microbiol.* 2:62. doi: 10.3389/fcimb.2012.00062

Hanses, F., Park, S., Rich, J., and Lee, J. C. (2011). Reduced neutrophil apoptosis in diabetic mice during staphylococcal infection leads to prolonged Tnfα production and reduced neutrophil clearance. *PLOS ONE* 6:e23633. doi: 10.1371/journal.pone.0023633

Heim, C. E., Vidlak, D., Scherr, T. D., Kozel, J. A., Holzapfel, M., Muirhead, D. E., et al. (2014). Myeloid-derived suppressor cells contribute to *Staphylococcus aureus* orthopedic biofilm infection. *J. Immunol.* 1950, 3778–3792. doi: 10.4049/jimmunol.1303408

Jain, R., and Weninger, W. (2013). Shedding light on cutaneous innate immune responses: the intravital microscopy approach. *Immunol. Cell Biol.* 91, 263–270. doi: 10.1038/icb.2012.76

Jakobsen, T. H., van Gennip, M., Phipps, R. K., Shanmugham, M. S., Christensen, L. D., Alhede, M., et al. (2012). Ajoene, a sulfur-rich molecule from garlic, inhibits genes controlled by quorum sensing. *Antimicrob. Agents Chemother.* 56, 2314–2325. doi: 10.1128/AAC.05919-11

Jakubzick, C. V., Randolph, G. J., and Henson, P. M. (2017). Monocyte differentiation and antigen-presenting functions. *Nat. Rev. Immunol.* 17, 349–362. doi: 10.1038/nri.2017.28

Jensen, P. Ø., Givskov, M., Bjarnsholt, T., and Moser, C. (2010). The immune system vs. *Pseudomonas aeruginosa* biofilms. *FEMS Immunol. Med. Microbiol.* 59, 292–305. doi: 10.1111/j.1574-695X.2010.00706.x

Jensen, P. Ø., Moser, C., Kobayashi, O., Hougen, H. P., Kharazmi, A., and Høiby, N. (2004). Faster activation of polymorphonuclear neutrophils in resistant mice during early innate response to *Pseudomonas aeruginosa* lung infection. *Clin. Exp. Immunol.* 137, 478–485. doi: 10.1111/j.1365-2249.2004.02554.x

Kashem, S. W., Haniffa, M., and Kaplan, D. H. (2017). Antigen-presenting cells in the skin. *Annu. Rev. Immunol.* 35, 469–499. doi: 10.1146/annurev-immunol-051116-052215

Kavanaugh, J. S., and Horswill, A. R. (2016). Impact of environmental cues on staphylococcal quorum sensing and biofilm development. *J. Biol. Chem.* 291, 12556–12564. doi: 10.1074/jbc.R116.722710

Lebeaux, D., Ghigo, J.-M., and Beloin, C. (2014). Biofilm-related infections: bridging the gap between clinical management and fundamental aspects of recalcitrance toward antibiotics. *Microbiol. Mol. Biol. Rev.* 78, 510–543. doi: 10.1128/MMBR.00013-14

Li, J. L., Goh, C. C., Keeble, J. L., Qin, J. S., Roediger, B., Jain, R., et al. (2012). Intravital multiphoton imaging of immune responses in the mouse ear skin. *Nat. Protoc.* 7, 221–234. doi: 10.1038/nprot.2011.438

Lindquist, R. L., Shakhar, G., Dudziak, D., Wardemann, H., Eisenreich, T., Dustin, M. L., et al. (2004). Visualizing dendritic cell networks *in vivo*. *Nat. Immunol.* 5, 1243–1250. doi: 10.1038/ni1139

Mac-Daniel, L., Buckwalter, M. R., Gueirard, P., and Ménard, R. (2016). Myeloid cell isolation from mouse skin and draining lymph node following intradermal immunization with live attenuated *Plasmodium* sporozoites. *J. Vis. Exp.* 111:e53796. doi: 10.3791/53796

Marquès, C., Tasse, J., Pracros, A., Collin, V., Franceschi, C., Laurent, F., et al. (2015). Effects of antibiotics on biofilm and unattached cells of a clinical *Staphylococcus aureus* isolate from bone and joint infection. *J. Med. Microbiol.* 64, 1021–1026. doi: 10.1099/jmm.0.000125

Mittal, R., Sharma, S., Chhibber, S., and Harjai, K. (2009). Evaluation of tumour necrosis factor-alpha and interleukin-1beta in an experimental pyelonephritis model induced with planktonic and biofilms cells of *Pseudomonas aeruginosa*. *Can. J. Infect. Dis. Med. Microbiol.* 20, e35–e42. doi: 10.1155/2009/810791

Moormeier, D. E., and Bayles, K. W. (2017). *Staphylococcus aureus* biofilm: a complex developmental organism. *Mol. Microbiol.* 104, 365–376. doi: 10.1111/mmi.13634

Moser, C., Pedersen, H. T., Lerche, C. J., Kolpen, M., Line, L., Thomsen, K., et al. (2017). Biofilms and host response - helpful or harmful. *APMIS* 125, 320–338. doi: 10.1111/apm.12674

Ng, L. G., Qin, J. S., Roediger, B., Wang, Y., Jain, R., Cavanagh, L. L., et al. (2011). Visualizing the neutrophil response to sterile tissue injury in mouse dermis reveals a three-phase cascade of events. *J. Invest. Dermatol.* 131, 2058–2068. doi: 10.1038/jid.2011.179

Nguyen, K. T., Seth, A. K., Hong, S. J., Geringer, M. R., Xie, P., Leung, K. P., et al. (2013). Deficient cytokine expression and neutrophil oxidative burst contribute to impaired cutaneous wound healing in diabetic, biofilm-containing chronic wounds. *Wound Repair Regen.* 21, 833–841. doi: 10.1111/wrr.12109

Nishitani, K., Sutipornpalangkul, W., de Mesy Bentley, K. L., Varrone, J. J., Bello-Irizarry, S. N., Ito, H., et al. (2015). Quantifying the natural history of biofilm formation in vivo during the establishment of chronic implant-associated *Staphylococcus aureus* osteomyelitis in mice to identify critical pathogen and host factors. *J. Orthop. Res.* 33, 1311–1319. doi: 10.1002/jor.22907

Niska, J. A., Meganck, J. A., Pribaz, J. R., Shahbazian, J. H., Lim, E., Zhang, N., et al. (2012). Monitoring bacterial burden, inflammation and bone damage longitudinally using optical and μCT imaging in an orthopaedic implant infection in mice. *PLOS ONE* 7:e47397. doi: 10.1371/journal.pone.0047397

Otto, M. (2008). Staphylococcal biofilms. *Curr. Top. Microbiol. Immunol.* 322, 207–228. doi: 10.1007/978-3-540-75418-3_10

Paharik, A. E., and Horswill, A. R. (2016). The staphylococcal biofilm: adhesins, regulation, and host response. *Microbiol. Spectr.* 4:VMBF-0022-2015. doi: 10.1128/microbiolspec.VMBF-0022-2015

Papenfort, K., and Bassler, B. L. (2016). Quorum sensing signal-response systems in Gram-negative bacteria. *Nat. Rev. Microbiol.* 14, 576–588. doi: 10.1038/nrmicro.2016.89

Pedersen, S. S., Kharazmi, A., Espersen, F., and Høiby, N. (1990). *Pseudomonas aeruginosa* alginate in cystic fibrosis sputum and the inflammatory response. *Infect. Immun.* 58, 3363–3368.

Periasamy, S., Joo, H.-S., Duong, A. C., Bach, T.-H. L., Tan, V. Y., Chatterjee, S. S., et al. (2012). How *Staphylococcus aureus* biofilms develop their characteristic structure. *Proc. Natl. Acad. Sci. U.S.A.* 109, 1281–1286. doi: 10.1073/pnas.1115006109

Peschel, A., and Otto, M. (2013). Phenol-soluble modulins and staphylococcal infection. *Nat. Rev. Microbiol.* 11, 667–673. doi: 10.1038/nrmicro3110

Peters, N. C., Egen, J. G., Secundino, N., Debrabant, A., Kimblin, N., Kamhawi, S., et al. (2008). In vivo imaging reveals an essential role for neutrophils in leishmaniasis transmitted by sand flies. *Science* 321, 970–974. doi: 10.1126/science.1159194

Prabhakara, R., Harro, J. M., Leid, J. G., Harris, M., and Shirtliff, M. E. (2011a). Murine immune response to a chronic *Staphylococcus aureus* biofilm infection. *Infect. Immun.* 79, 1789–1796. doi: 10.1128/IAI.01386-10

Prabhakara, R., Harro, J. M., Leid, J. G., Keegan, A. D., Prior, M. L., and Shirtliff, M. E. (2011b). Suppression of the inflammatory immune response prevents the development of chronic biofilm infection due to methicillin-resistant *Staphylococcus aureus*. *Infect. Immun.* 79, 5010–5018. doi: 10.1128/IAI.05571-11

Pribaz, J. R., Bernthal, N. M., Billi, F., Cho, J. S., Ramos, R. I., Guo, Y., et al. (2012). Mouse model of chronic post-arthroplasty infection: noninvasive in vivo bioluminescence imaging to monitor bacterial burden for long-term study. *J. Orthop. Res.* 30, 335–340. doi: 10.1002/jor.21519

Scherr, T. D., Hanke, M. L., Huang, O., James, D. B. A., Horswill, A. R., Bayles, K. W., et al. (2015). *Staphylococcus aureus* biofilms induce macrophage dysfunction through leukocidin AB and Alpha-toxin. *mBio* 6:e01021-15. doi: 10.1128/mBio.01021-15

Scherr, T. D., Heim, C. E., Morrison, J. M., and Kielian, T. (2014). Hiding in plain sight: interplay between staphylococcal biofilms and host immunity. *Front. Immunol.* 5:37. doi: 10.3389/fimmu.2014.00037

Secor, P. R., Michaels, L. A., Smigiel, K. S., Rohani, M. G., Jennings, L. K., Hisert, K. B., et al. (2017). Filamentous bacteriophage produced by *Pseudomonas aeruginosa* alters the inflammatory response and promotes noninvasive infection *in vivo*. *Infect. Immun.* 85: e00648-16. doi: 10.1128/IAI.00648-16

Shiels, S. M., Bedigrew, K. M., and Wenke, J. C. (2015). Development of a hematogenous implant-related infection in a rat model. *BMC Musculoskelet. Disord.* 16:255. doi: 10.1186/s12891-015-0699-7

Silva-Santana, G., Lenzi-Almeida, K. C., Lopes, V. G. S., and Aguiar-Alves, F. (2016). Biofilm formation in catheter-related infections by Panton-Valentine leukocidin-producing *Staphylococcus aureus*. *Int. Microbiol.* 19, 199–207. doi: 10.2436/20.1501.01.278

Snyder, D. T., Hedges, J. F., and Jutila, M. A. (2017). Getting "inside" type I IFNs: type I IFNs in intracellular bacterial infections. *J. Immunol. Res.* 2017:9361802. doi: 10.1155/2017/9361802

Sprangers, S., de Vries, T. J., and Everts, V. (2016). Monocyte heterogeneity: consequences for monocyte-derived immune cells. *J. Immunol. Res.* 2016:1475435. doi: 10.1155/2016/1475435

Sumaria, N., Roediger, B., Ng, L. G., Qin, J., Pinto, R., Cavanagh, L. L., et al. (2011). Cutaneous immunosurveillance by self-renewing dermal gammadelta T cells. *J. Exp. Med.* 208, 505–518. doi: 10.1084/jem.20101824

Tavares, J., Formaglio, P., Thiberge, S., Mordelet, E., Van Rooijen, N., Medvinsky, A., et al. (2013). Role of host cell traversal by the malaria sporozoite during liver infection. *J. Exp. Med.* 210, 905–915. doi: 10.1084/jem.20121130

Tay, S. S., Roediger, B., Tong, P. L., Tikoo, S., and Weninger, W. (2014). The skin-resident immune network. *Curr. Dermatol. Rep.* 3, 13–22. doi: 10.1007/s13671-013-0063-9

Teng, T.-S., Ji, A.-L., Ji, X.-Y., and Li, Y.-Z. (2017). Neutrophils and immunity: from bactericidal action to being conquered. *J. Immunol. Res.* 2017:9671604. doi: 10.1155/2017/9671604

Thurlow, L. R., Hanke, M. L., Fritz, T., Angle, A., Aldrich, A., Williams, S. H., et al. (2011). *Staphylococcus aureus* biofilms prevent macrophage phagocytosis and attenuate inflammation in vivo. *J. Immunol.* 1950, 6585–6596. doi: 10.4049/jimmunol.1002794

Tong, P. L., Roediger, B., Kolesnikoff, N., Biro, M., Tay, S. S., Jain, R., et al. (2015). The skin immune atlas: three dimensional analysis of cutaneous leukocyte subsets by multiphoton microscopy. *J. Invest. Dermatol.* 135, 84–93. doi: 10.1038/jid.2014.289

Torre, A., Bacconi, M., Sammicheli, C., Galletti, B., Laera, D., Fontana, M. R., et al. (2015). Four-component *Staphylococcus aureus* vaccine 4C-staph enhances Fcγ receptor expression in neutrophils and monocytes and mitigates *S. aureus* infection in neutropenic mice. *Infect. Immun.* 83, 3157–3163. doi: 10.1128/IAI.00258-15

Trøstrup, H., Thomsen, K., Christophersen, L. J., Hougen, H. P., Bjarnsholt, T., Jensen, P. Ø., et al. (2013). *Pseudomonas aeruginosa* biofilm aggravates skin inflammatory response in BALB/c mice in a novel chronic wound model. *Wound Repair Regen.* 21, 292–299. doi: 10.1111/wrr.12016

Valentini, M., and Filloux, A. (2016). Biofilms and cyclic di-GMP (c-di-GMP) signaling: lessons from *Pseudomonas aeruginosa* and other bacteria. *J. Biol. Chem.* 291, 12547–12555. doi: 10.1074/jbc.R115.711507

Valle, J., Solano, C., García, B., Toledo-Arana, A., and Lasa, I. (2013). Biofilm switch and immune response determinants at early stages of infection. *Trends Microbiol.* 21, 364–371. doi: 10.1016/j.tim.2013.05.008

Van Gennip, M., Christensen, L. D., Alhede, M., Qvortrup, K., Jensen, P. Ø., Høiby, N., et al. (2012). Interactions between polymorphonuclear leukocytes and *Pseudomonas aeruginosa* biofilms on silicone implants *in vivo*. *Infect. Immun.* 80, 2601–2607. doi: 10.1128/IAI.06215-11

van Gennip, M., Moser, C., Christensen, L. D., Bjarnsholt, T., Calum, H., Jensen, P. Ø., et al. (2009). Augmented effect of early antibiotic treatment in mice with experimental lung infections due to sequentially adapted mucoid strains of *Pseudomonas aeruginosa*. *J. Antimicrob. Chemother.* 64, 1241–1250. doi: 10.1093/jac/dkp352

Verdrengh, M., and Tarkowski, A. (1997). Role of neutrophils in experimental septicemia and septic arthritis induced by *Staphylococcus aureus*. *Infect. Immun.* 65, 2517–2521.

Vidlak, D., and Kielian, T. (2016). Infectious dose dictates the host response during *Staphylococcus aureus* orthopedic-implant biofilm infection. *Infect. Immun.* 84, 1957–1965. doi: 10.1128/IAI.00117-16

Voyich, J. M., Vuong, C., DeWald, M., Nygaard, T. K., Kocianova, S., Griffith, S., et al. (2009). The SaeR/S gene regulatory system is essential for innate immune evasion by *Staphylococcus aureus*. *J. Infect. Dis.* 199, 1698–1706. doi: 10.1086/598967

Wagner, C., Kondella, K., Bernschneider, T., Heppert, V., Wentzensen, A., and Hänsch, G. M. (2003). Post-traumatic osteomyelitis: analysis of inflammatory cells recruited into the site of infection. *Shock* 20, 503–510. doi: 10.1097/01.shk.0000093542.78705.e3

Wang, Y., Cheng, L. I., Helfer, D. R., Ashbaugh, A. G., Miller, R. J., Tzomides, A. J., et al. (2017). Mouse model of hematogenous implant-related *Staphylococcus aureus* biofilm infection reveals therapeutic targets. *Proc. Natl. Acad. Sci. U.S.A.* 114, E5094–E5102. doi: 10.1073/pnas.1703427114

Watters, C., DeLeon, K., Trivedi, U., Griswold, J. A., Lyte, M., Hampel, K. J., et al. (2013). *Pseudomonas aeruginosa* biofilms perturb wound resolution and antibiotic tolerance in diabetic mice. *Med. Microbiol. Immunol.* 202, 131–141. doi: 10.1007/s00430-012-0277-7

Watters, C., Everett, J. A., Haley, C., Clinton, A., and Rumbaugh, K. P. (2014). Insulin treatment modulates the host immune system to enhance *Pseudomonas aeruginosa* wound biofilms. *Infect. Immun.* 82, 92–100. doi: 10.1128/IAI.00651-13

Watters, C., Fleming, D., Bishop, D., and Rumbaugh, K. P. (2016). Host responses to biofilm. *Prog. Mol. Biol. Transl. Sci.* 142, 193–239. doi: 10.1016/bs.pmbts.2016.05.007

Yarwood, J. M., and Schlievert, P. M. (2003). Quorum sensing in *Staphylococcus* infections. *J. Clin. Invest.* 112, 1620–1625. doi: 10.1172/JCI20442

18

Role of Gut Microbiota on Cardio-Metabolic Parameters and Immunity in Coronary Artery Disease Patients with and without Type-2 Diabetes Mellitus

Lidia Sanchez-Alcoholado[1†], Daniel Castellano-Castillo[1,2†], Laura Jordán-Martínez[3], Isabel Moreno-Indias[1,2], Pilar Cardila-Cruz[3], Daniel Elena[3], Antonio J. Muñoz-Garcia[3], Maria I. Queipo-Ortuño[1,2] and Manuel Jimenez-Navarro[3]*

[1] Unidad de Gestión Clínica de Endocrinología y Nutrición, Instituto de Investigación Biomédica de Málaga, Hospital Universitario Virgen de la Victoria, Universidad de Málaga, Málaga, Spain, [2] CIBER Fisiopatología de la Obesidad y Nutrición, Instituto de Salud Carlos III, Madrid, Spain, [3] Unidad de Gestión Clínica Área del Corazón, Hospital Universitario Virgen de la Victoria, Instituto de Investigación Biomédica de Málaga, Universidad de Málaga, CIBERCV Enfermedades Cardiovasculares, Málaga, Spain

Correspondence:
Maria I. Queipo-Ortuño
maribelqo@gmail.com

† These authors have contributed equally to this work.

Gut microbiota composition has been reported as a factor linking host metabolism with the development of cardiovascular diseases (CVD) and intestinal immunity. Such gut microbiota has been shown to aggravate CVD by contributing to the production of trimethylamine *N*-oxide (TMAO), which is a pro-atherogenic compound. Treg cells expressing the transcription factor Forkhead box protein P3 (FoxP3) play an essential role in the regulation of immune responses to commensal microbiota and have an atheroprotective role. However, the aim of this study was to analyze the role of gut microbiota on cardio-metabolic parameters and immunity in coronary artery disease (CAD) patients with and without type-2 diabetes mellitus (DM2). The study included 16 coronary CAD-DM2 patients, and 16 age, sex, and BMI matched CAD patients without DM2 (CAD-NDM2). Fecal bacterial DNA was extracted and analyzed by sequencing in a GS Junior 454 platform followed by a bioinformatic analysis (QIIME and PICRUSt). The present study indicated that the diversity and composition of gut microbiota were different between the CAD-DM2 and CAD-NDM2 patients. The abundance of phylum *Bacteroidetes* was lower, whereas the phyla *Firmicutes* and *Proteobacteria* were higher in CAD-DM2 patients than those in the CAD-NDM2 group. CAD-DM2 patients had significantly less beneficial or commensal bacteria (such as *Faecalibacterium prausnitzii* and *Bacteroides fragilis*) and more opportunistic pathogens (such as *Enterobacteriaceae*, *Streptococcus*, and *Desulfovibrio).* Additionally, CAD-DM2 patients had significantly higher levels of plasma zonulin, TMAO, and IL-1B and significantly lower levels of IL-10 and FOXP3 mRNA expression than CAD-NDM2. Moreover, in the CAD-MD2 group, the increase in *Enterobacteriaceae* and the decrease in *Faecalibacterium prausnitzii* were significantly associated with the increase in serum TMAO levels, while the decrease in the abundance of *Bacteroides fragilis* was associated with the reduction in the FOXP3 mRNA expression, implicated in the development and function of Treg cells. These results suggest that the presence of DM2 is related to an impaired regulation of the immune system in CAD patients, mediated in part by the gut microbiota composition and functionality and the production and effects of their gut microbiota derived molecules.

Keywords: gut microbiota, coronary artery disease, zonulin levels, gut permeability increase, TMAO production, factor Forkhead box P3, type-2 diabetes mellitus, anti-inflammatory IL-10

INTRODUCTION

Previous studies have shown an important connection between metabolism, intestinal microbial composition and the development of cardiovascular risk (Tremaroli and Backhed, 2012; Tang and Hazen, 2014; Org et al., 2015). Several authors have strongly supported the contribution of intestinal microbiota in the conversion of L-carnitine and dietary phosphatidylcholine in trimethylamine (TMA), which is absorbed into the bloodstream and then oxidized to trimethylamine *N*-oxide (TMAO) (a pro-atherogenic compound) by the hepatic enzyme flavin-containing monooxygenase-3 (Ufnal et al., 2015; Stremmel et al., 2017). Independent of traditional CVD risk factors, this microbiota-dependent metabolite TMAO has been related with the development of clinical CVD in the general population (Koeth et al., 2013; Tang et al., 2013, 2014, 2015; Wang et al., 2014; Troseid et al., 2015). Furthermore, elevated TMAO plasma levels are associated with increased CVD (Wang et al., 2011; Tang et al., 2013, 2014; Koeth et al., 2014).

Nevertheless, the intestinal bacterial species responsible for phosphatidylcholine breakdown have not yet been completely described, however, some species of *Bacteroidetes* (such as, *B. thetaiotaomicron* and *B. fragilis*) may be involved in the formation of TMA since they express phospholipases which hydrolyse dietary phosphatidylcholine to choline (Sitaraman, 2013). In addition, it has been reported that bacteria of the Erysipelotrichia class (*Firmicutes* phylum) can produce TMA from choline whereby it imitates a choline deficiency (Serino et al., 2014), while several families of bacteria such as *Deferribacteraceae*, *Anaeroplasmataceae*, *Prevotellaceae* (Koeth et al., 2013), and *Enterobacteriaceae* (Craciun and Balskus, 2012; Zhu et al., 2014) have been also associated with TMA/TMAO production.

On the other hand, TMAO has also been suggested to be a strong candidate molecule to mediate the development of type-2 diabetes mellitus (DM2) in animal and human studies (Kim et al., 2015). Moreover, coronary artery disease (CAD) is an important determining factor of the long term prognosis among patients with DM2 and the prevalence of diabetes in patients with CAD is up to 50% in many countries. Patients with diabetes have a 2- to 4-fold greater risk of developing atherosclerotic CAD than non-diabetic patients (Aronson and Edelman, 2016; Hölscher et al., 2016). Accumulating evidence suggests that DM2 and cardiovascular diseases such as hypertension, atherosclerosis, or heart failure are associated with alterations in the integrity of the gut barrier and augmented gut permeability (Ufnal and Pham, 2017).

Finally, gut microbiota has been reported to be a factor that is able to link intestinal immunity and host metabolism. It has been suggested that the increase or decrease of the abundant quantities of some specific bacteria may result in an increased generation of Tregs or in the reduced differentiation of pathogenic T cells, which may prevent inflammatory diseases (Smith et al., 2013). Treg cells expressing the transcription factor Forkhead box protein P3 (FoxP3) play an essential role in the regulation of immune responses to commensal microbiota. Furthermore, metabolites of commensal bacteria might regulate Treg development (Pereira et al., 2017). The administration of *Bifidobacterium infantis* 35624 has been found to induce Foxp3 T regulatory cells in human peripheral blood (Konieczna et al., 2012). It has also been described that FOXP3 positive regulatory T cells play a crucial role in maintaining the immune balance having an atheroprotective role (Hasib et al., 2016).

Therefore, the aim of this study was to analyze the role of gut microbiota on cardio-metabolic parameters and immunity in CAD patients with and without DM2. Furthermore, we have also analyzed the association of the gut microbiota found in these patients with the glucose metabolism, inflammatory status, intestinal permeability, and serum levels of TMAO and FOXP3 gene expression in peripheral blood.

MATERIALS AND METHODS

Study Subjects

We included a total of 32 patients with CAD who were divided into two groups: 16 patients with DM2 (the CAD-DM2 group) and 16 patients without DM2 (the CAD-NDM2). The CAD group was defined by the presence of at least one coronary stenosis $\geq$50% of luminal diameter diagnosed by coronary angiogram. DM2 was defined by the history of diabetes diagnosed and/or the presence of treatment with medication (insulin or anti-diabetic drugs) and/or fasting blood glucose $\geq$126 mg/dl and/or glycated hemoglobin (HbA1c) $\geq$6.5%. Diabetic treatment of CAD patients with DM2 was the following: oral anti-diabetic (metformin $n = 8$ and glibenclamide $n = 3$) and insulin ($n = 5$).

All subjects underwent a complete physical examination, including measurements of height, weight, and blood pressure. The medical history of all patients was recorded, including the duration of diabetes, hypertension history, the history of taking anti-hypertensive and hypoglycemic drugs, and smoking history. The definition of systemic arterial hypertension was determined as a history of high blood pressure or treatment with anti-hypertensive medication. The definition of Dyslipidemia was determined as known but untreated dyslipidemia or currently undergoing treatment with lipid lowering medication. The family history of coronary heart disease was determined by interviewing the patients. The definition of a positive smoking history was determined as current smokers or cessation of smoking within the previous 3 months before the start of the study.

The following were considered as exclusion criteria: acute inflammatory disease, severe infective disease and/or cancer, chronic kidney disease (GFR < 45 mL/min/1.73 m^2), hepatic impairment and autoimmune disease. This study was carried out in accordance with the recommendations of the Ethical Committee of the Virgen de la Victoria Hospital. Written informed consent was obtained in all cases in accordance with the Declaration of Helsinki. The protocol was approved by the Ethical Committee of the Virgen de la Victoria Hospital.

Biochemical Variable Analysis

Serum was separated from blood samples which were collected after an overnight fast, aliquoted and immediately frozen at −80°C. Enzymatic methods (Randox Laboratories Ltd., United Kingdom) were employed to analyze the levels of serum cholesterol, triglycerides, HDL-cholesterol, glucose, and glycated hemoglobin (HbA1c) using a Dimension autoanalyzer (Dade Behring Inc., Deerfield, IL, United States). The Friedewald equation was used to calculate LDL-cholesterol. Standard enzymatic methods (Wako Bioproducts, Richmond, VA, United States) were used to measure gamma-glutamyl transpeptidase (GGT), glutamate-oxaloacetate transaminase (GOT), and glutamic pyruvic transaminase (GPT). RIA provided by BioSource S.A. (Nivelles, Belgium) was utilized for insulin quantification. The ELISA kit from BLK Diagnostics (Badalona, Spain) was employed to measure high sensitivity C-reactive protein (CRP) levels. To calculate the HOMA-IR we used the equation: HOMA-IR = fasting insulin (mIU/mL)/fasting glucose (mol/L)/22.5.

IL-10 and IL-1β cytokines were measured in serum samples using commercially available Novex® ELISA Kits (Life Technology), performed according to the manufacturer's instructions. The assay range was 7.8–500 pg/mL for IL-10 and 3.9–250 pg/mL for IL-1β.

Anthropometric Measures

Standardized procedures were used to measure body weight, height, waist, and hip circumferences (Lohman et al., 1988). BMI was calculated as weight (kilograms) divided by height (in meters) squared.

PCR Amplification and Analysis of 16S rDNA Sequences

DNA was extracted from fecal samples using the QIAamp DNA Stool Mini Kit (Qiagen, Hilden, Germany) following the manufacturer's protocol. Amplification of genomic DNA was performed using barcoded primers that targeted the V2 to V3 regions of the bacterial 16S rRNA gene. Amplification, sequencing, and basic analysis were performed by using a GS Junior 454 platform according to the manufacturer's protocols using a Titanium chemistry apparatus (Roche Applied Science, Indianapolis, IN, United States). For further details, see Moreno-Indias et al. (2015).

Bioinformatic Analysis

Quantitative Insights into Microbial Ecology (QIIME) 1.8.0 software was used to analyze the 454-pyrosequencing data sets as previously described by our group (Moreno-Indias et al., 2015). Raw reads were filtered first following the 454 amplicon processing pipeline. The pyrosequencing reads were de-multiplexed and filtered further by means of the split_library.py script of QIIME. Reads with an average quality score lower than 25, ambiguous base calls, primer mismatches or shorter than 100 bp were excluded from the analysis in order to increase the level of accuracy. After the quality filter, the pipeline analysis used to analyze the 16S gene reads was the following: sequences were denoised and singletons excluded. The operational taxonomic units (OTUs) were selected by clustering sequences with a similarity of >97% and the representative sequences, selected as the most abundant in each cluster, were passed on to the UCLUST to obtain the taxonomy assignment and the relative abundance of each OTU by means of using the Greengenes 16S rRNA gene database. QIIME was used to evaluate alpha and beta diversity, as described (De Filippis et al., 2013).

PICRUSt Analysis

The PICRUSt analysis was used to predict metagenome function by picking OTUs against the Greengenes database.[1] As has been previously described by Bhute et al. (2016), "a closed reference based OTU picking approach was utilized to bin the amplicon sequences using latest Greengenes database 13.5 at 97% sequence similarity cut-off. The normalization for 16S rRNA gene copy number was carried out before prediction of the metagenome. This OTU table was used for predicting metagenome at different KEGG levels." The R packages "pheatmap" were used for data analysis and plotting. Statistical analysis was done in R 3.3.3. *P*-values were corrected for multiple comparisons using the Benjamini–Hochberg method. A corrected $p < 0.05$ was considered as statistically significant.

Intestinal Permeability

The plasma level of zonulin was determined by means of the enzyme linked immunosorbent assay (ELISA) using commercial kits (Immundiagnostik AG, Bensheim, Germany). Measurements were made in duplicate, and the mean values were used for the analysis. The detection limit for zonulin was established at 0.22 ng/mL. Intra- and inter-assay coefficients of variation were between 3 and 10%.

Total RNA Extraction, cDNA Synthesis, and Real-Time Quantitative PCR (qRT-PCR)

The total RNA was extracted from peripheral blood mononuclear cells using TRIPURE Reagent (Sigma–Aldrich, United States) according to the manufacturer's protocol. RNA was diluted

[1] http://huttenhower.sph.harvard.edu/galaxy/

in 20 μl RNase-free water and was subsequently quantified with a spectrophotometer (Nanodrop N-100, Thermo Scientific). Reverse transcriptions were performed using 1 μg of total RNA with the Transcriptor First Strand cDNA Synthesis Kit (Roche) and random hexamers in 20 μl reactions. The amplifications were performed by means of a MicroAmpH Optical 96-well reaction plate (Applied Biosystems, Foster City, CA, United States) on an ABI 7500 Fast Real-Time PCR System (Applied Biosystems, Foster City, CA, United States). Pre-validated and commercially available TaqMan® primer/probe sets were used as follows: 18S rRNA (4319413E) used as the endogenous control for the target gene in each reaction and FOXP3 gene (RefSeq NM_001114377.1). A threshold cycle (*Ct* value) was obtained for each amplification curve and a ΔCt value was calculated first by subtracting the *Ct* value for human 18S rRNA cDNA from the *Ct* value for every sample and transcript. mRNA expression levels relative to 18S rRNA were calculated by means of the $2^{-\Delta Ct}$ method. All tests were performed in duplicate.

Quantification TMAO in Serum Samples

Trimethylamine *N*-oxide was quantified in serum samples using Nuclear Magnetic Resonance (NMR) (Embade et al., 2016). For NMR analysis, serum samples were thawed for 30 min and aliquots of 300 μL were mixed with 300 μL of phosphate buffer (pH 7.0) containing 5 mmol/L TSP (Trimethylsilyl propionate) and 5% v/v D2O. The final mixtures were gently shaken and transferred to NMR 96 rack tubes. NMR spectra were measured at 300 K on a Bruker Avance IVDr 600 MHz spectrometer (Bruker Biospin, Germany) and a Sample Jet Robot (Bruker Biospin, Germany) was used for automatization of the measurements. For each sample, three complementary NMR spectra were recorded. A standard ^1H spectrum with water suppression (NOESY) was assessed. We repeated the same experiment with an appended T2 relaxation filter implemented as a CPMG module to decrease broad signals from proteins and lipoproteins. Finally, a two dimensional $^1H,^1H$ JRES was measured to help with the identification of the metabolites. All spectra were acquired and processed within the TopSpin program (Bruker Biospin, Germany) applying an automatic phase correction and referenced against internal TSP ($\delta = 0.00$ ppm). To identify and quantify the desired metabolites (TMAO) different amounts of these compounds were added to the serum samples, were measured by NMR and the values of the intensity peaks were represented against concentration. The pure metabolite molecules used for referencing were all obtained from Sigma–Aldrich (St. Louis, MO, United States). For all the spectra we measured the intensity of the peaks corresponding to TMAO (singlets) and the concentrations in the samples were calculated with the power fitted calibration curves.

Statistical Analysis

Given that there are no previous studies assessing gut microbiota differences between patients with CAD with or without DM2, we have based our sample size estimation on a previous paper from Emoto et al. (2016). To calculate the sample size, we considered a difference in the mean relative abundance of *Bacteroidetes* between CAD patients and non-CAD controls with coronary risk factors of 0.084 and an estimated standard deviation between groups of 0.05, at least 9 patients in each study group were needed (90% power and a two-sided alpha level of 0.05). However, we increased the sample size to 16 samples per group.

The relative abundance of each OTU (taxa) were compared by a Wilcoxon test with a continuity correction using the Explicit software package specifically addressed to analyze microbiome data. α- and β-diversities were achieved by QIIME: α-diversity using a non-parametric *t*-test with a default number of Monte Carlo permutations of 999, and β-diversity using the ANOSIM statistical method with 99 permutations (Moreno-Indias et al., 2015). Continuous variables are summarized as mean ± SD. Discrete variables are presented as frequencies and percentages. Differences in clinical characteristics between two groups were analyzed using the Mann–Whitney *U* test. The Spearman correlation coefficients were calculated to estimate the correlations between variables. A lineal regression analysis was performed to identify individual bacteria as independent predictors for HOMA-IR, levels of inflammatory mediators, serum TMAO and plasma zonulin levels and relative expression of FOXP3 in the study groups. Statistical analyses were carried out with the statistical software package SPSS version 15.0 (SPSS Inc., Chicago, IL, United States). Values were considered to be statistically significant when the $p < 0.05$.

RESULTS

The general characteristics of the patients in both study groups are summarized in **Table 1**. There were no significant differences in age, sex, and body mass index (BMI) between the two study groups. The number of patients with dyslipidemia and hypertension was significantly higher in CAD-DM2 patients when compared with the CAD-NM2 patients. Triglyceride, glucose, and HbA1C were significantly higher and HDL-cholesterol was significantly lower in CAD-DM2 patients when compared with CAD-NM2 ($P < 0.05$). There was no significant difference in serum total cholesterol and LDL-cholesterol between the two study groups ($P > 0.05$). CAD-DM2 patients had significantly higher levels of inflammatory markers IL-1B and significantly lower levels of anti-inflammatory IL-10 when compared with non-diabetic patients. TMAO plasma levels were also significantly increased in CAD-DM2 patients when compared with CAD-NDM2 ($P < 0.05$). Finally, FOXP3 mRNA expression in PBMC was significantly lower (2.9-fold decrease) in CAD-DM2 patients when compared with CAD-NDM2 ($p < 0.001$).

Analysis of the Diversity and Similarity of Microbial Communities in the Study Patients

A total of 249.815 good quality 16S rRNA gene sequences with an average of 11.895 ± 6527 sequences per sample passed the filters, which were applied by means of QIIME. In order to obtain a detailed structural overview of the microbiome of each subject who was enrolled in this study, an analysis of OTU was developed. The microbiota of all fecal samples after QIIME was composed by 2701 OTUS with a relative abundance higher than 1% in at least two samples (97% similarity cut-off).

Before assessing alpha and beta diversity measures, samples were rarefied to 3119 sequences, which represents the lowest number of quality reads which were obtained from any individual sample in the data set. The CAD-DM2 group had a lower number of OTUs than the CAD no-diabetic group (mean = 925 versus 987, $P < 0.05$, respectively).

The Chao index and Shannon index were calculated to estimate the alpha diversity. The average of community richness (Chao 1) and Shannon index of each group suggested a significant decrease in bacterial richness and diversity in fecal samples of CAD-DM2 with respect to CAD-NDM2 ($P = 0.036$ and $P < 0.001$, respectively) (**Table 2**). The rarefaction curve of the OTUs observed started to plateau at approximately 100 reads which suggests that a greater number of reads per sample would not have supplied a more extensive catalog of bacterial taxa.

Principal coordinate analysis (PCoA) plots based on unweighted UniFrac metrics was used to evaluate the beta diversity. The present study showed that apart from a few samples from both study groups closer together in the ordination, a separation between the samples from the diabetic group and the non-diabetic group could be observed from PC1 and PC2 scores that accounted for 22.08 and 24.39% of total variations. ANOSIM with permutations suggested that the intestinal microflora composition of these two groups is significantly different ($P = 0.039$) (**Figure 1**).

TABLE 1 | Biochemical, clinical characteristics, TMAO and inflammatory mediators serum levels and PBMC relative expression of FOXP3 in both study groups.

	CAD-DM2 $N = 16$	CAD-NDM2 $N = 16$	P*
Age (years)	61.63 ± 9.15	58.75 ± 8.15	0.355
Gender, *n* (M/F)	13/3	13/3	0.652
BMI (kg/m^2)	31.89 ± 6.04	29.23 ± 3.28	0.132
Risk factors, *n* (%)			
Hypertension	13 (81.25%)	7 (43.75%)	0.070
Dyslipidemia	10 (62.5%)	4 (25%)	0.075
Diabetes	16 (100%)	0 (0)	<0.001
Current smoking	13 (81.25%)	12 (75%)	0.999
CVA	1 (6.25%)	1 (6.25%)	0.715
Medication, *n* (%)			
Aspirin	10 (62.5%)	6 (37.5%)	0.289
Statin	7 (43.75%)	4 (25%)	0.457
ACEI/ARB	8 (50%)	6 (37.5%)	0.722
Beta-blocker	10 (62.5%)	8 (50%)	0.722
Biochemical data			
Total cholesterol (mg/dl)	179.0 ± 30.28	163.63 ± 29.05	0.153
HDL cholesterol (mg/dl)	28.68 ± 7.32	36.81 ± 8.68	0.008
LDL cholesterol (mg/dl)	104.7 ± 22.42	98.85 ± 23.51	0.192
Triglycerides (mg/dl)	200.37 ± 32.57	136.39 ± 35.9	0.001
HbA1c	7.70 ± 1.35	5.05 ± 0.56	0.001
Glucose (mg/dl)	153.40 ± 13.69	100.42 ± 16.02	0.001
HOMA-IR	9.91 ± 2.89	3.89 ± 0.98	0.001
GOT (U/l)	34.25 ± 6.70	30.21 ± 5.77	0.078
GPT (U/l)	45.0 ± 8.05	41.68 ± 6.60	0.135
GGT (U/l)	47.27 ± 16.00	44.20 ± 13.84	0.566
CRP (mg/L)	9.65 ± 1.59	9.50 ± 2.82	0.854
TMAO (ng/ml)	31.64 ± 8.5	16.26 ± 5.42	0.001
IL-1B (pg/ml)	120.41 ± 39.75	90.75 ± 37.23	0.037
IL-10 (pg/ml)	134.32 ± 36.24	162.31 ± 34.75	0.033
Foxp3 relative expression	0.27 ± 0.07	0.80 ± 0.15	<0.001

*BMI, body mass index; CVA, cerebrovascular accident; ACEI, angiotensin converting enzyme inhibitor; ARB, angiotensin II receptor blocker; LDL, low density lipoprotein; HDL, high density lipoprotein; HbA1c, glycated hemoglobin; GGT, gamma-glutamyl transferase; GOT, glutamic oxaloacetic transaminase; GPT, glutamic pyruvic transaminase, TMAO: trimethylamine N-oxide; L-1β, interleukin-1β; CRP, C-reactive protein; Foxp3, Forkhead box P3. Values are expressed as mean ± SD. *P < 0.05.*

16S rRNA Gene Pyrosequencing in Fecal Samples from CAD-DM2 and CAD-NDM2 Patients

In this study, variations in the composition of fecal microbiota of CAD-DM2 and CAD-NDM2 groups were observed at different bacterial levels. At the phyla level the majority of the OTUS were found to belong to *Bacteroidetes* (53.87% CAD-DM2 vs. 63.42% CAD-NDM2, $P < 0.001$), *Firmicutes* was the next most abundant (25.69% CAD-DM2 vs. 23.29% CAD-NDM2, $P = 0.49$) followed by *Proteobacterias* (3.67% CAD-DM2 vs. 2.05% CAD-NDM2, $P = 0.04$), but only *Bacteroidetes* and *Proteobacterias* exhibited significant differences between both, the CAD-DM2 and the CAD-NDM2 study groups. The remaining bacterial population belonged to the other four phyla (*Fusobacteria, Actinobacteria, Verrucomicrobia,* and *Tenericutes*) that had a relative abundance lower than 1% in at least two samples (**Figure 2**).

Twenty-two families were detected among all groups. We found a significant increase in *Veillonellaceae* (28.93% CAD-DM2 vs. 16.97% CAD-NDM2, $P < 0.001$), *Enterobacteriaceae* (19.53% CAD-DM2 vs. 4.73% CAD-NDM2, $P = 0.016$), *Rikenellaceae* (11.13% CAD-DM2 vs. 9.92% CAD-NDM2, $P = 0.023$, *Streptococcaceae* (6.64% CAD-DM2 vs. 2.55% CAD-NDM2, $P < 0.001$), and *Desulfovibrionaceae* (13.95% CAD-DM2 vs. 10.69% CAD-NDM2, $P < 0.001$) in CAD-DM2 group. Furthermore, a significant decrease in the abundance was found in CAD-DM2 when compared with CAD-NDM2 for *Bacteroidaceae* (49.02% CAD-DM2 vs. 60.48% CAD-NDM2, $P < 0.001$), *Lachnospiraceae* (14.67% CAD-DM2 vs. 20.56% CAD-NDM2, $P < 0.001$), *Prevotellaceae* (5.06% CAD-DM2 vs. 8.85% CAD-NDM2, $P = 0.05$), *S24-7* (1.59% CAD-DM2 vs. 2.38% CAD-NDM2, $P = 0.023$, $P < 0.001$),

TABLE 2 | Estimate richness (Chao1) and diversity index (Shannon) indices among microbial communities obtained from fecal samples from CAD-DM2 and CAD-NDM2 patients.

	CAD-DM2 patients ($n = 16$)	CAD-NDM2 patients ($n = 16$)	P*
Chao 1	374.01 ± 50.52	328.37 ± 66.20	0.036
Shannon	4.59 ± 0.68	5.90 ± 0.57	<0.001

*The richness estimator Chao and diversity estimator Shannon were calculated at 3% distance. *P < 0.05.*

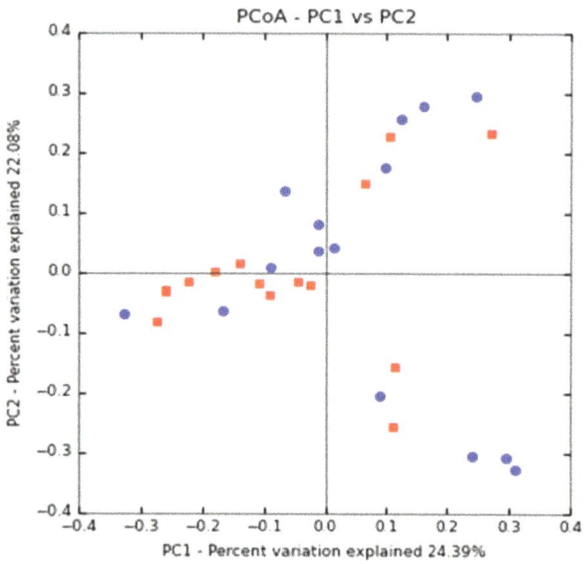

FIGURE 1 | Clustering of fecal bacterial communities according to the different study groups by principal coordinate analysis (PCoA) using unweighted UniFrac distances. Each point corresponds to a community coded according to the patient group. The percentage of variation explained by the plotted principal coordinates is indicated on the axes. CAD-DM2 (red dots) and CAD-NDM2 (blue dots).

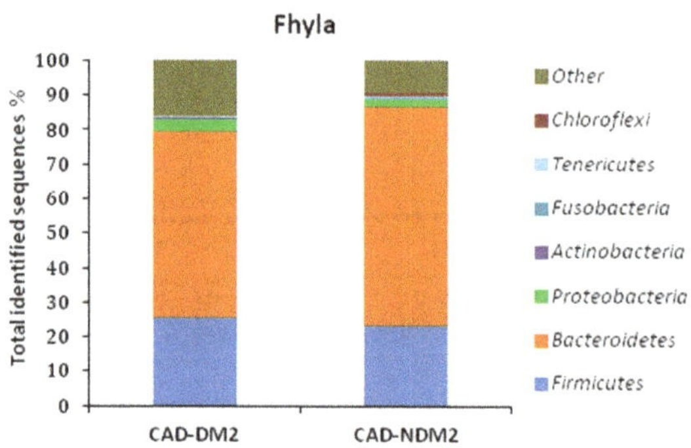

FIGURE 2 | Pyrosequencing analysis of phyla in CAD-DM2 and CAD-NDM2 groups. Data are shown as a percentage of the total identified sequences per group.

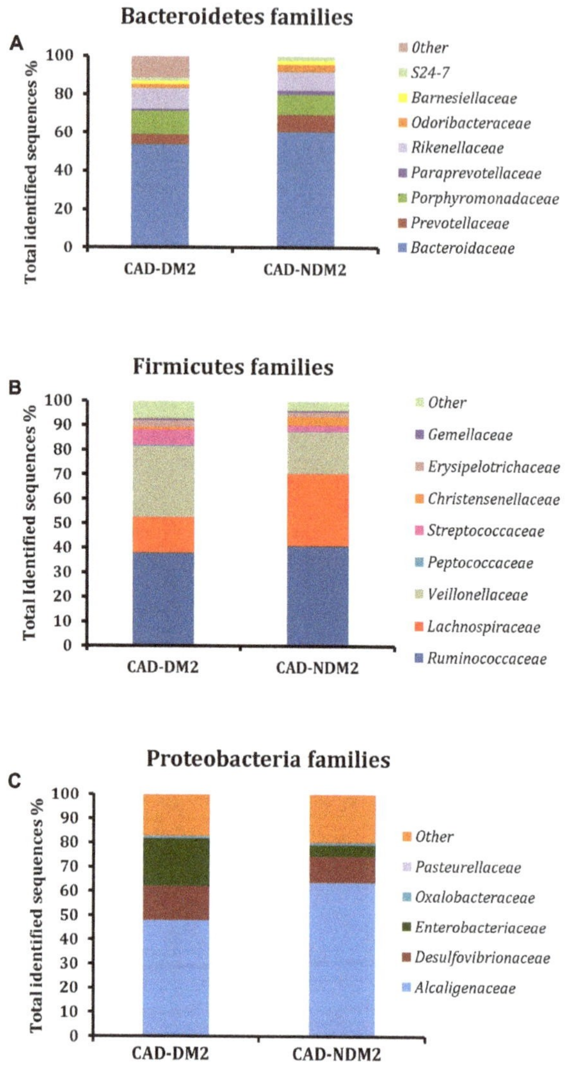

FIGURE 3 | Microbial community structure at the family level using 454 sequence data in fecal samples of CAD-DM2 and CAD-NDM2 patients. Data are shown as a percentage of the total identified sequences per group. **(A)** Bacteroidetes families; **(B)** Firmicutes families and **(C)** Proteobacteria families.

Odoribacteraceae (1.90% CAD-DM2 vs. 3.57% CAD-NDM2, $P = 0.02$), and *Paraprevotellaceae* (0.79% CAD-DM2 vs. 1.81% CAD-NDM2, $P < 0.05$). In addition, no significant differences between the two study groups were found in other abundant families, such as *Ruminococcaceae* (37.87% CAD-DM2 vs. 40.91% CAD-NDM2, $P > 0.05$), *Alcaligenaceae* (48.10% CAD-DM2 vs. 63.63% CAD-NDM2, $P > 0.05$), *Porphyromonadaceae* (12.38% CAD-DM2 vs. 11.02% CAD-NDM2, $P > 0.05$), and *Erysipelotrichaceae* (2.63% CAD-DM2 vs. 1.75% CAD-NDM2, $P > 0.05$) (**Figure 3**).

Significant differences between the study groups were also found in the microbial composition at the genus level. A total of 40 genera were identified among the 32 fecal samples, with only significant differences in eight genera between the CAD-DM2 and the CAD-NDM2 groups. Thus, the genera *Enterobacter*, *Streptococcus*, *Dialister*, *Megasphaera*, and *Desulfovibrio* were significantly higher in the CAD-DM2 group when compared with the CAD-NDM2 group. On the other hand, we found in the CAD-NDM2 group a significant rise in the abundance of *Bacteroides*, *Faecalibacterium*, and *Prevotella* when compared with the CAD-DM2 patients. No significant differences in the abundance of *Sutterella*, *Phascolarctobacterium*, *Parabacteroides*, *Oscillospira*, *Roseburia*, *Ruminococcus*, *Odoribacter*, *Blautia*, and other minority genera were found between the two study groups (**Table 3** and **Figure 4**).

At a specie levels, we found a significant decrease in the abundance of *Bacteroides fragilis* (0.43% CAD-DM2 vs. 1.38% CAD-NDM2, $P < 0.05$), *Bacteroides ovatus* (0.99% CAD-DM2 vs.

1.86% CAD-NDM2, $P < 0.05$), and *Faecalibacterium prausnitzii* (2.03% CAD-DM2 vs. 3.72% CAD-NDM2, $P < 0.05$) in the CAD-DM2 group when compared with the CAD-NDM2 patients.

Increased Circulating Zonulin Levels in CAD-DM2 Patients

The circulating zonulin levels were measured by means of the ELISA method. In the CAD-DM2 patients, circulating zonulin levels were significantly higher than in CAD-NDM2 patients (5.98 ± 1.4 vs. 3.34 ± 1.6 ng/ml, $P < 0.001$).

Relationship between the Gut Microbiota Composition and Glucose Metabolism, Serum Levels of Inflammatory Mediators, Serum TMAO and Plasma Zonulin Levels and Relative Expression of FOXP3

In the CAD-DM2 patients, *Firmicutes* was positively correlated with HbA1c and fasting triglycerides ($r = 0.849$, $P = 0.030$, and $r = 0.648$, $P = 0.043$, respectively) and *Proteobacteria* was positively correlated with HOMA-IR ($r = 0.754$, $P = 0.012$), while *Bacteroidetes* was negatively associated with HOMA-IR ($r = -0.849$, $P = 0.03$). The abundance of *Streptococcus* was negatively associated with the serum HDL-cholesterol levels ($r = -0.728$, $P = 0.017$). We also confirmed a positive association between serum TMAO and the abundance of *Enterobacteriaceae* ($r = 0.711$, $P = 0.021$) and *Desulfovibrio* ($r = 0.849$, $P = 0.03$) and a negative association between TMAO and the abundance of the common gut commensals *Faecalibacterium prausnitzii* ($r = -0.681$, $P = 0.030$) and *Ruminococcaceae* ($r = -0.699$, $P = 0.04$). Likewise, the abundance of *Faecalibacterium prausnitzii* was negatively associated with plasma zonulin ($r = -0.642$, $P = 0.045$) and was positively associated with serum IL-10 levels ($r = 0.663$, $P = 0.037$). Finally, FOXP3 mRNA expression in PBMC was positively associated with the abundance of *Bacteroides fragilis* ($r = 0.742$, $P = 0.037$) and *Butyricimonas* ($r = 0.717$, $P = 0.020$).

In CAD-NDM2 patients, plasma zonulin levels were positively associated with the abundance of *Prevotella* ($r = 0.681$, $P = 0.030$) and *Rikenellaceae* ($r = 0.669$, $P = 0.035$), while serum TMAO was positively associated with *Bacteroides* ($r = 0.742$, $P = 0.014$) and negatively related to *Faecalibacterium prausnitzii* ($r = -0.669$, $P = 0.035$). Furthermore, there was a positive association between IL-10 and *Bifidobacterium* ($r = 0.794$, $P = 0.006$).

Subsequent lineal regression analysis including all the bacterial groups showed that the increase in *Proteobacterias* ($p = 0.029$, $\beta = 0.548$, $r^2 = 0.83$) was associated with the higher HOMA-IR found in CAD-DM2. On the other hand, in the CAD-DM2 group the increase in *Enterobacteriaceae* ($p = 0.005$, $\beta = 0.945$, $r^2 = 0.96$) and the decrease in *Faecalibacterium prausnitzii* ($p = 0.041$, $\beta = -0.911$, $r^2 = 0.91$) were associated with the increase in serum TMAO levels, while the decrease in the abundance of *Bacteroides fragilis* ($p = 0.039$, $\beta = 0.911$, $r^2 = 0.91$) was associated with the reduction in the FOXP3 mRNA expression.

TABLE 3 | Complete list of genus level microbial abundance (OTUs) in both study groups.

Genus	Average bacteria abundance (OTUs) %		
	CAD-DM2 $N = 16$	CAD-NDM2 $N = 16$	P^*
Enterobacter	14.25	8.29	0.03
Streptococcus	6.64	2.55	<0.001
Dialister	4.88	1.26	<0.001
Megasphaera	3.61	2.10	0.001
Desulfovibrio	3.23	1.85	0.001
Bacteroides	59.02	65.48	<0.001
Faecalibacterium	6.13	12.29	0.01
Prevotella	0.35	1.33	0.03
Sutterella	63.68	48.10	>0.05
Phascolarctobacterium	14.27	11.50	>0.05
Parabacteroides	12.20	11.55	>0.05
Oscillospira	6.39	5.10	>0.05
Roseburia	5.95	7.63	>0.05
Ruminococcus	3.28	3.51	>0.05
Odoribacter	1.43	2.72	>0.05
Blautia	1.05	2.12	>0.05

Data are shown as a percentage of the total identified sequences per group.
$^*P < 0.05$.

Functional Differences in Gut Microbiota between Both Study Groups

The PICRUSt analysis indicated that the genes for the metabolism of carbohydrates, lipids, amino acids, and energy were significantly over represented in CAD-NDM2 in comparision with CAD-DM2 ($P < 0.05$). Moreover, in the microbiota of CAD-NDM2 patients, we found inside the carbohydrate metabolism, significantly enriched for the proportion of genes related to glycolysis/gluconeogénesis ($P = 0.036$), pyruvate metabolism ($P = 0.029$), inositol phosphate metabolism ($P = 0.027$), pentose phosphate pathway ($P = 0.016$), propanoate metabolism ($P = 0.020$), butanoate metabolism ($P = 0.023$), and starch and sucrose metabolism ($P = 0.016$), additionally, in the lipid metabolism pathways we observed an increase in the proportions of genes for fatty acid biosynthesis ($P = 0.013$), fatty acid metabolism ($P = 0.021$), glycerophospholipid metabolism ($P = 0.036$), sphingolipid metabolism ($P = 0.008$), biosynthesis of unsaturated fatty acids ($P = 0.020$), and secondary bile acid metabolism ($P = 0.005$).

Furthermore, the metagenomic comparison between CAD-DM2 and CAD-NDM2 groups showed that gene families linked to amino acid metabolism [including the metabolism of glycine ($P = 0.022$), alanine ($P = 0.043$), and glutamine ($P = 0.029$)] and energy metabolism such as sulfur ($P = 0.036$) and nitrogen metabolism ($P = 0.016$) were significantly depleted in the CAD-DM2 group.

Finally, the microbiota from CAD-NDM2 patients were also significantly more enriched with genes for antigen processing and presentation ($P = 0.006$) and siderophore biosynthesis ($P = 0.036$) when compared with CAD-DM2 patients (**Figure 5**).

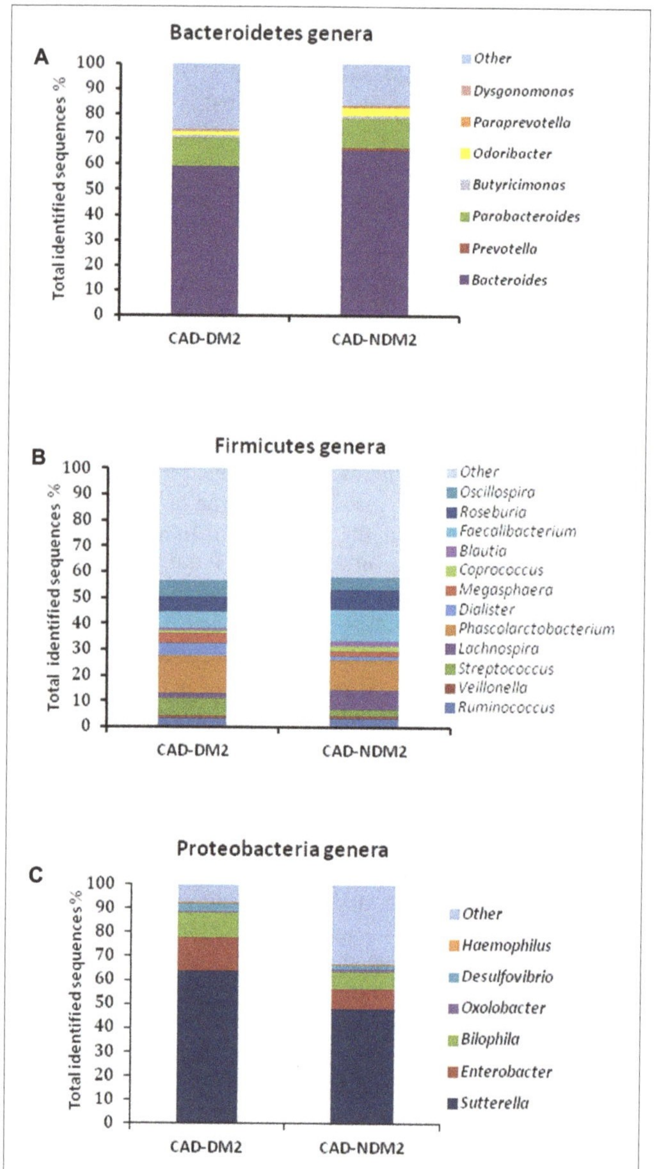

FIGURE 4 | Relative abundance of predominant genera in the microbiota of CAD-DM2 and CAD-NDM2 patients. Data are shown as a percentage of the total identified sequences per group. **(A)** Bacteroidetes genera; **(B)** Firmicutes genera and **(C)** Proteobacteria genera.

DISCUSSION

The present study in which we used 16S ribosomal RNA of gut microbiota for high throughput sequencing has demonstrated that the diversity and gut microbial composition were different between CAD-DM2 and CAD-NDM2. We also observed that the CAD-DM2 patients had significantly higher levels of zonulin, TMAO, and IL-1B and significantly lower levels of IL-10 and FOXP3 mRNA expression than CAD-NDM2.

Microbiota diversity is essential to maintain ecosystem stability and efficiency. The α-diversity analysis in this study showed that the Shannon and Chao 1 indices were significantly lower in the CAD-DM2 patient group when compared with the CAD-NDM2 group. These data revealed that bacterial communities in diabetic patients with CAD had lower taxa richness than those in the non-diabetic group. These results may suggest that the decrease in gut microbiota diversity in CAD-DM2 patients might be related to the presence of DM2. In addition, the unweighted UniFrac PCoA plot analysis indicated a clustering of the microbial populations of the CAD-DM2 patients away from that of the CAD-NDM2, confirming that the presence of DM2 in patients with CAD can significantly alter intestinal microbial populations.

On the other hand, the taxonomy based analysis of the assigned sequences showed that the presence of DM2 in patients from CAD is related to a decrease in the phylum *Bacteroidetes* and an increase in the phyla *Firmicutes* and *Proteobacteria*. Moreover, at genera level the CAD-DM2 patients had more opportunistic pathogens such as *Enterobacteriaceae*, *Megasphaera*, *Streptococcus*, *Dialister*, and *Desulfovibrio*, and lower beneficial or commensal bacteria including *Bacteroides* (*Bacteroides fragilis*), *Faecalibacterium* (*Faecalibacterium prausnitzii*), and *Prevotella* when compared with CAD-NDM2. Previous studies using terminal restriction fragment length polymorphism (T-RFLP) analysis demonstrated a decrease in the phylum *Bacteroidetes* and an increase in the phylum *Firmicutes* in CAD patients when compared with healthy subjects. Moreover, they observed that the order Lactobacillales, in which *Streptococcus* genus is included, was significantly increased in the CAD group when compared with healthy subjects (Emoto et al., 2016, 2017). Cui et al. (2017) revealed that the phyla *Bacteroidetes* and *Proteobacteria* were decreased, while the phyla *Firmicutes* and *Fusobacteria* were increased in coronary heart disease patients when compared with healthy controls by high throughput sequencing. In our study, the significant decrease in the phylum *Bacteroidetes* and the increase in the abundance of the phylum *Proteobacteria* in the CAD-DM2 group possibly reflected the fact of suffering from DM2, one of the major risk factors for CAD.

After using PICRUSt, we were able to predict that the gut microbiome of CAD-DM2 patients showed a depletion in genes involved in metabolic functions such as the metabolism of carbohydrates, lipids, amino acids, and energy as well as in genes of antigen processing and presentation related to inflammation and immune response and siderophore biosynthesis. The enrichment in this siderophore pathway could suggest a higher intra- or inter-species communication in CAD-NDM2 patients, due to the fact that siderophore act as quorum sensing molecules for gram-negative organisms (McHardy et al., 2013). These results indicate that the presence of DM2 in CAD patients may also influence the functional diversity.

Koren et al. (2011) compared the microbiota among the gut, oral cavities, and the atherosclerotic plaque in patients with aterosclerosis. This study suggested that the bacteria which is present in the atherosclerotic plaque may be derived from the gut or the oral cavities (Koren et al., 2011). Furthermore, the gut microbiota is essential to bioconvert cholesterol into bile acids, which are necessary for the excretion and the absorption of cholesterol (Fagerberg et al., 2010). Thus, the significantly

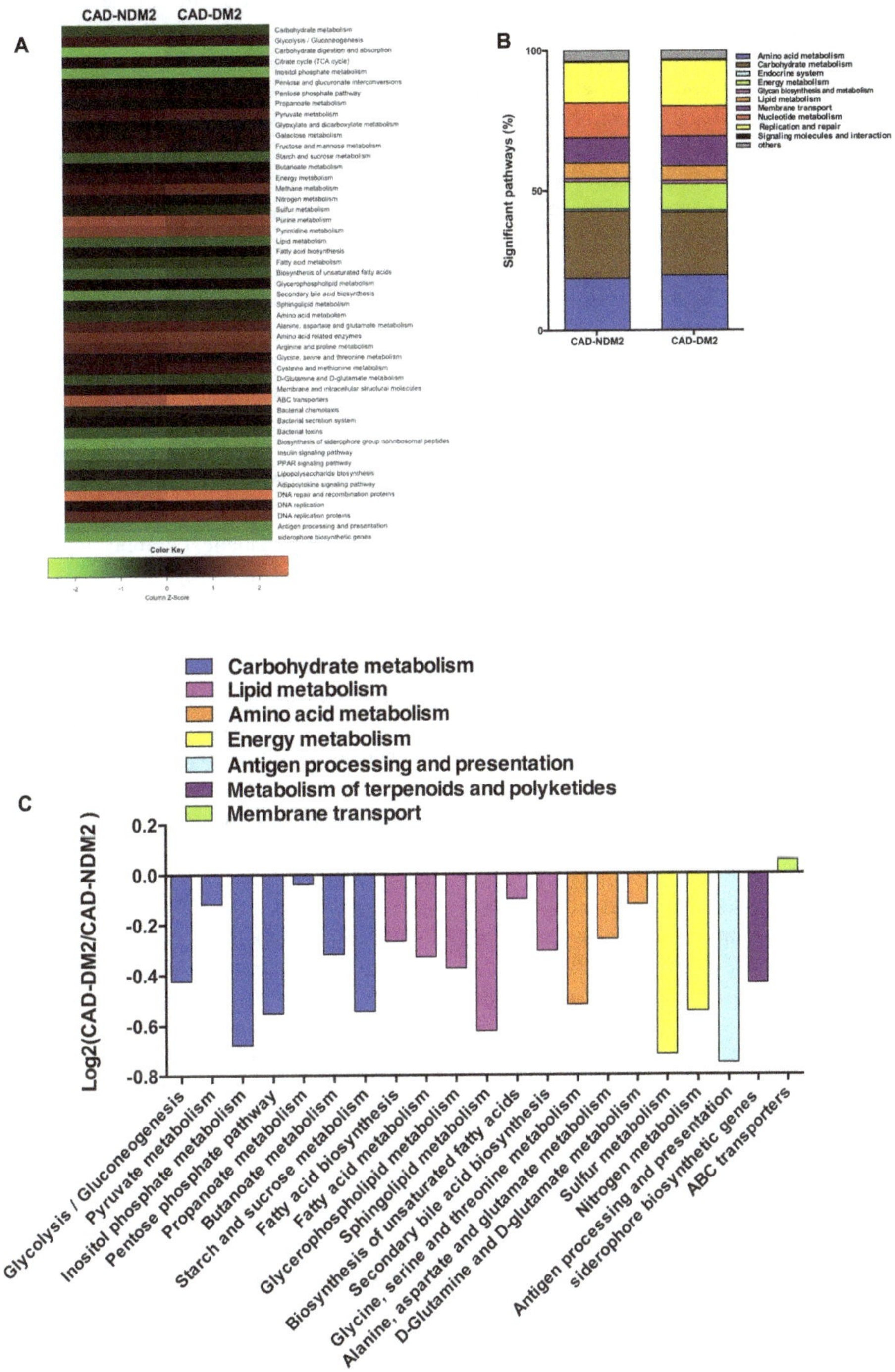

FIGURE 5 | Predicted functional composition of metagenomes based on 16S rRNA gene sequencing data of CAD-DM2 and CAD-NDM2 groups. **(A)** Heatmap of differentially abundant KEGG pathways identified in both study groups. The values of color in the heatmap represent the normalized relative abundance of KEGG pathways. **(B)** Relative abundances of significant predicted functions of each study group. **(C)** Log2-fold change of the abundances of KEGG categories showing significant difference between CAD-DM2 and CAD-NDM2 groups.

higher levels of *Streptococcus* (a common oral and gut taxón) found in CAD-DM2 patients when compared with CAD-NDM2 patients, which were negatively correlated with HDL cholesterol levels in these diabetic patients, could be influencing CAD evolution through the regulation of the lipid metabolism in the host.

The present study has demonstrated that CAD-DM2 patients had significantly higher plasma levels of TMAO when compared with CAD-NDM2. Tang et al. (2015) also found that the presence of diabetes in those patients belonging to a heart failure cohort was associated with elevations in plasma TMAO which were statistically relevant. Moreover, Gao et al. (2014) described that dietary TMAO supplementation in mice increases impaired glucose tolerance, insulin signaling, and promotes the inflammation of adipose tissue. Additionally, we found that the presence of certain specific bacterial taxa in human feces was associated with the concentration of plasma TMAO in both study groups. We observed that the plasma TMAO concentrations were significantly and negatively associated with the abundance of *Faecalibacterium prausnitzii* in CAD-DM2 patients. Moreover, we found a significant positive correlation of plasma TMAO concentrations with *Enterobacteriaceae* and *Desulfovibrio.* According to our results, other human and animal studies have suggested that several families of bacteria are involved in the production of TMA/TMAO such as *Prevotellaceae* (Koeth et al., 2013) and *Enterobacteriaceae* (Craciun and Balskus, 2012; Zhu et al., 2014). Additionally, it has been previously reported that the increase in the conversion of choline to TMA can be caused by the expression of the *cutC* gene by bacteria such as *Desulfovibrio* (Craciun and Balskus, 2012).

On the other hand, in order to enter the bloodstream, the microbiota derived molecules TMAO need to pass the gut-blood barrier. Accordingly, we observed that plasma zonulin levels were significantly higher in CAD-DM2 patients. Recent research has revealed that circulating zonulin levels are significantly higher in patients with diabetes, polycystic ovary syndrome, obesity, non-alcoholic fatty liver disease, all of which are regarded as traditional risk factors of atherosclerosis (Li et al., 2016).

Therefore, in our study, CAD-DM2 patients presented an alteration in gut microbiota equilibrium (dysbiosis), a disruption of gut barrier function and an increase in gut permeability which altogether may result in aberrant production and absorption of microbe derived metabolites such as TMAO, which can exert their atherogenic effect through alterations in cholesterol and bile acid metabolism, activation of inflammatory pathways, and promotion of foam cells formation. This situation could contribute to an increased risk of major adverse cardiovascular events and death in the CAD-DM2 group.

The pathological basis of CAD is aterosclerosis. Furthermore, inflammation plays a decisive role in atherosclerotic plaque progression, plaque rupture, and thrombosis, which are the initial factors in acute coronary syndrome (Min et al., 2017). In addition, intestinal permeability may contribute to CAD through the production of inflammatory cytokines and the weakening of the stability of plaque. Thus, in this study the significantly higher serum IL-1B levels generated in the gut epithelium during the systematic or localized inflammation in CAD-DM2 patients could also raise intestinal permeability and facilitate intestinal translocation of microbial components and metabolites into the circulation. Moreover, IL-1β enhance cholesterol uptake from human macrophages by upregulation of their oxidized LDL receptors, resulting in foam cell formation and plaque growth (Ikonomidis et al., 1999). In a previous study, IL-1β levels were associated with a less favorable prognosis after acute coronary syndrome (Van Tassell et al., 2013).

Additionally, the significant decrease in the peripheral FOXP3 mRNA expression and serum IL-10 in the CAD-DM2 when compared with the CAD-NDM2 group was significatively associated with the decrease in the abundance of *Bacteroides fragilis* and *Faecalibacterium prausnitzii*, respectively. *Bacteroides fragilis* plays an important role in mucosal T cell homeostasis by means of regulating the function of T cells (Mazmanian et al., 2008). The immunomodulatory molecule polysaccharide A derived from the human commensal *Bacteroides fragilis* mediates the conversion of CD4+ T cells into Foxp3+ Treg cells that produce IL-10 during commensal colonization, stimulating immunological development within mammalian hosts (Round and Mazmanian, 2010). At the same time, IL-10 is a key cytokine in Treg-mediated suppression (Wang et al., 2001). It has been described as a decreased percentage of peripheral CD4 + CD25 + Foxp3 + Treg and serum IL-10 level in patients with DM2. Furthermore, the percentages of peripheral CD4 + CD25 + Foxp3 + Treg and serum IL-10 level were influenced by diabetic complications such as cardiovascular diseases (Qiao et al., 2016).

On the other hand, the commensal bacteria *Faecalibacterium prausnitzii* is an important supplier of butyrate to the colonic epithelium. Butyrate is a short chain fatty acid (SCFA) that promotes the integrity of gut epithelial tight junctions as well as increases the release of the anti-inflammatory and anti-atherogenic cytokine IL-10 (Caligiuri et al., 2003) and promotes Foxp3 + Treg induction (Furusawa et al., 2013). So, the significant reduction in the abundance of *Faecalibacterium prausnitzii* and in the predicted proportion of genes related to the butanoate metabolism that we found in the CAD-DM2 patients when compared with CAD-NDM2 may partially explain the significantly lower levels of zonulin and serum IL-10 and the significantly higher levels of serum IL-1β and plasma TMAO in the CAD-DM2 patients.

Our study has certain limitations but also some important strengths. The limitations include the number of patients which was small and the possible influence of conflicting factors such as diabetes medication over gut microbiota. The strengths of our study lie in the well matched cohorts and the next generation sequencing of the microbiome.

CONCLUSION

We have demonstrated that the presence of DM2 in CAD patients is associated with a gut microbiota change and reduced diversity together with functional metagenomic differences. CAD-DM2 patients had less beneficial or commensal bacteria (such as *Faecalibacterium prausnitzii,* and *Bacteroides fragilis*) and more opportunistic pathogens (such as *Enterobacteriaceae, Streptococcus,* and *Desulfovibrio*) that may impair intestinal barrier function (increasing zonulin levels), enhance the serum levels of TMAO, and may therefore contribute to inflammatory processes related to CAD by means of increasing the production of inflammatory cytokines (such as IL-1B). Moreover, the significant reduction in the abundance of *Faecalibacterium prausnitzii* and *Bacteroides fragilis* found in CAD-DM2 patients was associated with the decrease in the release of the anti-inflammatory and anti-atherogenic cytokine IL-10 and the peripheral FOXP3 mRNA expression, respectively, both implicated in the development and function of Treg cells. These results suggest that the presence of DM2 is related to an impaired regulation of the immune system in CAD patients, mediated in part by the gut microbiota composition and functionality and the production and effects of their gut microbiota derived molecules. Thus, gut microbiota may represent a new target for therapeutic manipulation, treatment, and prevention of complex cardiometabolic diseases through regulation of the immune system.

AUTHOR CONTRIBUTIONS

MQ-O, AM-G, and MJ-N: Conceived the study and developed the experimental design. LJ-M, PC-C, DE, AM-G, MQ-O, and MJ-N: Were responsible for the acquisition and selection of all samples utilized in this study. LS-A, DC-C, IM-I, and MQ-O: Performed all laboratory assays. LS-A, IM-I, DC-C, MJ-N, and MQ-O: Compiled the database and performed the statistical analysis and data interpretation. LS-A, DC-C, IM-I, LJ-M, PC-C, DE, MJ-N, and MQ-O: Wrote the paper. LJ-M, PC-C, AM-G, MJ-N, and MQ-O: Provided critical revision. All authors read and approved the final manuscript.

FUNDING

This work was supported by the Fundación Andaluza de Cardiología and a grant from the Spanish Ministry of Health (FIS) (PI13/02542), co-founded by Fondo Europeo de Desarrollo Regional (FEDER). The research group belongs to the "Centros de Investigación en Red" CIBERobn "Fisiopatología de la Obesidad y Nutrición" (CB06/03/0018) and CIBERCV "Enfermedades Cardiovasculares" (CB16/11/00360) of the "Instituto de Salud Carlos III". Isabel Moreno-Indias and María Isabel Queipo-Ortuño acknowledges support from the "Miguel Servet Type I" program (CP16/00163) and (CP13/00065) respectively) from the Instituto de Salud Carlos III, Madrid, Spain, co-founded by Fondo Europeo de Desarrollo Regional (FEDER). Daniel Castellano-Castillo acknowledges support from the "FPU" program (FPU13/04211) from the Ministerio de Educacion, Cultura y Deporte.

REFERENCES

Aronson, D., and Edelman, E. R. (2016). Coronary artery disease and diabetes mellitus. *Heart Fail. Clin.* 12, 117–133.

Bhute, S., Pande, P., Shetty, S. A., Shelar, R., Mane, S., Kumbhare, S. V., et al. (2016). Molecular characterization and meta-analysis of gut microbial communities illustrate enrichment of prevotella and *Megasphaera* in Indian subjects. *Front. Microbiol.* 7:660. doi: 10.3389/fmicb.2016.00660

Caligiuri, G., Rudling, M., Ollivier, V., Jacob, M. P., Michel, J. B., Hansson, G. K., et al. (2003). Interleukin-10 deficiency increases atherosclerosis, thrombosis, and low-density lipoproteins in apolipoprotein E knockout mice. *Mol. Med.* 9, 10–17.

Craciun, S., and Balskus, E. P. (2012). Microbial conversion of choline to trimethylamine requires a glycyl radical enzyme. *Proc. Natl. Acad. Sci. U.S.A.* 109, 21307–21312. doi: 10.1073/pnas.1215689109

Cui, L., Zhao, T., Hu, H., Zhang, W., and Hua, X. (2017). Association study of gut flora in coronary heart disease through high-throughput sequencing. *Biomed. Res. Int.* 2017:3796359. doi: 10.1155/2017/3796359

De Filippis, F., La Storia, A., Villani, F., and Ercolini, D. (2013). Exploring the sources of bacterial spoilers in beefsteaks by culture-independent high-throughput sequencing. *PLOS ONE* 8:e70222. doi: 10.1371/journal.pone.0070222

Embade, N., Mariño, Z., Diercks, T., Cano, A., Lens, S., and Cabrera, D. (2016). Metabolic characterization of advanced liver fibrosis in HCV patients as studied by serum 1H-NMR spectroscopy. *PLOS ONE* 11:e0155094. doi: 10.1371/journal.pone.0155094

Emoto, T., Yamashita, T., Kobayashi, T., Sasaki, N., Hirota, Y., Hayashi, T., et al. (2017). Characterization of gut microbiota profiles in coronary artery disease patients using data mining analysis of terminal restriction fragment length polymorphism: gut microbiota could be a diagnostic marker of coronary artery disease. *Heart Vessels* 32, 39–46. doi: 10.1007/s00380-016-0841-y

Emoto, T., Yamashita, T., Sasaki, N., Hirota, Y., Hayashi, T., So, A., et al. (2016). Analysis of gut microbiota in coronary artery disease patients: a possible link between gut microbiota and coronary artery disease. *J. Atheroscler. Thromb.* 23, 908–921. doi: 10.5551/jat.32672

Fagerberg, B., Ryndel, M., Kjelldahl, J., Akyürek, L. M., Rosengren, L., Karlström, L., et al. (2010). Differences in lesion severity and cellular composition between in vivo assessed upstream and downstream sides of human symptomatic carotid atherosclerotic plaques. *J. Vasc. Res.* 47, 221–230. doi: 10.1159/000255965

Furusawa, Y., Obata, Y., Fukuda, S., Endo, T. A., Nakato, G., Takahashi, D., et al. (2013). Commensal microbe derived butyrate induces the differentiation of colonic regulatory T cells. *Nature* 504, 446–450. doi: 10.1038/nature12721

Gao, X., Liu, X., Xu, J., Xue, C., Xue, Y., and Wang, Y. (2014). Dietary trimethylamine N-oxide exacerbates impaired glucose tolerance in mice fed a high fat diet. *J. Biosci. Bioeng.* 118, 476–481. doi: 10.1016/j.jbiosc.2014.03.001

Hasib, L., Lundberg, A. K., Zachrisson, H., Ernerudh, J., and Jonasson, L. (2016). Functional and homeostatic defects of regulatory T cells in patients with coronary artery disease. *J. Intern. Med.* 279, 63–77. doi: 10.1111/joim.12398

Hölscher, M. E., Bode, C., and Bugger, H. (2016). Diabetic cardiomyopathy: does the type of diabetes matter? *Int. J. Mol. Sci.* 17:E2136. doi: 10.3390/ijms17122136

Ikonomidis, I., Andreotti, F., Economou, E., Stefanadis, C., Toutouzas, P., and Nihoyannopoulos, P. (1999). Increased proinflammatory cytokines in patients with chronic stable angina and their reduction by Aspirin. *Circulation* 100, 793–798.

Kim, Y., Keogh, J., and Clifton, P. (2015). A review of potential metabolic etiologies of the observed association between red meat consumption and development of type 2 diabetes mellitus. *Metabolism* 64, 768–779. doi: 10.1016/j.metabol.2015.03.008

Koeth, R. A., Levison, B. S., Culley, M. K., Buffa, J. A., Wang, Z., Gregory, J. C., et al. (2014). γ-Butyrobetaine is a proatherogenic intermediate in gut microbial metabolism of L-carnitine to TMAO. *Cell Metab.* 20, 799–812. doi: 10.1016/j.cmet.2014.10.006

Koeth, R. A., Wang, Z., Levison, B. S., Buffa, J. A., Org, E., Sheehy, B. T., et al. (2013). Intestinal microbiota metabolism of L-carnitine, a nutrient in red meat, promotes atherosclerosis. *Nat. Med.* 19, 576–585. doi: 10.1038/nm.3145

Konieczna, P., Groeger, D., Ziegler, M., Frei, R., Ferstl, R., Shanahan, F., et al. (2012). Bifidobacterium infantis 35624 administration induces Foxp3 T regulatory cells in human peripheral blood: potential role for myeloid and plasmacytoid dendritic cells. *Gut* 61, 354–366. doi: 10.1136/gutjnl-2011-300936

Koren, O., Spor, A., Felin, J., Fåk, F., Stombaugh, J., Tremaroli, V., et al. (2011). Human oral, gut, and plaque microbiota in patients with atherosclerosis. *Proc. Natl. Acad. Sci. U.S.A.* 108, 4592–4598. doi: 10.1073/pnas.1011383107

Li, C., Gao, M., Zhang, W., Chen, C., Zhou, F., Hu, Z., et al. (2016). Zonulin regulates intestinal permeability and facilitates enteric bacteria permeation in coronary artery disease. *Sci. Rep.* 6:29142. doi: 10.1038/srep29142

Lohman, T. G., Roche, A. F., and Martorell, R. (1988). *Anthropometric Standardization Reference Manual.* Champaign, IL: Human Kinetics Books.

Mazmanian, S. K., Round, J. L., and Kasper, D. L. (2008). A microbial symbiosis factor prevents intestinal inflammatory disease. *Nature* 453, 620–625. doi: 10.1038/nature07008

McHardy, I. H., Li, X., Tong, M., Ruegger, P., Jacobs, J., and Borneman, J. (2013). HIV Infection is associated with compositional and functional shifts in the rectal mucosal microbiota. *Microbiome* 1:26. doi: 10.1186/2049-2618-1-26

Min, X., Lu, M., Tu, S., Wang, X., Zhou, C., Wang, S., et al. (2017). Serum cytokine profile in relation to the severity of coronary artery disease. *Biomed. Res. Int.* 2017:4013685. doi: 10.1155/2017/4013685

Moreno-Indias, I., Torres, M., Montserrat, J. M., Sanchez-Alcoholado, L., Cardona, F., Tinahones, F. J., et al. (2015). Intermittent hypoxia alters gut microbiota diversity in a mouse model of sleep apnoea. *Eur. Respir. J.* 45, 1055–1065. doi: 10.1183/09031936.00184314

Org, E., Mehrabian, M., and Lusis, A. J. (2015). Unraveling the environmental and genetic interactions in atherosclerosis: central role of the gut microbiota. *Atherosclerosis* 241, 387–399. doi: 10.1016/j.atherosclerosis.2015.05.035

Pereira, L. M. S., Gomes, S. T. M., Ishak, R., and Vallinoto, A. C. R. (2017). Regulatory T cell and forkhead box protein 3 as modulators of immune homeostasis. *Front. Immunol.* 8:605. doi: 10.3389/fimmu.2017.00605

Qiao, Y. C., Shen, J., He, L., Hong, X. Z., Tian, F., Pan, Y. H., et al. (2016). Changes of regulatory T cells and of proinflammatory and immunosuppressive cytokines in patients with type 2 diabetes mellitus: a systematic review and meta-analysis. *J. Diabetes. Res.* 2016, 3694957.

Round, J. L., and Mazmanian, S. K. (2010). Inducible Foxp3+ regulatory T-cell development by a commensal bacterium of the intestinal microbiota. *Proc. Natl. Acad. Sci. U.S.A.* 107, 12204–12209. doi: 10.1073/pnas.0909122107

Serino, M., Blasco-Baque, V., Nicolas, S., and Burcelin, R. (2014). Far from the eyes, close to the heart: dysbiosis of gut microbiota and cardiovascular consequences. *Curr. Cardiol. Rep.* 16:540. doi: 10.1007/s11886-014-0540-1

Sitaraman, R. (2013). Phospholipid catabolism by gut microbiota and the risk of cardiovascular disease. *J. Med. Microbiol.* 62, 948–950.

Smith, P. M., Howitt, M. R., Panikov, N., Michaud, M., Gallini, C. A., Bohlooly-Y, M., et al. (2013). The microbial metabolites, short chain fatty acids, regulate colonic Treg cell homeostasis. *Science* 341, 569–573. doi: 10.1126/science.1241165

Stremmel, W., Schmidt, K. V., Schuhmann, V., Kratzer, F., Garbade, S. F., Langhans, C. D., et al. (2017). Blood Trimethylamine-N-Oxide originates from microbiota mediated breakdown of phosphatidylcholine and absorption from small intestine. *PLOS ONE* 12:e0170742. doi: 10.1371/journal.pone.0170742

Tang, W. H., and Hazen, S. L. (2014). The contributory role of gut microbiota in cardiovascular disease. *J. Clin. Invest.* 124, 4204–4211. doi: 10.1172/JCI72331

Tang, W. H., Wang, Z., Fan, Y., Levison, B., Hazen, J. E., Donahue, L. M., et al. (2014). Prognostic value of elevated levels of intestinal microbe-generated metabolite trimethylamine-N-oxide in patients with heart failure: refining the gut hypothesis. *J. Am. Coll. Cardiol.* 64, 1908–1914. doi: 10.1016/j.jacc.2014.02.617

Tang, W. H., Wang, Z., Levison, B. S., Koeth, R. A., Britt, E. B., Fu, X., et al. (2013). Intestinal microbial metabolism of phosphatidylcholine and cardiovascular risk. *N. Engl. J. Med.* 368, 1575–1584. doi: 10.1056/NEJMoa1109400

Tang, W. H., Wang, Z., Shrestha, K., Borowski, A. G., Wu, Y., Troughton, R. W., et al. (2015). Intestinal microbiota-dependent phosphatidylcholine metabolites, diastolic dysfunction, and adverse clinical outcomes in chronic systolic heart failure. *J. Card. Fail.* 21, 91–96. doi: 10.1016/j.cardfail.2014.11.006

Tremaroli, V., and Backhed, F. (2012). Functional interactions between the gut microbiota and host metabolism. *Nature* 489, 242–249. doi: 10.1038/nature11552

Troseid, M., Ueland, T., Hov, J. R., Svardal, A., Gregersen, I., Dahl, C. P., et al. (2015). Microbiota-dependent metabolite trimethylamine-N-oxide is associated with disease severity and survival of patients with chronic heart failure. *J. Intern. Med.* 277, 717–726. doi: 10.1111/joim.12328

Ufnal, M., and Pham, K. (2017). The gut-blood barrier permeability - A new marker in cardiovascular and metabolic diseases? *Med. Hypotheses* 98, 35–37. doi: 10.1016/j.mehy.2016.11.012

Ufnal, M., Zadlo, A., and Ostaszewski, R. (2015). TMAO: a small molecule of great expectations. *Nutrition* 31, 1317–1323. doi: 10.1016/j.nut.2015.05.006

Van Tassell, B. W., Toldo, S., Mezzaroma, E., and Abbate, A. (2013). Targeting interleukin-1 in heart disease. *Circulation* 128, 1910–1923.

Wang, Q., Fang, C. H., and Hasselgren, P. O. (2001). Intestinal permeability is reduced and IL-10 levels are increased in septic IL-6 knockout mice. *Am. J. Physiol. Regul. Integr. Comp. Physiol.* 281, R1013–R1023.

Wang, Z., Klipfell, E., Bennett, B. J., Koeth, R., Levison, B. S., Dugar, B., et al. (2011). Gut flora metabolism of phosphatidylcholine promotes cardiovascular disease. *Nature* 472, 57–63. doi: 10.1038/nature09922

Wang, Z., Tang, W. H., Buffa, J. A., Fu, X., Britt, E. B., Koeth, R. A., et al. (2014). Prognostic value of choline and betaine depends on intestinal microbiota-generated metabolite trimethylamine-N-oxide. *Eur. Heart. J.* 35, 904–910. doi: 10.1093/eurheartj/ehu002

Zhu, Y., Jameson, E., Crosatti, M., Schafer, H., Rajakumar, K., Bugg, T. D., et al. (2014). Carnitine metabolism to trimethylamine by an unusual Rieske-type oxygenase from human microbiota. *Proc. Natl. Acad. Sci. U.S.A.* 111, 4268–4273. doi: 10.1073/pnas.1316569111

19

Mast Cell Chymase/Mcpt4 Suppresses the Host Immune Response to Plasmodium yoelii, Limits Malaria-Associated Disruption of Intestinal Barrier Integrity and Reduces Parasite Transmission to Anopheles stephensi

Nora Céspedes [1], Erinn L. Donnelly [2], Casey Lowder [1], Gretchen Hansten [1], Delaney Wagers [1], Anna M. Briggs [1], Joseph Schauer [3], Lori Haapanen [3], Magnus Åbrink [4], Judy Van de Water [3] and Shirley Luckhart [1,2]*

[1] Department of Entomology, Plant Pathology and Nematology, University of Idaho, Moscow, ID, United States, [2] Department of Biological Sciences, University of Idaho, Moscow, ID, United States, [3] Division of Rheumatology, Allergy and Clinical Immunology, University of California, Davis, Davis, CA, United States, [4] Section of Immunology, Department of Biomedical Sciences & Veterinary Public Health, Swedish University of Agricultural Sciences, Uppsala, Sweden

***Correspondence:**
Shirley Luckhart
sluckhart@uidaho.edu

An increase in mast cells (MCs) and MCs mediators has been observed in malaria-associated bacteremia, however, the role of these granulocytes in malarial immunity is poorly understood. Herein, we studied the role of mouse MC protease (Mcpt) 4, an ortholog of human MC chymase, in malaria-induced bacteremia using *Mcpt4* knockout (*Mcpt4*$^{-/-}$) mice and *Mcpt4*$^{+/+}$ C57BL/6J controls, and the non-lethal mouse parasite *Plasmodium yoelii yoelii* 17XNL. Significantly lower parasitemia was observed in *Mcpt4*$^{-/-}$ mice compared with *Mcpt4*$^{+/+}$ controls by day 10 post infection (PI). Although bacterial 16S DNA levels in blood were not different between groups, increased intestinal permeability to FITC-dextran and altered ileal adherens junction E-cadherin were observed in *Mcpt4*$^{-/-}$ mice. Relative to infected *Mcpt4*$^{+/+}$ mice, ileal MC accumulation in *Mcpt4*$^{-/-}$ mice occurred two days earlier and IgE levels were higher by days 8-10 PI. Increased levels of circulating myeloperoxidase were observed at 6 and 10 days PI in *Mcpt4*$^{+/+}$ but not *Mcpt4*$^{-/-}$ mice, affirming a role for neutrophil activation that was not predictive of parasitemia or bacterial 16S copies in blood. In contrast, early increased plasma levels of TNF-α, IL-12p40 and IL-3 were observed in *Mcpt4*$^{-/-}$ mice, while levels of IL-2, IL-10 and MIP1β (CCL4) were increased over the same period in *Mcpt4*$^{+/+}$ mice, suggesting that the host response to infection was skewed toward a type-1 immune response in *Mcpt4*$^{-/-}$ mice and type-2 response in *Mcpt4*$^{+/+}$ mice. Spearman analysis revealed an early (day 4 PI) correlation of *Mcpt4*$^{-/-}$ parasitemia with TNF-α and IFN-γ, inflammatory cytokines known for their roles in pathogen clearance, a pattern that was observed in *Mcpt4*$^{+/+}$ mice much later (day 10 PI). Transmission success of *P. y. yoelii*

17XNL to *Anopheles stephensi* was significantly higher from infected *Mcpt4*$^{-/-}$ mice compared with infected *Mcpt4*$^{+/+}$ mice, suggesting that Mcpt4 also impacts transmissibility of sexual stage parasites. Together, these results suggest that early MCs activation and release of Mcpt4 suppresses the host immune response to *P. y. yoelii* 17XNL, perhaps *via* degradation of TNF-α and promotion of a type-2 immune response that concordantly protects epithelial barrier integrity, while limiting the systemic response to bacteremia and parasite transmissibility.

Keywords: malaria, bacteremia, mast cells, Mcpt4, chymase, *Plasmodium yoelii*, *Anopheles stephensi*, intestinal permeability

INTRODUCTION

Malaria is a vector-borne parasitic disease caused by infection with protozoa of the genus *Plasmodium*. The disease is endemic in tropical and sub-tropical regions worldwide and affects about 45% of the global population. In 2019, there were an estimated of 229 million malaria cases and 409,000 deaths, mainly due to *Plasmodium falciparum*, with 67% of malaria deaths in children under 5 years (1). Numerous studies have indicated that children with acute falciparum malaria are predisposed to developing concomitant bacteremia, resulting in increased risk of mortality (2). In contrast, a lower prevalence of bacteremia has been reported in adults with severe malaria (3). However, as observed in children with malaria, adult bacteremic patients present with increased disease severity and have a greater risk of death than non-bacteremic patients regardless of parasitemia levels (4; 5).

Our studies with malaria in mouse and non-human primate models have demonstrated that intestinal permeability and bacteremia are functionally associated with increased intestinal infiltration of mast cells (MCs) or intestinal mastocytosis (6–8). MCs are rare granulocytes that can respond to and synthesize a large number of effectors including prostaglandin D2, cytokines, chemokines, heparin and histamine as well as a variety of proteases such as tryptases, carboxypeptidase A3 and chymases (9–11). In previous work, we demonstrated that L-arginine and L-citrulline supplementation reversed murine malaria-induced intestinal mastocytosis, significantly reduced bacteremia, and improved epithelial barrier morphology (6). Further, we showed that MC-deficient mice with malaria exhibited reduced gut permeability and bacteremia relative to controls, with histamine contributing to some but not all of this pathology (7), supporting the involvement of MCs in malaria-induced gut barrier disruption. In recent studies with the nonlethal mouse parasite *Plasmodium yoelii yoelii* 17XNL, we observed increased circulating MC protease-4 (Mcpt4) at 4 days post infection (PI) (10-fold above control) and 8 days PI (6-fold above control) and sharply increased numbers of intestinal MCs on those same days. Infection was also associated with rising levels of IgE and the MC-activating type-2 cytokines interleukin (IL)-3, -4, -5, -9, -10 and -13 as well as increased intestinal permeability and bacteremia through 10 days PI (8).

Mouse Mcpt4 is functionally homologous to human chymase and has been associated with MC-dependent regulation of intestinal epithelial cell migration and barrier function (12), the extravascular coagulation system (13), survival in models of sepsis and traumatic spinal cord injury and recruitment of leukocytes in a variety of inflammatory contexts (10). Together with our data showing high circulating levels of Mcpt4 during *P. y. yoelii* 17XNL infection (8), these observations suggested that Mcpt4 could contribute to early intestinal epithelial barrier damage and regulation of the observed type-2 immune response shift in this model. To test these hypotheses, we used *P. y. yoelii* 17XNL-infected *Mcpt4*$^{-/-}$ and *Mcpt4*$^{+/+}$ C57BL/6J mice as well as uninfected controls. Our data demonstrate for the first time that this human chymase ortholog orchestrates the regulation of malarial parasitemia and sexual stage parasite transmissibility as well as intestinal barrier function and host immunity to both infection and bacteremia.

MATERIALS AND METHODS

Mouse Strains

Female, 7-8 week old *Mcpt4*$^{-/-}$ (13) and *Mcpt4*$^{+/+}$ C57BL/6J mice (Jackson Laboratory 000664) were housed in ventilated micro-isolator caging and provided food and water *ad libitum*. All procedures were approved by the Institutional Animal Care and Use Committee of the University of Idaho (IACUC Protocol 2020-10, approved 30 March 2020).

Mouse Infection and Monitoring

Mcpt4$^{-/-}$ (n=44) and *Mcpt4*$^{+/+}$ (n=44) mice, distributed in three biological replicates, were injected intraperitoneally with 150 μL of *P. y. yoelii* 17XNL-infected red blood cells (iRBCs, 1×10^6 parasites) as described (8). Control *Mcpt4*$^{-/-}$ (n=11) and *Mcpt4*$^{+/+}$ (n=10) mice were injected with equivalent numbers of uninfected RBCs. Infected mice were distributed into subgroups (n=11), in three replicates of 4, 4 and 3 mice, respectively, that were sacrificed at 4, 6, 8, or 10 days PI. Daily parasitemias were recorded from microscopic examination of Giemsa-stained thin blood films. Blood, plasma and ileum samples were collected and processed as described below.

Bacterial 16S qPCR

Bacterial 16S copy numbers were determined by qPCR as described (8) for individual infected and uninfected mice from the three replicate studies (n=109). Briefly, whole blood was collected into EDTA on the day of necropsy and DNA was isolated using DNeasy Blood and Tissue kit (Qiagen) according to the manufacturer's protocol. Samples were analyzed in triplicate using DNA SYBR Green/ROX qPCR Master Mix (2X) (Bio-Rad) with 16S primers and quantified against a 16S bacterial DNA plasmid standard curve using a QuantStudio 6 Flex Applied Biosystems qPCR as described (8).

Intestinal Permeability

Intestinal permeability was determined as described (8) for individual mice in the third replicate (n=30), with 15 Mcpt4$^{-/-}$ and 15 Mcpt4$^{+/+}$ mice distributed in 5 subgroups each of 3 mice. Four subgroups were infected and sacrificed at 4, 6, 8 and 10 days PI and one subgroup served as uninfected controls. Briefly, fasted mice were orally gavaged with 4 kDa fluorescein isothiocyanate (FITC)-dextran and blood samples collected into EDTA at 3 h after gavage were analyzed using a microplate reader (Molecular Devices LLC, San Jose, CA) at excitation/emission wavelengths of 490/520 nm.

Cytokines and Chemokines in Plasma and Ileum Samples

Plasma cytokine and chemokine concentrations (IL-1α, -1β, -2, -3, -4, -5, -6, -9, -10, -12p70, -12p40, -13, -17, IFN-γ, TNF-α, MCP-1, MIP-1α, MIP-1β, RANTES, eotaxin, GM-CSF, KC) were determined for individual infected and uninfected control mice in the three replicates (n=109) using a Bio-Plex Pro™ Luminex assay and analyzed on a Bio-Plex 200 system (Bio-Rad Laboratories) using Bio-Plex Manager software (Bio-Rad Laboratories) as described (8).

Ileum tissue sections (~2 cm long) collected at necropsy were weighed and processed for protein isolation using the Bio-Plex cell lysis kit (Bio-Rad, Hercules, CA). A lysing solution containing Bio-Plex cell lysis buffer and factors 1 and 2, along with a complete protease inhibitor cocktail (Millipore Sigma) was prepped and stored on ice until use. Tissue samples were kept on dry ice prior to lysing. Each tissue was rinsed thoroughly with 500 μL wash buffer provided in the lysis kit. The wash buffer was discarded and replaced with 500 μL of lysis solution. Ileum tissue was then lysed by sonication with a probe sonicator (Branson SFX150, Danbury, CT) using 8-12 pulses at 75 sec with 50% amplitude and 1 sec pause between each pulse. Once ileum tissue was homogenized, samples were transferred to dry ice for minimum of 10 min, then placed on ice to thaw slowly. After thawing, samples were sonicated in a water bath for 3 min then centrifuged at 4500 x g for 4 min at 4 ° C. Supernatant was collected and placed on ice. Protein concentration was determined using Pierce BCA assay (ThermoFisher) based on the manufacturer's protocol. Each sample was diluted 1:20 and absorbance was determined at 595 nm on an iMark Bio-Rad Microplate reader (Bio-Rad, Hercules, CA). Cytokine/chemokine profiles of the supernatants were determined by Bio-Plex Pro™ Luminex as for plasma samples and run in duplicate (14).

ELISAs

Levels of plasma IgE (eBioscience; Thermo Fisher Scientific, Inc.), Mcpt1 (eBioscience) neutrophil elastase (NE) (Abcam) and myeloperoxidase (MPO) (eBioscience; Thermo Fisher Scientific, Inc.) were determined for individual mice in the three replicates (n=109) using commercial ELISAs according to manufacturer's instructions and a microplate reader (Molecular Devices, LLC).

Ileum Histochemistry

Ileum samples from individual mice in the first two replicates (n=79) were formalin-fixed and embedded in paraffin at the Washington Animal Disease Diagnostic Laboratory, Washington State University, and then subjected to detection of MC chymase activity by naphthol AS-D chloroacetate esterase (NASDCE) activity (Sigma-Aldrich) as described (8).

Immunofluorescence of Mouse Ileum Sections

Paraffin-embedded ileum sections from three mice per time point (n=15) were heated for 20 min at 50°C in a dry oven to soften the paraffin and then treated with xylene (three exchanges, 5 min each) to remove paraffin, followed by a wash/incubation sequence (100%, 90% and 70% ethanol, 5 min each) at room temperature to rehydrate the tissues, then the slides were rinsed in distilled water for 5 min. To enhance antigen retrieval, the slides were steamed for 40 min in Epitope Retrieval Solution (IHC WORLD). Slides were then washed with phosphate-buffered saline (PBS) and incubated for 1 h at room temperature in 5% bovine serum albumin (BSA) to block nonspecific binding sites. After three PBS washes, primary antibodies or isotype controls (1:100 rabbit anti-ZO-1, 1:100 monoclonal rat anti-E-cadherin, 1:100 rabbit primary isotype control, 1:100 mouse primary isotype control, eBioscience) were added, and the slides incubated overnight in a humidified chamber at 4°C. Following this incubation, slides were washed three time with PBS and fluorochrome-labeled secondary antibodies (1:150 chicken anti-rat Alexa Fluor 488 or 1:150 goat anti-rabbit Alexa Fluor 568; Invitrogen) were applied, and the slides were incubated for 1 h in a humidified chamber in the dark. After three PBS washes, coverslips were mounted with ProLong Gold antifade reagent (Invitrogen). Slides were viewed using a Nikon ECLIPSE Ti confocal microscope with a 40x objective. Quantitative analysis of immunofluorescence was performed by densitometry using NIH ImageJ software. A total of 10 to 15 high-power fields (HPF) per section were evaluated for each mouse from three independent biological replicates per time point.

Mosquito Infection

Anopheles stephensi Liston were reared and allowed to feed on *P. y. yoelii* 17XNL-infected mice as described (15). Briefly, *Mcpt4*$^{-/-}$ (n=7) and *Mcpt4*$^{+/+}$ (n=7) mice from three biological replicates were infected as described above. At 3 days after mouse infection, levels of blood-stage parasitemia, gametocytemia and exflagellation were recorded and each mouse was used to infect 3-5 day old female *A. stephensi* (~60 mosquitoes per mouse). At least 30 fed mosquitoes per mouse were dissected and microscopically examined for the presence of oocysts in the midgut at 10 days post-feeding. Midgut oocysts were counted by microscopic examination at 20X magnification.

Statistical Analyses

Parasitemia and bacterial 16S DNA copies per µL of blood were analyzed by one-way ANOVA followed by Dunnett's multiple comparisons test of each time point with the control group, or Šidák's multiple comparisons test between *Mcpt4*$^{-/-}$ and *Mcpt4*$^{+/+}$ at 4, 6, 8 and 10 days PI. Plasma FITC-dextran, Mcpt1, IgE and NE, ileal MCs per HPF, plasma and ileal cytokines and chemokines and fluorescence intensity of E-cadherin and ZO-1 were analyzed with the Kruskal-Wallis test followed by Dunn's multiple comparison of infected versus uninfected controls or *Mcpt4*$^{-/-}$ versus *Mcpt4*$^{+/+}$ mice at 4, 6, 8, and 10 days PI. Plasma MPO levels and percentages of infected mosquitoes were analyzed using Fisher's exact test of *Mcpt4*$^{-/-}$ versus *Mcpt4*$^{+/+}$ mice. The numbers of oocysts per midgut from mosquitoes fed on *Mcpt4*$^{-/-}$ and *Mcpt4*$^{+/+}$ infected mice were compared using the Mann Whitney test. Parasitemia and gametocytemia at day 3 PI were analyzed using an unpaired t test of *Mcpt4*$^{-/-}$ versus *Mcpt4*$^{+/+}$ mice. P values ≤ 0.05 were considered significant. Correlations among parasitemia, blood 16S copies, plasma and ileal cytokines and chemokines as well as plasma IgE, Mcpt1, NE and MPO were assessed by Spearman test at 4, 6, 8, and 10 days PI. Network analysis was performed with Cytoscape® software (www.cytoscape.org) version 3.8.2 using significant Spearman correlation coefficients (P ≤ 0.05) with parasitemia and 16S copies as main targets and MCs and immune factors as sources. Immune factors with a fold-change >1.5 relative to uninfected control were included in the network visualization analyses.

RESULTS

Mcpt4 Deficiency Was Associated With Decreased *P. y. yoelii* 17XNL Parasitemia and Elevated Intestinal Permeability, But Unaltered Bacteremia Relative to *Mcpt4*$^{+/+}$ Mice

Previous studies showed that *Mcpt4*$^{-/-}$ mice exhibit increased basal intestinal barrier integrity relative to *Mcpt4*$^{+/+}$ mice (12), while *Mcpt4*$^{-/-}$ mice infected with the protozoan parasite *Giardia intestinalis* showed significantly reduced intestinal cytokine and alarmin expression and increased weight loss over time that was both more rapid and more severe relative to weight loss in infected *Mcpt4*$^{+/+}$ mice (16). Together with our data affirming the role of MCs in malaria-induced bacteremia (6, 7), we sought to determine whether Mcpt4 deficiency in the context of malaria was associated with alterations in parasitemia, intestinal permeability and infection-induced bacteremia over time.

In our studies, *Mcpt4*$^{-/-}$ mice exhibited a trend towards reduced mean *P. y. yoelii* 17XNL parasitemia by 6 days PI (*Mcpt4*$^{-/-}$ mice = 3.9%, *Mcpt4*$^{+/+}$ mice = 4.6%) and 8 days PI (*Mcpt4*$^{-/-}$ mice = 12%, *Mcpt4*$^{+/+}$ mice = 15%) that was significantly lower relative to *Mcpt4*$^{+/+}$ mice by 10 days PI (*Mcpt4*$^{-/-}$ mice = 18%, *Mcpt4*$^{+/+}$ mice = 32%) (**Figure 1A**). Intestinal permeability, as measured by FITC-dextran translocation *in vivo* across the gut barrier (**Figure 1B**), was significantly increased in *Mcpt4*$^{+/+}$ mice relative to control at days 4 and 10 PI as previously observed (8). In *Mcpt4*$^{-/-}$ mice, FITC-dextran levels were significantly increased relative to control at 6 and 8 days PI, with a trend toward higher levels in *Mcpt4*$^{-/-}$ mice compared to *Mcpt4*$^{+/+}$ mice at 4 and 6 days PI that was significant at 8 days PI (**Figure 1B**). Levels in *Mcpt4*$^{-/-}$ mice decreased to control at 10 days PI (**Figure 1B**). Despite a pattern of increased intestinal permeability in *Mcpt4*$^{-/-}$ mice, infected *Mcpt4*$^{-/-}$ and *Mcpt4*$^{+/+}$ mice exhibited similarly increased bacterial 16S DNA levels in blood over time (**Figure 1C**). In contrast to Mcpt4-dependent host resistance to *G. intestinalis*-induced pathology, our data suggested that Mcpt4 suppresses the host immune response to *P. y. yoelii* 17XNL with alterations in parasitemia that overlapped with Mcpt4-dependent changes in intestinal permeability.

P. y. yoelii 17XNL-Infected *Mcpt4*$^{-/-}$ Mice Exhibited Earlier Increases in Infection-Associated Ileal MCs and Higher Circulating Levels of IgE Relative to Infected *Mcpt4*$^{+/+}$ Mice

Together with data showing that Mcpt4 controls intestinal barrier function (12) and the potential for autocrine regulation

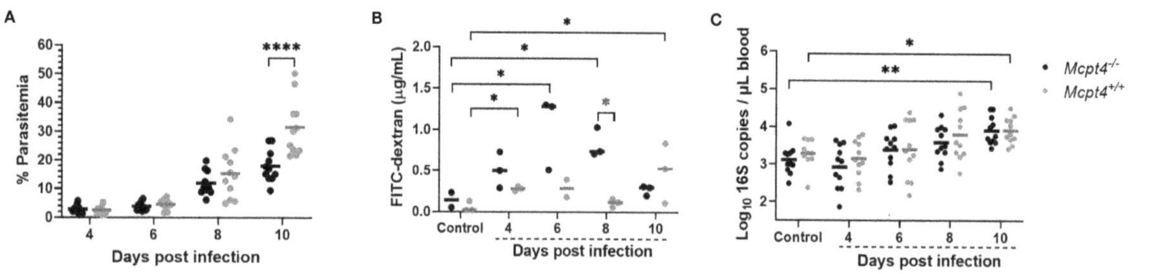

FIGURE 1 | *Plasmodium y. yoelii* 17XNL parasitemia was decreased, intestinal permeability to FITC-dextran was increased, but bacteremia over time was not different in *Mcpt4*$^{-/-}$ relative to *Mcpt4*$^{+/+}$ mice. **(A)** Peripheral parasitemia following *P. y. yoelii* 17XNL infection, **(B)** intestinal permeability quantified as FITC-dextran in plasma of infected and uninfected mice after oral gavage and **(C)** bacterial 16S DNA copies/µL of blood in infected and uninfected mice. Each dot represents a single mouse. Parasitemia and bacterial 16S copies were determined for the three replicates (n=11 per group, per time point), while FITC-dextran was determined using the last replicate of mice only (n=3 mice per group per time point). Parasitemia and log 16S copies per µL of blood were analyzed using one-way ANOVA followed by Dunnett's or Šidák's multiple comparisons test; lines represent the mean. FITC-dextran data were analyzed with the Kruskal-Wallis test followed by Dunn's test for multiple comparisons for each time point versus control or between *Mcpt4*$^{-/-}$ and *Mcpt4*$^{+/+}$ mice at specific time points; lines represent the median. P values ≤ 0.05 were considered significant. *P ≤ 0.05, **P ≤ 0.01, ****P ≤ 0.0001.

of MCs by chymase/Mcpt4 (17), our observations of MC-dependent malaria-induced disruption of the intestinal barrier suggested that Mcpt4 might mediate intestinal MC accumulation and activation during *P. y. yoelii* 17XNL infection. To test this hypothesis, we counted NASDCE-positive ileal MC and quantified plasma Mcpt1 as an additional marker of MC activation in control uninfected and *P. y. yoelii* 17XNL-infected *Mcpt4*$^{-/-}$ and *Mcpt4*$^{+/+}$ mice.

An infection-associated increase in ileal MCs was observed in *Mcpt4*$^{-/-}$ mice at 6 days PI relative to uninfected controls, while no increase was noted in *Mcpt4*$^{+/+}$ mice at this time point (**Figures 2A, D**). By 8 and 10 days PI, both infected *Mcpt4*$^{+/+}$ and *Mcpt4*$^{-/-}$ mice exhibited significantly increased ileal MCs relative to uninfected controls (**Figures 2A, D** and **Figure 1S**). While Mcpt1 levels rose over time with infection, there were no differences in plasma Mcpt1 levels between *Mcpt4*$^{+/+}$ and *Mcpt4*$^{-/-}$ mice at any time point PI (**Figures 2A, B**). Elevated levels of IgE were observed at 8 days PI in both *Mcpt4*$^{+/+}$ and *Mcpt4*$^{-/-}$ mice relative to control uninfected mice with a trend towards higher levels in *Mcpt4*$^{-/-}$ mice (**Figure 2C**). By 10 days PI, IgE levels dropped in both groups and were no longer significant relative to control uninfected mice, but IgE levels in infected *Mcpt4*$^{-/-}$ mice were significantly higher than levels in infected *Mcpt4*$^{+/+}$ mice (**Figure 2C**). Mcpt4 deficiency has been associated with increased serum IgE levels in a model of airway allergic inflammation (18), suggesting an effect of Mcpt4 that is conserved in our model. Overall, our data indicate that significantly increased intestinal MCs appeared earlier in infected *Mcpt4*$^{-/-}$ mice. Further, contrary to our hypothesis, MC activation is not disabled by *Mcpt4* depletion, a state which is also associated with a stronger and more sustained IgE response later in infection.

Mcpt4 Deficiency Was Associated With Altered Patterns of Ileal Adherens Junctions During *P. y. yoelii* 17XNL Infection Relative to *Mcpt4*$^{+/+}$ Mice

Differences in intestinal permeability can be positively associated with physical structure of the intestinal epithelial barrier and MCs are important regulators of the integrity of this barrier (19, 20). Accordingly, we evaluated distribution and intensity of zonula occludens 1 (ZO-1) and E-cadherin in the ileal epithelium as indicators of the integrity of intracellular tight junctions (TJs) and adherens junctions (AJs), respectively, in tissue sections from uninfected and infected *Mcpt4*$^{-/-}$ and *Mcpt4*$^{+/+}$ mice (**Figures 3A, B**).

In uninfected control mice, E-cadherin and ZO-1 staining intensities were significantly lower in *Mcpt4*$^{-/-}$ relative to *Mcpt4*$^{+/+}$ mice (**Figures 3C, D**). E-cadherin staining was significantly increased by parasite infection in *Mcpt4*$^{-/-}$ mice at 4 and 6 days PI and these increases were significant relative to infected *Mcpt4*$^{+/+}$ mice within these time points (**Figure 3C**). E-cadherin staining in infected *Mcpt4*$^{-/-}$ mice was significantly lower than in infected *Mcpt4*$^{+/+}$ mice at days 8 and 10 PI, but staining intensities at these time points were not different from uninfected controls. ZO-1 staining was significantly increased in

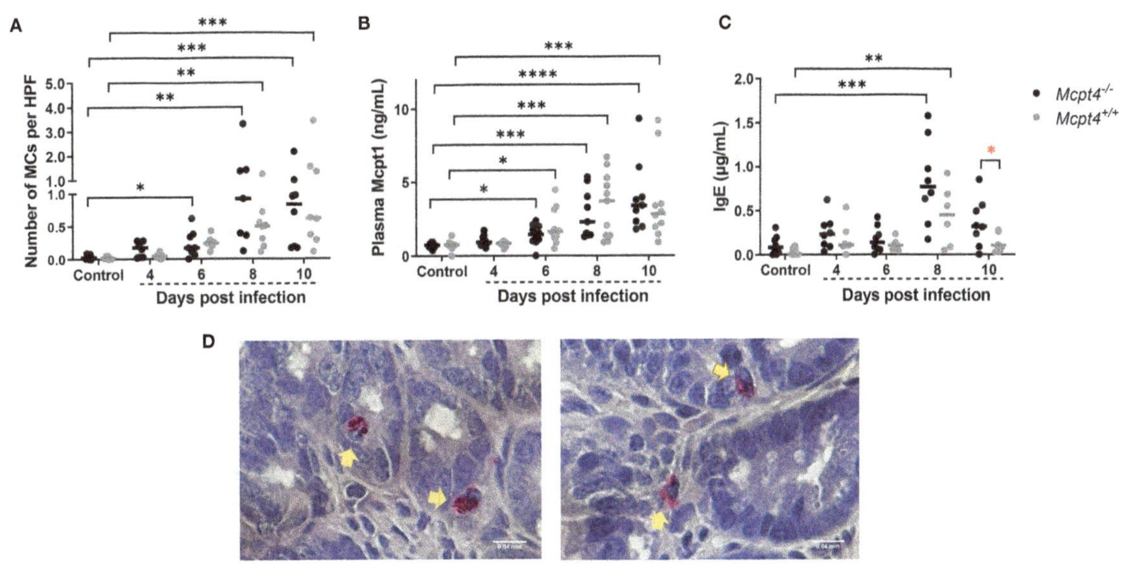

FIGURE 2 | *Plasmodium y. yoelii* 17XNL-infected *Mcpt4*$^{-/-}$ mice exhibited earlier infection-associated increases in ileal MCs and higher circulating levels of IgE relative to infected *Mcpt4*$^{+/+}$ mice. **(A)** Numbers of ileal MCs per high-powered field (HPF) from naphthol AS-D chloroacetate esterase (NASDCE) stained sections from uninfected control mice and infected *Mcpt4*$^{-/-}$ and *Mcpt4*$^{+/+}$ mice. **(B)** Plasma MC protease 1 (Mcpt1) concentrations as determined by ELISA. **(C)** Plasma IgE concentrations as determined by ELISA. **(D)** Representative stained MCs (pink cells indicated by yellow arrows) in ileum of *Mcpt4*$^{-/-}$ (left) and *Mcpt4*$^{+/+}$ (right) mice at 8 days PI. Number of MCs and IgE levels in plasma were determined for biological replicates 1 and 2 (n=8 mice per group per time point), while plasma Mcpt1 levels were determined for the three replicates (n=11 mice per group per time point). Data were analyzed with the Kruskal-Wallis test followed by Dunn's multiple comparison for each time point versus control or between *Mcpt4*$^{-/-}$ and *Mcpt4*$^{+/+}$ mice at specific time points; lines represent the median. P values ≤ 0.05 were considered significant. *P ≤ 0.05, **P ≤ 0.01; ***P ≤ 0.001, ****P ≤ 0.0001.

Mcpt4$^{-/-}$ mice at 4, 6, and 8 days PI relative to uninfected controls, but staining intensity was not different from infected *Mcpt4*$^{+/+}$ mice within these time points (**Figure 3D**). ZO-1 staining in *Mcpt4*$^{-/-}$ mice was reduced relative to infected *Mcpt4*$^{+/+}$ mice at day 10 PI, but staining intensity at this time point was not different from uninfected controls. In looking more closely at the patterns of staining in infected *Mcpt4*$^{-/-}$ versus infected *Mcpt4*$^{+/+}$ mice, intracellular E-cadherin staining was more evident in infected *Mcpt4*$^{-/-}$ versus infected *Mcpt4*$^{+/+}$ mice at 4 and 6 days PI, while ZO-1 staining remained localized to the cell surface (merge, **Figures 3A, B** and **Figure 2S**). Further, intracellular E-cadherin staining at days 4 and 6 PI in *Mcpt4*$^{-/-}$ mice corresponded with trends toward increased permeability to FITC-dextran relative to *Mcpt4*$^{+/+}$ at days 4 and 6 PI that were followed by a significant infection-associated increase at 8 days PI (**Figure 1B**). In a mouse model of irritable bowel disease (IBD; *C1orf106* -/-), intestinal epithelial cells from mutant mice showed increased intracellular versus cell surface staining of E-cadherin in the absence of significant changes in the distribution of ZO-1 (21). Although this pattern was not associated with increased permeability to FITC-dextran *in vivo*, the *C1orf106* -/- intestinal epithelium was significantly more permeable *in vitro* to the smaller compound lucifer yellow and *C1orf106* -/- mice exhibited significantly increased extraintestinal translocation of the enteric pathogen *Citrobacter rodentium* relative to *C1orf106* +/+ mice (21). Taken together with these observations, the shift in intensity and localization of ileal E-cadherin staining in infected *Mcpt4*$^{-/-}$ mice relative to infected *Mcpt4*$^{+/+}$ mice provide an interesting foundation for future studies.

Mcpt4 Deficiency Was Associated With Decreased Neutrophil Activation During *P. y. yoelii* 17XNL Infection

The association of altered ileal adherens junctions in a mouse model of IBD with both increased intestinal permeability and increased extraintestinal translocation of gut bacteria (21) pointed to a clear difference compared with our data. That is, relative to *Mcpt4*$^{+/+}$ mice, parasitemia was reduced in *Mcpt4*$^{-/-}$ mice (**Figure 1A**), adherens junctions were altered (**Figures 3A–C**) and intestinal permeability to FITC-dextran was markedly increased (**Figure 1B**), but there were no differences in blood 16S copies over time between infected *Mcpt4*$^{-/-}$ and *Mcpt4*$^{+/+}$ mice (**Figure 1C**). Human chymase and mouse Mcpt4 can induce the inflammatory recruitment and accumulation of neutrophils (10), cells which could provide protection against infection but also contribute to disease pathology (22). To examine neutrophil

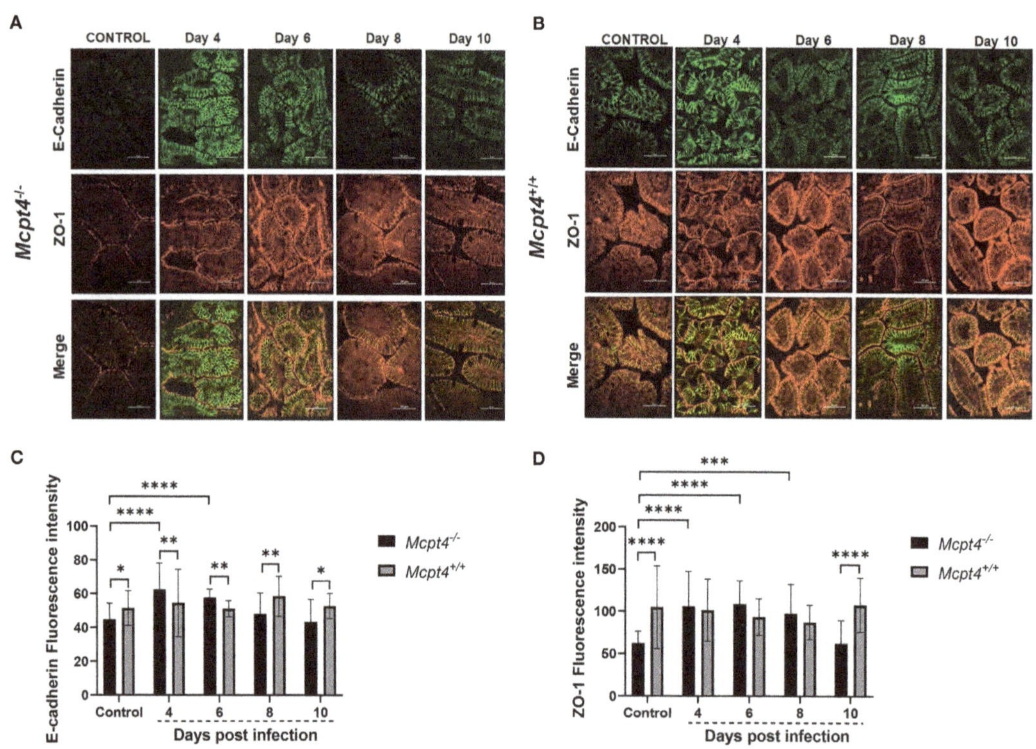

FIGURE 3 | *Mcpt4*$^{-/-}$ mice exhibited altered patterns of ileal adherens junctions during *P. y. yoelii* 17XNL infection relative to *Mcpt4*$^{+/+}$ mice. Representative images from *P. y. yoelii* 17XNL-infected *Mcpt4*$^{-/-}$ **(A)** and *Mcpt4*$^{+/+}$ **(B)** mice and uninfected controls. The top, middle and bottom rows contain images of E-cadherin (green) and ZO-1 (red) staining and merged images. Scale bars represent 50 µm length. Quantitation of E-cadherin **(C)** and ZO-1 **(D)**. Quantitative analysis of fluorescence was performed using NIH ImageJ software. Data are represented as mean ± SD from 10-15 HPF per mouse from three independent biological replicates (n=5 *Mcpt4*$^{-/-}$ mice and n=5 *Mcpt4*$^{+/+}$ mice per replicate). Data were analyzed with the Kruskal-Wallis test followed by Dunn's multiple comparison for each time point versus control or between *Mcpt4*$^{-/-}$ and *Mcpt4*$^{+/+}$ mice at specific time points. P values ≤ 0.05 were considered significant. *P ≤ 0.05, **P ≤ 0.01, ***P ≤ 0.001, ****P ≤ 0.0001.

activation in the context of parasite infection and Mcpt4 deficiency, we examined levels of plasma myeloperoxidase (MPO) and neutrophil elastase (NE) (23), antimicrobial effectors frequently used as markers for neutrophil activation (24, 25). The proportions of MPO-positive mice varied across infection with no difference at 4 days PI, decreased MPO detection in *Mcpt4*$^{-/-}$ versus *Mcpt4*$^{+/+}$ mice at 6 days PI, low MPO detection in *Mcpt4*$^{-/-}$ mice relative to no detection in *Mcpt4*$^{+/+}$ mice at 8 days PI and decreased MPO detection in *Mcpt4*$^{-/-}$ versus *Mcpt4*$^{+/+}$ mice at 10 days PI (**Figure 4A**). Levels of plasma NE were not different between *Mcpt4*$^{-/-}$ and *Mcpt4*$^{+/+}$ mice, with elevated levels in both groups at 4, 8, and 10 days PI relative to uninfected controls (**Figure 4B**). While robust MPO detection at 6 and 10 days PI in infected *Mcpt4*$^{+/+}$ mice relative to *Mcpt4*$^{-/-}$ mice affirmed a role for Mcpt4 in neutrophil activation, these observations were not consistent with increased parasitemia in *Mcpt4*$^{+/+}$ mice relative to the *Mcpt4*$^{-/-}$ mice at 10 days PI (**Figure 1A**) and with the lack of differences in blood 16S copies in *Mcpt4*$^{-/-}$ and *Mcpt4*$^{+/+}$ mice over time (**Figure 1C**).

Cytokine Profiles During *P. y. yoelii* 17XNL Infection Suggested an Earlier Type-1 Immune Response in *Mcpt4*$^{-/-}$ Mice and a Type-2 Response in *Mcpt4*$^{+/+}$ Mice

Given that Mcpt4 can degrade a variety of pro-inflammatory cytokines (10), we hypothesized that a deficiency in this protease could be correlated with increased levels of cytokines associated with host protection against parasite infection and bacteremia. To test this hypothesis, we examined cytokine and chemokine levels in both plasma and ileum tissue over time to reveal patterns of systemic and local responses, respectively, following *P. y. yoelii* 17XNL infection in *Mcpt4*$^{-/-}$ and *Mcpt4*$^{+/+}$ mice.

The pro-inflammatory cytokines IL-12p40 (**Figure 5A**) and TNF-α (**Figure 5B**) as well as the MC growth factor IL-3 (**Figure 5C**) were significantly increased in plasma of *Mcpt4*$^{-/-}$ mice compared to uninfected controls early after infection (4 days PI). In *Mcpt4*$^{+/+}$ mice, IL-2 (**Figure 5D**), IL-10 (**Figure 5E**) and MIP-1β/CCL4 (**Figure 5F**) were significantly increased compared to uninfected controls by the same days PI as observed previously (8). Pro-inflammatory IL-6 (**Figure 5G**), IFN-γ (**Figure 5H**) and IL-1β (**Figure 5I**), the type 1 chemokine MIP-1α/CCL3 (**Figure 5J**), the type 2 regulatory cytokine IL-4 (**Figure 5K**), MCP-1/CCL2 (**Figure 5L**), RANTES/CCL5 (**Figure 5M**) and the granulocytic growth factor GM-CSF (**Figure 5N**) were increased in plasma at 4 days PI in both *Mcpt4*$^{-/-}$ and *Mcpt4*$^{+/+}$ mice. Within time points, MCP-1/CCL2 was significantly different between *Mcpt4*$^{-/-}$ and *Mcpt4*$^{+/+}$ mice at 10 days PI (**Figure 5L**). Increased plasma levels of IL-9 (**Figure 5O**) and IL-13 (**Figure 5P**), both of which are associated with type 2 immunity and MC activation, were observed at 6 and 8 days PI, respectively, in both *Mcpt4*$^{-/-}$ and *Mcpt4*$^{+/+}$ mice. Eotaxin/CCL11 was significantly decreased relative to control by 10 days PI in both *Mcpt4*$^{-/-}$ and *Mcpt4*$^{+/+}$ mice (**Figure 5Q**). No differences relative to control were observed for IL-12p70 (**Figure 5R**), IL-17 (**Figure 5S**) and KC (CXCL1) (**Figure 5T**). Overall, these results suggested an early type 1 response in infected *Mcpt4*$^{-/-}$ mice and skewing towards a type-2 response in infected *Mcpt4*$^{+/+}$ mice over the same time period. Based on MCP-1/CCL2 regulation of the migration and infiltration of monocytes and macrophages (26), an early type-1 response and elevated MCP-1/CCL2 in *Mcpt4*$^{-/-}$ relative to *Mcpt4*$^{+/+}$ mice could explain the significant reduction in parasitemia in *Mcpt4*$^{-/-}$ mice.

In the ileum, early expression (4 days PI) of IL-12p40 (**Figure 6A**) and IL-4 (**Figure 6B**) were observed in *Mcpt4*$^{-/-}$ mice, while increased expression of IL-12p70 (**Figure 6C**) (antagonist of IL-12p40), IL-10 (**Figure 6D**) and the neutrophil chemoattractant KC/CXCL1 (**Figure 6E**) were observed in *Mcpt4*$^{+/+}$ mice at the same time point, followed by RANTES/CCL5 (**Figure 6F**) at 6 days PI in the same group of animals. Early (4 days PI) increases in MCP-1/CCL2 (**Figure 6G**) and MIP-1α/CCL3 (**Figure 6H**) were observed in both *Mcpt4*$^{-/-}$

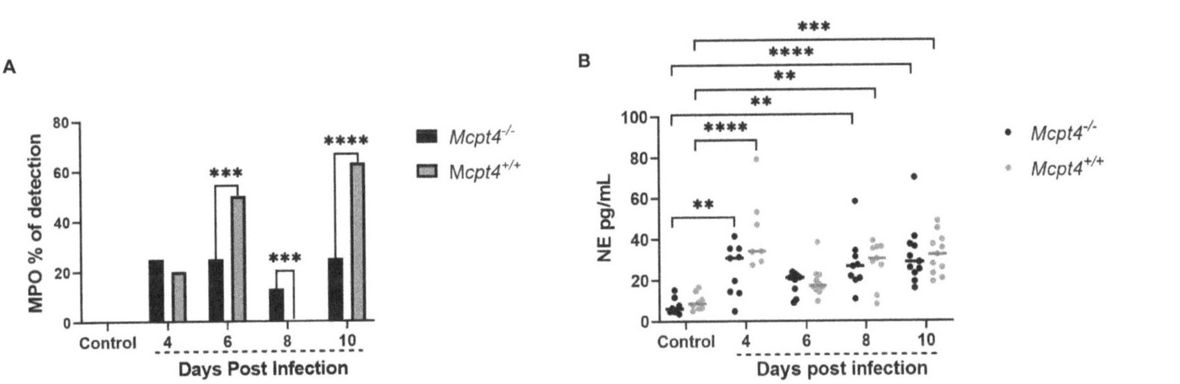

FIGURE 4 | *Mcpt4*$^{-/-}$ mice exhibited significantly decreased neutrophil activation at 6 and 10 days following *P. y. yoelii* 17XNL infection. **(A)** Plasma myeloperoxidase (MPO) detection by ELISA, represented as percentage of positive plasma samples at 4, 6, 8, and 10 days PI. **(B)** Plasma neutrophil elastase (NE) as determined by ELISA. MPO and NE were determined for the three biological replicates (n=11 mice per group per time point). MPO data were analyzed with Fisher's exact test and NE data were analyzed with the Kruskal-Wallis test followed by Dunn's multiple comparison for each time point versus control or between *Mcpt4*$^{-/-}$ and *Mcpt4*$^{+/+}$ mice at specific time points. P values ≤ 0.05 were considered significant. **P ≤ 0.01; ***P ≤ 0.001, ****P ≤ 0.0001.

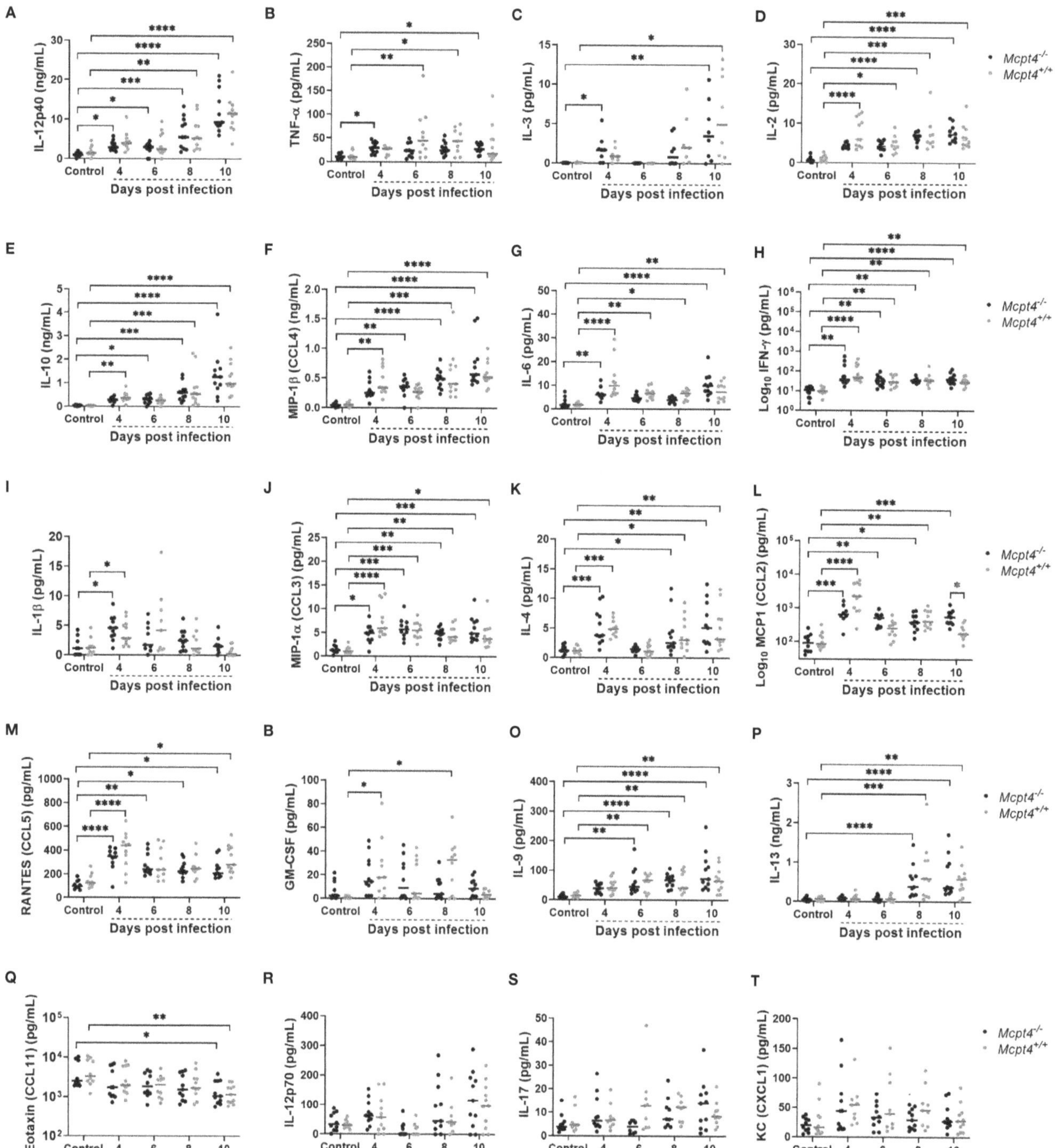

FIGURE 5 | Plasma cytokines and chemokines in *P. y. yoelii* 17XNL-infected *Mcpt4*$^{-/-}$ and *Mcpt4*$^{+/+}$ mice and uninfected controls. **(A–T)** The x axis represents the time points in days after infection, and the y axis represents the concentrations of IL-12p40 **(A)**, TNF-α **(B)**, IL-3 **(C)**, IL-2 **(D)**, IL-10 **(E)**, MIP1β (CCL4) **(F)**, IL-6 **(G)**, IFN-γ **(H)**, IL-1β **(I)**, MIP1α (CCL3) **(J)**, IL-4 **(K)**, MCP-1 (CCL2) **(L)**, RANTES (CCL5) **(M)**, GM-CSF **(N)**, IL-9 **(O)** IL-13 **(P)** Eotaxin (CCL11) **(Q)**, IL-12p70 **(R)**, IL-17 **(S)** and KC (CXCL1) **(T)**. Each dot represents a single mouse. Plasma cytokines were determined for the three biological replicates (n=11 mice per group per time point). Data were analyzed with the Kruskal-Wallis test followed by Dunn's multiple comparison for each time point versus control or between *Mcpt4*$^{-/-}$ and *Mcpt4*$^{+/+}$ mice at specific time points. P values ≤ 0.05 were considered significant. *P ≤ 0.05, **P ≤ 0.01; ***P ≤ 0.001, **** P ≤ 0.0001.

and *Mcpt4*$^{+/+}$ mice, followed by later (8 days PI) increases in MIP-1β/CCL4 (**Figure 6I**) in *Mcpt4*$^{-/-}$ mice and IL-6 (**Figure 6J**) in both *Mcpt4*$^{-/-}$ and *Mcpt4*$^{+/+}$ mice. No differences relative to control were observed for IL-17 (**Figure 6K**) and IL-2 (**Figure 6L**). In general, ileum cytokine levels were lower than plasma levels, but as observed in plasma samples, the local ileal immune response in *Mcpt4*$^{-/-}$ mice was more consistent with a type-1 immune response (IL-12p40), while the local response in *Mcpt4*$^{+/+}$ mice was more type-2 (IL-12p70, IL-10).

Correlation Analyses and Network Visualization Affirmed a Stronger Earlier Immune Response in *Mcpt4*$^{-/-}$ Mice Relative to *Mcpt4*$^{+/+}$ Mice

To visualize the networked host response, we first constructed correlation matrices for *Mcpt4*$^{-/-}$ and *Mcpt4*$^{+/+}$ mice to identify significant positive and negative relationships over time between parasitemia and blood 16S copies with ileal MC numbers, levels of plasma and ileal cytokines and chemokines, plasma IgE, plasma Mcpt1, MPO and NE (**Figure S3**). Significant correlations ($P \leq 0.05$) with fold changes > 1.5 relative to uninfected controls were used to build interaction networks by day to better understand these complex host responses (**Figure 7**).

At 4 days PI, *Mcpt4*$^{-/-}$ mice exhibited a more balanced type-1/type-2 immune response relative to *Mcpt4*$^{+/+}$ mice as evidenced by the presence of IFN-γ at the center of the host response network and the presence of plasma IL-17. In *Mcpt4*$^{-/-}$ mice, MCs were also networked directly and negatively correlated with parasitemia, suggesting early MC regulation of parasitemia. In *Mcpt4*$^{+/+}$ mice, no correlations between parasitemia and any cytokines or chemokines were observed at 4 days PI, and the host response appears to be driven primarily by blood 16S copies at the level of the ileum. Plasma IgE was positively correlated with parasitemia in both *Mcpt4*$^{-/-}$ and *Mcpt4*$^{+/+}$ mice, with this being the only direct correlation with parasitemia in *Mcpt4*$^{+/+}$ mice.

By 6 days PI, no correlations were observed between parasitemia and any cytokines or chemokines in *Mcpt4*$^{-/-}$ or *Mcpt4*$^{+/+}$ mice. The host responses in both *Mcpt4*$^{-/-}$ and *Mcpt4*$^{+/+}$ mice were 16S-dependent with blood 16S copies directly and positively correlated with plasma MCP-1/CCL2 and eotaxin/CCL11 and ileal MIP-1β/CCL4 as well as NE and MPO in

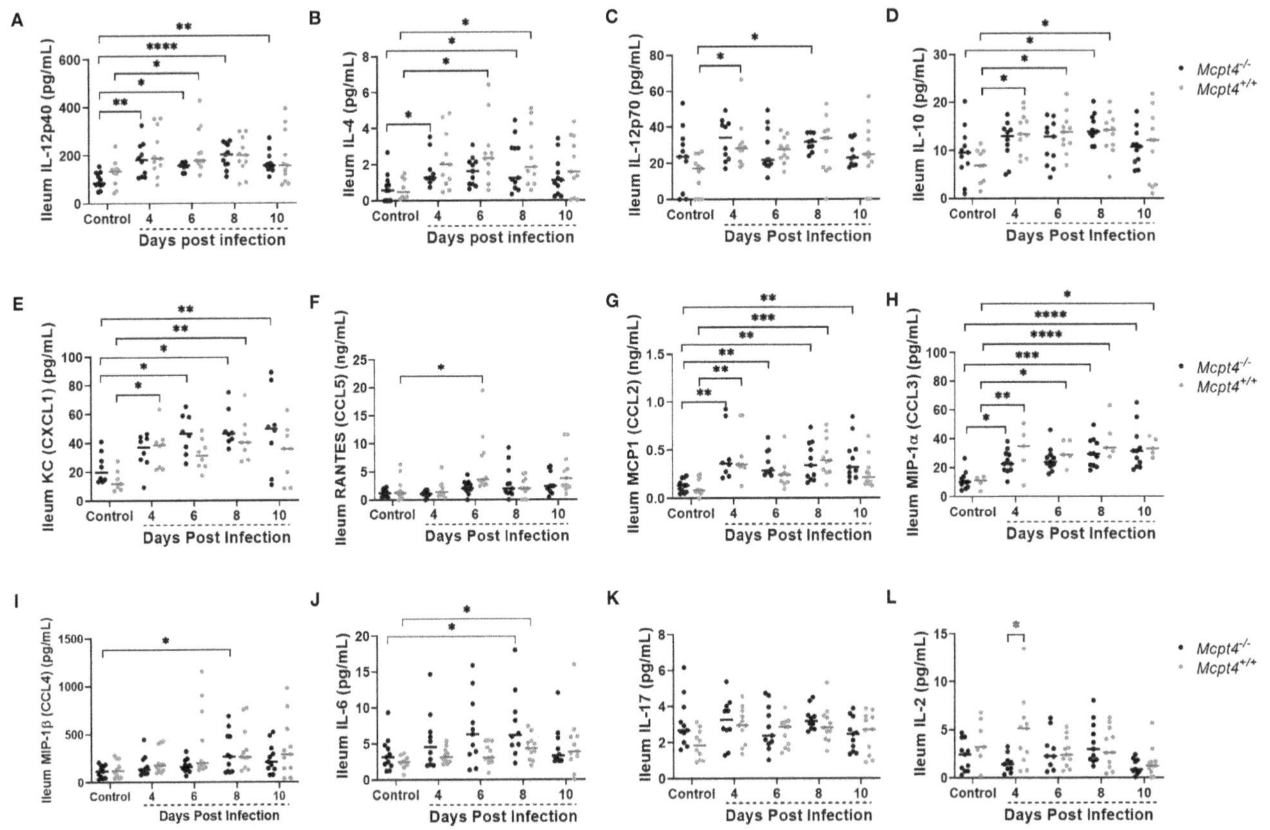

FIGURE 6 | Ileal cytokines and chemokines in *P. y. yoelii* 17XNL-infected *Mcpt4*$^{-/-}$ and *Mcpt4*$^{+/+}$ mice and uninfected controls. **(A–L)** The x axis represents the time points in days after infection, and the y axis represents the concentrations of IL-12p40 **(A)**, IL-4 **(B)**, IL-12p40 **(C)**, IL-10 **(D)**, KC (CXCL1) **(E)**, RANTES (CCL5) **(F)**, MCP-1 (CCL2) **(G)**, MIP1α (CCL3) **(H)**, MIP1β (CCL4) **(I)**, IL-6 **(J)**, IL-17 **(K)** and IL-2 **(L)**. Each dot represents a single mouse. Cytokines levels in ileum were determined for the three biological replicates (n=11 mice per group per time point). Data were analyzed with the Kruskal-Wallis test followed by Dunn's multiple comparison for each time point versus control or between *Mcpt4*$^{-/-}$ and *Mcpt4*$^{+/+}$ mice at specific time points. P values ≤ 0.05 were considered significant. *$P \leq 0.05$, **$P \leq 0.01$, ***$P \leq 0.001$, ****$P \leq 0.0001$.

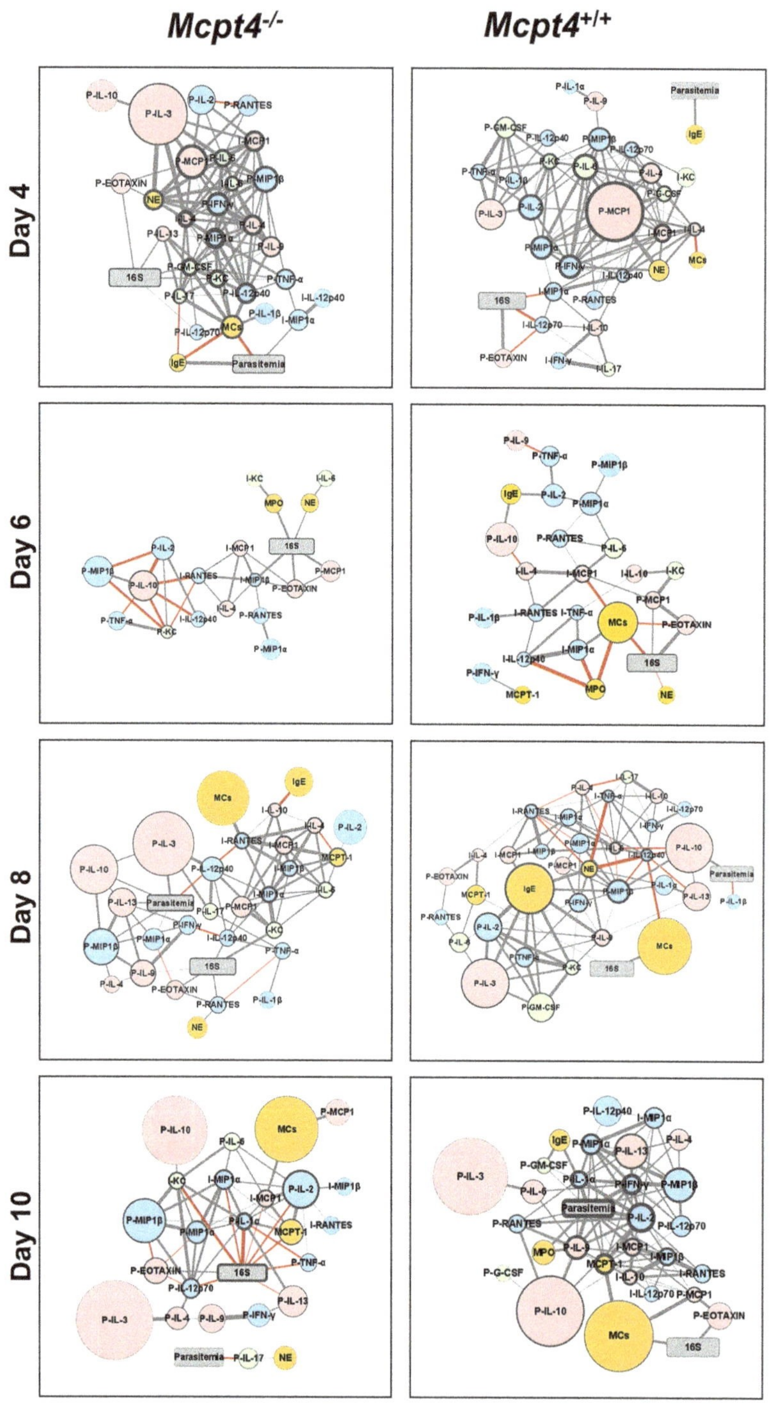

FIGURE 7 | Network visualization of *Mcpt4*$^{-/-}$ and *Mcpt4*$^{+/+}$ mouse phenotypes during *P. y. yoelii* 17XNL infection. Network visualization of significant correlations (**Figure S3**) at different times post-infection in *Mcpt4*$^{-/-}$mice (left) and *Mcpt4*$^{+/+}$ mice (right). The size of a circular node represents relative fold change (larger circle = larger fold change) of a parameter calculated as average levels in infected mice/average levels in control uninfected mice. The border width represents the degree or number of connections (the higher the number of connected edges, the thicker the edge). Parasitemia and 16S nodes are presented in gray, blue nodes are pro-inflammatory cytokines and chemokines (type-1 immune response), pink nodes are anti-inflammatory or regulatory cytokines and chemokines (type-2 immune response), green nodes are type-17 immunity-related cytokines and chemokines, orange nodes represent cells and cells markers (MCs, Mcpt1, MPO and NE). Gray strokes connect nodes with positive correlations and red strokes reflect negative correlations. Increasing stroke line width reflects increasing Spearman's correlation value.

Mcpt4$^{-/-}$ mice. In *Mcpt4*$^{+/+}$ mice, blood 16S copies were negatively correlated with NE and MCs and positively correlated with plasma eotaxin/CCL11 and MCP-1/CCL2.

By 8 days PI, parasitemia in *Mcpt4*$^{-/-}$ was correlated with larger fold changes in plasma type-2 cytokines (IL-3, IL-13 and IL-10) and chemokines (MIP-1α/CCL3 and MIP-1β/CCL4), while blood 16S copies were correlated directly and positively with plasma eotaxin/CCL11, IL-9, MCP-1/CCL2 and RANTES/CCL5 and ileal KC/CXCL1. Plasma MCP-1/CCL2 and ileal KC/CXCL1 connected blood 16S copies with a series of ileal cytokines and chemokines (IL-6, IL-10, MCP-1/CCL2, MIP-1α/CCL3, MIP-1β/CCL4 and RANTES/CCL5) and with MCs. In *Mcpt4*$^{+/+}$ mice, parasitemia was positively correlated with plasma IL-10 and negatively with plasma IL-1β while blood 16S copies were positively correlated with MCs and Mcpt1

By 10 days PI, parasitemia in *Mcpt4*$^{-/-}$ mice was correlated only with the pro-inflammatory cytokine IL-17 in the plasma and this correlation was negative. The overall host response in *Mcpt4*$^{-/-}$ mice appears to be driven by blood 16S copies, with a notable number of direct negative correlations with plasma and ileal cytokines and chemokines. In *Mcpt4*$^{+/+}$ mice, parasitemia is the overwhelming focal point of the host immune response, with correlations between type 1 (IFN-γ) and type 2 (IL-10 and IL-13) cytokines and chemokines as well as MPO. In *Mcpt4*$^{+/+}$ mice, MCs connect with parasitemia through Mcpt1 and are positively correlated with blood 16S copies.

Mcpt4 Deficiency Was Associated With Increased *P. y. yoelii* 17XNL Transmission to *Anopheles stephensi*

The interruption of malaria parasite transmission from infected humans to mosquitoes is one of the main challenges for malaria control and elimination programs. It has been established that naturally acquired immune responses to gametocytes can affect parasite infectiousness to *Anopheles* mosquitoes (27). To identify the effects of Mcpt4 on gametocytemia and parasite transmission in our model, we exposed infected *Mcpt4*$^{-/-}$ and *Mcpt4*$^{+/+}$ mice to 3-5 day old female *A. stephensi*. In three biological replicates, midgut oocyst numbers were modestly, but significantly higher in *A. stephensi* fed on *Mcpt4*$^{-/-}$ mice relative to mosquitoes fed on infected *Mcpt4*$^{+/+}$ mice (**Figure 8A**). Similarly, a higher percentage of mosquitoes were infected following feeding on *Mcpt4*$^{-/-}$ versus *Mcpt4*$^{+/+}$ mice (**Figure 8B**). Surprisingly, there were no differences in exflagellation (not shown), parasitemia (**Figure 8C**) or gametocytemia (**Figure 8D**) between infected *Mcpt4*$^{-/-}$ and *Mcpt4*$^{+/+}$ mice on the day of mosquito infection. Taken together, these results suggest that the mouse chymase Mcpt4 alters parasite transmissibility without discernable effects on peripheral gametocytemia.

DISCUSSION

In a previous study, we observed that circulating levels of mouse Mcpt4 were significantly increased at 4 days (10-fold above control) and 8 days (6-fold above control) after *P. y. yoelii* 17XNL infection (8) with sharply increased intestinal MCs relative to control on the same days. Mcpt4 has been associated with MC-dependent regulation and homeostasis of the intestinal epithelium (12), limiting inflammation in a sepsis model (28), modulating scar development (29, 30) and regulation of the intestinal inflammatory response to *G. intestinalis* (16), but the role of Mcpt4 in malaria has not been studied. Here we provide data that suggest for the first time that Mcpt4, the ortholog of human chymase, promotes a type-2 immune response, regulates alterations to the intestinal barrier associated with the development of parasitemia and bacteremia and restricts parasite transmission to *A. stephensi*.

In general, our network analyses revealed patterns and complexity over time that were consistent with an interpretation of temporally accelerated control of parasitemia and a stronger systemic response to bacteremia in *Mcpt4*$^{-/-}$ mice relative to *Mcpt4*$^{+/+}$ mice. The *Mcpt4*$^{-/-}$ interaction network had a substantially larger number of nodes around parasitemia at days 4 and 8 PI and around blood 16S copies at 4, 8, and 10 days PI than observed in *Mcpt4*$^{+/+}$ mice. At 4 days PI, the *Mcpt4*$^{+/+}$

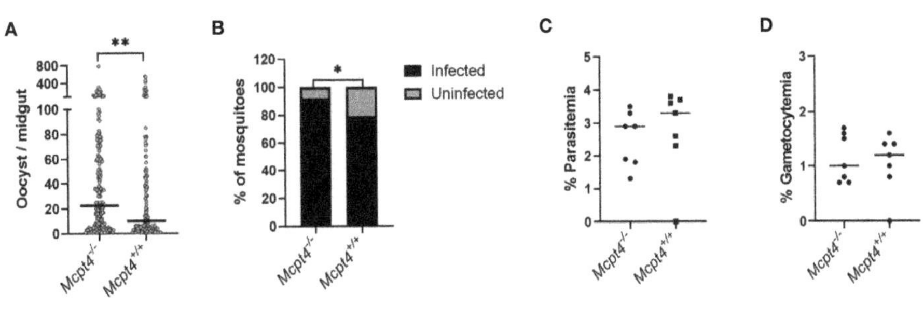

FIGURE 8 | Transmission of *P. y. yoelii* 17XNL from infected *Mcpt4*$^{-/-}$ and *Mcpt4*$^{+/+}$ mice to *Anopheles stephensi*. Panels **(A, B)**, respectively, represent the numbers of oocysts per midgut and proportions of infected mosquitoes in three independent biological replicates. Panels **(C, D)**, respectively, illustrate the percentages of mouse erythrocytes infected with asexual stage *P. y. yoelii* 17XNL and sexual stage gametocytes on the day of mosquito infection (day 3 PI). Parasite transmission was determined in three biological replicates (n=7 mice per group, 30 fed mosquitoes per mouse). The numbers of midgut oocysts in mosquitoes fed on *Mcpt4*$^{-/-}$ and *Mcpt4*$^{+/+}$ infected mice were analyzed by Mann Whitney test. The percentages of infected mosquitoes (mosquitoes with zero oocysts excluded) were analyzed with Fisher's exact test. Parasitemia and gametocytemia data were analyzed using unpaired t tests. P values ≤ 0.05 were considered significant. *P ≤ 0.05, **P ≤ 0.01.

network had a single node connected with parasitemia; a strong network focus on parasitemia was delayed in *Mcpt4*$^{+/+}$ mice until 10 days PI. In contrast, blood 16S copies were the major network focus in *Mcpt4*$^{-/-}$ mice at 10 days PI, while parasitemia was separated from the primary network with only a few interacting nodes, a pattern consistent with significantly reduced parasitemia in *Mcpt4*$^{-/-}$ mice at this time (**Figure 1A**). Intriguingly, the networks for both *Mcpt4*$^{-/-}$ mice and *Mcpt4*$^{+/+}$ mice at 6 days PI were relatively small and lacked nodes correlated with parasitemia. We previously inferred that this time point is associated with a shift between innate and adaptive immunity in our infection model (8), which appears to be the case herein given the significant increase in IgE for both *Mcpt4*$^{-/-}$ and *Mcpt4*$^{+/+}$ mice at 8 days PI (**Figure 2C**). However, the nearly identical levels of parasitemia preceding (4 days) and coinciding with this shift (6 days; **Figure 1A**) suggested that another insult was responsible for the divergence of the *Mcpt4*$^{-/-}$ and *Mcpt4*$^{+/+}$ networks over time. Based on our data, we suggest that this insult was increased intestinal permeability in *Mcpt4*$^{-/-}$ mice that trended higher than *Mcpt4*$^{+/+}$ mice at 4 and 6 days PI, a pattern that was significantly increased by 8 days PI (**Figure 1B**). We infer from our network analyses that this barrier disruption likely contributed to an earlier and broader systemic immune response in the *Mcpt4*$^{-/-}$ mice relative to the *Mcpt4*$^{+/+}$ mice that maintained blood 16S copies at levels that were not different with *Mcpt4*$^{+/+}$ levels at any time point and that significantly reduced parasitemia by 10 days PI in *Mcpt4*$^{-/-}$ mice. We discuss these patterns and complexity in more detail below to support our inferences.

In contrast to previous studies that showed that *Mcpt4*$^{-/-}$ mice exhibited increased basal intestinal barrier integrity relative to *Mcpt4*$^{+/+}$ mice (12), we observed an infection-associated decrease in intestinal barrier integrity in *Mcpt4*$^{-/-}$ mice (**Figure 1B**) and altered ileal E-cadherin staining (**Figures 3C, D**) that was similar to a pattern associated with increased enteric bacterial translocation in another mouse model (21). Ileal MC numbers in *Mcpt4*$^{-/-}$ mice were significantly increased relative to control at 6 days PI, two days earlier than observed in *Mcpt4*$^{+/+}$ mice, but both *Mcpt4*$^{-/-}$ and *Mcpt4*$^{+/+}$ mice exhibited significantly increased ileal MCs relative to control at 8 and 10 days PI (**Figure 2A**). The trend toward increased IgE levels in *Mcpt4*$^{-/-}$ mice relative to *Mcpt4*$^{+/+}$ at 8 days PI became significant by 10 days PI (**Figure 2C**) and could predict increasingly greater MC activation in *Mcpt4*$^{-/-}$ versus *Mcpt4*$^{+/+}$ mice. Intestinal permeability in *Mcpt4*$^{-/-}$ mice returned to baseline by 10 days PI, however, with a trend towards reduced permeability relative to *Mcpt4*$^{+/+}$ mice at this time point (**Figure 1C**), suggesting a homeostatic correction in *Mcpt4*$^{-/-}$ mice later in infection. The role of MCs as key modulators of barrier function and homeostasis of the intestinal mucosa has been previously established (20) and we can now add that a leaky gut in *Mcpt4*$^{-/-}$ mice is associated with substantial changes in the host immune response to malaria parasite infection.

The observed reduction in parasitemia in *Mcpt4*$^{-/-}$ mice was associated with an earlier type 1 immune response relative to *Mcpt4*$^{+/+}$ mice, with increased plasma IL-12p40 (**Figure 5A**) and TNF-α (**Figure 5B**) by 4 days PI. Both of these cytokines, as well as IFN-γ, were indirectly correlated with parasitemia through MCs, GM-CSF, KC/CXCL1 and IL-17 at the same time point (**Figure 7**). In contrast to *Mcpt4*$^{-/-}$ mice, plasma IL-10 in *Mcpt4*$^{+/+}$ mice was significantly increased relative to controls at 4 days PI, two days earlier than in *Mcpt4*$^{-/-}$mice (**Figure 5E**), suggesting earlier immune down-regulation in *Mcpt4*$^{+/+}$ mice. By 8 days PI, parasitemia in *Mcpt4*$^{-/-}$ mice was correlated mainly with type-2 cytokines including large fold-changes in IL-3 and IL-10, which were also notable in *Mcpt4*$^{+/+}$ mice. However, the *Mcpt4*$^{-/-}$ network also included indirect correlations with the chemokines MIP-1α/CCL3 and MIP-1β/CCL4, as well as persistence of IL-12p40, IFN-γ and TNF-α (**Figure 7**). Pro-inflammatory cytokines, particularly IL-12 and INF-γ, have been associated with protection and parasite clearance in malaria (31, 32). While the role of IL-17 in parasite clearance is not clear, MCs are reported to be an important source of this cytokine in addition to Th17 cells (33–35) and IL-17 levels has been associated with protection against *Plasmodium berghei* (ANKA strain) (36) and severe disease in falciparum malaria (37). Moreover, tryptase co-released from stimulated human MCs following FcεRI cross-linking has been associated with *in vitro* degradation of MCP-1/CCL2 (38), an important chemoattractant of monocytes and macrophages (26) that could also participate in parasite clearance. Some studies have suggested that Mcpt4 also cleaves MCP-1 (39), but others have not shown this (40–42), leaving this biology unclear. IgE levels trended higher at 8 days PI in *Mcpt4*$^{-/-}$ mice and were significantly higher than *Mcpt4*$^{+/+}$ levels at 10 days PI (**Figure 2C**), suggesting an association between IgE, activated MCs and elevated MCP-1/CCL2 in *Mcpt4*$^{-/-}$ mice. Together, our data suggest that early MC synthesis of Mcpt4 suppresses the host immune response to *P. y. yoelii* 17XNL infection, perhaps *via* degradation of pro-inflammatory TNF-α, IFN-γ and MCP-1/CCL2 (28, 39) and promotion of a type-2 immune response.

Inflammatory cytokines and chemokines can enhance neutrophil responsiveness to circulating bacteria, but in the context of malaria, this response can be compromised (43), so we monitored circulating levels of MPO and NE as markers of neutrophil activation in *Mcpt4*$^{-/-}$ and *Mcpt4*$^{+/+}$ mice over the course of *P. y. yoelii* 17XNL infection. Surprisingly, MPO detection was reduced in *Mcpt4*$^{-/-}$ versus *Mcpt4*$^{+/+}$ mice at 6 and 10 days PI (**Figure 4A**), while circulating NE levels gradually increased with infection but were not different between *Mcpt4*$^{-/-}$ and *Mcpt4*$^{+/+}$ mice at any time point (**Figure 4B**). In our network analyses (**Figure 7**), MPO was absent in *Mcpt4*$^{-/-}$ mice at 4 days PI and NE was indirectly correlated with blood 16S copies through plasma eotaxin. At 6 days PI, MPO and NE were positively correlated with blood 16S copies in *Mcpt4*$^{-/-}$ mice and negatively correlated in *Mcpt4*$^{+/+}$ mice. By 8 days PI, MPO was absent in *Mcpt4*$^{-/-}$ mice and NE was associated with blood 16S copies through RANTES/CCL5. MPO was not detected in the *Mcpt4*$^{+/+}$ network, previously, were observed significant increases in neutrophils by day 4 PI that declined to control levels by day 8 PI that could explain the lower levels of MPO at this time point (8). In ileum, NE was negatively associated with

IL-12p40, TNF-α and RANTES/CCL5, and positively with plasma IL-9, IFN-γ and IgE. By 10 days PI in *Mcpt4*$^{-/-}$ mice, NE was positively correlated with IL-17, which was negatively correlated with parasitemia, while MPO in *Mcpt4*$^{+/+}$ mice was positively correlated with parasitemia. These results suggest very different roles of neutrophils in bacterial clearance and potential effects on parasitemia in *Mcpt4*$^{-/-}$ and *Mcpt4*$^{+/+}$ mice, perhaps through different activation mechanisms. Reactive oxygen species (ROS)-dependent signaling activation of neutrophil NETosis in response to microbial infections is well established (44). However, NET formation can occur through different signaling pathways depending on the stimulus (45), and NE and MPO have different functions and mechanisms of action. For example, MPO can inactivate NE through HOCl but not H_2O_2 (46). Mcpt4 has been associated with control of neutrophil extravasation and activation and with limiting associated damage in renal ischemia reperfusion injury (47). The distinct correlations of NE with bacterial 16S copies as well as the differences in MPO expression between the *Mcpt4*$^{-/-}$ and *Mcpt4*$^{+/+}$ mice suggest a novel role for Mcpt4 in neutrophil regulation in the context of malaria.

There is evidence in human malaria that an antibody response to gametocyte surface proteins can influence transmission to mosquitoes (27). It also has been suggested that enhanced transmission can be associated with low antibody titers and low inherent gametocyte infectivity (i.e. low gametocyte densities) (48–50). Relative to *Mcpt4*$^{+/+}$ mice, we observed modestly but significantly higher parasite transmission from *Mcpt4*$^{-/-}$ mice to *A. stephensi*. This was not reflected in differences in exflagellation, gametocytemia or parasitemia in *Mcpt4*$^{-/-}$ versus *Mcpt4*$^{+/+}$ mice. Transmission success has also been associated with male to female gametocyte ratio (50, 51) and gametocyte maturation (52). Moreover, although the effects of cellular immune responses to sexual stages and associated changes in transmission to mosquitoes is not clear (53), CD4 + T cells have been shown to respond to gametocyte antigens (54, 55). In the mosquito host, ingested mammalian blood factors can significantly and profoundly affect transmission success of both mouse and human malaria parasites to *A. stephensi*, independently of patterns of gametocytemia and exflagellation (56–59). While it is clear that Mcpt4-dependent host responses can impact parasite transmission to the mosquito host, additional studies are required to define mechanisms that may affect parasite development and maturation in both mammalian and mosquito hosts.

In conclusion, our studies show that Mcpt4 plays a role in sustaining *P. y. yoelii* 17XNL infection by promoting a type-2 immune response that concordantly protects intestinal epithelial barrier integrity and limits the systemic response to bacteremia. One possible explanation is that iRBC sequestration in the intestine (60), which is well known in falciparum malaria (11) and also reported by us for *P. yoelii* infection (60), triggers an early inflammatory response that induces local tissue damage and bacterial translocation. This in turn could induce MC activation and degranulation to control the immune response and initially protect intestinal barrier integrity, thereby delaying the immune response to the parasite and allowing parasite replication to proceed. Several studies indicate that MC proteases can inactivate pro-inflammatory mediators *via* degradation (16, 18, 28, 39), thereby restricting the early pro-inflammatory response to the parasite. This study provides novel findings regarding the contribution of Mcpt4 in promoting acute malaria while concordantly regulating intestinal barrier integrity and parasite transmission.

AUTHOR CONTRIBUTIONS

SL contributed to conception, design of the study and funding acquisition. NC coordinated the research activities, organized the data, performed data analyses, and wrote the first draft of the manuscript. NC, ED, CL, GH, DW, AB, JS and LH contributed to performing the experiments and data collection. SL and JW wrote sections of the manuscript. MÅ provided the Mcpt4-/- mutant mouse line. All authors read the manuscript, contributed to revision and approved the submitted version.

FUNDING

This work was funded by NIH NIAID RO1 AI131609 to SL. The funders had no role in study design, data collection and interpretation, or the decision to submit the work for publication.

ACKNOWLEDGMENTS

Authors acknowledge the members of the Luckhart lab as well as the staff of the Laboratory Animal Research Facility (LARF), University of Idaho.

REFERENCES

WHO. "*World Malaria Report 2020: 20 Years of Global Progress and Challenges*". Geneva: World Health Organization (2020).

Church J, Maitland K. Invasive Bacterial Co-Infection in African Children With Plasmodium Falciparum Malaria: A Systematic Review. *BMC Med* (2014) 12:31. doi: 10.1186/1741-7015-12-31

Imwong M, Stepniewska K, Tripura R, Peto TJ, Lwin KM, Vihokhern B, et al. Numerical Distributions of Parasite Densities During Asymptomatic Malaria. *J Infect Dis* (2016) 213(8):1322–9. doi: 10.1093/infdis/jiv596

Aung NM, Nyein PP, Htut TY, Htet ZW, Kyi TT, Anstey NM, et al. Antibiotic Therapy in Adults With Malaria (ANTHEM): High Rate of Clinically Significant Bacteremia in Hospitalized Adults Diagnosed With Falciparum Malaria. *Am J Trop Med Hyg* (2018) 99(3):688–96. doi: 10.4269/ajtmh.18- 0378

Phu NH, Day NPJ, Tuan PQ, Mai NTH, Chau TTH, Van Chuong L, et al. Concomitant Bacteremia in Adults With Severe Falciparum Malaria. *Clin Infect Dis* (2020) 71(9):e465–70. doi: 10.1093/cid/ciaa191

Chau JY, Tiffany CM, Nimishakavi S, Lawrence JA, Pakpour N, Mooney JP, et al. Malaria-Associated L-Arginine Deficiency Induces Mast Cell-Associated Disruption to Intestinal Barrier Defenses Against Nontyphoidal Salmonella Bacteremia. *Infect Immun* (2013) 81(10):3515–26. doi: 10.1128/IAI.00380-13

Potts RA, Tiffany CM, Pakpour N, Lokken KL, Tiffany CR, Cheung K, et al. Mast Cells and Histamine Alter Intestinal Permeability During Malaria Parasite Infection. *Immunobiology* (2016) 221(3):468–74. doi: 10.1016/j.imbio.2015.11.003

C'espedes N, Donnelly E, Garrison S, Haapanen L, Van De Water J, Luckhart S. Nonlethal *Plasmodium Yoelii* Infection Drives Complex Patterns of Th2-Type Host Immunity and Mast Cell-Dependent Bacteremia. *Infect Immun* (2020) 88(12):e00427. doi: 10.1128/IAI.00427-20

Krystel-Whittemore M, Dileepan KN, Wood JG. Mast Cell: A Multi- Functional Master Cell. *Front Immunol* (2015) 6:620. doi: 10.3389/ fimmu.2015.00620

Pejler G. Novel Insight Into the *In Vivo* Function of Mast Cell Chymase: Lessons From Knockouts and Inhibitors. *J Innate Immun* (2020) 12(5):357– 72. doi: 10.1159/000506985

Donnelly E, Vande Water J, Luckhart S. Malaria-Induced Bacteremia as a Consequence of Multiple Parasite Survival Strategies. *Curr Res Microbial Sci* (2021) 2:100036. doi: 10.1016/j.crmicr.2021.100036

Groschwitz KR, Ahrens R, Osterfeld H, Gurish MF, Han X, Abrink M, et al. Mast Cells Regulate Homeostatic Intestinal Epithelial Migration and Barrier Function by a Chymase/Mcpt4-Dependent Mechanism. *Proc Natl Acad Sci USA* (2009) 106(52):22381–6. doi: 10.1073/pnas.0906372106

Tchougounova E, Pejler G, Abrink M. The Chymase, Mouse Mast Cell Protease 4, Constitutes the Major Chymotrypsin-Like Activity in Peritoneum and Ear Tissue. A Role for Mouse Mast Cell Protease 4 in Thrombin Regulation and Fibronectin Turnover. *J Exp Med* (2003) 198 (3):423–31. doi: 10.1084/jem.20030671

Matelski L, Keil Stietz KP, Sethi S, Taylor SL, Van de Water J, Lein PJ. The Influence of Sex, Genotype, and Dose on Serum and Hippocampal Cytokine Levels in Juvenile Mice Developmentally Exposed to a Human-Relevant Mixture of Polychlorinated Biphenyls. *Curr Res Toxicol* (2020) 1:85–103. doi: 10.1016/j.crtox.2020.09.001

Rodriguez AM, Hambly MG, Jandu S, Simao-Gurge R, Lowder C, Lewis EE, et al. Histamine Ingestion by Anopheles Stephensi Alters Important Vector Transmission Behaviors and Infection Success With Diverse Plasmodium Species. *Biomolecules* (2021) 11(5):719. doi: 10.3390/biom11050719

Li Z, Peirasmaki D, Svard S, Abrink M. The Chymase Mouse Mast Cell Protease-4 Regulates Intestinal Cytokine Expression in Mature Adult Mice Infected With *Giardia Intestinalis*. *Cells* (2020) 9(4):925. doi: 10.3390/cells9040925

Pejler G, Abrink M, Ringvall M, Wernersson S. Mast Cell Proteases. *Adv Immunol* (2007) 95:167–255. doi: 10.1016/S0065-2776(07)95006-3

Waern I, Lundequist A, Pejler G, Wernersson S. Mast Cell Chymase Modulates IL-33 Levels and Controls Allergic Sensitization in Dust-Mite Induced Airway Inflammation. *Mucosal Immunol* (2013) 6(5):911–20. doi: 10.1038/mi.2012.129

Bischoff SC, Kramer S. Human Mast Cells, Bacteria, and Intestinal Immunity. *Immunol Rev* (2007) 217:329–37. doi: 10.1111/j.1600-065X.2007.00523.x

Albert-Bayo M, Paracuellos I, Gonzalez-Castro AM, Rodriguez-Urrutia A, Rodriguez-Lagunas MJ, Alonso-Cotoner C, et al. Intestinal Mucosal Mast Cells: Key Modulators of Barrier Function and Homeostasis. *Cells* (2019) 8 (2):135. doi: 10.3390/cells8020135

Mohanan V, Nakata T, Desch AN, Levesque C, Boroughs A, Guzman G, et al. C1orf106 Is a Colitis Risk Gene That Regulates Stability of Epithelial Adherens Junctions. *Science* (2018) 359(6380):1161–6. doi: 10.1126/science.aan0814

Aitken EH, Alemu A, Rogerson SJ. Neutrophils and Malaria. *Front Immunol* (2018) 9:3005. doi: 10.3389/fimmu.2018.03005

Castanheira FVS, Kubes P. Neutrophils and NETs in Modulating Acute and Chronic Inflammation. *Blood* (2019) 133(20):2178–85. doi: 10.1182/blood-2018-11-844530

Otterdal K, Berg A, Michelsen AE, Patel S, Tellevik MG, Haanshuus CG, et al. Soluble Markers of Neutrophil, T-Cell and Monocyte Activation Are Associated With Disease Severity and Parasitemia in Falciparum Malaria. *BMC Infect Dis* (2018) 18(1):670. doi: 10.1186/s12879-018-3593-8

Boettcher M, Esser M, Trah J, Klohs S, Mokhaberi N, Wenskus J, et al. Markers of Neutrophil Activation and Extracellular Traps Formation Are Predictive of Appendicitis in Mice and Humans: A Pilot Study. *Sci Rep* (2020) 10(1):18240. doi: 10.1038/s41598-020-74370-9

Deshmane SL, Kremlev S, Amini S, Sawaya BE. Monocyte Chemoattractant Protein-1 (MCP-1): An Overview. *J Interferon Cytokine Res* (2009) 29(6):313 26. doi: 10.1089/jir.2008.0027

de Jong RM, Tebeje SK, Meerstein-Kessel L, Tadesse FG, Jore MM, Stone W, et al. Immunity Against Sexual Stage Plasmodium Falciparum and *Plasmodium Vivax* Parasites. *Immunol Rev* (2020) 293(1):190–215. doi: 10.1111/imr.12828

Piliponsky AM, Chen CC, Rios EJ, Treuting PM, Lahiri A, Abrink M, et al. The Chymase Mouse Mast Cell Protease 4 Degrades TNF, Limits Inflammation, and Promotes Survival in a Model of Sepsis. *Am J Pathol* (2012) 181(3):875–86. doi: 10.1016/j.ajpath.2012.05.013

Succar J, Giatsidis G, Yu N, Hassan K, Khouri RJr., Gurish MF, et al. Mouse Mast Cell Protease-4 Rrecruits Leukocytes in the Inflammatory Phase of Surgically Wounded Skin. *Adv Wound Care (New Rochelle)* (2019) 8(10):469 75. doi: 10.1089/wound.2018.0898

Vangansewinkel T, Lemmens S, Geurts N, Quanten K, Dooley D, Pejler G, et a–l. Mouse Mast Cell Protease 4 Suppresses Scar Formation After Traumatic Spinal Cord Injury. *Sci Rep* (2019) 9(1):3715. doi: 10.1038/s41598-019-39551-1

Torre D, Speranza F, Martegani R. Role of Proinflammatory and Anti-Inflammatory Cytokines in the Immune Response to Plasmodium falciparum malaria. *Lancet Infect Dis* (2002) 2(12):719–20. doi: 10.1016/s1473-3099(02)00449-8

Oyegue-Liabagui SL, Bouopda-Tuedom AG, Kouna LC, Maghendji-Nzondo S, Nzoughe H, Tchitoula-Makaya N, et al. Pro- and Anti-Inflammatory Cytokines in Children With Malaria in Franceville, Gabon. *Am J Clin Exp Immunol* (2017) 6(2):9–20.

Lin AM, Rubin CJ, Khandpur R, Wang JY, Riblett M, Yalavarthi S, et al. Mast Cells and Neutrophils Release IL-17 Through Extracellular Trap Formation in– Psoriasis. *J Immunol* (2011) 187(1):490–500. doi: 10.4049/jimmunol.1100123

Tu JF, Pan HY, Ying XH, Lou J, Ji JS, Zou H. Mast Cells Comprise the Major of Interleukin 17-Producing Cells and Predict a Poor Prognosis in Hepatocellular Carcinoma. *Med (Baltimore)* (2016) 95(13):e3220. doi: 10.1097/MD.0000000000003220

Dowell AC, Cobby E, Wen K, Devall AJ, During V, Anderson J, et al. Interleukin-17-Positive Mast Cells Influence Outcomes From BCG for Patients With CIS: Data From a Comprehensive Characterisation of the Immune Microenvironment of Urothelial Bladder Cancer. *PloS One* (2017) 12 (9):e0184841. doi: 10.1371/journal.pone.0184841

Helegbe GK, Huy NT, Yanagi T, Shuaibu MN, Kikuchi M, Cherif MS, et al. Elevated IL-17 Levels in Semi-Immune Anaemic Mice Infected With Plasmodium Berghei ANKA. *Malar J* (2018) 17(1):169. doi: 10.1186/s12936-018-2257-x

Herbert F, Tchitchek N, Bansal D, Jacques J, Pathak S, Becavin C, et al. Evidence of IL-17, IP-10, and IL-10 Involvement in Multiple-Organ Dysfunction and IL-17 Pathway in Acute Renal Failure Associated to Plasmodium Falciparum Malaria. *J Transl Med* (2015) 13:369. doi: 10.1186/ s12967-015-0731-6

Tam IYS, Ng CW, Lau HYA, Tam SY. Degradation of Monocyte Chemoattractant Protein-1 by Tryptase Co-Released in Immunoglobulin E- Ddependent Activation of Primary Human Cultured Mast Cells. *Int Arch Allergy Immunol* (2018) 177(3):199–206. doi: 10.1159/000490533

Nelissen S, Vangansewinkel T, Geurts N, Geboes L, Lemmens E, Vidal PM, et al. Mast Cells Protect From Post-Traumatic Spinal Cord Damage in Mice by Degrading Inflammation-Associated Cytokines *via* Mouse Mast Cell Protease 4. *Neurobiol Dis* (2014) 62:260 72. doi: 10.1016/j.nbd.2013.09.012

Roy A, Ganesh G, Sippola H, Bolin S, Sawesi O, Dagalv A, et al. Mast Cell Chymase Degrades the Alarmins Heat Shock Protein 70, Biglycan, HMGB1, and Interleukin-33 (IL-33) and Limits Danger-Induced Inflammation. *J Biol Chem* (2014) 289(1):237–50. doi: 10.1074/jbc.M112.435156

Fu Z, Thorpe M, Alemayehu R, Roy A, Kervinen J, de Garavilla L, et al. Highly Selective Cleavage of Cytokines and Chemokines by the Human Mast Cell Chymase and Neutrophil Cathepsin G. *J Immunol* (2017) 198(4):1474–83. doi: 10.4049/jimmunol.1601223

Fu Z, Akula S, Thorpe M, Hellman L. Highly Selective Cleavage of Th2-Promoting Cytokines by the H– uman and the Mouse Mast Cell Tryptases, Indicating a Potent Negative Feedback Loop on Th2 Immunity. *Int J Mol Sci* (2019) 20(20):5147. doi: 10.3390/ijms20205147

Mooney JP, Galloway LJ, Riley EM. Malaria, Anemia, and Invasive Bacterial Disease: A Neutrophil Problem? *J Leukoc Biol* (2019) 105(4):645–55. doi: 10.1002/JLB.3RI1018-400R

Papayannopoulos V, Metzler KD, Hakkim A, Zychlinsky A. Neutrophil Elastase and Myeloperoxidase Regulate the Formation of Neutrophil Extracellular Traps. *J Cell Biol* (2010) 191(3):677–91. doi: 10.1083/jcb.201006052

Kenny EF, Herzig A, Kruger R, Muth A, Mondal S, Thompson PR, et al. Diverse Stimuli Engage Different Neutrophil Extracellular Trap Pathways. W*Elife* (2017) 6:e24437. doi: 10.7554/eLife.24437

Hirche TO, Gaut JP, Heinecke JW, Belaaouaj A. Myeloperoxidase Plays Critical Roles in Killing Klebsiella Pneumoniae and Inactivating Neutrophil Elastase: Effects on Host Defense. *J Immunol* (2005) 174(3):1557–65. doi: 10.4049/jimmunol.174.3.1557

Madjene LC, Danelli L, Dahdah A, Vibhushan S, Bex-Coudrat J, Pacreau E, et al. Mast Cell Chymase Protects Against Acute Ischemic Kidney Injury by Limiting Neutrophil Hyperactivation and Recruitment. *Kidney Int* (2020) 97 (3):516–27. doi: 10.1016/j.kint.2019.08.037

Naotunne TD, Rathnayake KD, Jayasinghe A, Carter R, Mendis KN. *Plasmodium Cynomolgi*: Serum-Mediated Blocking and Enhancement of Infectivity to Mosquitoes During Infections in the Natural Host, Macaca Sinica. *Exp Parasitol* (1990) 71(3):305–13. doi: 10.1016/0014-4894(90)90035-b

Carter R, Mendis KN. Immune Responses Against Sexual Stages of Plasmodium Vivax During Human Malarial Infections in Sri Lanka. *Parassitologia* (1991) 33(1):67–70.

Bradley J, Stone W, Da DF, Morlais I, Dicko A, Cohuet A, et al. Predicting the Likelihood and Intensity of Mosquito Infection From Sex Specific Plasmodium Falciparum Gametocyte Density. *Elife* (2018) 7. doi: 10.7554/eLife.34463

Paul RE, Brey PT, Robert V. Plasmodium Sex Determination and Transmission to Mosquitoes. *Trends Parasitol* (2002) 18(1):32–8. doi: 10.1016/s1471-4922(01)02122-5

Hallett RL, Dunyo S, Ord R, Jawara M, Pinder M, Randall A, et al. Chloroquine/sulphadoxine-Pyrimethamine for Gambian Children With Malaria: Transmission to Mosquitoes of Multidrug-Resistant Plasmodium Falciparum. *PloS Clin Trials* (2006) 1(3):e15. doi: 10.1371/journal.pctr.0010015

Healer J, Graszynski A, Riley E. Phagocytosis Does Not Play a Major Role in Naturally Acquired Transmission-Blocking Immunity to Plasmodium Falciparum Malaria. *Infect Immun* (1999) 67(5):2334–9. doi: 10.1128/IAI.67.5.2334-2339.1999

Riley EM, Ong CS, Olerup O, Eida S, Allen SJ, Bennett S, et al. Cellular and Humoral Immune Responses to Plasmodium Falciparum Gametocyte Antigens in Malaria-Immune Individuals. Limited Response to the 48/45-Kilodalton Surface Antigen Does Not Appear to be Due to MHC Restriction. *J Immunol* (1990) 144(12):4810–6.

Goodier MR, Targett GA. Evidence for CD4+ T Cell Responses Common to Plasmodium Falciparum and Recall Antigens. *Int Immunol* (1997) 9 (12):1857–65. doi: 10.1093/intimm/9.12.1857

Pakpour N, Akman-Anderson L, Vodovotz Y, Luckhart S. The Effects of Ingested Mammalian Blood Factors on Vector Arthropod Immunity and Physiology. *Microbes Infect* (2013) 15(3):243–54. doi: 10.1016/j.micinf.2013.01.003

Pakpour N, Riehle MA, Luckhart S. Effects of Ingested Vertebrate-Derived Factors on Insect Immune Responses. *Curr Opin Insect Sci* (2014) 3:1–5. doi: 10.1016/j.cois.2014.07.001

Luckhart S, Pakpour N, Giulivi C. Host-Pathogen Interactions in Malaria: Cross-Kingdom Signaling and Mitochondrial Regulation. *Curr Opin Immunol* (2015) 36:73–9. doi: 10.1016/j.coi.2015.07.002

Luckhart S, Riehle MA. Midgut Mitochondrial Function as a Gatekeeper for Malaria Parasite Infection and Development in the Mosquito Host. *Front Cell Infect Microbiol* (2020) 10:593159. doi: 10.3389/fcimb.2020.593159

Mooney JP, Lokken KL, Byndloss MX, George MD, Velazquez EM, Faber F, et al. Inflammation-Associated Alterations to the Intestinal Microbiota Reduce Colonization Resistance Against non-Typhoidal Salmonella During Concurrent Malaria Parasite Infection. *Sci Rep* (2015) 5:14603. doi: 10.1038/srep14603

Permissions

All chapters in this book were first published by Frontiers; hereby published with permission under the Creative Commons Attribution License or equivalent. Every chapter published in this book has been scrutinized by our experts. Their significance has been extensively debated. The topics covered herein carry significant findings which will fuel the growth of the discipline. They may even be implemented as practical applications or may be referred to as a beginning point for another development.

The contributors of this book come from diverse backgrounds, making this book a truly international effort. This book will bring forth new frontiers with its revolutionizing research information and detailed analysis of the nascent developments around the world.

We would like to thank all the contributing authors for lending their expertise to make the book truly unique. They have played a crucial role in the development of this book. Without their invaluable contributions this book wouldn't have been possible. They have made vital efforts to compile up to date information on the varied aspects of this subject to make this book a valuable addition to the collection of many professionals and students.

This book was conceptualized with the vision of imparting up-to-date information and advanced data in this field. To ensure the same, a matchless editorial board was set up. Every individual on the board went through rigorous rounds of assessment to prove their worth. After which they invested a large part of their time researching and compiling the most relevant data for our readers.

The editorial board has been involved in producing this book since its inception. They have spent rigorous hours researching and exploring the diverse topics which have resulted in the successful publishing of this book. They have passed on their knowledge of decades through this book. To expedite this challenging task, the publisher supported the team at every step. A small team of assistant editors was also appointed to further simplify the editing procedure and attain best results for the readers.

Apart from the editorial board, the designing team has also invested a significant amount of their time in understanding the subject and creating the most relevant covers. They scrutinized every image to scout for the most suitable representation of the subject and create an appropriate cover for the book.

The publishing team has been an ardent support to the editorial, designing and production team. Their endless efforts to recruit the best for this project, has resulted in the accomplishment of this book. They are a veteran in the field of academics and their pool of knowledge is as vast as their experience in printing. Their expertise and guidance has proved useful at every step. Their uncompromising quality standards have made this book an exceptional effort. Their encouragement from time to time has been an inspiration for everyone.

The publisher and the editorial board hope that this book will prove to be a valuable piece of knowledge for researchers, students, practitioners and scholars across the globe.

List of Contributors

Adriele Scopel-Guerra and Natália Callai-Silva
Center of Biotechnology, Universidade Federal do Rio Grande do Sul, Porto Alegre, Brazil

Deiber Olivera-Severo
Center of Biotechnology, Universidade Federal do Rio Grande do Sul, Porto Alegre, Brazil
Department of Biology, Universidade Regional Integrada do Alto Uruguai e das Missões, São Luiz Gonzaga, Brazil

Fernanda Staniscuaski
Center of Biotechnology, Universidade Federal do Rio Grande do Sul, Porto Alegre, Brazil
Department of Molecular Biology and Biotechnology, Institute of Biosciences, Universidade Federal do Rio Grande do Sul, Porto Alegre, Brazil

Augusto F. Uberti
Center of Biotechnology, Universidade Federal do Rio Grande do Sul, Porto Alegre, Brazil
Institute of Biology, Universidade Federal de Pelotas, Pelotas, Brazil

Natália Jaeger and Bárbara N. Porto
Institute of Biomedical Research, Pontifícia Universidade Católica do Rio Grande do Sul, Porto Alegre, Brazil

Miguel S. Marques and Céu Figueiredo
i3S, Instituto de Investigação e Inovação em Saúde, University of Porto, Porto, Portugal
Ipatimup-Institute of Molecular Pathology and Immunology of the University of Porto, Porto, Portugal
Faculty of Medicine of the University of Porto, Porto, Portugal

Marta T. Pinto and Marina Leite
i3S, Instituto de Investigação e Inovação em Saúde, University of Porto, Porto, Portugal
Ipatimup-Institute of Molecular Pathology and Immunology of the University of Porto, Porto, Portugal

Maria Gomez-Lazaro
i3S, Instituto de Investigação e Inovação em Saúde, University of Porto, Porto, Portugal
INEB - Instituto Nacional de Engenharia Biomédica, University of Porto, Porto, Portugal

Christiane Forestier and Pascale Gueirard
CNRS UMR 6023, Laboratoire Microorganismes: Génome et Environnement, Université Clermont-Auvergne Clermont-Ferrand, France

Célia R. Carlini
Center of Biotechnology, Universidade Federal Rio Grande do Sul, Porto Alegre, Brazil
Brain Institute (BRAINS-InsCer), Pontifícia Universidade Católica do Rio Grande do Sul, Porto Alegre, Brazil

Maria C. Opazo and Claudia A. Riedel
Laboratorio de Biología Celular y Farmacología, Departamento de Ciencias Biológicas, Facultad de Ciencias Biológicas, Millennium Institute on Immunology and Immunotherapy, Universidad Andres Bello, Santiago, Chile
Facultad de Medicina, Millennium Institute on Immunology and Immunotherapy, Universidad Andres Bello, Santiago, Chile

Elizabeth M. Ortega-Rocha
Laboratorio de Inmunobiología, Facultad de Medicina, Departamento de Biología Celular y Tisular, Universidad Nacional Autónoma de México, Mexico City, Mexico

Irenice Coronado-Arrázola and Susan M. Bueno
Departamento de Genética Molecular y Microbiología, Facultad de Ciencias Biológicas, Millennium Institute on Immunology and Immunotherapy, Pontificia Universidad Católica de Chile, Santiago, Chile

Laura C. Bonifaz
Unidad de Investigación Médica en Inmunoquímica Hospital de Especialidades Centro Médico Nacional Siglo XXI, Instituto Mexicano del Seguro Social, Mexico City, Mexico

Helene Boudin and Michel Neunlist
Institut National de la Santé et de la Recherche Médicale U1235, Institut des Maladies de l'Appareil Digestif, Université de Nantes, Nantes, France

Alexis M. Kalergis
Departamento de Genética Molecular y Microbiología, Facultad de Ciencias Biológicas, Millennium Institute on Immunology and Immunotherapy, Pontificia Universidad Católica de Chile, Santiago, Chile
Departamento de Endocrinología, Facultad de Medicina, Pontificia Universidad, Metropolitana, Chile

Khalit S. Khaertynov, Vladimir A. Anokhin, Irina V. Nicolaeva, Svetlana V. Khalioullina and Dina R. Semyenova
Department of Children Infectious Diseases, Kazan State Medical University, Kazan, Russia

Melissa J. Blumenthal, Sylvia Ujma, Arieh A. Katz and Georgia Schäfer
Receptor Biology Research Unit, Division of Medical Biochemistry and Structural Biology, Institute of Infectious Disease and Molecular Medicine, Department of Integrative Biomedical Sciences, Faculty of Health Sciences, SA-MRC Gynecology Cancer Research Centre, University of Cape Town, Cape Town, South Africa

Yuri N. Davidyuk
Institute of Fundamental Medicine and Biology, Kazan Federal University, Kazan, Russia

Evgeny Y. Alatyrev and Natalia N. Skvortsova
Intensive Care Unit No 2, Republican Clinical Infectious Diseases Hospital, Kazan, Russia

Levon G. Abrahamyan
Laboratory for Animal Molecular Virology, Research Group on Infectious Diseases in Production Animals and Swine and Poultry Infectious Diseases Research Center, Faculty of Veterinary Medicine, Université de Montréal, Saint-Hyacinthe, QC, Canada

Aaron Lerner
The Ruth and Bruce Rappaport Faculty of Medicine, Technion Israel Institute of Technology, Haifa, Israel
Department of Research, AESKU.KIPP Institute, Wendelsheim, Germany

Marina Arleevskaya
Central Research Laboratory, Kazan State Medical Academy Kazan, Kazan, Russia

Andreas Schmiedl and Torsten Matthias
Department of Research, AESKU.KIPP Institute, Wendelsheim, Germany

Renée N. Douville
Department of Biology, University of Winnipeg, Winnipeg, MB, Canada
Department of Immunology, University of Manitoba, Winnipeg, MB, Canada

Avindra Nath
Section of Infections of the Nervous System, National Institute of Neurological Diseases and Stroke, National Institutes of Health, Bethesda, MD, United States

Emma T. Saltzman, Talia Palacios, Michael Thomsen and Luis Vitetta
Sydney Medical School, University of Sydney, Sydney, NSW, Australia
Medlab Clinical, Sydney, NSW, Australia

Marlena Kłak
Research and Development Center, Regional Specialist Hospital, Wrocław, Poland

Jingshu Zhang and Yun Lan
HKU-Pasteur Research Pole, School of Public Health, Li Ka Shing Faculty of Medicine, University of Hong Kong, Hong Kong, China

Sumana Sanyal
HKU-Pasteur Research Pole, School of Public Health, Li Ka Shing Faculty of Medicine, University of Hong Kong, Hong Kong, China
School of Biomedical Sciences, Li Ka Shing Faculty of Medicine, University of Hong Kong, Hong Kong, China

Anna Kłopot, Adriana Zakrzewska, Dorota Lecion, Joanna M. Majewska, Marek A. Harhala, Karolina Lahutta and Zuzanna Kaźmierczak
Bacteriophage Laboratory, Institute of Immunology and Experimental Therapy, Polish Academy of Sciences, Wrocław, Poland

Łukasz Łaczmański and Krystyna Dąbrowska
Bacteriophage Laboratory, Institute of Immunology and Experimental Therapy, Polish Academy of Sciences, Wrocław, Poland
Research and Development Center, Regional Specialist Hospital, Wrocław, Poland

Andrea Picchianti-Diamanti and Raffaele D'Amelio
Department of Clinical and Molecular Medicine, Sant'Andrea University Hospital, Sapienza University of Rome, Rome, Italy

Maria M. Rosado
Independent Researcher, Rome, Italy

Jana Pindjakova and Oriana Lo Re
Center for Translational Medicine, International Clinical Research Center, St. Anne's University Hospital, Brno, Czechia

Claudio Sartini
Department of Primary Care and Population Health, University College London, London, United Kingdom

Francesca Rappa
Section of Human Anatomy, Department of Experimental Biomedicine and Clinical Neurosciences, University of Palermo, Palermo, Italy

Berengere Coupe and Benjamin Lelouvier
Vaiomer, Labège, France

Manlio Vinciguerra
Center for Translational Medicine, International Clinical Research Center, St. Anne's University Hospital, Brno, Czechia
Division of Medicine, Institute for Liver and Digestive Health, University College London, London, United Kingdom

Valerio Pazienza
Gastroenterology Unit, IRCCS "Casa Sollievo della Sofferenza" Hospital, San Giovanni Rotondo, Italy

Eduardo Mendes, Caroline M. Ferreira and Willian R. Ribeiro
Department of Pharmaceutics Sciences, Institute of Environmental, Chemistry and Pharmaceutical Sciences, Universidade Federal de São Paulo, Diadema, Brazil

Beatriz G. Acetturi
Department of Pharmacology, Institute of Biomedical Sciences I, University of São Paulo, São Paulo, Brazil

Andrew M. Thomas
Medical Genomics Laboratory, CIPE/A.C.Camargo Cancer Center, São Paulo, Brazil
Department of Biochemistry, Institute of Chemistry, University of São Paulo, São Paulo, Brazil
Bioinformatics Graduate Program, University of São Paulo, São Paulo, Brazil

Flaviano dos S. Martins
Department of Microbiology, Institute of Biological Sciences, Federal University of Minas Gerais, Belo Horizonte, Brazil

Amanda R. Crisma and Gilson Murata
Department of Physiology and Biophysics, Institute of Biomedical Sciences, University of São Paulo, São Paulo, Brazil

Adriana L. dos S. Franco
Post Graduate Program in Biophotonics Applied to Health Sciences, Universidade Nove de Julho, São Paulo, Brazil

João C. Setubal
Department of Biochemistry, Institute of Chemistry, University of São Paulo, São Paulo, Brazil

Claudete J. Valduga
Department of Pharmacy and Biotechnology, Universidade de Anhanguera de São Paulo, São Paulo, Brazil

Rui Curi
Department of Physiology and Biophysics, Institute of Biomedical Sciences, University of São Paulo, São Paulo, Brazil

Emmanuel Dias-Neto
Medical Genomics Laboratory, CIPE/A.C.Camargo Cancer Center, São Paulo, Brazil
Laboratory of Neurosciences (LIM-27), Institute of Psychiatry, Medical School University of São Paulo, São Paulo, Brazil

TárcioT. Braga and Niels O. S. Camâra
Department of Immunology, Institute of Biomedical Sciences IV, University of São Paulo, São Paulo, Brazil

Wothan Tavares-de-Lima
Department of Pharmacology, Institute of Biomedical Sciences I, University of São Paulo, São Paulo, Brazil

Giulia Freer
Retrovirus Center, Department of Translational Research, University of Pisa, Pisa, Italy

Fabrizio Maggi
Virology Unit, University Hospital of Pisa, Pisa, Italy

Massimo Pifferi, Maria E. Di Cicco and Diego G. Peroni
Department of Clinical and Experimental Medicine, Section of Pediatrics, University of Pisa, Pisa, Italy

Mauro Pistello
Retrovirus Center, Department of Translational Research, University of Pisa, Pisa, Italy
Virology Unit, University Hospital of Pisa, Pisa, Italy

Klara Klimesova, Zuzana Jiraskova Zakostelska and Helena Tlaskalova-Hogenova
Laboratory of Cellular and Molecular Immunology, Institute of Microbiology of the CAS, Prague, Czechia

Alexander Swidsinski
Laboratory for Molecular Genetics, Polymicrobial Infections and Biofilms, Section of Gastroenterology and Hepatology, Department of Medicine, Charité Universitätsmedizin Berlin, Berlin, Germany
Institute of Molecular Medicine, Sechenov First Moscow State Medical University, Moscow, Russia

Yvonne Dörffel
Outpatient Clinic, Charité Universitätsmedizin Berlin, Berlin, Germany

Vera Loening-Baucke, Christoph Gille, Önder Göktas and Anne Reißhauer
Laboratory for Molecular Genetics, Polymicrobial Infections and Biofilms, Section of Gastroenterology and Hepatology, Department of Medicine, Charité Universitätsmedizin Berlin, Berlin, Germany

Jürgen Neuhaus
Faculty of Veterinary Medicine, Centre for Infectious Diseases, University of Leipzig, Leipzig, Germany

Karsten-Henrich Weylandt
Charité Universitätsmedizin Berlin, Campus Virchow, Gastroenterology Berlin, Berlin, Germany

Alexander Guschin
Laboratory of Molecular Diagnostics, Russian Research Center for Molecular Diagnostics and Therapy, Central Research Institute, Moscow, Russia

Markus Bock
Experimental and Clinical Research Center, A Joint Cooperation between the Charité Medical Faculty and the Max-Delbrueck Center for Molecular Medicine, Berlin, Germany

Elisabeth Billard
INRA USC 2018, Inserm U1071, Laboratoire Microbes Intestin Inflammation et Susceptibilité de l'Hôte, Université Clermont-Auvergne, Clermont-Ferrand, France

Geneviève Milon
Institut Pasteur, Paris, France

Lidia Sanchez-Alcoholado
Unidad de Gestión Clínica de Endocrinología y Nutrición, Instituto de Investigación Biomédica de Málaga, Hospital Universitario Virgen de la Victoria, Universidad de Málaga, Málaga, Spain

Daniel Castellano-Castillo, Isabel Moreno-Indias and Maria I. Queipo-Ortuño
Unidad de Gestión Clínica de Endocrinología y Nutrición, Instituto de Investigación Biomédica de Málaga, Hospital Universitario Virgen de la Victoria, Universidad de Málaga, Málaga, Spain
CIBER Fisiopatología de la Obesidad y Nutrición, Instituto de Salud Carlos III, Madrid, Spain

Laura Jordán-Martínez, Pilar Cardila-Cruz, Daniel Elena, Antonio J. Muñoz-Garcia and Manuel Jimenez-Navarro
Unidad de Gestión Clínica Área del Corazón, Hospital Universitario Virgen de la Victoria, Instituto de Investigación Biomédica de Málaga, Universidad de Málaga, CIBERCV Enfermedades Cardiovasculares, Málaga, Spain

Nora Céspedes, Casey Lowder, Gretchen Hansten, Delaney Wagers and Anna M. Briggs
Department of Entomology, Plant Pathology and Nematology, University of Idaho, Moscow, ID, United States

Erinn L. Donnelly
Department of Biological Sciences, University of Idaho, Moscow, ID, United States

Joseph Schauer, Lori Haapanen and Judy Van de Water
Division of Rheumatology, Allergy and Clinical Immunology, University of California, Davis, Davis, CA, United States

Magnus Åbrink
Section of Immunology, Department of Biomedical Sciences & Veterinary Public Health, Swedish University of Agricultural Sciences, Uppsala, Sweden

Shirley Luckhart
Department of Entomology, Plant Pathology and Nematology, University of Idaho, Moscow, ID, United States
Department of Biological Sciences, University of Idaho, Moscow, ID, United States

Index

www.ingramcontent.com/pod-product-compliance
Lightning Source LLC
LaVergne TN
LVHW082150200926
848484LV00008B/2131
9798887402529